A color atlas of sectional anatomy

CHEST, ABDOMEN, AND PELVIS

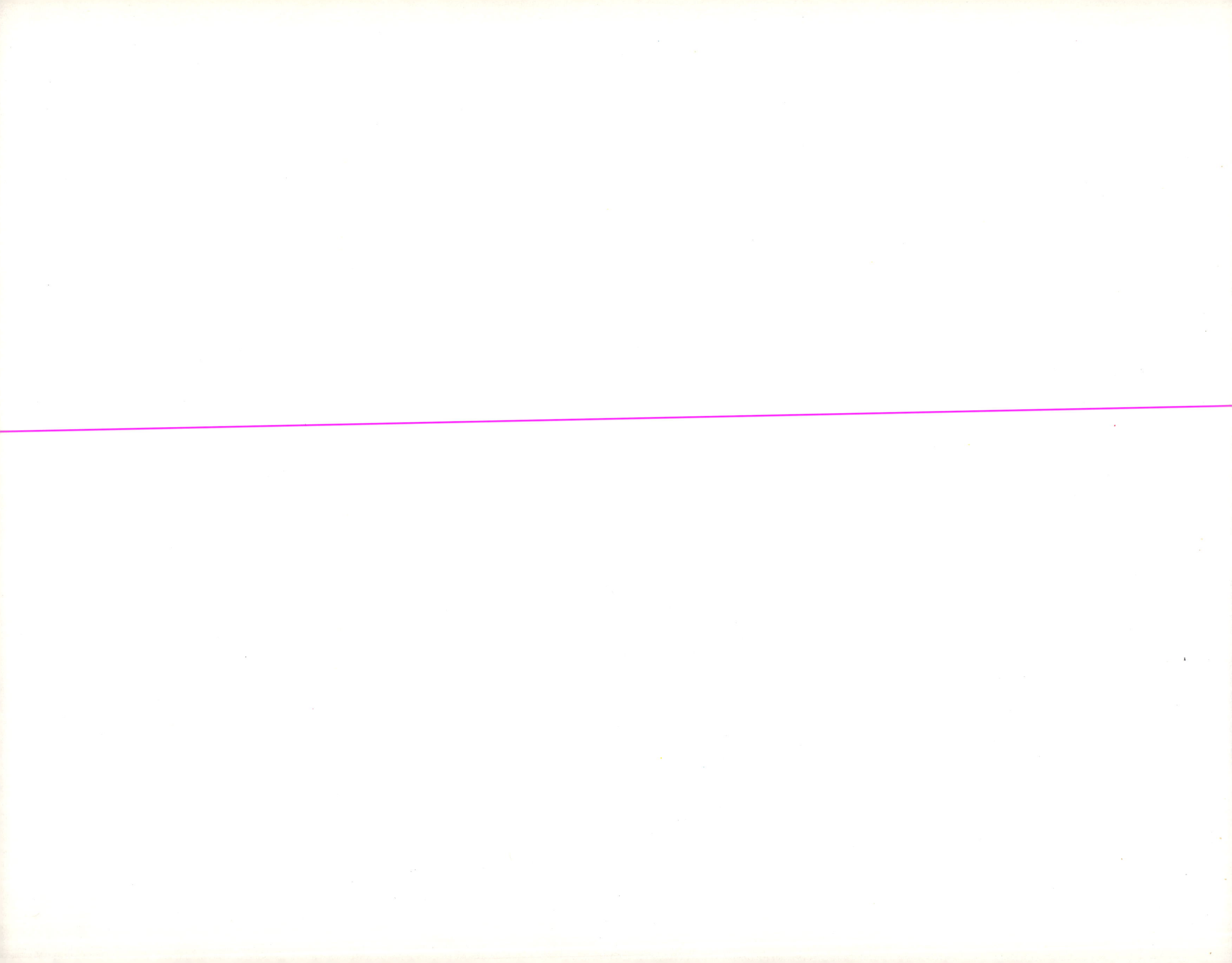

A color atlas of sectional anatomy

CHEST, ABDOMEN, AND PELVIS

E. A. Lyons, M.D., F.R.C.P.(C)

Director, Section of Diagnostic Ultrasound,
Health Sciences Centre;
Associate Professor of Medicine,
University of Manitoba:
Winnipeg, Manitoba,
Canada

Photography
ROB MATHIESON

Artist
DAVID LEE

Professional assistance
SYD BRADBURY and RAY St. HILAIRE

Anatomical collaboration
R. E. GRAHAME, M.D., and RUVIN LYONS, M.D.

with **283** illustrations and **138** color plates

The C. V. Mosby Company

Saint Louis   1978

The C. V. Mosby Company
11830 Westline Industrial Drive, St. Louis, Missouri 63141

Library of Congress Cataloging in Publication Data

Lyons, Edward Arthur, 1943-
   Color atlas of sectional anatomy: chest, abdomen, and pelvis.

   Includes index.
   1. Chest—Atlases.   2. Abdomen—Atlases.
3. Pelvis—Atlases.   4. Anatomy, Surgical and topographical—Atlases.   I.   Title.
QM540.L95   611'.9   78-15746
ISBN 0-8016-3052-5

GW/U/B 9 8 7 6 5 4 3 2 1

To Har and Mara

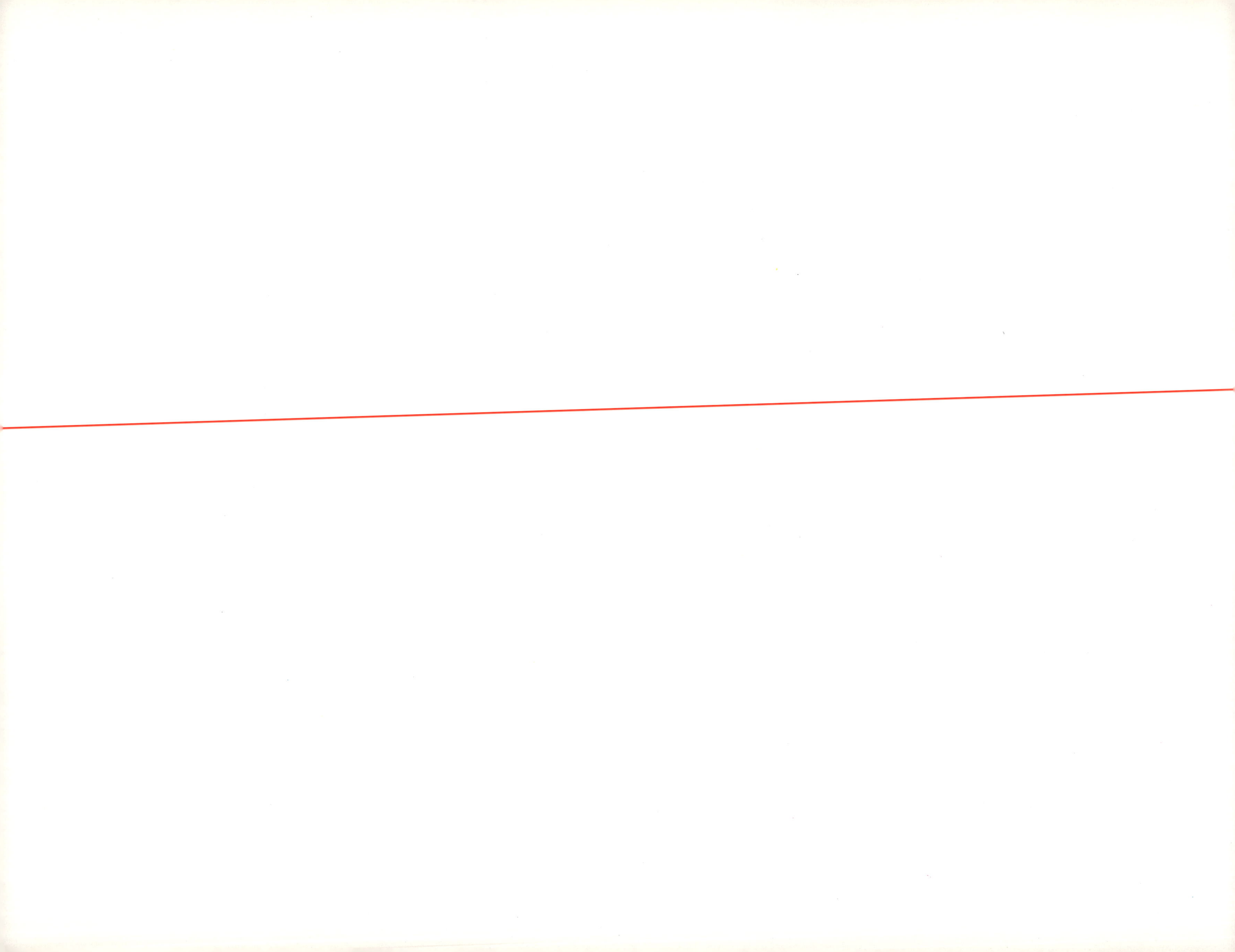

Acknowledgments

As with every undertaking, there are a number of people whose contributions must be acknowledged, for without their presence the task would have been more difficult if not impossible.

My parents provided the initial stimulus in my medical career, especially my father, also a physician. He established a high personal standard in his own field of obstetrics, which he continues to maintain after 40 years of practice. My goals are to achieve, in some small measure, some of his professional fulfillment. It was on his insistence that I spent my summers of undergraduate medical training in research, which led directly to my career in ultrasound and to this anatomical undertaking.

The late Dr. M. G. Saunders was my first mentor in ultrasound and was followed by Dr. Ross E. Brown and Prof. I. Donald. I am grateful for their early guidance. Dr. D. W. MacEwan, professor of radiology, has been a continuous source of encouragement.

The book began as a means of teaching sectional anatomy to my staff and students. Their day-to-day stimulation and inquisitiveness provided the impetus to continue. My thanks to Shael Harris, Darrel Barkman, Kathy McDiarmid, Denis Gratton, Bruce Goalen, Gene Charney, Gerry Ballard, Julie Hay, and Doug Shaw.

My colleagues in the Department of Anatomy at the University of Manitoba—Dr. K. Moore, Dr. R. E. Grahame, and Dr. T. V. Persaud—assisted me in every way, and without their complete cooperation this book would not have been possible.

The technical aspect of preparing and sectioning the cadavers fell to Syd Bradbury and Ray St. Hilaire. Their willingness to assist and their expertise have been much appreciated. We were fortunate enough to be able to utilize the facilities of the Provincial Veterinary Lab, for which I am truly grateful.

The sections were photographed by Rob Mathieson, a master at his craft. He did an outstanding job in capturing the color and detail of the original sections. I was also fortunate to have the support of the Department of Medical Photography at the Health Sciences Centre as a whole and of its director, Ken McGregor, in particular.

All of the art work was done by David Lee, who did an admirable job on all of the line diagrams.

In the arduous task of labeling all pertinent structures, I received tremendous assistance and support from Dr. Ruvin Lyons and Dr. R. E. Grahame. I am indebted to them for their help.

Finally, for the thread that held the whole thing together— my wife Har—words cannot express my gratitude.

E. A. Lyons

Contents

Introduction

The purpose of this atlas is to portray normal anatomy and anatomical relationships in as simplistic a manner as possible. To accomplish this, serial sections 1 cm thick were prepared using frozen cadavers not previously embalmed. The major arterial and venous systems were injected with red and blue latex solutions respectively. Each section can therefore be presented in such a way as to preserve the natural color of all the organs with some artificial accentuation of the vascular tree. In addition to the use of color as an aid to rapid identification, a large number of sections are presented in a serial fashion so as to provide a sense of continuity as well as for the sake of completeness. Using this kind of presentation, I have tried to present as detailed an atlas as possible. It was not feasible to identify some of the small yet significant structures in each and every section. In such instances, it is hoped that the reader will refer to the sections before and after the one of interest to find the structure in question. If one remembers that each section is only 1 cm thick, the relative position of all structures should be satisfactorily locatable. Every attempt has been made to be honest, so that where a structure could not accurately be identified, its label was omitted from that section but may be found in subsequent ones.

Sections were cut in the three major anatomical planes: *transverse* or *cross* sections, *parasagittal* or *longitudinal* sections, and *coronal* sections. Again, to provide a continuum of sections, the general layout of the book emphasizes the *plane of sections* rather than the general anatomical region. For example, transverse sections of the chest, abdomen, and pelvis are presented one after the other. This was most important for the transverse plane where the chest and abdominal sections were from the same cadaver. A definite continuity is maintained throughout the body.

I felt that it was more important to provide an atlas using this layout rather than the more conventional format where all three major anatomical planes of a specific region are presented together in one chapter. In this atlas, for example, there is not a chapter on *chest* presenting transverse, parasagittal, and coronal sections in a sequential manner.

In the fields of diagnostic radiology, computed tomography, and ultrasound, a single study often spans two or even three major anatomical regions (for example, chest, abdomen, and pelvis)—hence the rationale for this mode of presentation.

Putting together an atlas such as this becomes very much like piecing together a complex puzzle; the beauty and detail that it offers when finally assembled make the task worthwhile. In the January 1978 issue of *Scientific American,* I was struck by the same intricate beauty of a mathematical puzzle sculpture entitled "Mini-David" by the Spanish artist Miguel Berrocal. He created a "body" out of numerous complex and intricate pieces encompassing many very different planes. This book consists of bodies sectioned in different planes to reveal the "intricate puzzle" hidden within.

In keeping with a basically simplistic approach, I have purposely not included ultrasonic or computed tomographic images. These have been excluded mainly for two reasons. First, I have tried to provide as large a format for the color photographs and line diagrams as possible. Any additional information would have reduced the available space and therefore the effectiveness of their presentation. Second, it takes a year to collect satisfactory comparative scans plus an additional 8 months or so to put a manuscript into print. When such a book would be ready for distribution, the quality of the scans would be far below that which is currently acceptable and therefore of little or no value to the reader. This kind of comparative anatomical demonstration is dealt with periodically in the literature; therefore, current information with state-of-the-art scans on this subject is always available.

In this same vein, I have limited the textual matter in the atlas to this introduction. The information that is often provided in the form of lengthy footnotes generally expresses features of current interest and in time proves to be only of limited value. With the provision of a continuum of thin sections, the need for continual orientation is negated. Finally, as I am not noted for my literary accomplishments, I have left that task to others. There are, in fact, numerous excellent texts and monographs verbalizing anatomy in exquisite detail. *Gray's Anatomy* is one such example.

Nomenclature is always a problem. There does not appear to be any accepted standard that is used exclusively; instead, one finds the formal nomenclature of Nomina Anatomica combined with some traditionally acceptable variants. For some reason, people are comfortable with the Latin form for certain structures and the English form for others. To provide an easily readable text, I have, for the most part, followed the nomenclature used in the thirty-fifth edition of *Gray's Anatomy,* which combines the formal nomenclature with accepted colloquialisms.

The sections presented in this atlas are the result of an examination in a sectional manner of approximately 18 cadavers. It would have been wonderful to have been able to present sections of three or four perfect specimens, each of which were built identically, embalmed perfectly, and sectioned without flaw. Such sections, however, can only be accomplished through an artist's impression of anatomy, such as has been presented in other atlases. Slight normal variations may exist in some of the sections presented here and, where appropriate, these have been indicated.

As often as possible, one body was used to provide sections of several anatomical regions. For example, the same body was used for the transverse sections of the chest and abdomen. However, the pelvic anatomy had to be provided by different cadavers. The parasagittal sections utilize four cadavers, one for each area (chest; abdomen and pelvis—male; pelvis—female; and abdominal aortic aneurysm). Fortunately the coronal sections were obtained entirely from one body, which should make a nice anatomical demonstration.

The technique used to prepare the cadavers for sectioning is described as follows.

Preparation of the body

SYD BRADBURY

The technique described here is for injecting two colors into fresh cadavers that will be frozen for thin abdominal sectioning.

Subjects chosen are as young as possible, of medium body habitus, and free of anatomically distorting diseases. In general, the major arterial and venous systems are flushed of blood and injected with a colored compound.

A 6-inch incision is made bilaterally in the neck to expose the internal jugular veins and internal carotid arteries. A similar bilateral incision is made in the groin, exposing the femoral arteries and veins. The vessels are elevated, fixated with a ligature, and then opened through a 4-mm incision, just large enough to insert a glass T-tube or plastic cannula. The tubes are secured with linen thread, and a section of rubber tubing is added to connect the cannulas to a Turner PE-7 Portabay embalming machine. Two bottles of clot disperser (Champion Co.)* are placed in the machine with a gallon of cold tap water and allowed to mix for 2 minutes. Under a pressure of 30 pounds per square inch (psi), the machine is attached to the right femoral artery and fluid is injected for 2 minutes with all other veins and arteries clamped off. In a similar manner, the right carotid artery is then injected for 2 minutes. The same procedure is performed on the left side until half of the declotting fluid has been used. Then all veins are opened, and injection is continued in a pulsatile fashion; at

*Champion Company, Toronto, Ontario.

this time blood should begin to drain. To enhance drainage, embalmer's forceps can be used to remove clots from the femoral and jugular veins. It is advisable to wait 15 to 20 minutes before opening the jugular and femoral veins to facilitate the dispersion and softening of the blood.

When as much blood as possible has been drained from the veins, they are clamped off and injected at 30 psi under pulsating pressure with 1 gallon of formalin mixed with 3 gallons of cold water. This will harden the tissues to prevent decay and will enhance proper freezing prior to sectioning. Then each of the carotid and femoral arteries is injected with 1 pint of red coloring fluid with the veins firmly occluded. When this is done, 1 pint of blue coloring fluid is injected into each of the jugular and femoral veins with the arteries securely clamped off. The coloring fluid (see below for formulas) is injected at 20 psi.

Formula (red)
> Water 8,000 ml
> Laundry starch 2,400 gm
> Aluminum acetate 25 gm

Stir thoroughly.
Add
> Congo red 25 gm $\Big\}$ previously mixed
> Erythrosine 15 gm

Stir until dissolved.
Then add
> Water 1,000 ml
> Phenol 100 ml
to prevent mold.

Formula (blue)
> Same as above but delete congo red and erythrosine and add 50 gm "Luxol" fast blue MBS.*

On completion of the dye injection, all arteries and veins are securely clamped off and the **T** tubes and cannulas removed. The cadaver is then placed in an open plastic bag and a cardboard coffin and frozen at −10° C for 1 month.

*Dupont Organic Chemicals Dept., Wilmington 98, Del.

Anatomical sectioning

The frozen cadavers utilized in this atlas were sectioned on a stainless steel band saw with a specially designed aluminum gate to maintain evenness of the sections. It was important to regulate the speed with which one cut the sections. If one went too slowly, the sections melted and then refroze, making separation difficult; if one went too fast, the blade would "wander," providing uneven sections. The individual sections were placed immediately on Plexiglas plates, cleaned with an alcohol mixture, and returned to the freezer without significant thawing having occurred. They were then photographed within 24 hours.

Some explanation is necessary regarding each of the cadavers utilized in the individual sections.

TRANSVERSE OR CROSS SECTIONS

Chest and abdomen. Sections were from a 53-year-old woman, cause of death unknown. The one cadaver provided a continuous series of sections from the level of the aortic arch down to the aortic bifurcation. Because of distortion in our initial attempts to freeze the body, the region above the aortic arch and below the bifurcation were unacceptable.

In this cadaver there are two features that resulted in some distortion of anatomical landmarks. The most significant is the relatively large amount of mesenteric and retroperitoneal fat that is present. This woman was by no means obese; however, she may have been regarded as slightly heavier than average. This is useful for our presentation in that major organs are "outlined" in fat, making identification easier. In some ways this is a disadvantage in that the separation between organs such as the kidney and the suprarenals may tend to distort the anatomical relationships. In classical texts the cadavers utilized seldom had excess fat, and organs were therefore presented in direct apposition to one another. In the average living individual this is not the case, and varying amounts of fat will separate organs to a varying degree. We should therefore think of the body more as a highly variable organ system with relatively wide variations of "normal" organ relationships rather than as one in which only a "fixed" simplistic relationship exists.

The other feature in this cadaver that should be noted is the presence of a left suprarenal cyst with only a small rim of residual glandular tissue. The sections are identified accordingly; and although the left suprarenal gland is not nicely displayed on transverse section, its demonstration in parasagittal and coronal section more than compensates for the loss.

Pelvis—female. Sections were from a 60-year-old woman who died of a myocardial infarct. The sections extend from the level of the aortic bifurcation through the entire pelvis and external genitalia.

Pelvis—male. Sections were from a middle-aged man who died of coronary artery disease. Although sections were obtained throughout the entire abdomen and were utilized in the labeling process, I have included sections beginning at the level of the fundus of the bladder and the bifurcation of the common iliac arteries and extending through the complete pelvis and external genitalia.

PARASAGITTAL OR LONGITUDINAL SECTIONS

Chest. Sections were from a 50-year-old woman, cause of death unknown. Only 12 sections were used out of the complete series in order to highlight important anatomical landmarks. The parasagittal chest sections are the ones I am least satisfied with, despite repeated attempts. In some cases, it was extremely difficult to completely remove the postmortem clot from all the cardiac chambers and adequately distend them with the dye solution, while in other cases a major vessel or chamber was ruptured in the process of instilling declotting or dye solution, making the specimen totally unacceptable.

In this particular specimen there was some leakage of blue solution into the tissues around the internal jugular vein as well as incomplete removal of clot from the right and left sides of the heart. Ideally, the left side of the heart would fill in a retrograde fashion with red solution and the right side, in an antegrade manner with blue solution. This was achieved in the cadaver used for transverse chest sections but not satisfactorily in any others.

Computerized axial tomography has generated an immediate need for a better understanding of the transverse anatomy of the chest. With a presentation of all three of the major anatomical planes, it is hoped that the deficiencies of each will be overcome.

Abdomen and pelvis—male. This complete series of sections 1 cm thick through the entire abdomen and pelvis of a middle-aged man are among the best in the book. All of the important organs and vessels are well injected, and the anatomical landmarks are easily recognizable. If it were not for the normal tortuosity of the abdominal aorta, we might have been more successful in bisecting it so as to demonstrate all of the major anterior branches. We found through experience that this type of result is seldom, if ever, possible to achieve. The cardiac anatomy in this individual was grossly distorted because of a large pericardial effusion; hence, no labeling of structures above the diaphragm was attempted.

Pelvis—female. Sections were from a 55-year-old woman who died of a myocardial infarct. Serial sections were obtained extending just beyond the lateral pelvic walls on each side. The pertinent pelvic anatomy is readily identifiable.

Abdominal aortic aneurysm. Sections were from a 60-year-old man who was found, at the time of sectioning, to have a large, unruptured abdominal aortic aneurysm. Two representative midline sections were included in this atlas of otherwise normal anatomy because it is a reasonably common condition and it demonstrates the normal and abnormal anatomy rather nicely. The normal male pelvic anatomy is also well seen.

CORONAL SECTIONS

Sections were from a 60-year-old man who died of a myocardial infarct. In our hands it was technically impossible to evenly and uniformly section the cadaver coronally without first bisecting it in the midsagittal plane. The relatively thin blade of the band saw wanders because of the various stresses put on it by different tissue densities; and if the throat of the saw is excessively large, the degree of blade wandering is unacceptable. In bisecting the body, we reduced the throat of the saw to 9 inches and were able to satisfactorily section the cadaver with little or no distortion. Each half was sectioned; the corresponding sections were then placed side by side on a Plexiglas plate and subsequently photographed. It appears that some of the sections do not match exactly, and this can only be the result of some inaccuracies in the cutting technique. Seldom does this cause confusion or detract from the beauty of the sections.

Photographic process

ROB MATHIESON

The color photographs were produced over a period of about 2 years, during which time only minor changes in the original photographic technique were necessary. A modified copy stand was used, but, finding that photoflood lamps caused the frozen sections to melt more quickly than was desirable, I resorted to electronic flash for all subsequent exposures. The film used was Ektachrome-X, processed using E-4 chemicals in a Colenta model 130 processor.

The photographs were made in a room set aside in the Anatomy Department of the University of Manitoba Medical School. Each section, on an individual piece of Plexiglas, was taken from a freezer, one at a time (Fig. 1) and placed on a tray, where a small amount of embalming fluid was poured on and spread as evenly as possible to remove the top layer of frost and allow the colors of the specimen to stand out more vividly (Fig. 2). Sections were then transferred quickly to a piece of glass 100 × 60 cm, which was resting on a piece of black velvet in turn supported on a piece of plywood. To overcome some of the reflections of the light sources, polarizing screens over the lights and a polarizing filter over the camera

lens were used. This technique resulted in a marked reduction in the number of reflections, but the reflective points now present as purple dots, which may be somewhat more distracting. Viewing and focusing were made more difficult because of the loss of light through the lens. For the smaller specimens, such as the transverse sections, use of polarizing materials did not result in any worthwhile improvement.

Two cameras mounted side by side on a versatile Linhof camera stand were used, and all were masked appropriately

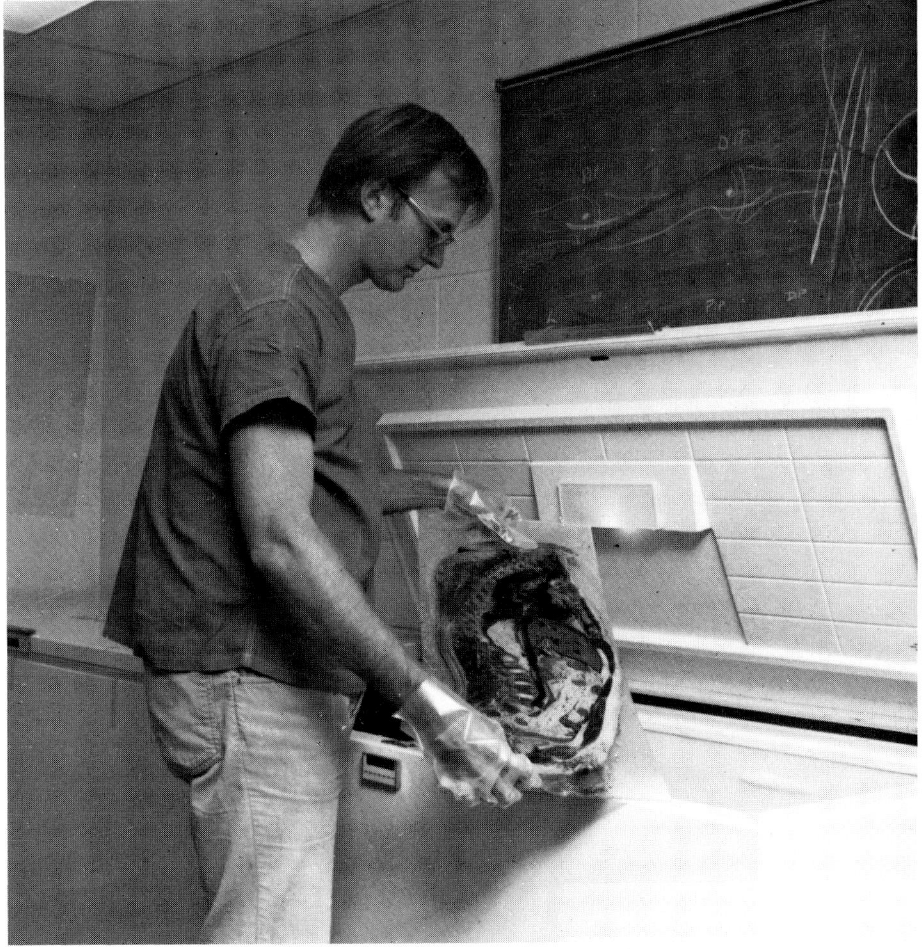

Fig. 1

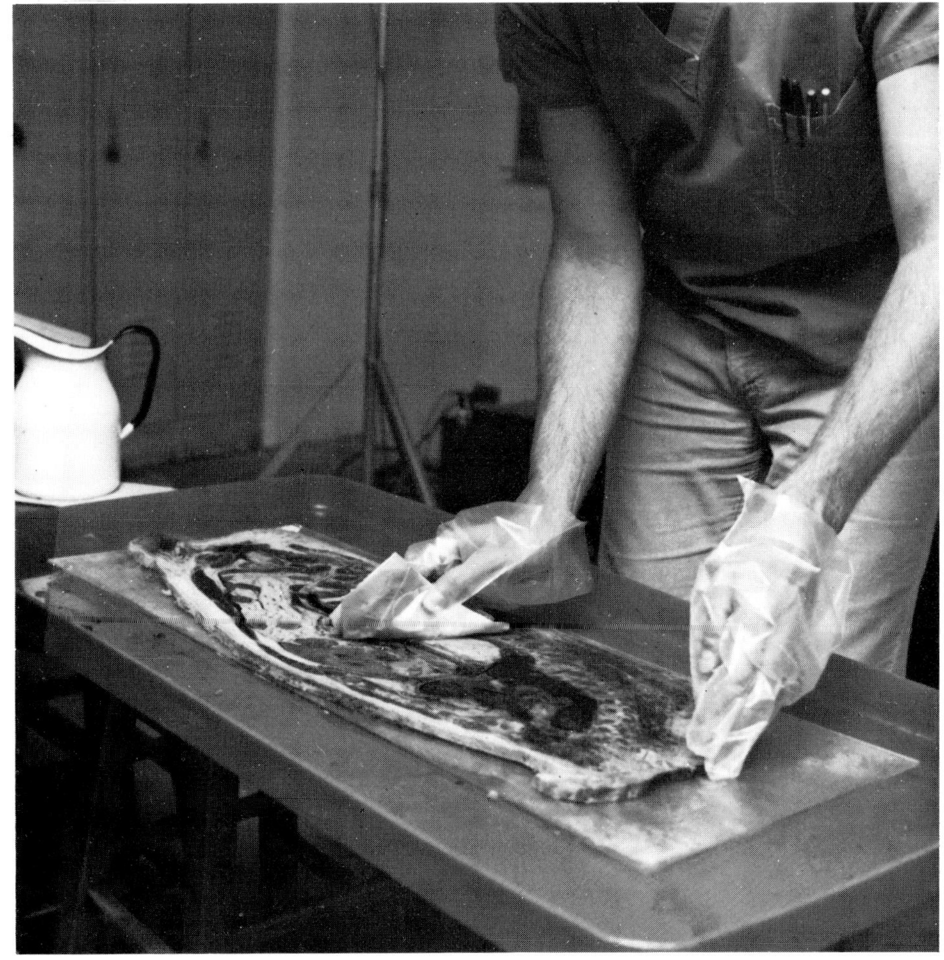

Fig. 2

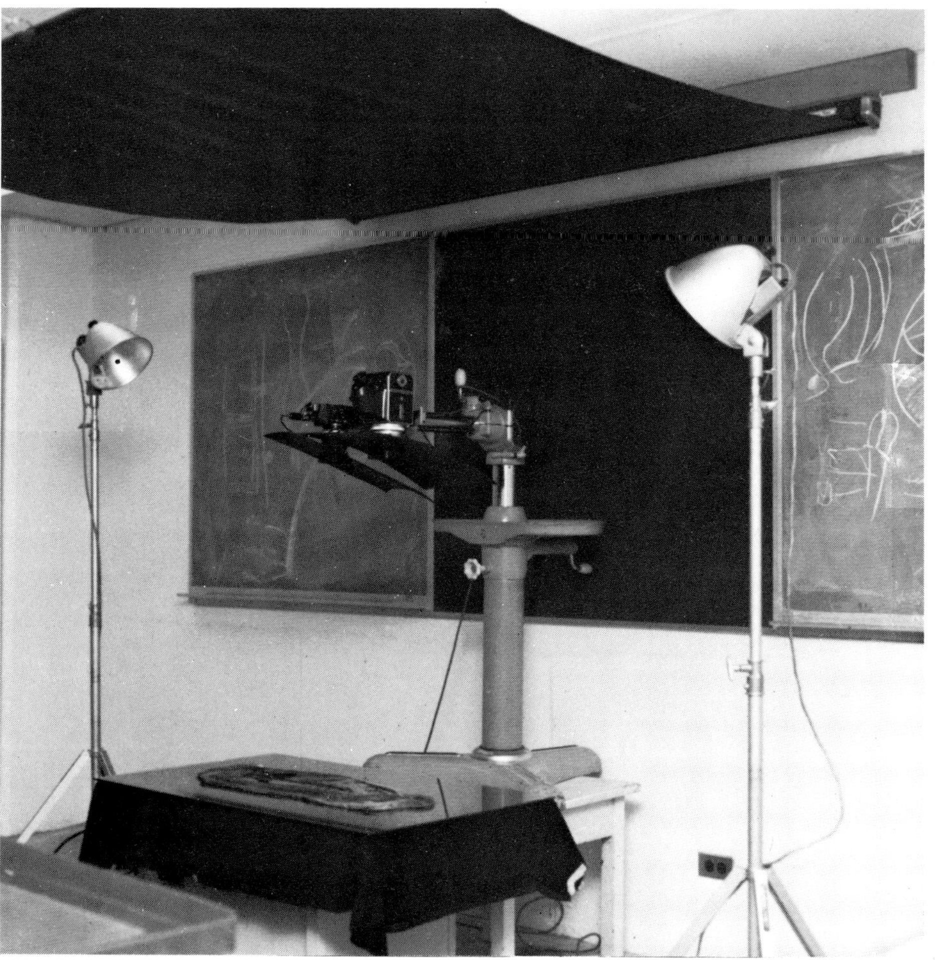

Fig. 3

to eliminate reflections in the glass. In Fig. 3, the draping has been removed to reveal the camera stand with its horizontal arm. A Nikkormat FTn with a 55-mm micro-Nikkor lens was used to make 35-mm color slides. A Hasselblad 500 C/M with an 80-mm lens (and a Proxar close-up lens as required) was used to make color negatives and 4 × 6 cm color positives. The negatives were used to make 8 × 10 prints, from which the line diagrams were generated. The positives were used in making the color plates for the book.

Because the room was light colored with a low ceiling, there were significant difficulties in light reflection. The use of a wall-hung projection screen with a black backing reduced overhead reflection (Fig. 3).

Preparation of line diagrams

Each section was reproduced on an 8 × 10 color print. An exact tracing of each section was made using a light box and onion skin tracing paper. These tracings were subsequently redone on heavier paper with more prominent outlines. Color was added to highlight three general tissue types. Yellow was used for all bony structures. Solid organs were colored red, and blue was used to identify the gastrointestinal tract. This was done to make it easier for the observer to rapidly identify significant landmarks. Following this, each section was labeled, with as many pertinent structures identified as possible.

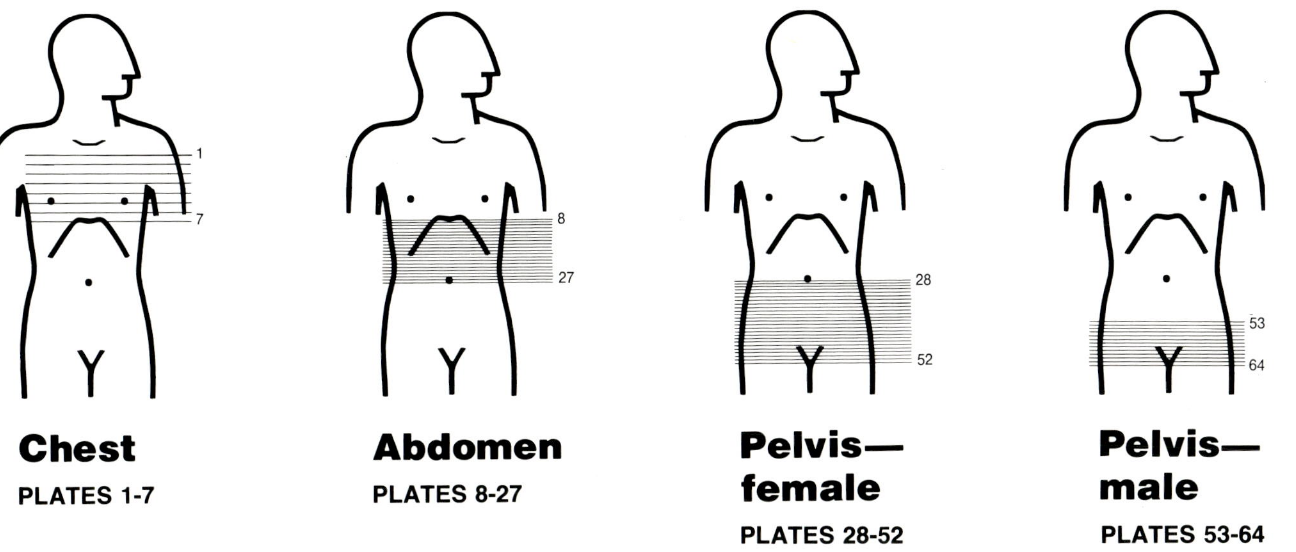

Chest

PLATES 1-7

Abdomen

PLATES 8-27

Pelvis— female

PLATES 28-52

Pelvis— male

PLATES 53-64

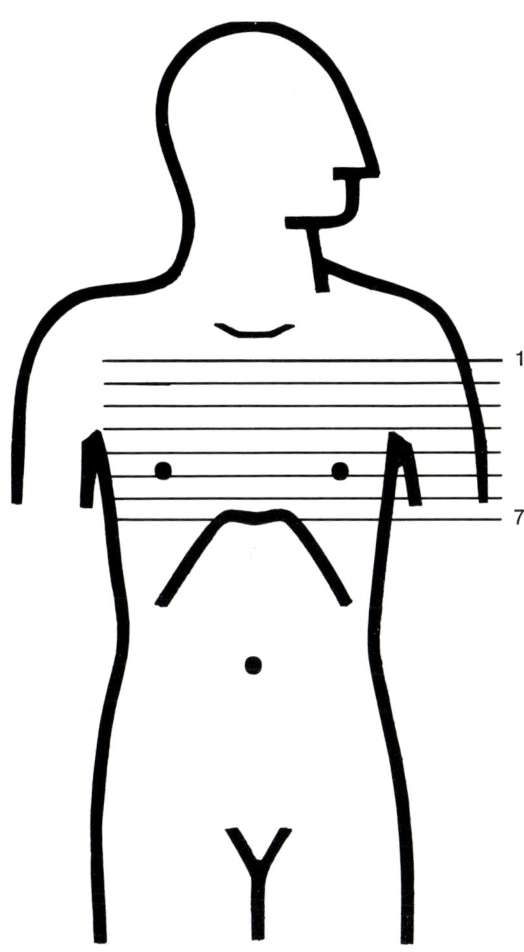
1
7

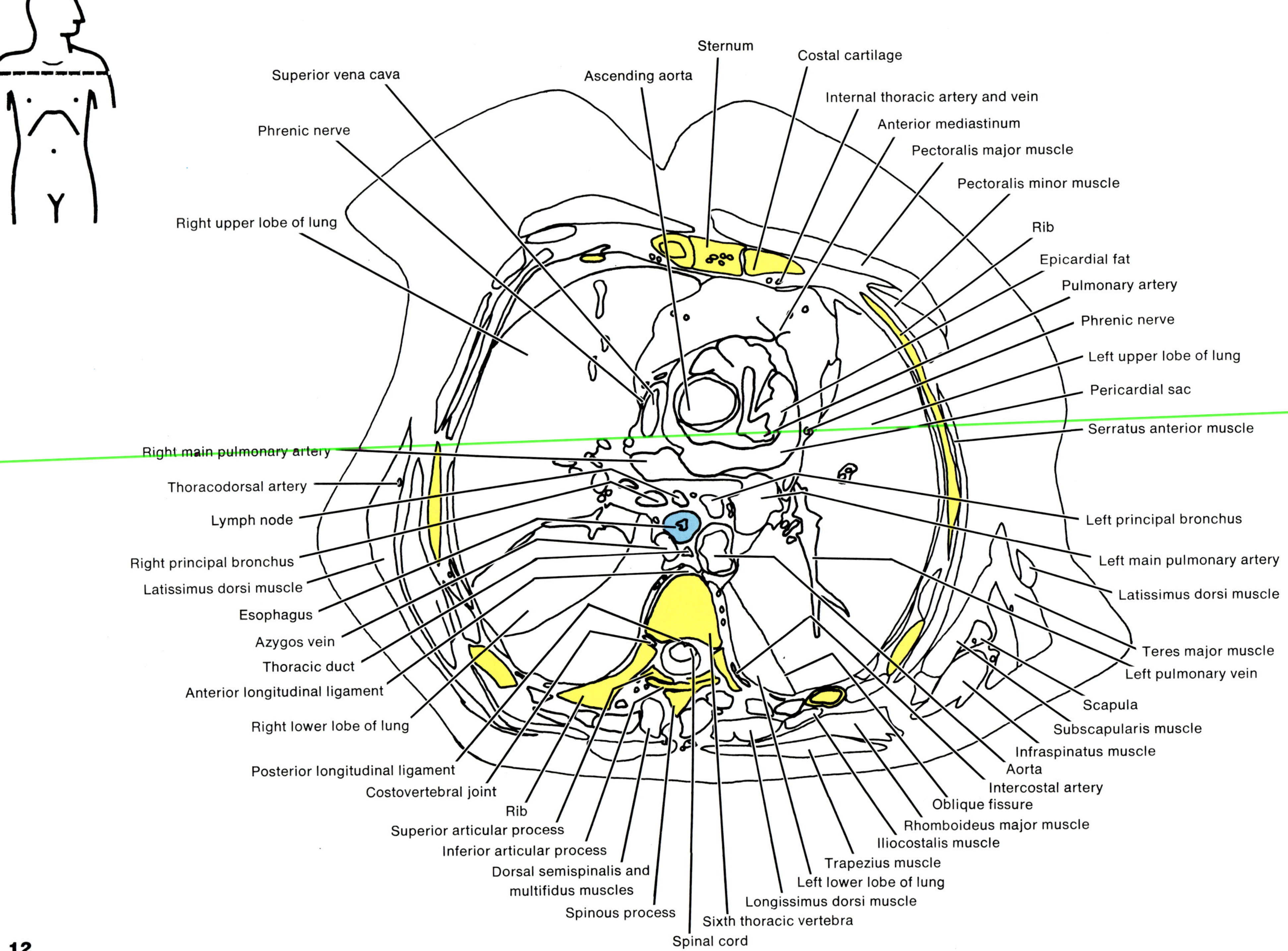

PLATE 1
Y
Superior vena cava
Phrenic nerve
Right upper lobe of lung
Sternum
Ascending aorta
Costal cartilage
Internal thoracic artery and vein
Anterior mediastinum
Pectoralis major muscle
Pectoralis minor muscle
Rib
Epicardial fat
Pulmonary artery
Phrenic nerve
Left upper lobe of lung
Pericardial sac
Serratus anterior muscle
Right main pulmonary artery
Thoracodorsal artery
Lymph node
Right principal bronchus
Latissimus dorsi muscle
Esophagus
Azygos vein
Thoracic duct
Anterior longitudinal ligament
Right lower lobe of lung
Posterior longitudinal ligament
Costovertebral joint
Rib
Superior articular process
Inferior articular process
Dorsal semispinalis and
multifidus muscles
Spinous process
Spinal cord
Sixth thoracic vertebra
Longissimus dorsi muscle
Left lower lobe of lung
Trapezius muscle
Iliocostalis muscle
Rhomboideus major muscle
Oblique fissure
Intercostal artery
Aorta
Infraspinatus muscle
Subscapularis muscle
Scapula
Left pulmonary vein
Teres major muscle
Latissimus dorsi muscle
Left main pulmonary artery
Left principal bronchus

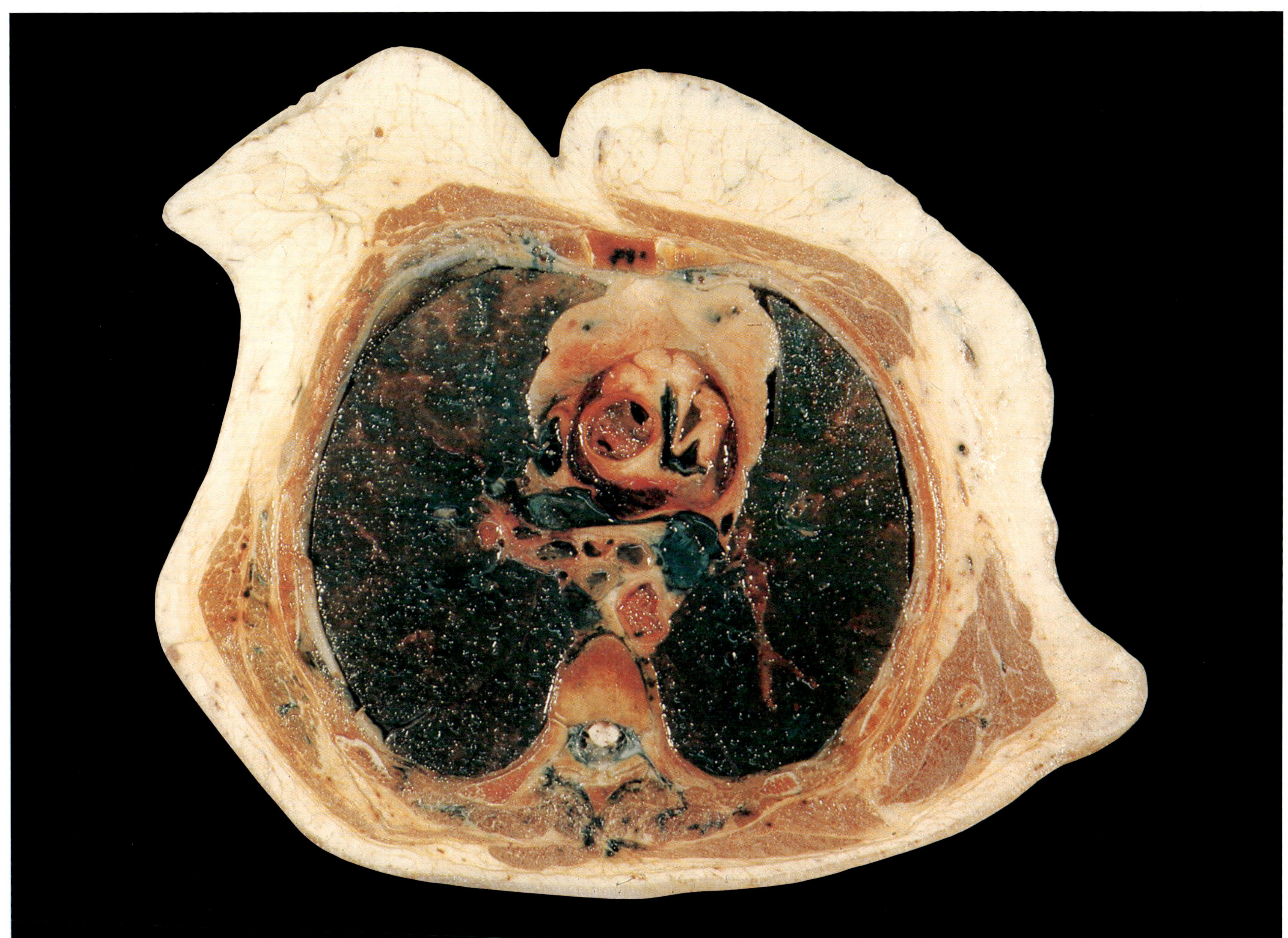

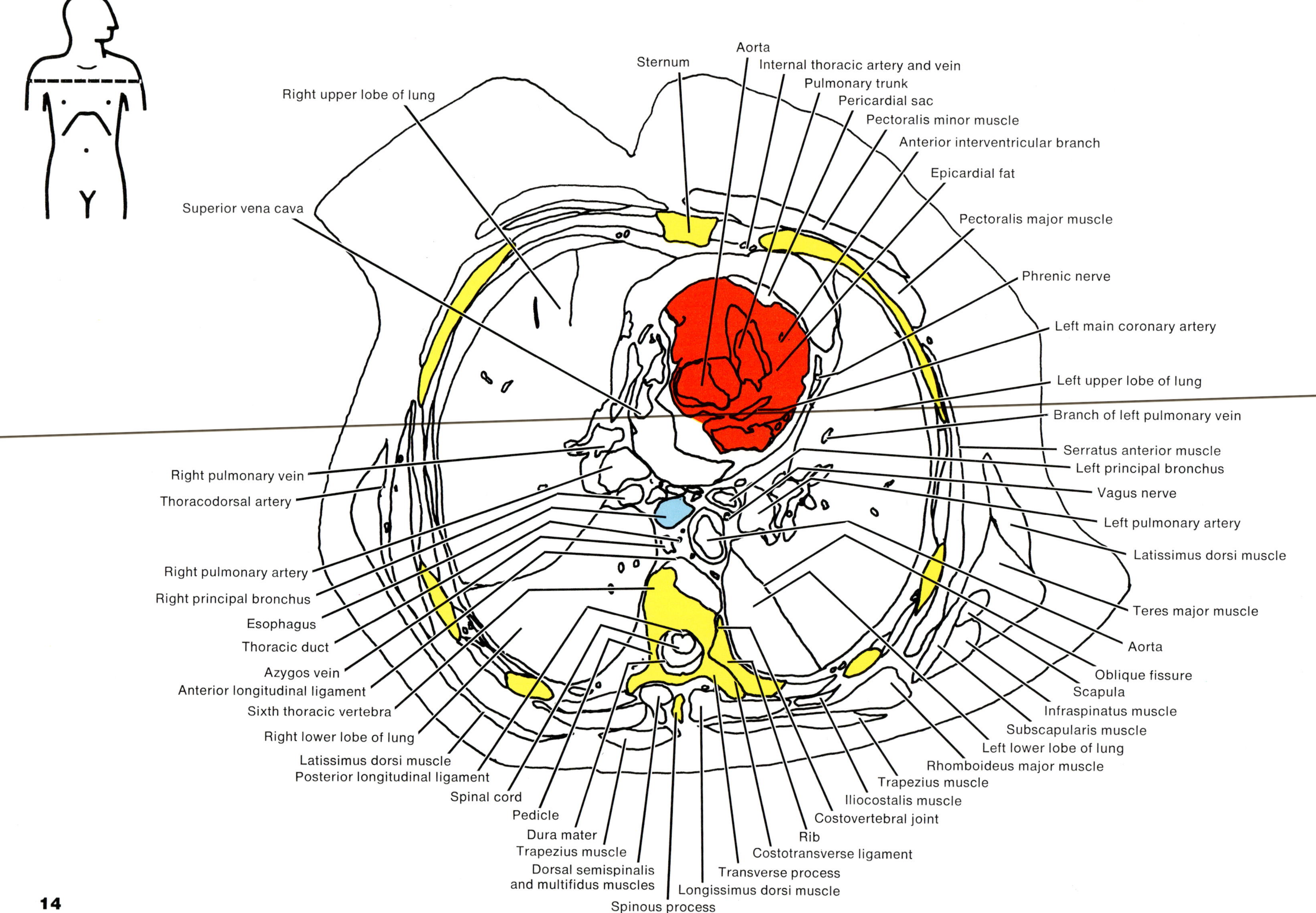

Sternum
Aorta
Internal thoracic artery and vein
Pulmonary trunk
Pericardial sac
Pectoralis minor muscle
Anterior interventricular branch
Epicardial fat
Pectoralis major muscle
Phrenic nerve
Left main coronary artery
Left upper lobe of lung
Branch of left pulmonary vein
Serratus anterior muscle
Left principal bronchus
Vagus nerve
Left pulmonary artery
Latissimus dorsi muscle
Teres major muscle
Aorta
Oblique fissure
Scapula
Infraspinatus muscle
Subscapularis muscle
Left lower lobe of lung
Rhomboideus major muscle
Trapezius muscle
Iliocostalis muscle
Costovertebral joint
Rib
Costotransverse ligament
Transverse process
Longissimus dorsi muscle
Spinous process
Dorsal semispinalis
and multifidus muscles
Trapezius muscle
Dura mater
Pedicle
Spinal cord
Posterior longitudinal ligament
Latissimus dorsi muscle
Right lower lobe of lung
Sixth thoracic vertebra
Anterior longitudinal ligament
Azygos vein
Thoracic duct
Esophagus
Right principal bronchus
Right pulmonary artery
Thoracodorsal artery
Right pulmonary vein
Superior vena cava
Right upper lobe of lung

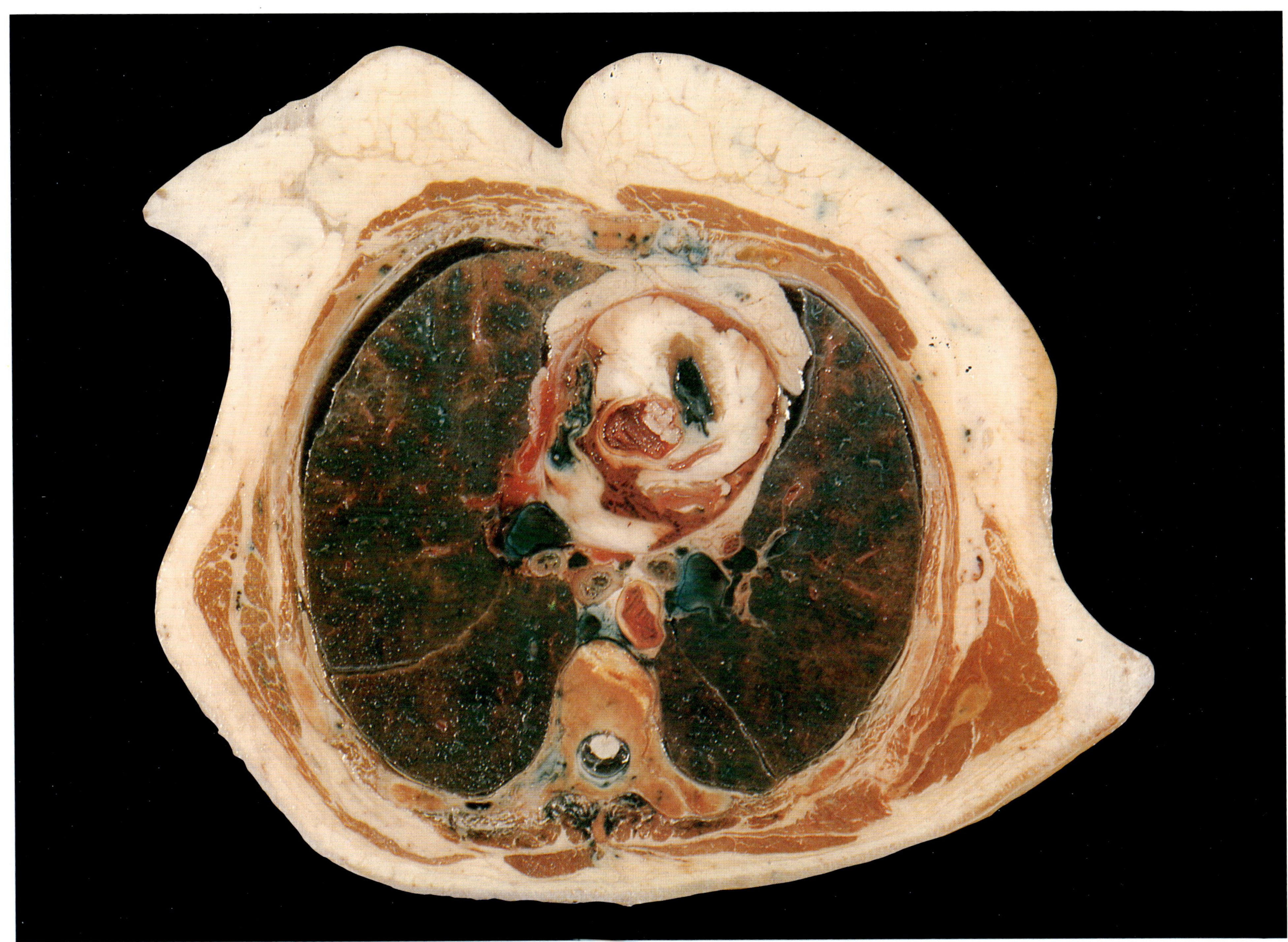

Right coronary artery
Right coronary cusp
Noncoronary cusp
Right main coronary artery
Phrenic nerve
Costal cartilage
Superior vena cava
Right upper lobe of lung
Right pulmonary vein
Anterior esophageal plexus
Right pulmonary artery
Latissimus dorsi muscle
Oblique fissure
Right bronchus
Serratus anterior muscle
Esophagus
Thoracic duct
Azygos vein
Anterior longitudinal ligament
Right lower lobe of lung
Costovertebral joint
Dura mater
Rib
Longissimus dorsi muscle
Dorsal semispinalis and multifidus muscles
Trapezius muscle
Spinous process
Sternum
Pectoralis major muscle
Internal thoracic artery and vein
Pericardial sac
Right ventricular outflow tract
Anterior interventricular branch
Great cardiac vein
Pectoralis minor muscle
Epicardial fat
Phrenic nerve
Left coronary cusp
Coronary sinus
Left upper lobe of lung
Circumflex branch
Left atrium
Latissimus dorsi muscle
Left pulmonary vein
Thoracodorsal artery
Left upper lobe bronchus
Serratus anterior muscle
Teres major muscle
Left pulmonary artery
Subscapularis muscle
Scapula
Infraspinatus muscle
Oblique fissure
Rhomboideus major muscle
Left lower lobe of lung
Trapezius muscle
Aorta
Intercostal artery
Longissimus dorsi muscle
Seventh thoracic vertebra
Posterior longitudinal ligament
Spinal cord

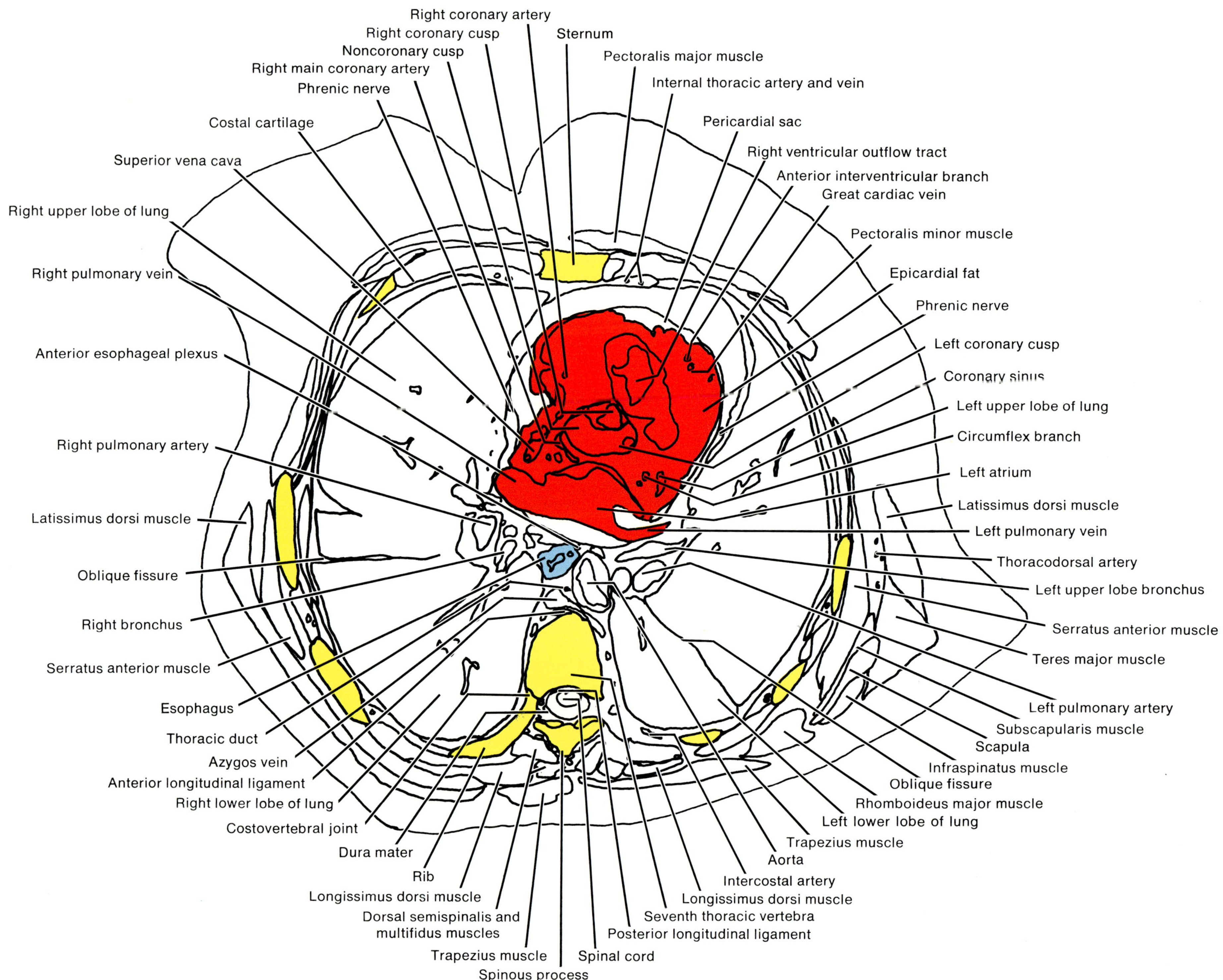

16

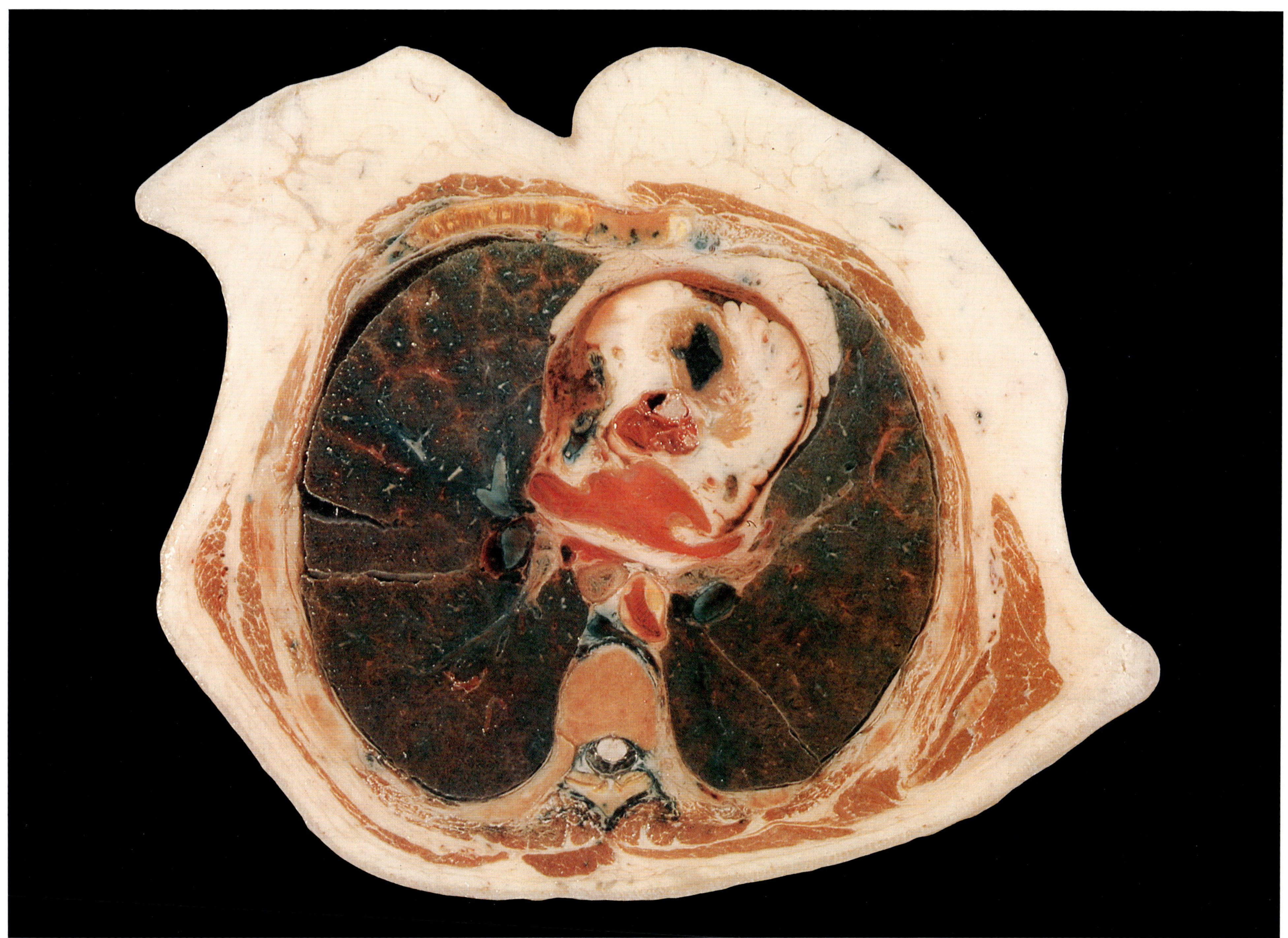

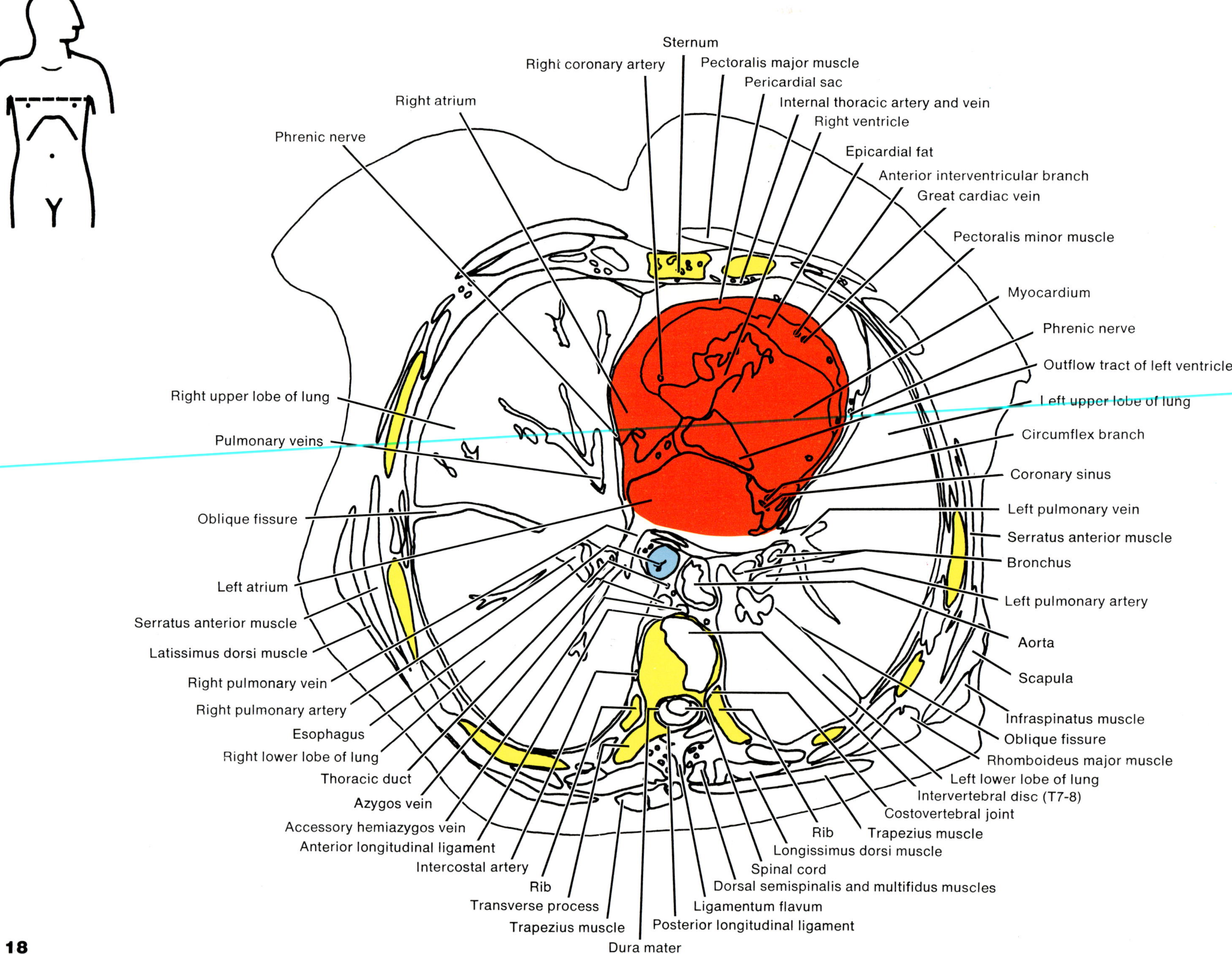
Y
Sternum
Right coronary artery
Pectoralis major muscle
Pericardial sac
Internal thoracic artery and vein
Right ventricle
Right atrium
Epicardial fat
Anterior interventricular branch
Great cardiac vein
Phrenic nerve
Pectoralis minor muscle
Myocardium
Phrenic nerve
Outflow tract of left ventricle
Right upper lobe of lung
Left upper lobe of lung
Circumflex branch
Pulmonary veins
Coronary sinus
Left pulmonary vein
Serratus anterior muscle
Oblique fissure
Bronchus
Left atrium
Left pulmonary artery
Serratus anterior muscle
Aorta
Latissimus dorsi muscle
Scapula
Right pulmonary vein
Right pulmonary artery
Infraspinatus muscle
Esophagus
Oblique fissure
Right lower lobe of lung
Rhomboideus major muscle
Thoracic duct
Left lower lobe of lung
Azygos vein
Intervertebral disc (T7-8)
Accessory hemiazygos vein
Costovertebral joint
Anterior longitudinal ligament
Rib
Trapezius muscle
Intercostal artery
Longissimus dorsi muscle
Rib
Spinal cord
Transverse process
Dorsal semispinalis and multifidus muscles
Trapezius muscle
Ligamentum flavum
Posterior longitudinal ligament
Dura mater

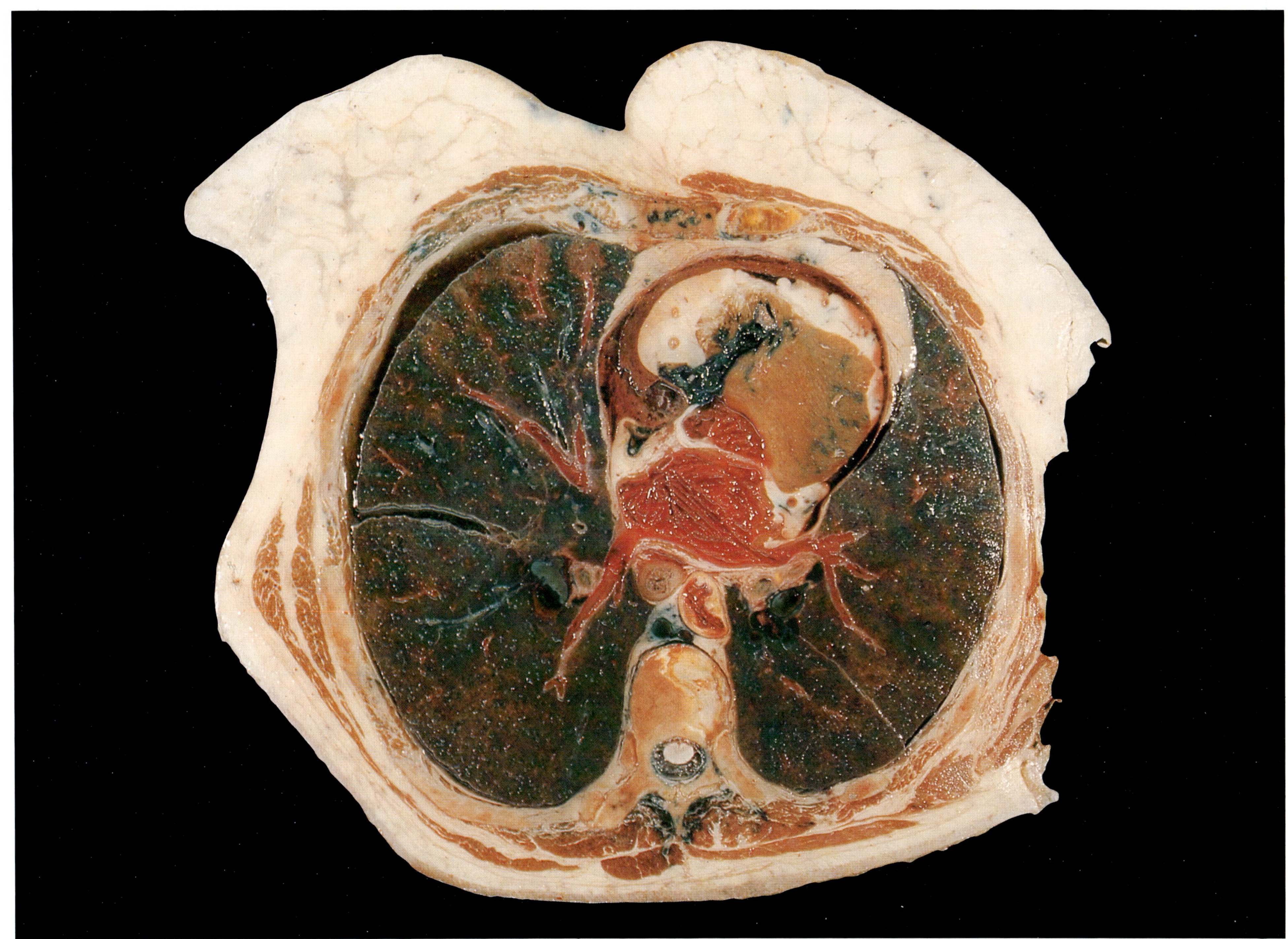

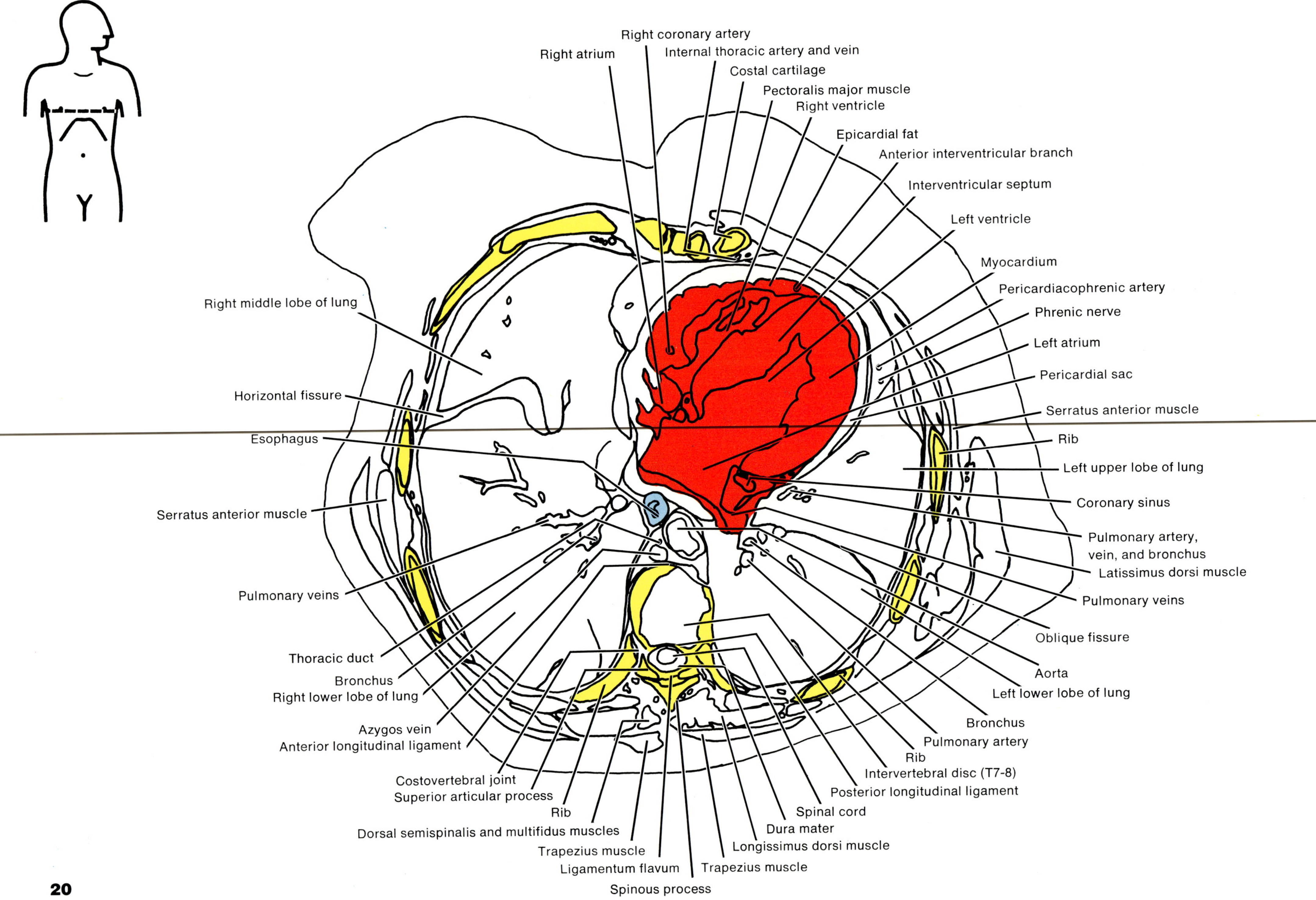

Right atrium
Right coronary artery
Internal thoracic artery and vein
Costal cartilage
Pectoralis major muscle
Right ventricle
Epicardial fat
Anterior interventricular branch
Interventricular septum
Left ventricle
Myocardium
Pericardiacophrenic artery
Phrenic nerve
Left atrium
Pericardial sac
Serratus anterior muscle
Rib
Left upper lobe of lung
Coronary sinus
Pulmonary artery, vein, and bronchus
Latissimus dorsi muscle
Pulmonary veins
Oblique fissure
Aorta
Left lower lobe of lung
Bronchus
Pulmonary artery
Rib
Intervertebral disc (T7-8)
Posterior longitudinal ligament
Spinal cord
Dura mater
Longissimus dorsi muscle
Trapezius muscle
Trapezius muscle
Ligamentum flavum
Spinous process
Ligamentum flavum
Rib
Dorsal semispinalis and multifidus muscles
Superior articular process
Costovertebral joint
Anterior longitudinal ligament
Azygos vein
Right lower lobe of lung
Bronchus
Thoracic duct
Pulmonary veins
Serratus anterior muscle
Esophagus
Horizontal fissure
Right middle lobe of lung

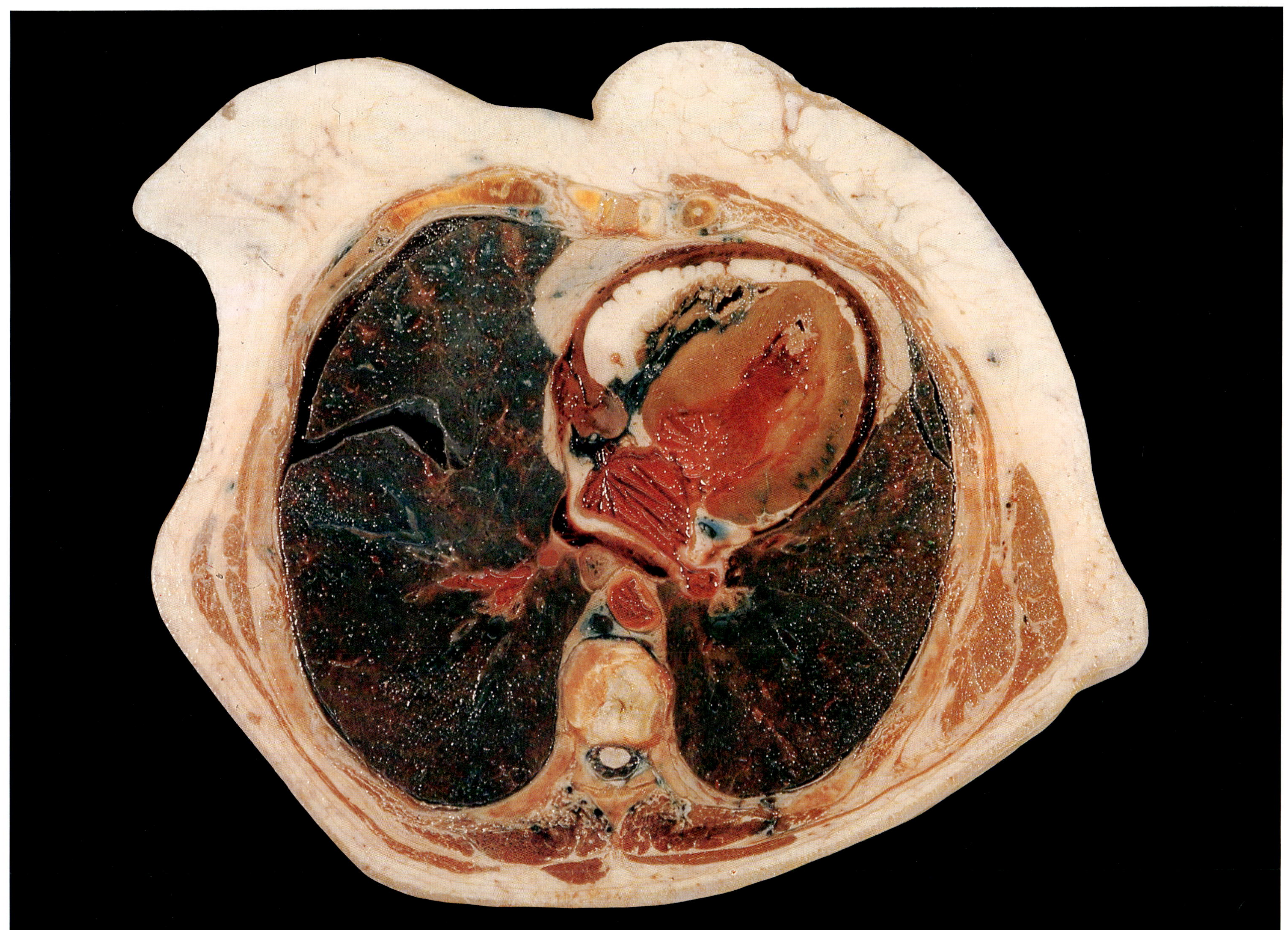

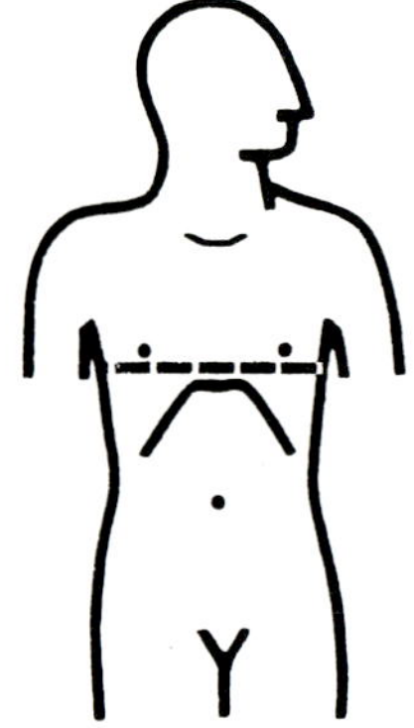

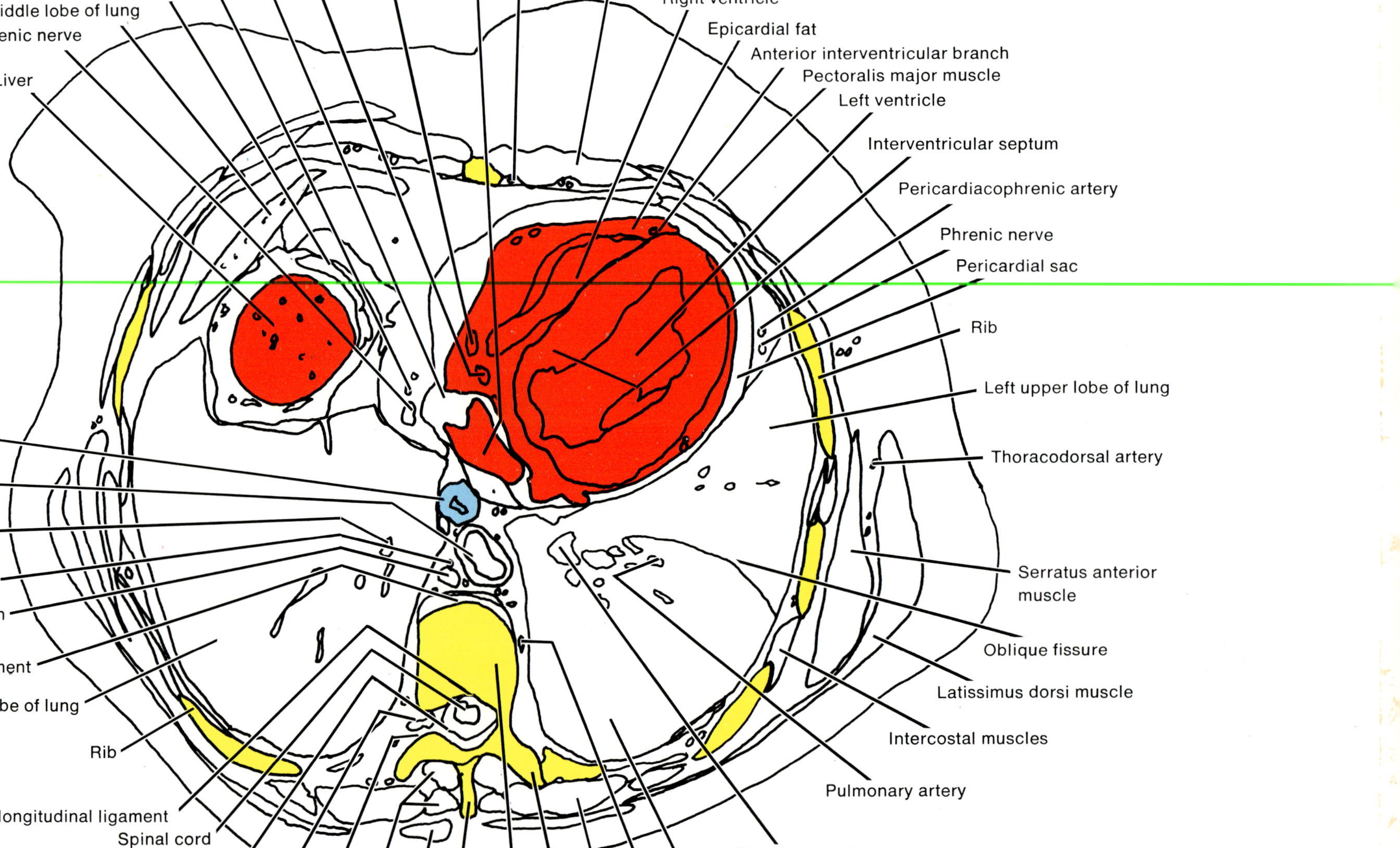

Marginal branch of right coronary artery
Posterior interventricular branch
Coronary sinus
Inferior vena cava
Internal thoracic artery and vein
Pericardiacophrenic artery
Costal cartilage
Diaphragm
Right ventricle
Right middle lobe of lung
Epicardial fat
Phrenic nerve
Anterior interventricular branch
Pectoralis major muscle
Liver
Left ventricle
Interventricular septum
Pericardiacophrenic artery
Phrenic nerve
Pericardial sac
Rib
Left upper lobe of lung
Esophagus
Thoracodorsal artery
Aorta
Pulmonary vein
Thoracic duct
Serratus anterior muscle
Azygos vein
Anterior longitudinal ligament
Oblique fissure
Right lower lobe of lung
Latissimus dorsi muscle
Intercostal muscles
Rib
Posterior longitudinal ligament
Spinal cord
Pulmonary artery
Dura mater
Dorsal root ganglion
Intervertebral foramen
Pulmonary vein
Dorsal semispinalis and multifidus muscles
Left lower lobe of lung
Intercostal artery
Longissimus dorsi muscle
Trapezius muscle
Transverse process
Spinous process
Eighth thoracic vertebra

TRANSVERSE **Chest**

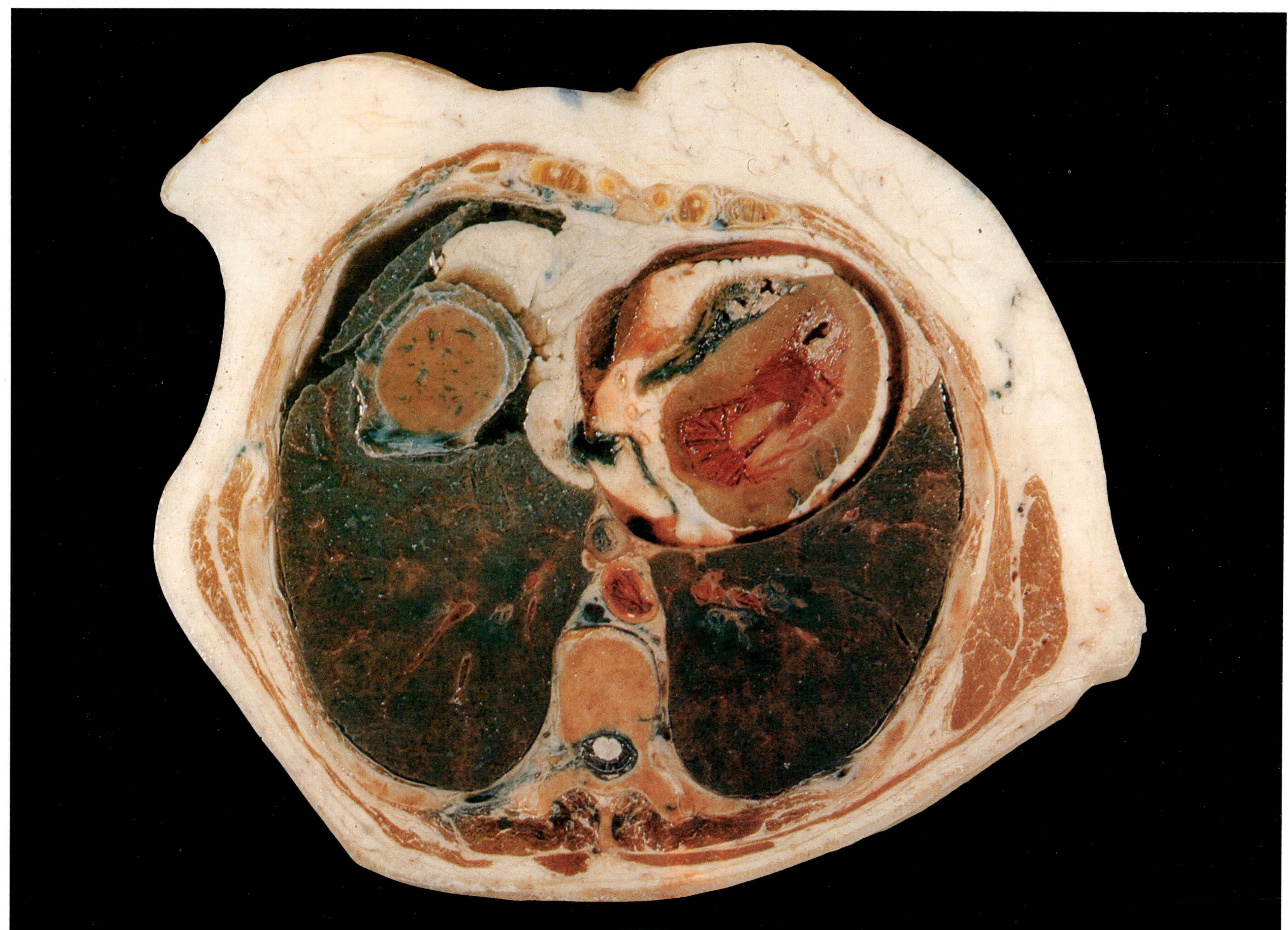

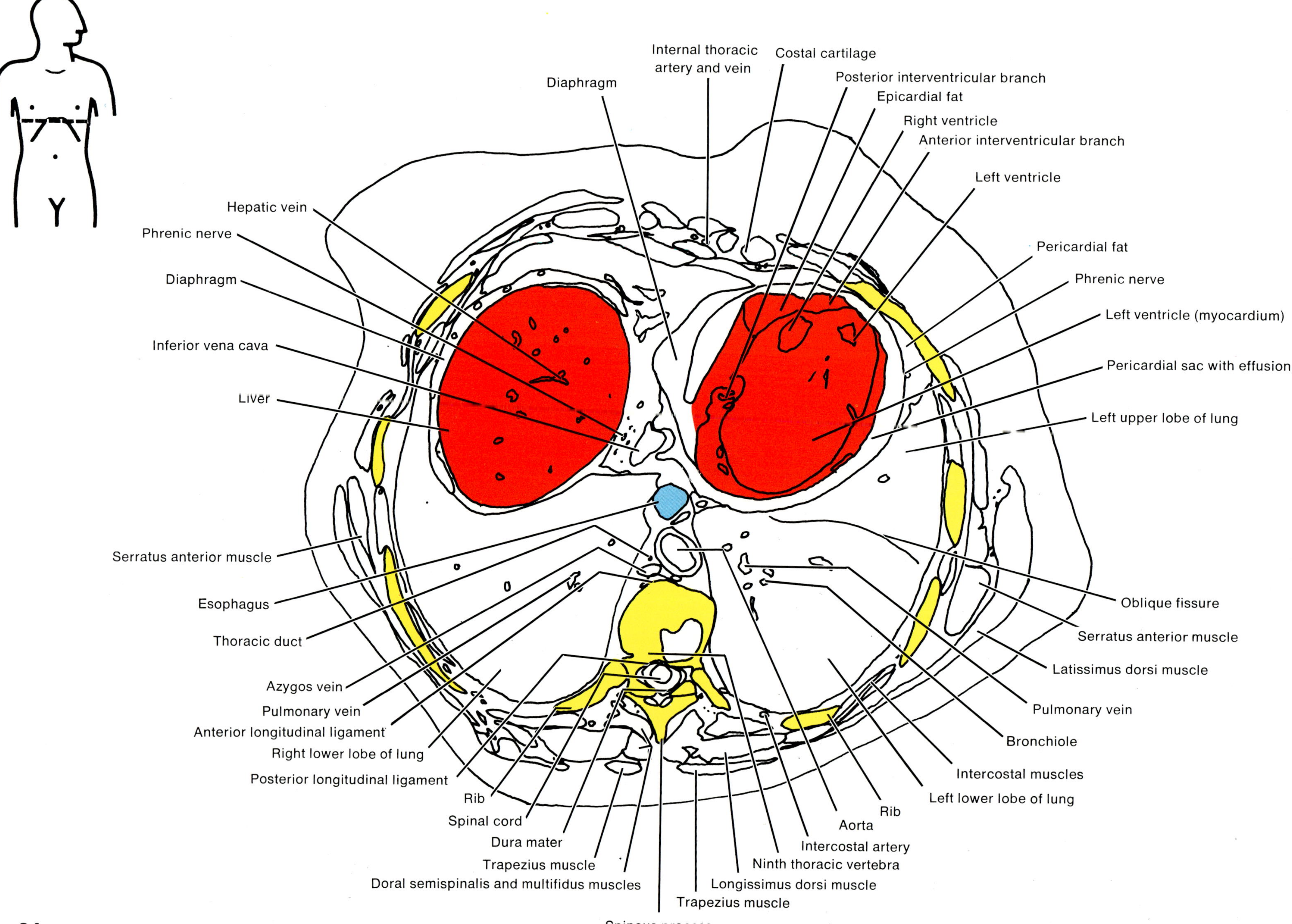

Internal thoracic artery and vein
Costal cartilage
Posterior interventricular branch
Epicardial fat
Right ventricle
Anterior interventricular branch
Left ventricle
Diaphragm
Hepatic vein
Phrenic nerve
Diaphragm
Inferior vena cava
Liver
Pericardial fat
Phrenic nerve
Left ventricle (myocardium)
Pericardial sac with effusion
Left upper lobe of lung
Serratus anterior muscle
Esophagus
Thoracic duct
Azygos vein
Pulmonary vein
Anterior longitudinal ligament
Right lower lobe of lung
Posterior longitudinal ligament
Oblique fissure
Serratus anterior muscle
Latissimus dorsi muscle
Pulmonary vein
Bronchiole
Intercostal muscles
Left lower lobe of lung
Rib
Spinal cord
Dura mater
Trapezius muscle
Doral semispinalis and multifidus muscles
Rib
Aorta
Intercostal artery
Ninth thoracic vertebra
Longissimus dorsi muscle
Trapezius muscle
Spinous process

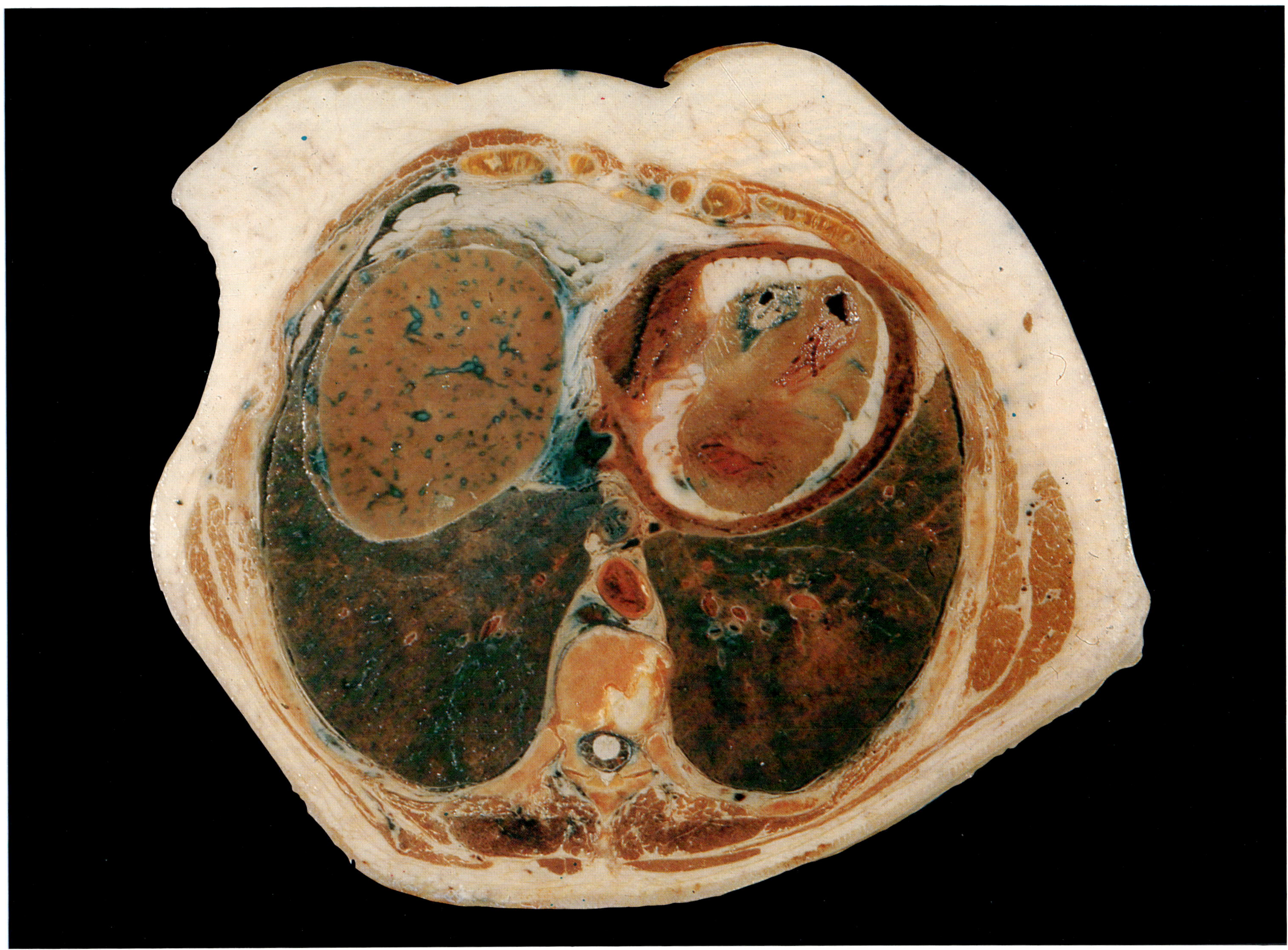

TRANSVERSE **Abdomen**
PLATES 8-27

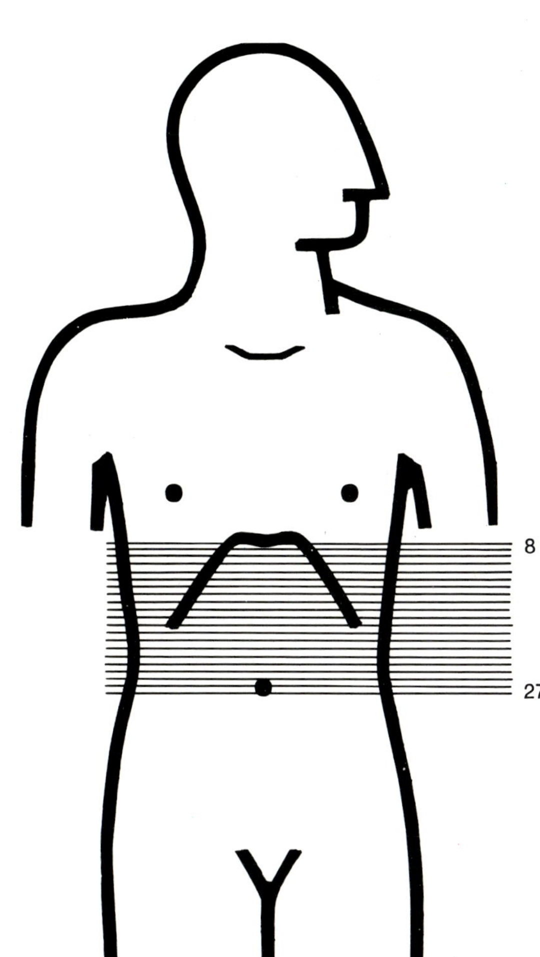

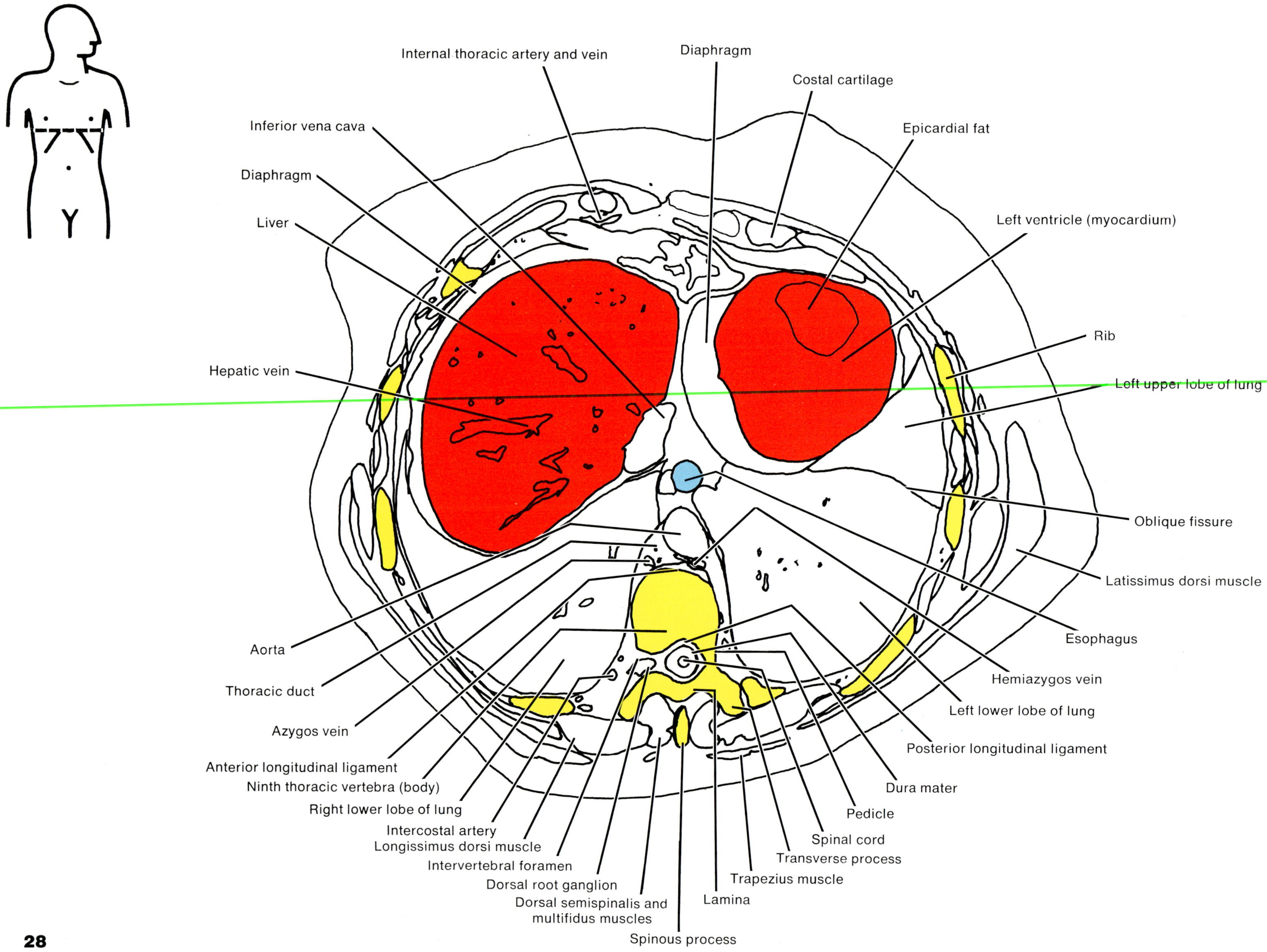

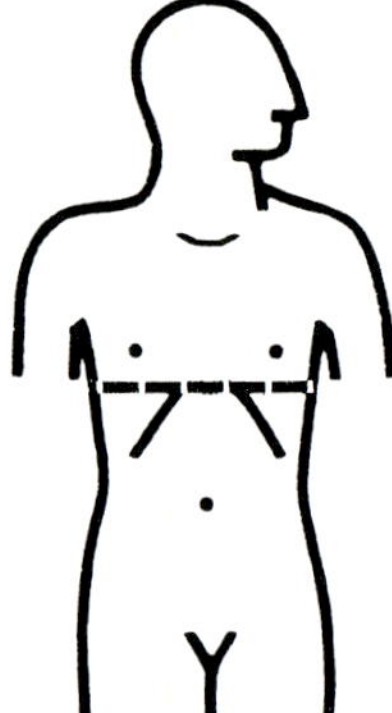

Internal thoracic artery and vein
Diaphragm
Costal cartilage
Epicardial fat
Inferior vena cava
Left ventricle (myocardium)
Diaphragm
Liver
Rib
Hepatic vein
Left upper lobe of lung
Oblique fissure
Latissimus dorsi muscle
Esophagus
Aorta
Hemiazygos vein
Thoracic duct
Left lower lobe of lung
Azygos vein
Posterior longitudinal ligament
Anterior longitudinal ligament
Dura mater
Ninth thoracic vertebra (body)
Pedicle
Right lower lobe of lung
Spinal cord
Intercostal artery
Transverse process
Longissimus dorsi muscle
Intervertebral foramen
Trapezius muscle
Dorsal root ganglion
Lamina
Dorsal semispinalis and
multifidus muscles
Spinous process

TRANSVERSE **Abdomen**

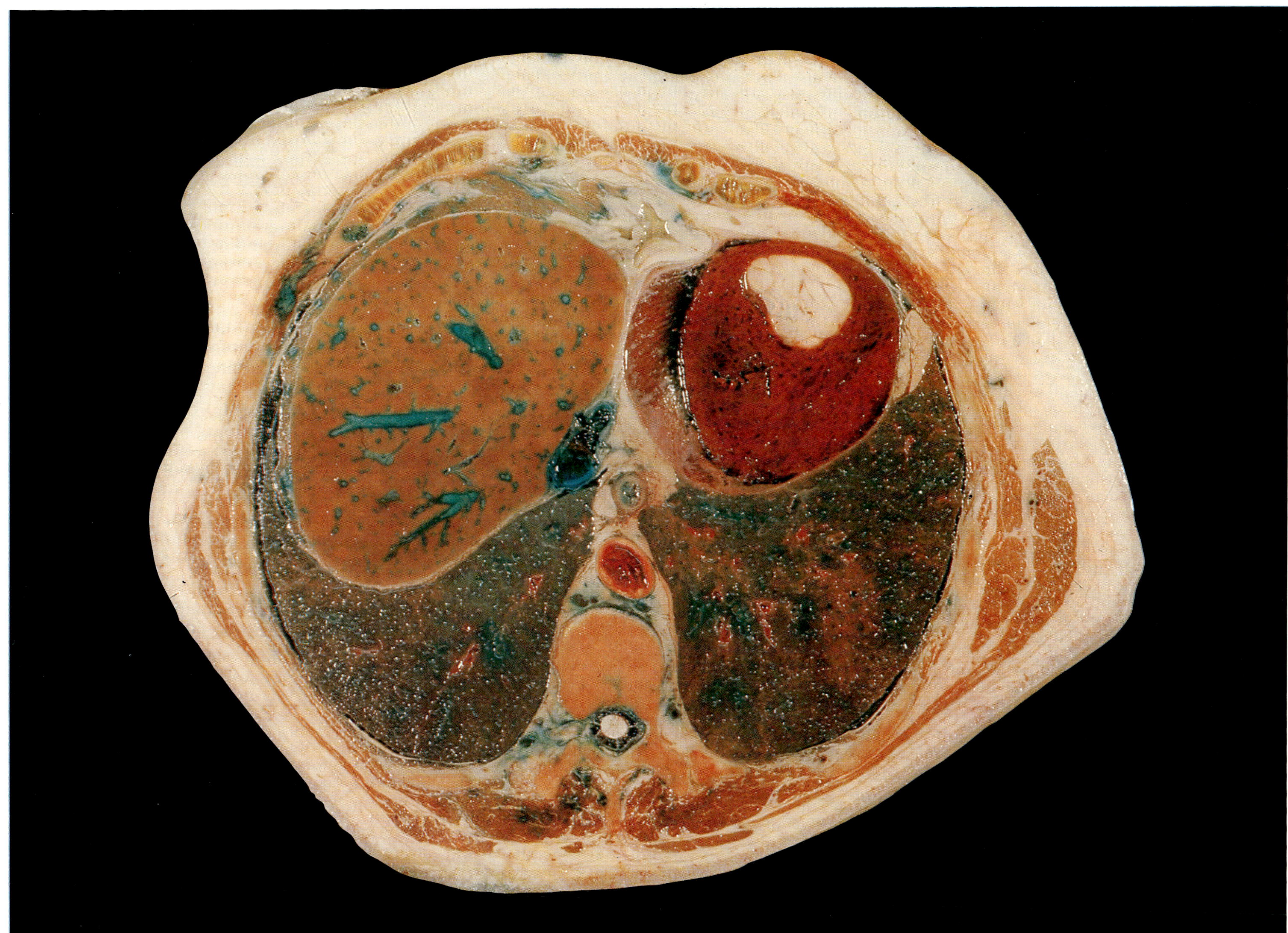

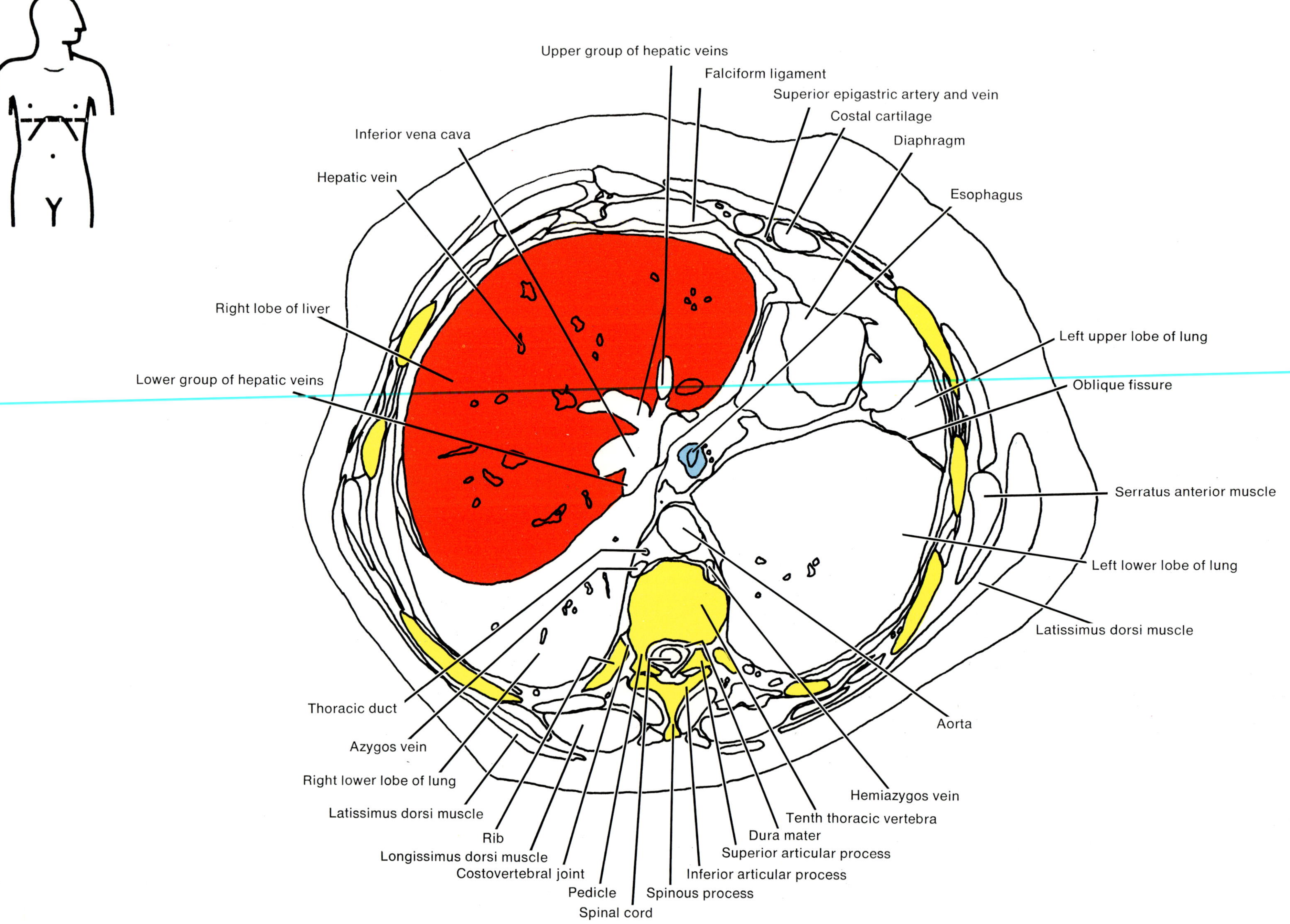

Upper group of hepatic veins
Falciform ligament
Superior epigastric artery and vein
Costal cartilage
Diaphragm
Esophagus
Inferior vena cava
Hepatic vein
Right lobe of liver
Left upper lobe of lung
Lower group of hepatic veins
Oblique fissure
Serratus anterior muscle
Left lower lobe of lung
Latissimus dorsi muscle
Aorta
Thoracic duct
Azygos vein
Hemiazygos vein
Right lower lobe of lung
Tenth thoracic vertebra
Latissimus dorsi muscle
Dura mater
Rib
Superior articular process
Longissimus dorsi muscle
Inferior articular process
Costovertebral joint
Pedicle
Spinous process
Spinal cord

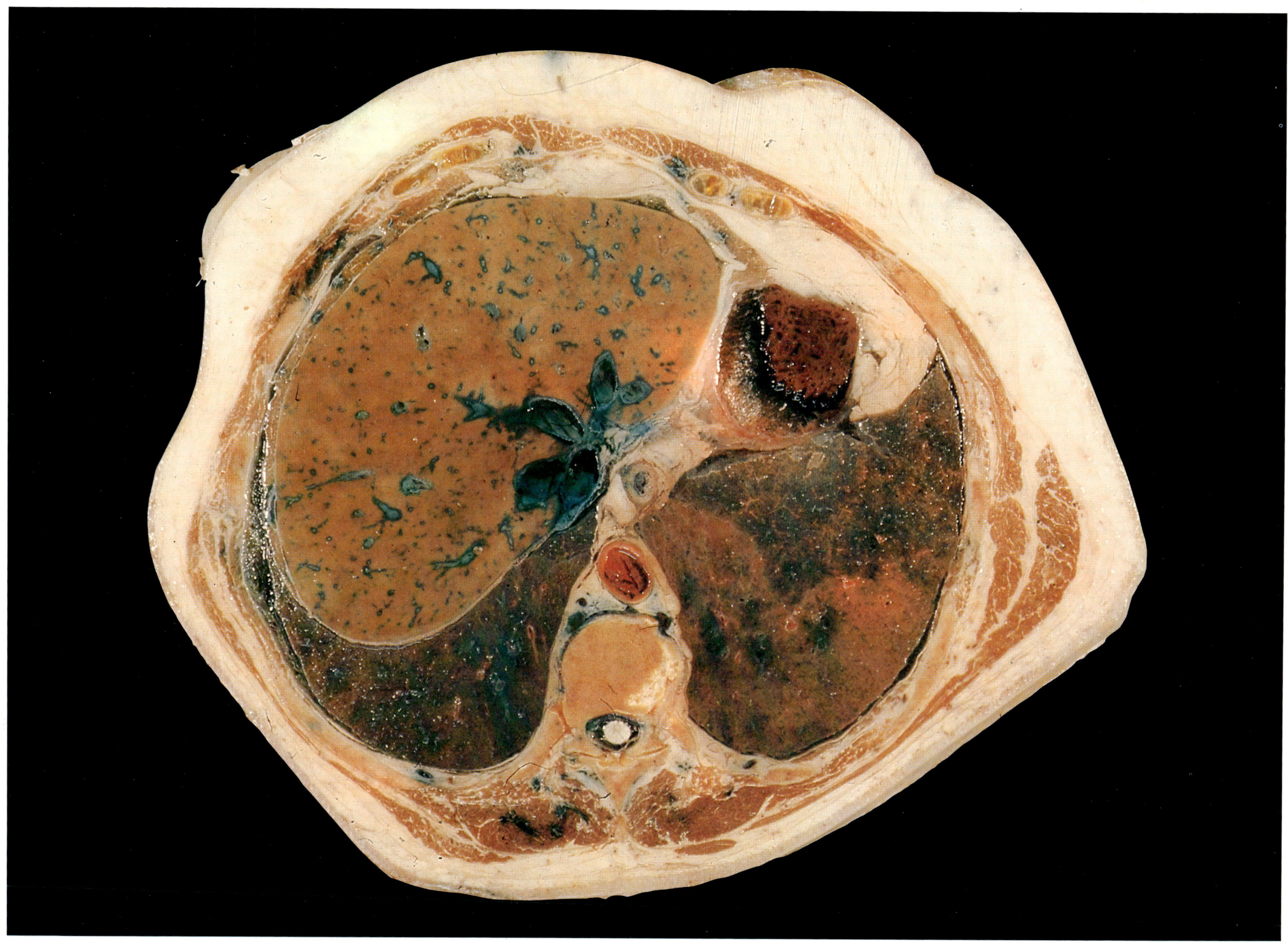

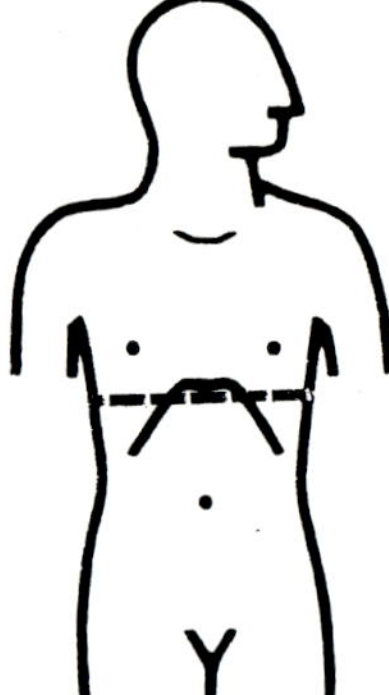

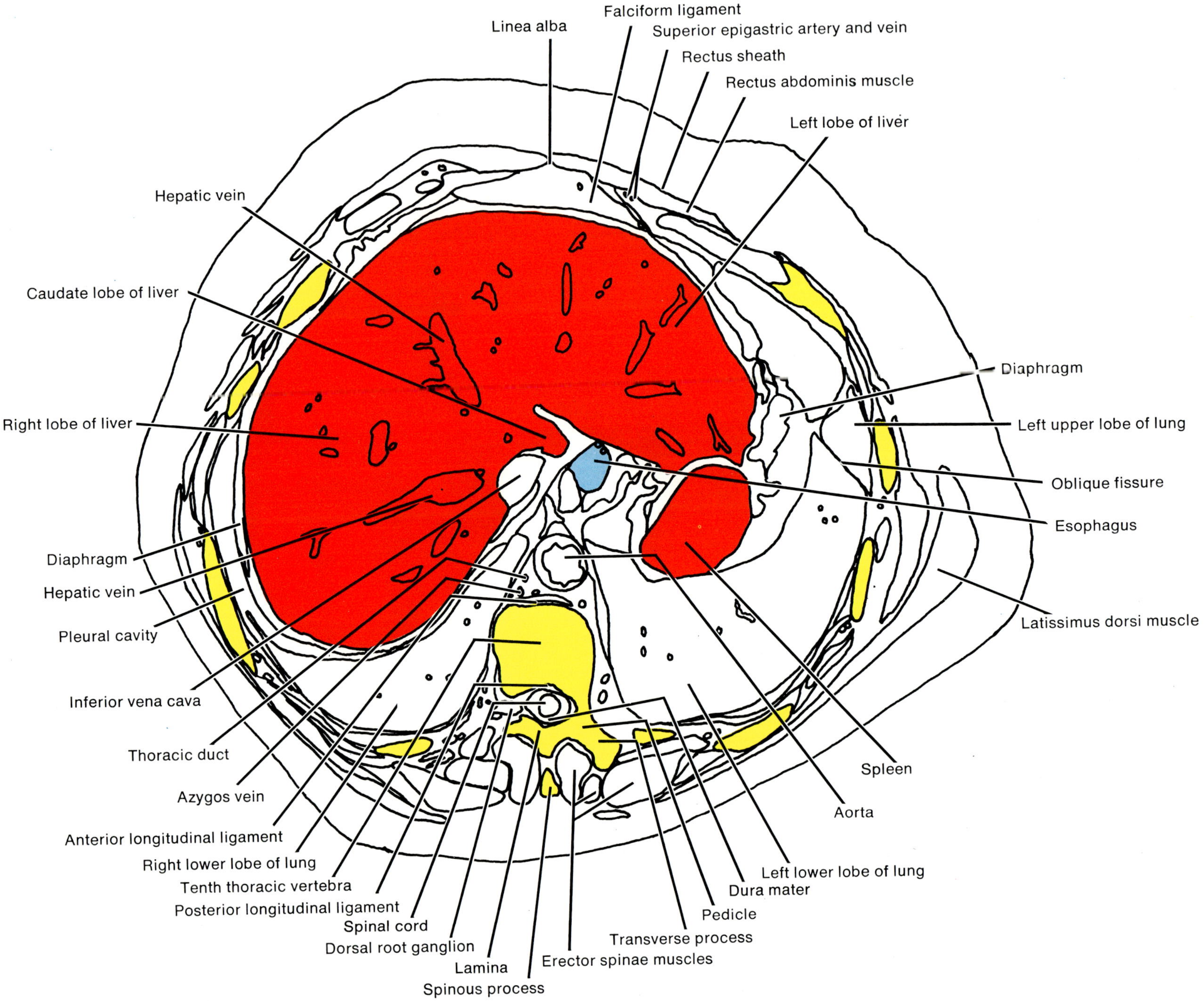

Linea alba
Falciform ligament
Superior epigastric artery and vein
Rectus sheath
Rectus abdominis muscle
Left lobe of liver
Hepatic vein
Caudate lobe of liver
Diaphragm
Right lobe of liver
Left upper lobe of lung
Oblique fissure
Esophagus
Diaphragm
Hepatic vein
Pleural cavity
Inferior vena cava
Latissimus dorsi muscle
Thoracic duct
Azygos vein
Spleen
Anterior longitudinal ligament
Aorta
Right lower lobe of lung
Left lower lobe of lung
Tenth thoracic vertebra
Dura mater
Posterior longitudinal ligament
Pedicle
Spinal cord
Transverse process
Dorsal root ganglion
Erector spinae muscles
Lamina
Spinous process

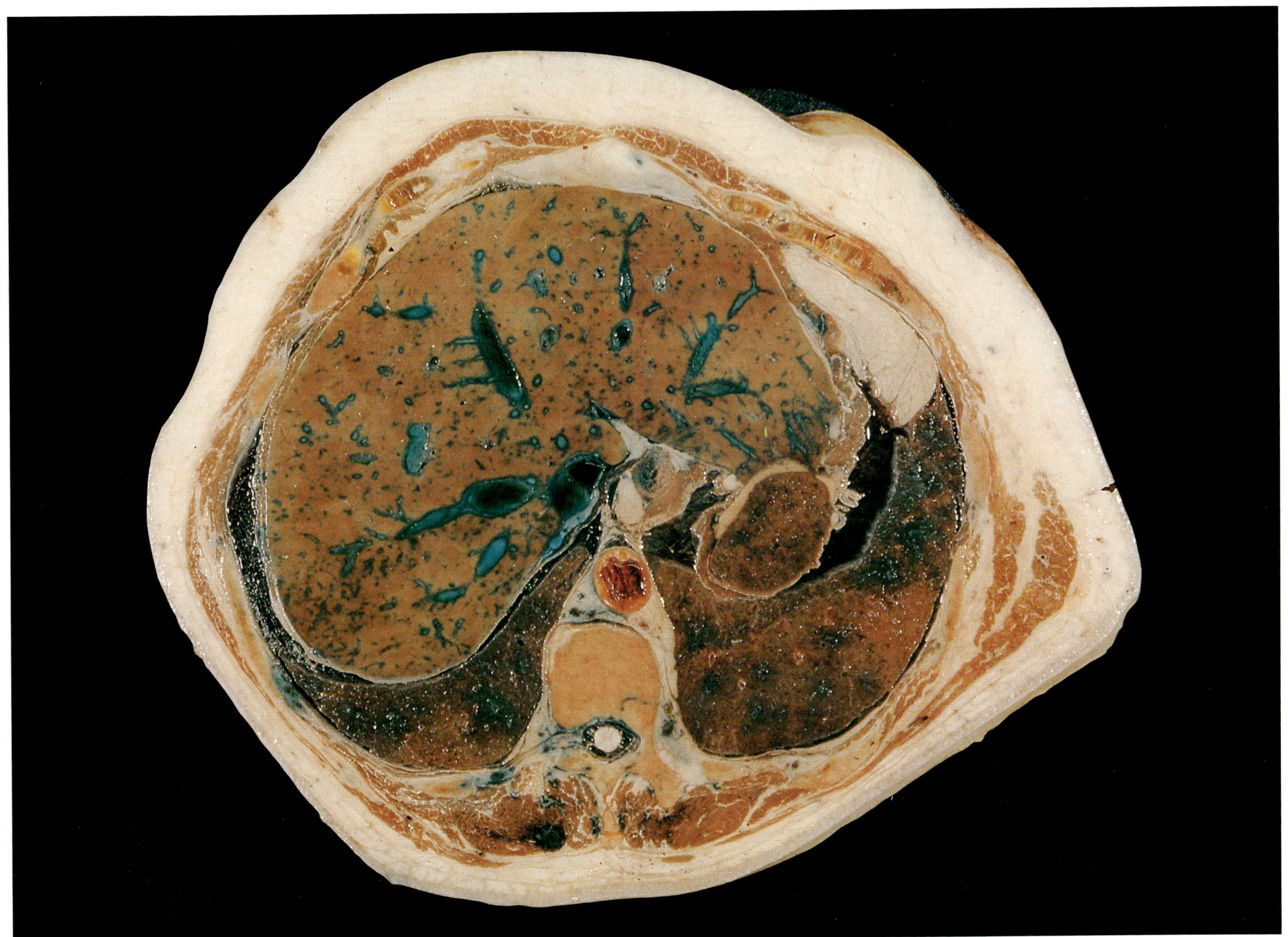

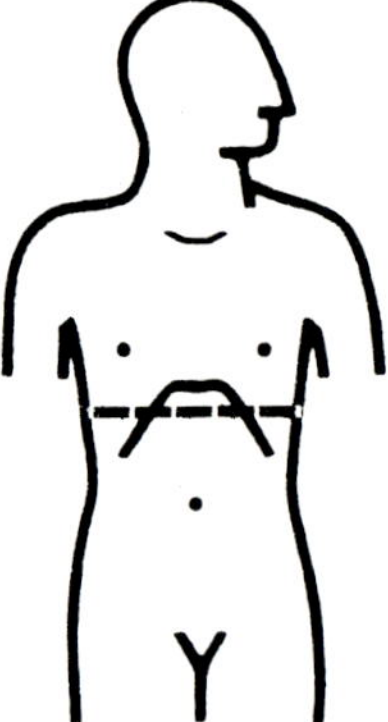

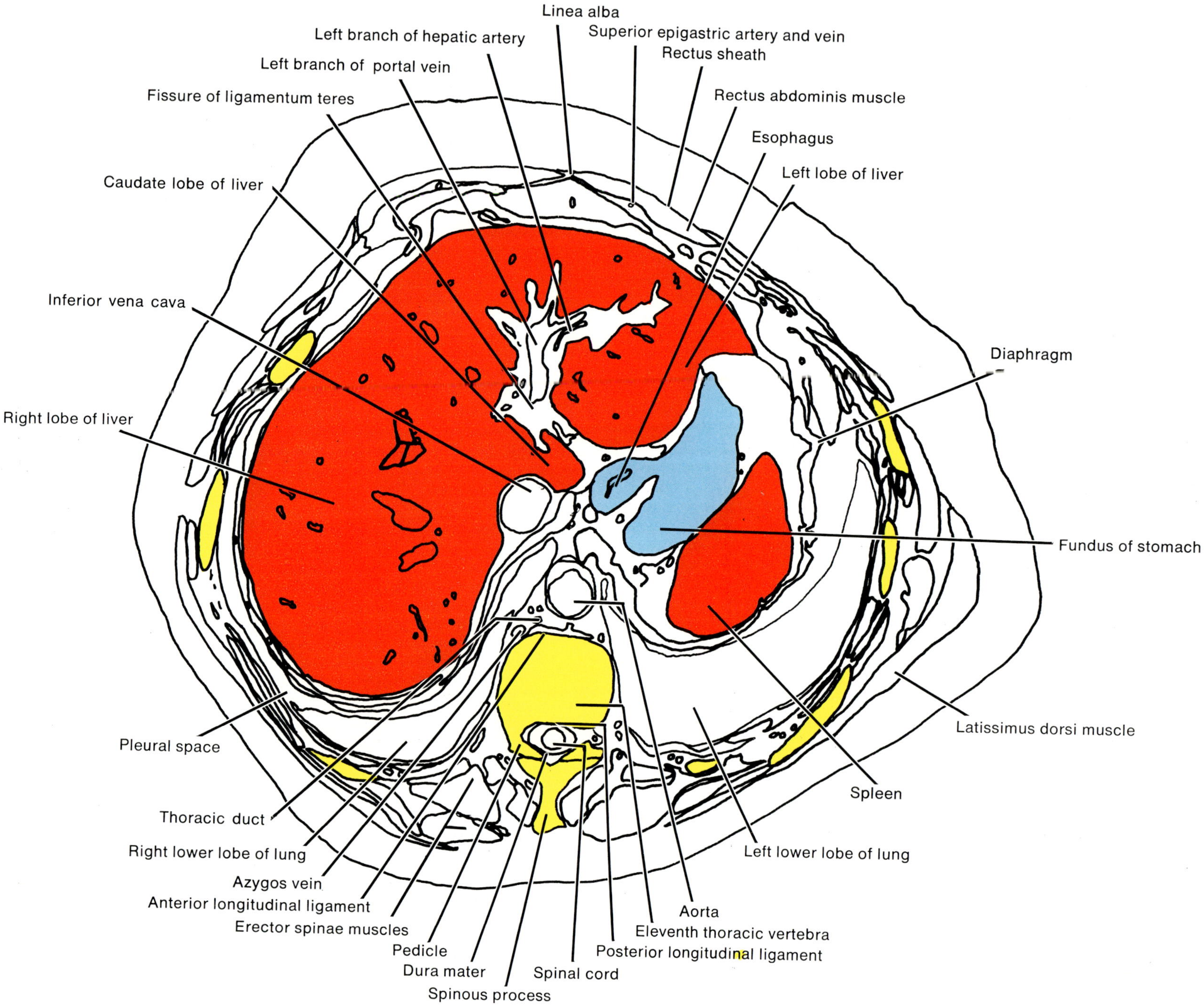

Linea alba
Left branch of hepatic artery
Superior epigastric artery and vein
Left branch of portal vein
Rectus sheath
Fissure of ligamentum teres
Rectus abdominis muscle
Caudate lobe of liver
Esophagus
Left lobe of liver
Inferior vena cava
Diaphragm
Right lobe of liver
Fundus of stomach
Pleural space
Latissimus dorsi muscle
Thoracic duct
Spleen
Right lower lobe of lung
Left lower lobe of lung
Azygos vein
Anterior longitudinal ligament
Aorta
Erector spinae muscles
Eleventh thoracic vertebra
Pedicle
Posterior longitudinal ligament
Dura mater
Spinal cord
Spinous process

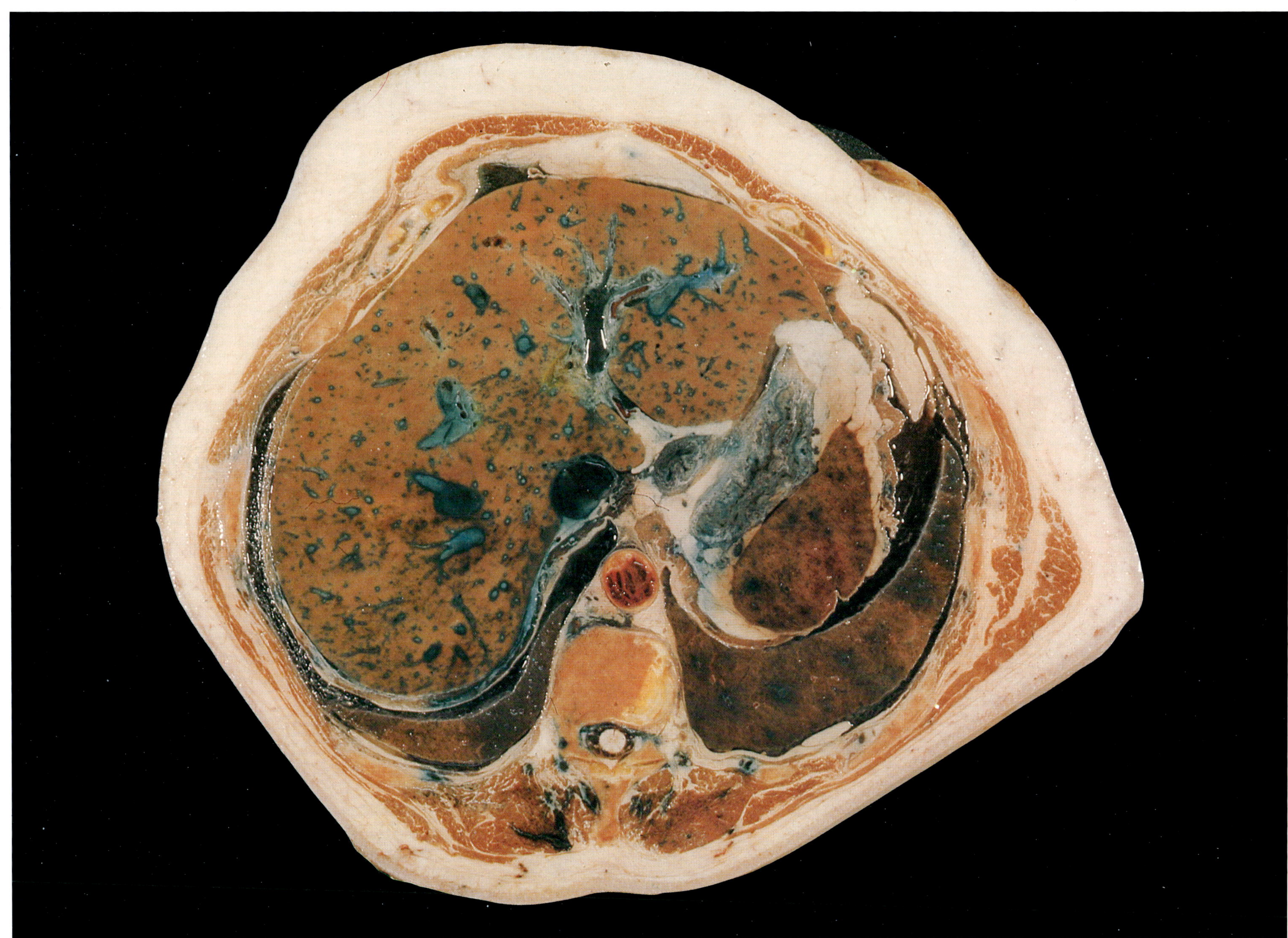

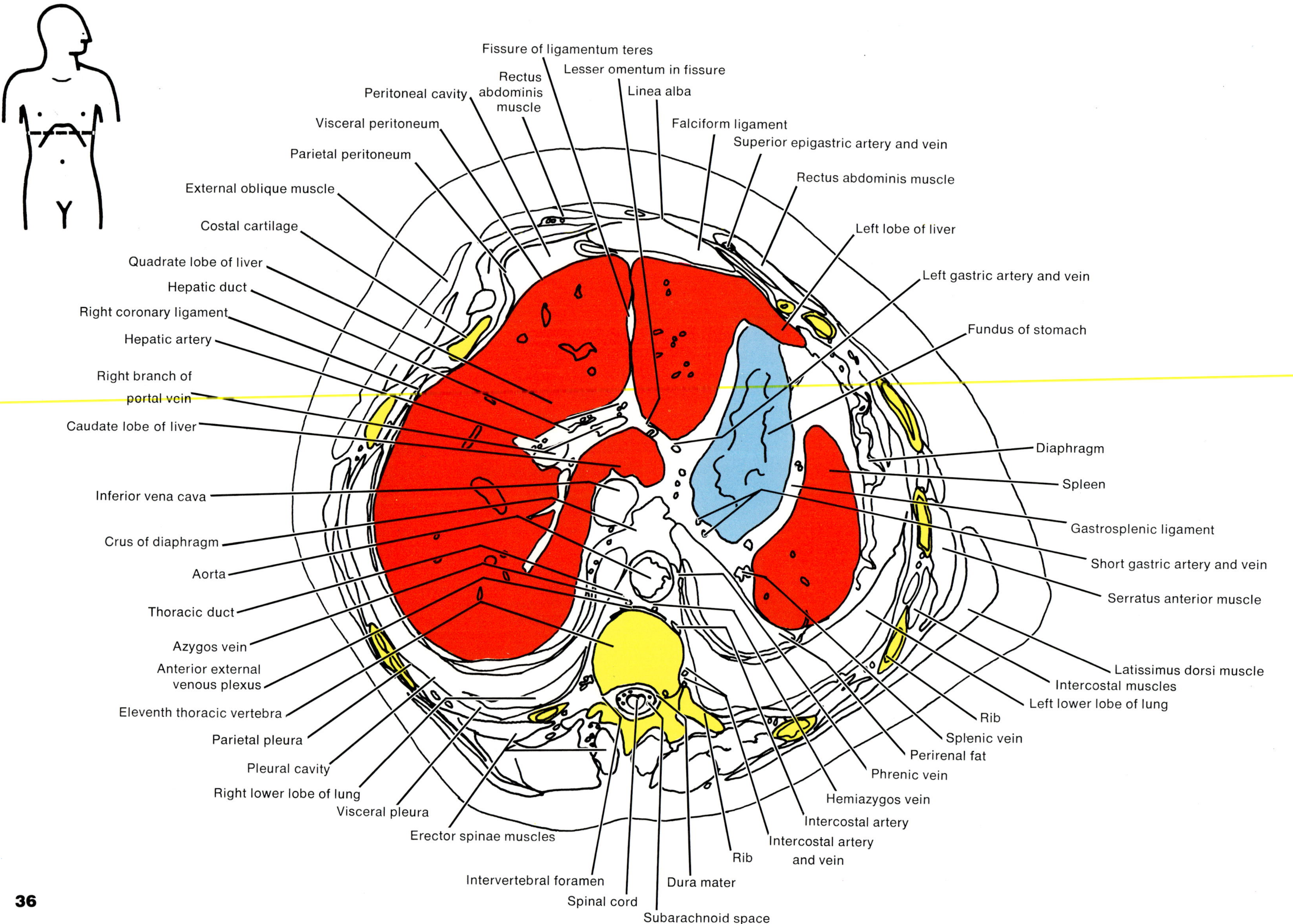

Fissure of ligamentum teres
Lesser omentum in fissure
Rectus abdominis muscle
Linea alba
Peritoneal cavity
Falciform ligament
Superior epigastric artery and vein
Visceral peritoneum
Rectus abdominis muscle
Parietal peritoneum
External oblique muscle
Left lobe of liver
Costal cartilage
Left gastric artery and vein
Quadrate lobe of liver
Hepatic duct
Fundus of stomach
Right coronary ligament
Hepatic artery
Right branch of portal vein
Caudate lobe of liver
Diaphragm
Inferior vena cava
Spleen
Crus of diaphragm
Gastrosplenic ligament
Aorta
Short gastric artery and vein
Thoracic duct
Serratus anterior muscle
Azygos vein
Anterior external venous plexus
Latissimus dorsi muscle
Intercostal muscles
Eleventh thoracic vertebra
Left lower lobe of lung
Parietal pleura
Rib
Pleural cavity
Splenic vein
Right lower lobe of lung
Perirenal fat
Visceral pleura
Phrenic vein
Erector spinae muscles
Hemiazygos vein
Intercostal artery
Intervertebral foramen
Intercostal artery and vein
Rib
Spinal cord
Dura mater
Subarachnoid space

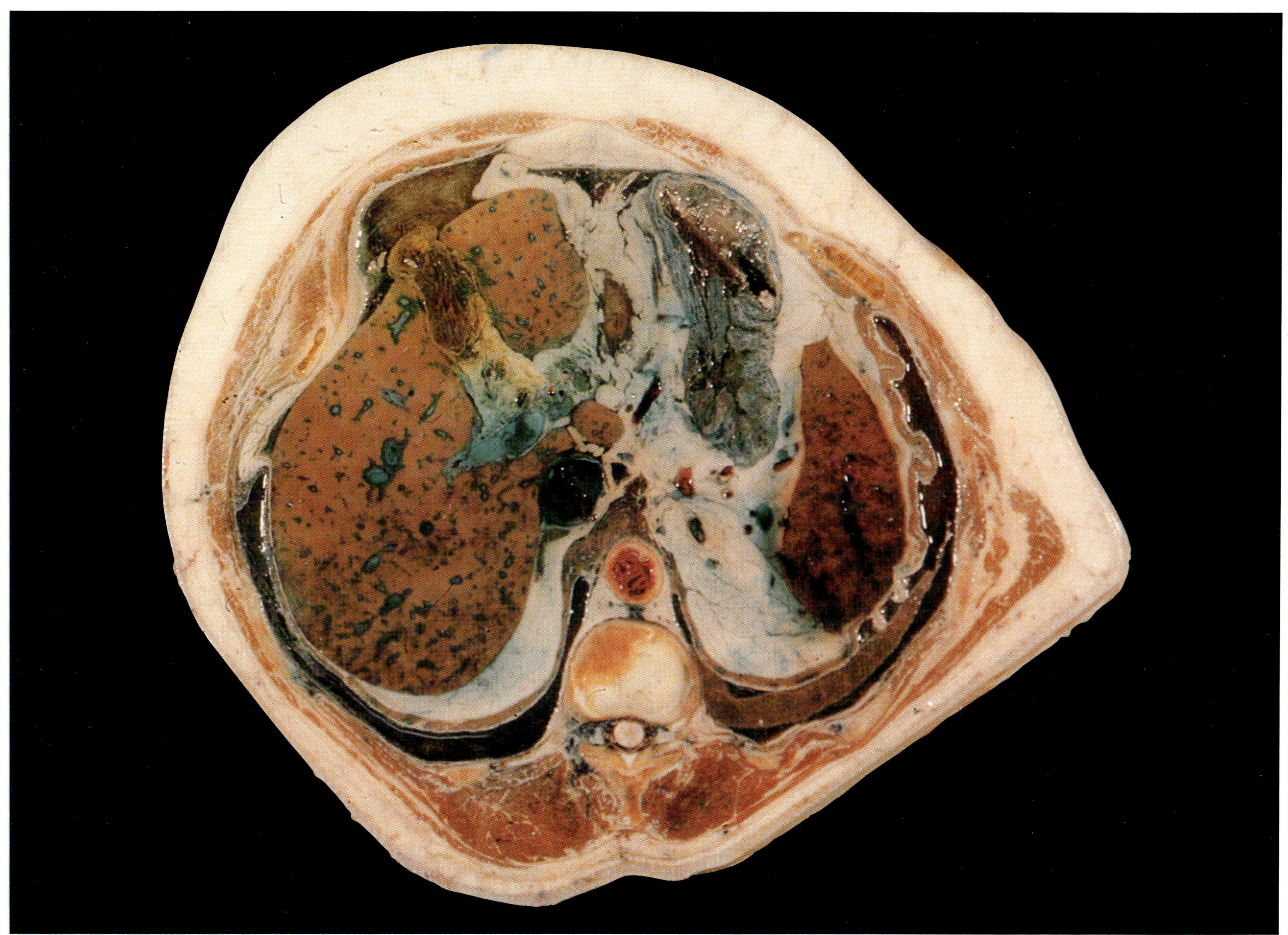

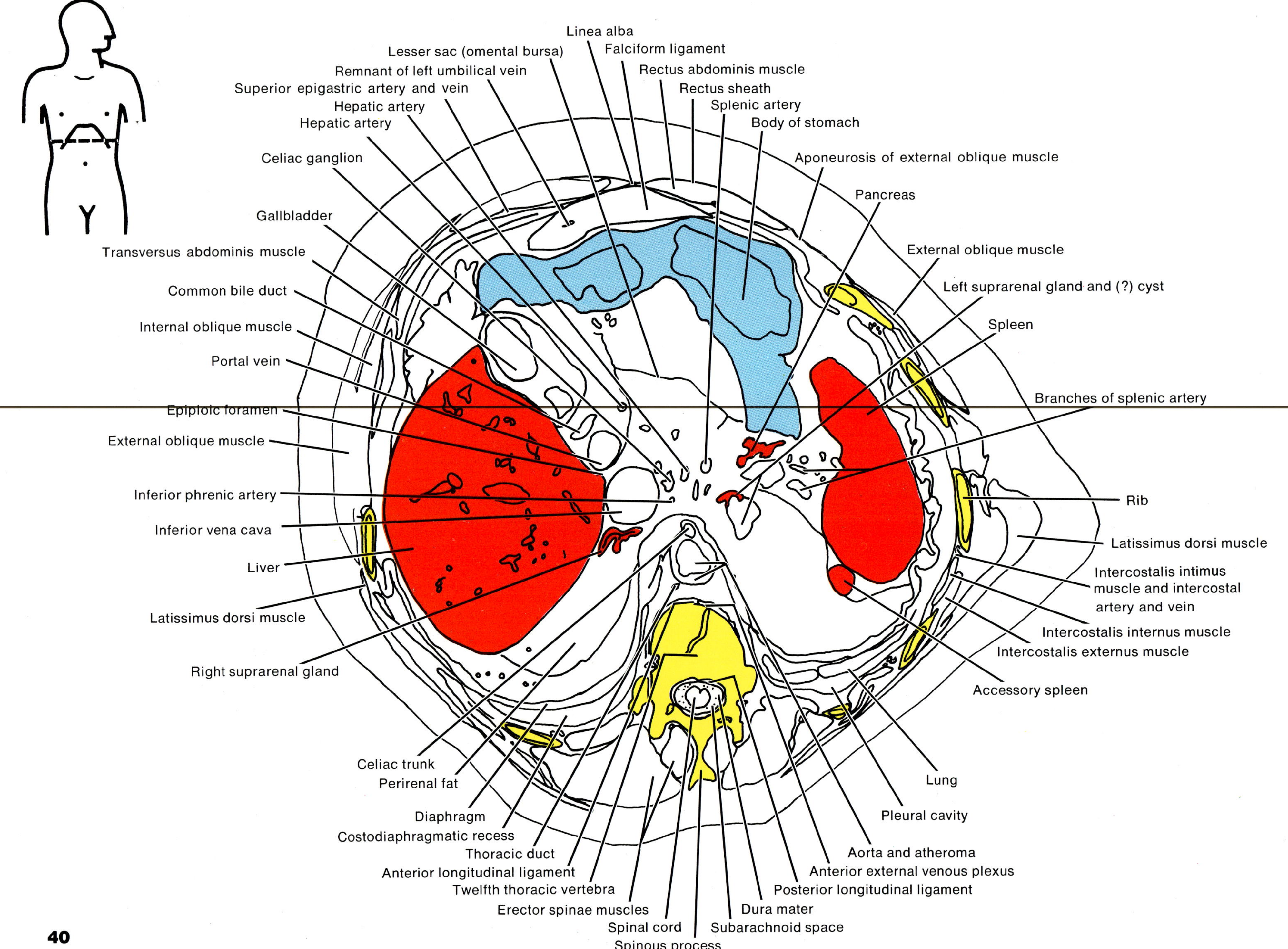

Linea alba
Lesser sac (omental bursa)
Falciform ligament
Remnant of left umbilical vein
Rectus abdominis muscle
Superior epigastric artery and vein
Rectus sheath
Hepatic artery
Splenic artery
Hepatic artery
Body of stomach
Celiac ganglion
Aponeurosis of external oblique muscle
Pancreas
Gallbladder
Transversus abdominis muscle
External oblique muscle
Common bile duct
Left suprarenal gland and (?) cyst
Internal oblique muscle
Spleen
Portal vein
Epiploic foramen
Branches of splenic artery
External oblique muscle
Inferior phrenic artery
Rib
Inferior vena cava
Latissimus dorsi muscle
Liver
Intercostalis intimus muscle and intercostal artery and vein
Latissimus dorsi muscle
Intercostalis internus muscle
Intercostalis externus muscle
Right suprarenal gland
Accessory spleen
Celiac trunk
Lung
Perirenal fat
Diaphragm
Pleural cavity
Costodiaphragmatic recess
Thoracic duct
Aorta and atheroma
Anterior longitudinal ligament
Anterior external venous plexus
Twelfth thoracic vertebra
Posterior longitudinal ligament
Erector spinae muscles
Dura mater
Spinal cord
Subarachnoid space
Spinous process

TRANSVERSE **Abdomen**

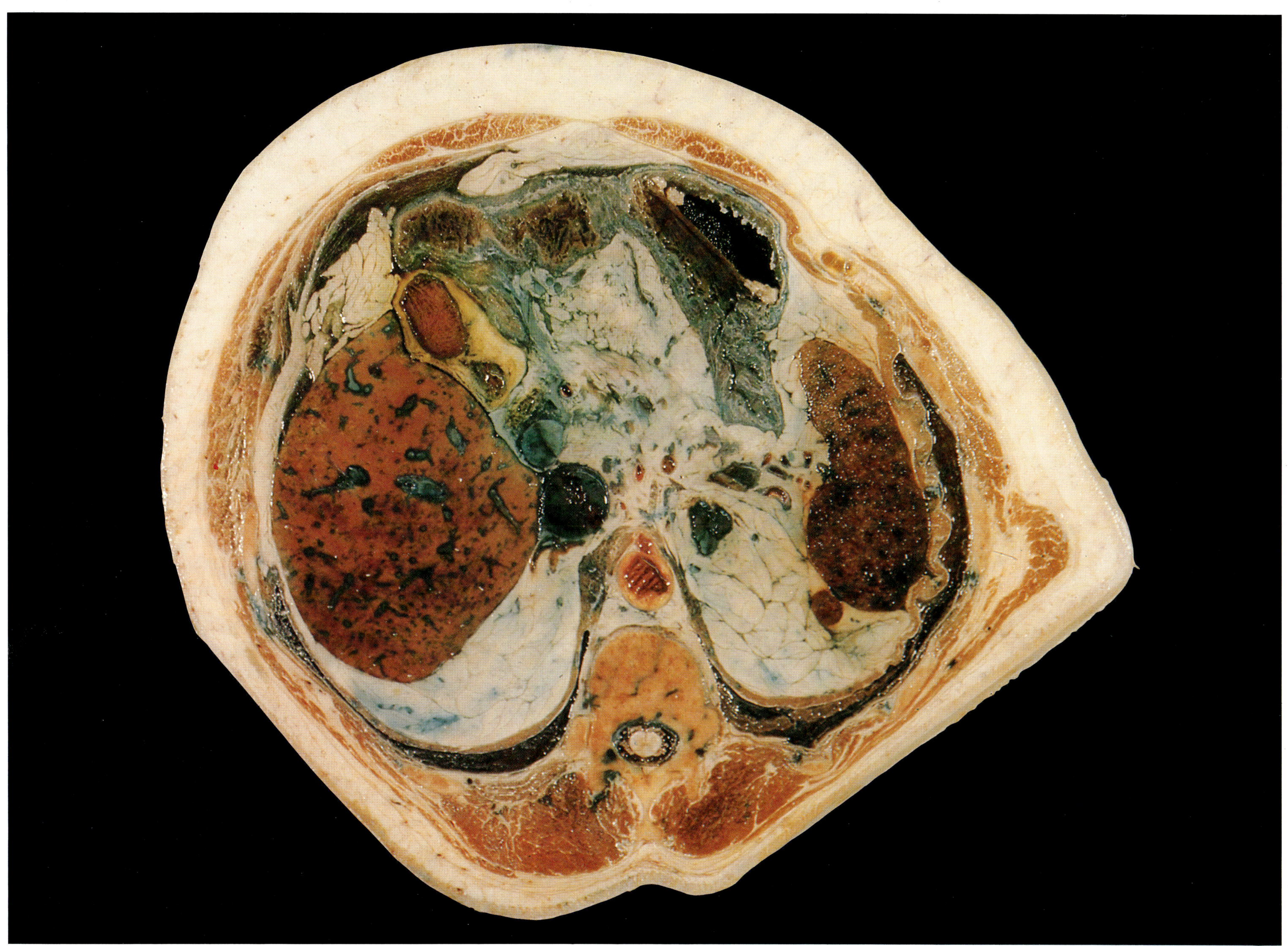

Linea alba
Falciform ligament
Rectus sheath
Pyloric antrum
Rectus abdominis muscle
Pyloric canal
Body of pancreas
Hepatic artery
Superior epigastric artery and vein
Pyloric sphincter
Body of stomach
Superior part of duodenum
Lesser sac (omental bursa)
Common bile duct
Splenic artery
Portal vein
Superior mesenteric artery
External oblique muscle
Internal oblique muscle
Splenic artery
Transversus abdominis muscle
Pancreatic duct of Wirsung
Branches of portal vein
Splenic vein
Right lobe of liver
Inferior vena cava
Spleen
Celiac ganglion
Left suprarenal cyst *
Diaphragm
Latissmus dorsi muscle
Right suprarenal gland
Rib
Perirenal fat
Left kidney
Intercostal muscles
Right kidney
Celiac ganglion
Thoracic duct
Anterior longitudinal ligament
Aorta
Intervertebral disc (T12-L1)
Erector spinae muscles
Twelfth thoracic vertebra
Dura mater
Dorsal root ganglion
Posterior longitudinal ligament
Spinal cord
Spinous process

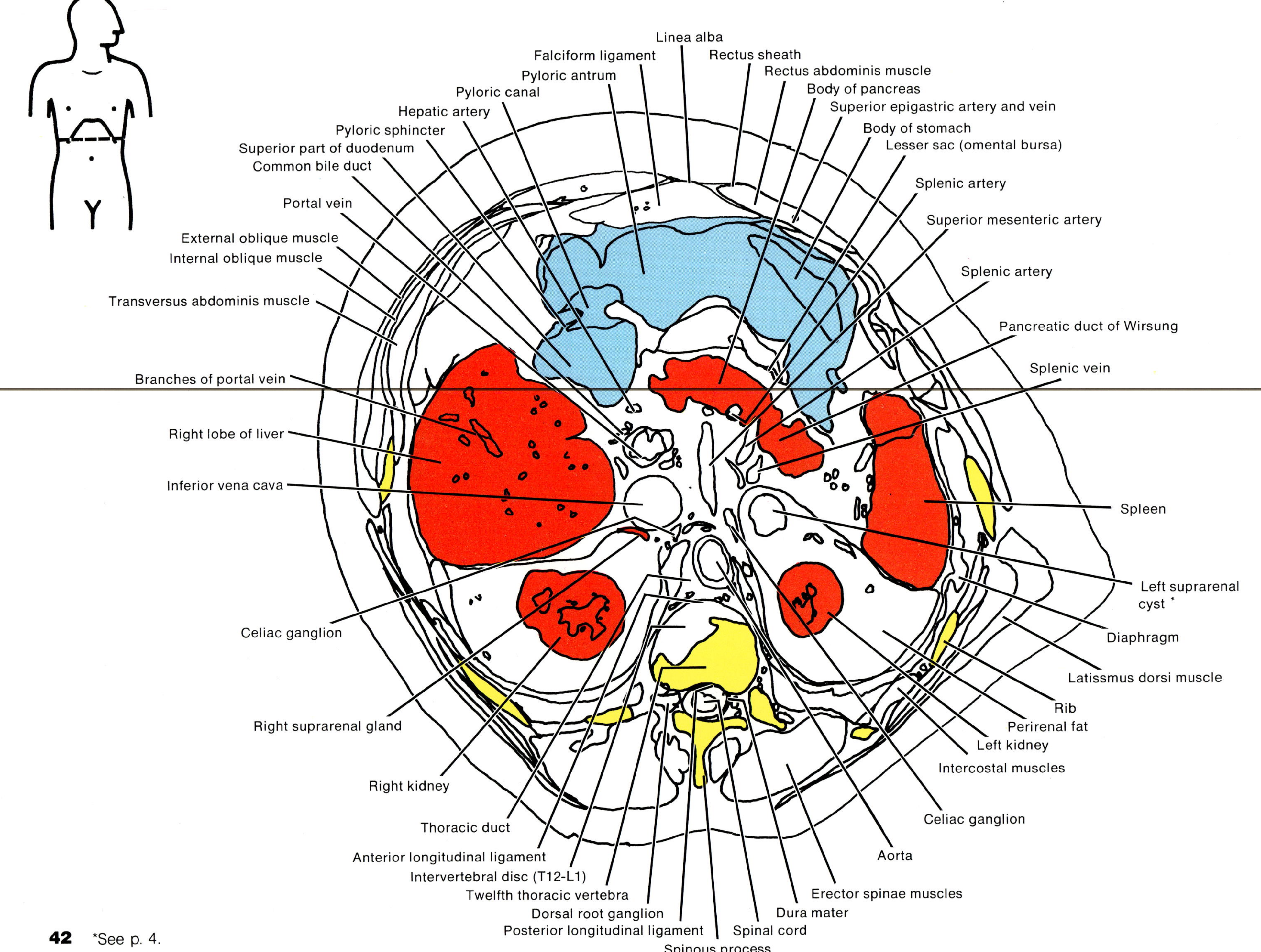

 *See p. 4.

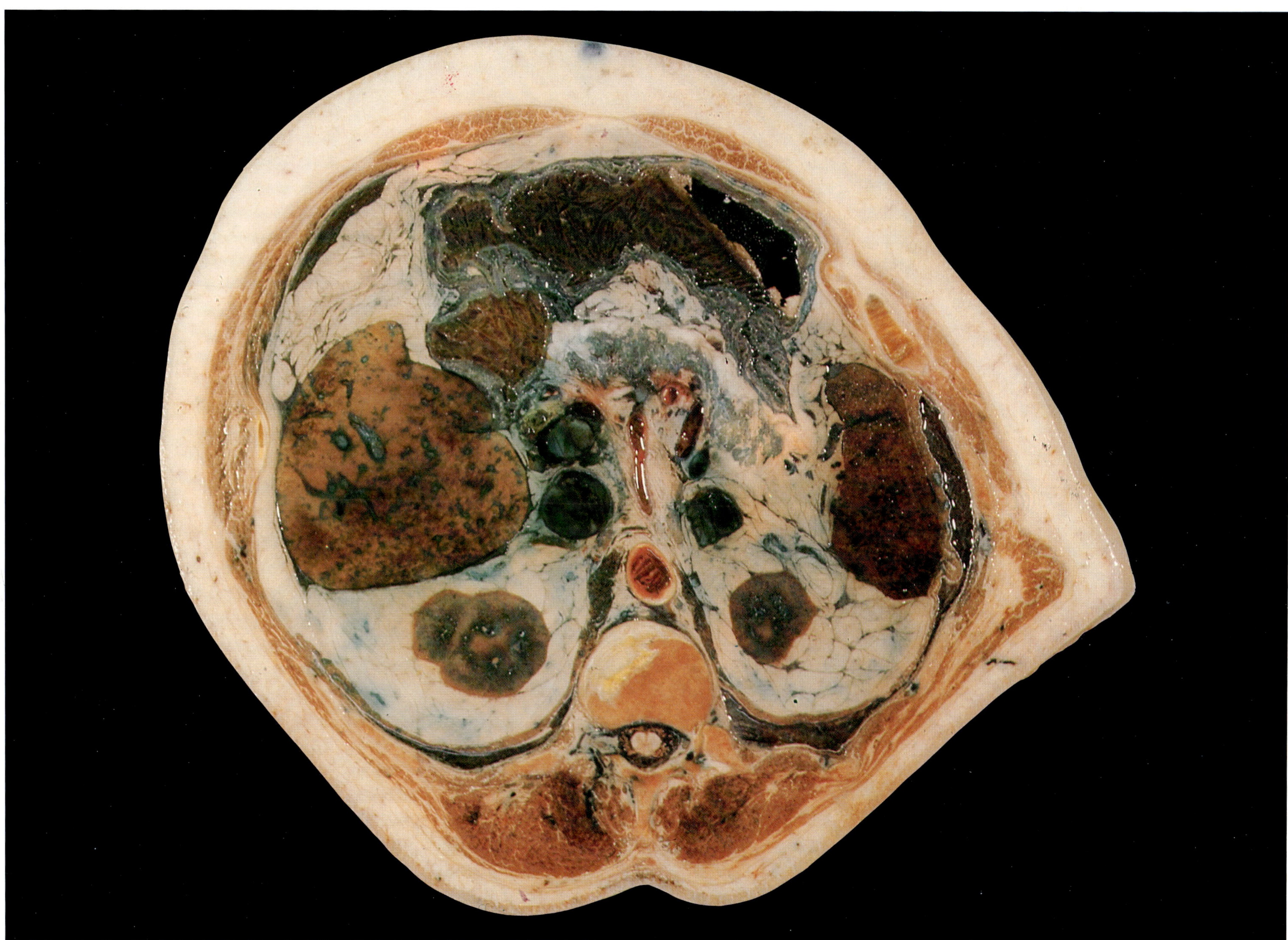

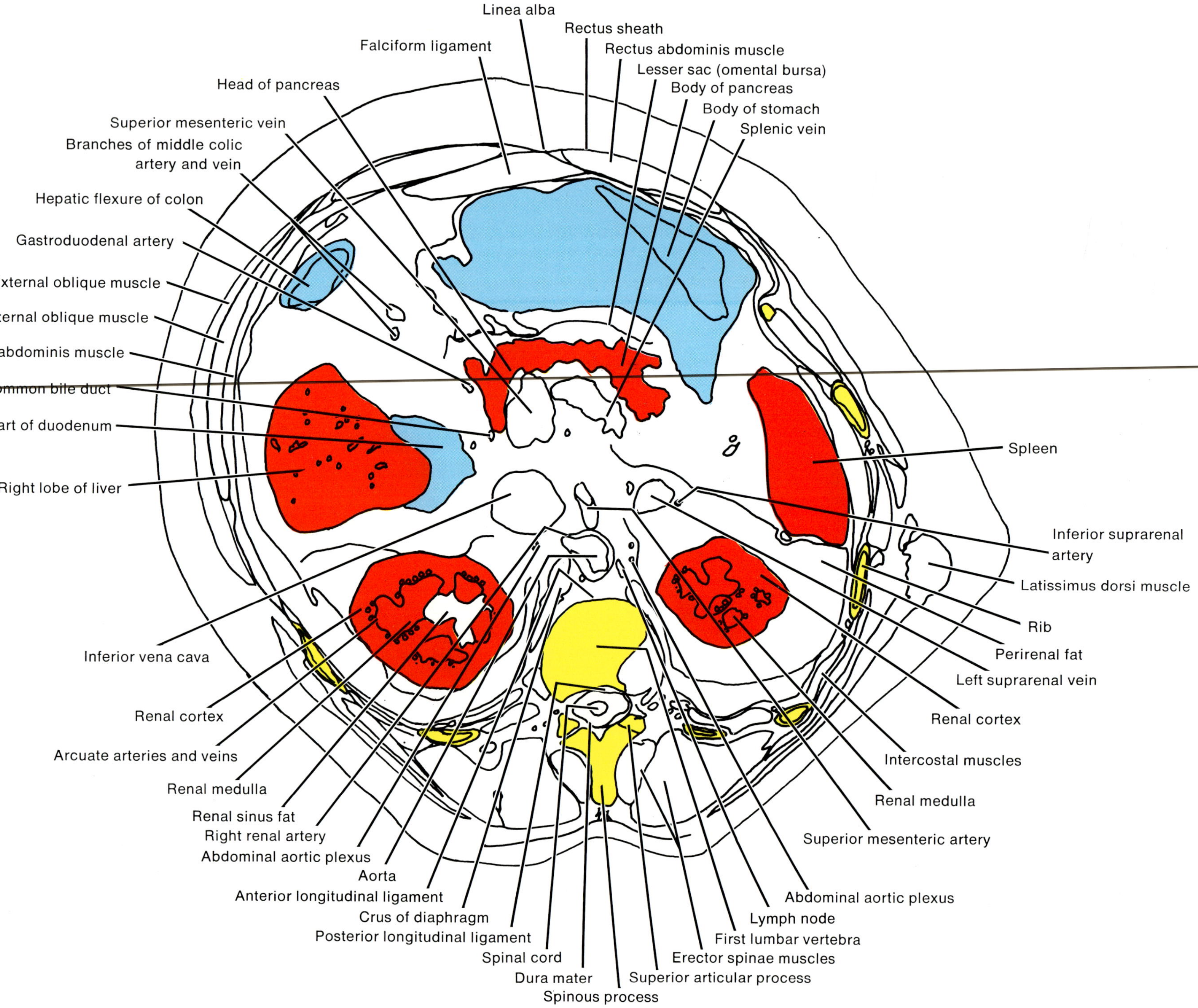

Linea alba
Rectus sheath
Rectus abdominis muscle
Lesser sac (omental bursa)
Body of pancreas
Body of stomach
Splenic vein
Falciform ligament
Head of pancreas
Superior mesenteric vein
Branches of middle colic artery and vein
Hepatic flexure of colon
Gastroduodenal artery
External oblique muscle
Internal oblique muscle
Transversus abdominis muscle
Common bile duct
Descending part of duodenum
Right lobe of liver
Spleen
Inferior suprarenal artery
Latissimus dorsi muscle
Rib
Perirenal fat
Left suprarenal vein
Renal cortex
Intercostal muscles
Renal medulla
Superior mesenteric artery
Abdominal aortic plexus
Lymph node
First lumbar vertebra
Erector spinae muscles
Superior articular process
Inferior vena cava
Renal cortex
Arcuate arteries and veins
Renal medulla
Renal sinus fat
Right renal artery
Abdominal aortic plexus
Aorta
Anterior longitudinal ligament
Crus of diaphragm
Posterior longitudinal ligament
Spinal cord
Dura mater
Spinous process

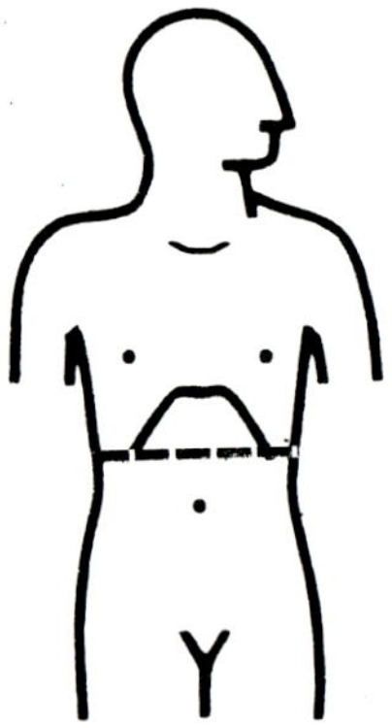

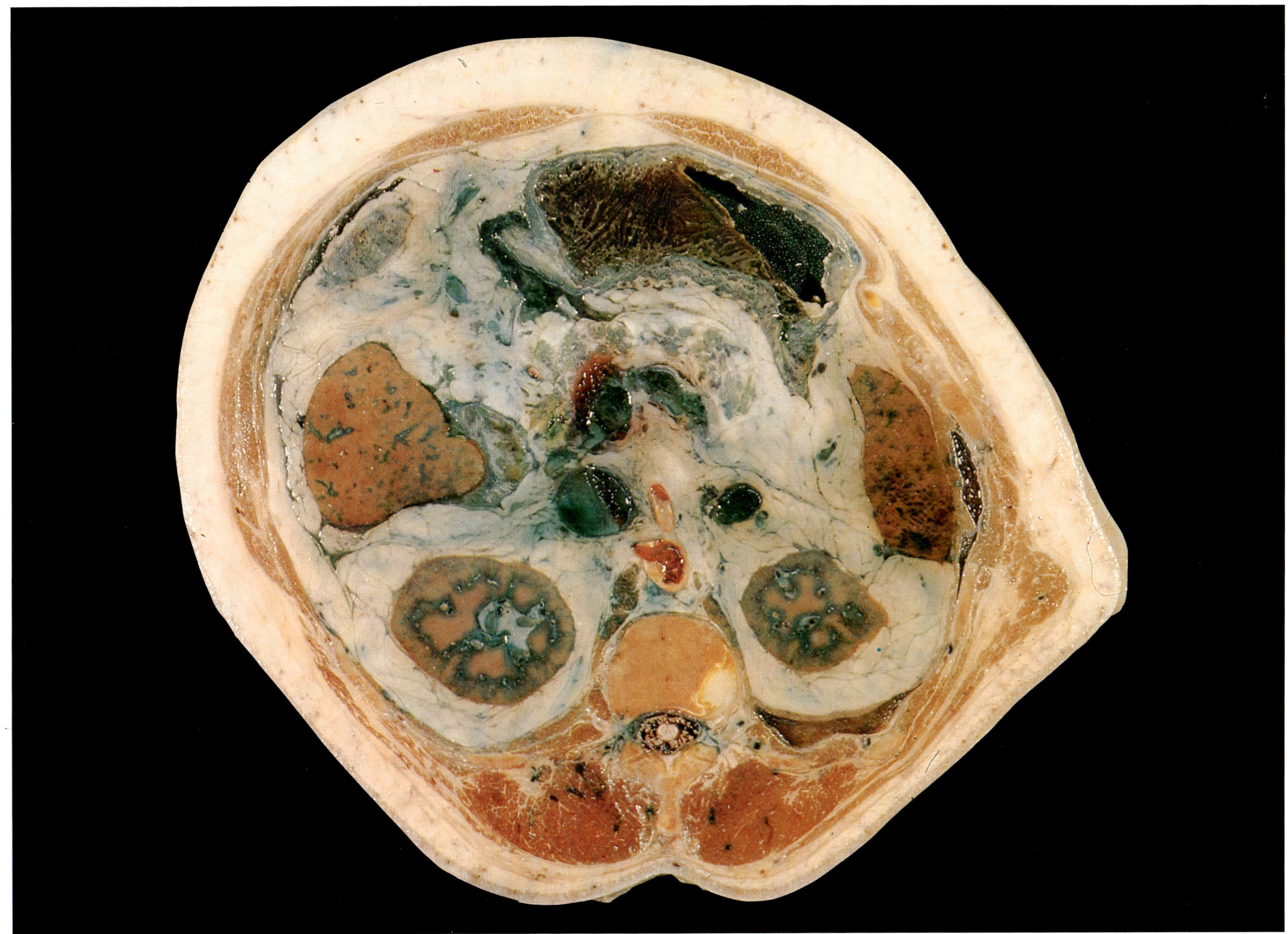

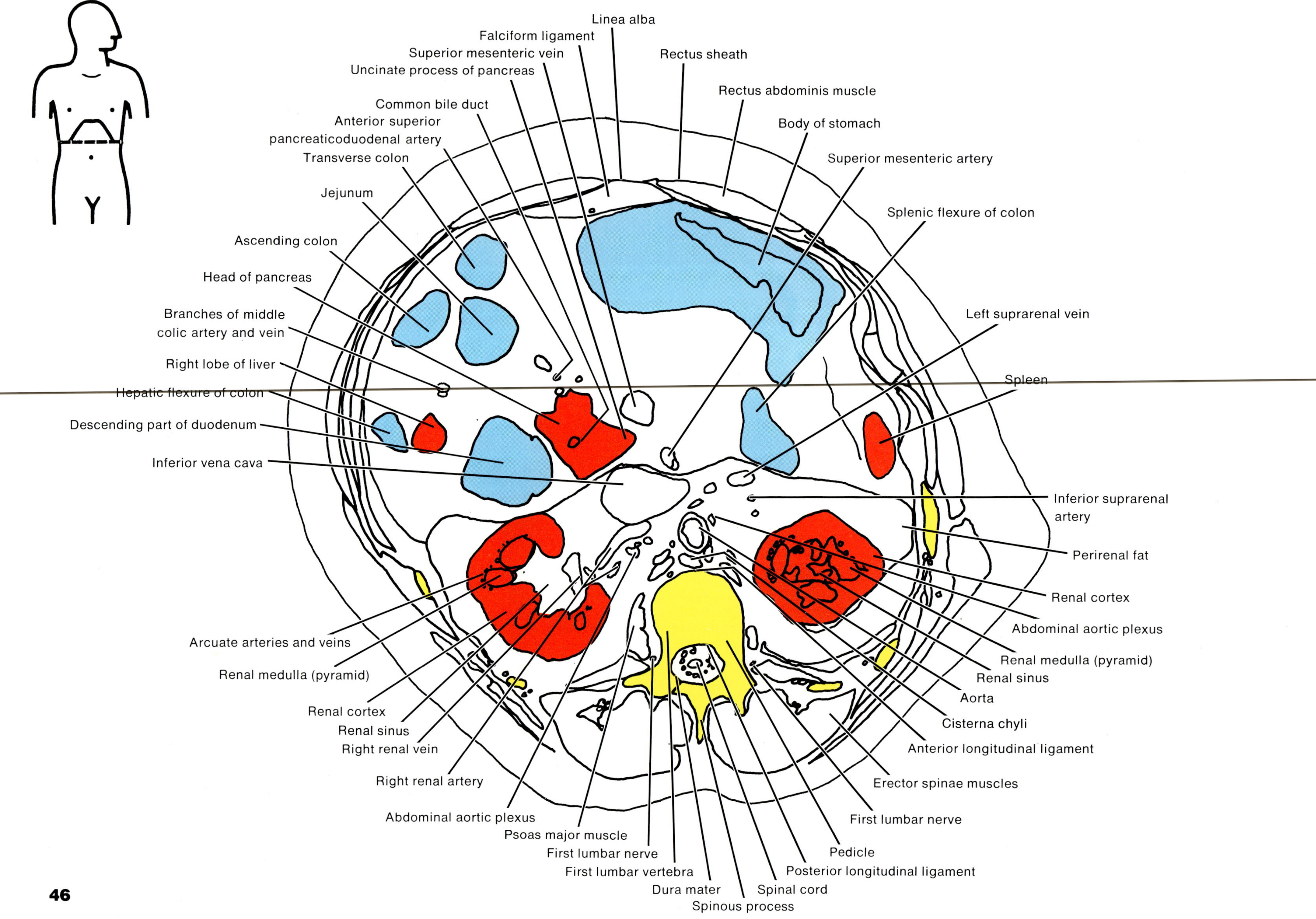

Linea alba
Falciform ligament
Superior mesenteric vein
Uncinate process of pancreas
Common bile duct
Anterior superior pancreaticoduodenal artery
Transverse colon
Jejunum
Ascending colon
Head of pancreas
Branches of middle colic artery and vein
Right lobe of liver
Hepatic flexure of colon
Descending part of duodenum
Inferior vena cava
Arcuate arteries and veins
Renal medulla (pyramid)
Renal cortex
Renal sinus
Right renal vein
Right renal artery
Abdominal aortic plexus
Psoas major muscle
First lumbar nerve
First lumbar vertebra
Dura mater
Spinous process
Spinal cord
Posterior longitudinal ligament
Pedicle
First lumbar nerve
Erector spinae muscles
Anterior longitudinal ligament
Cisterna chyli
Aorta
Renal sinus
Renal medulla (pyramid)
Abdominal aortic plexus
Renal cortex
Perirenal fat
Inferior suprarenal artery
Spleen
Left suprarenal vein
Splenic flexure of colon
Superior mesenteric artery
Body of stomach
Rectus abdominis muscle
Rectus sheath

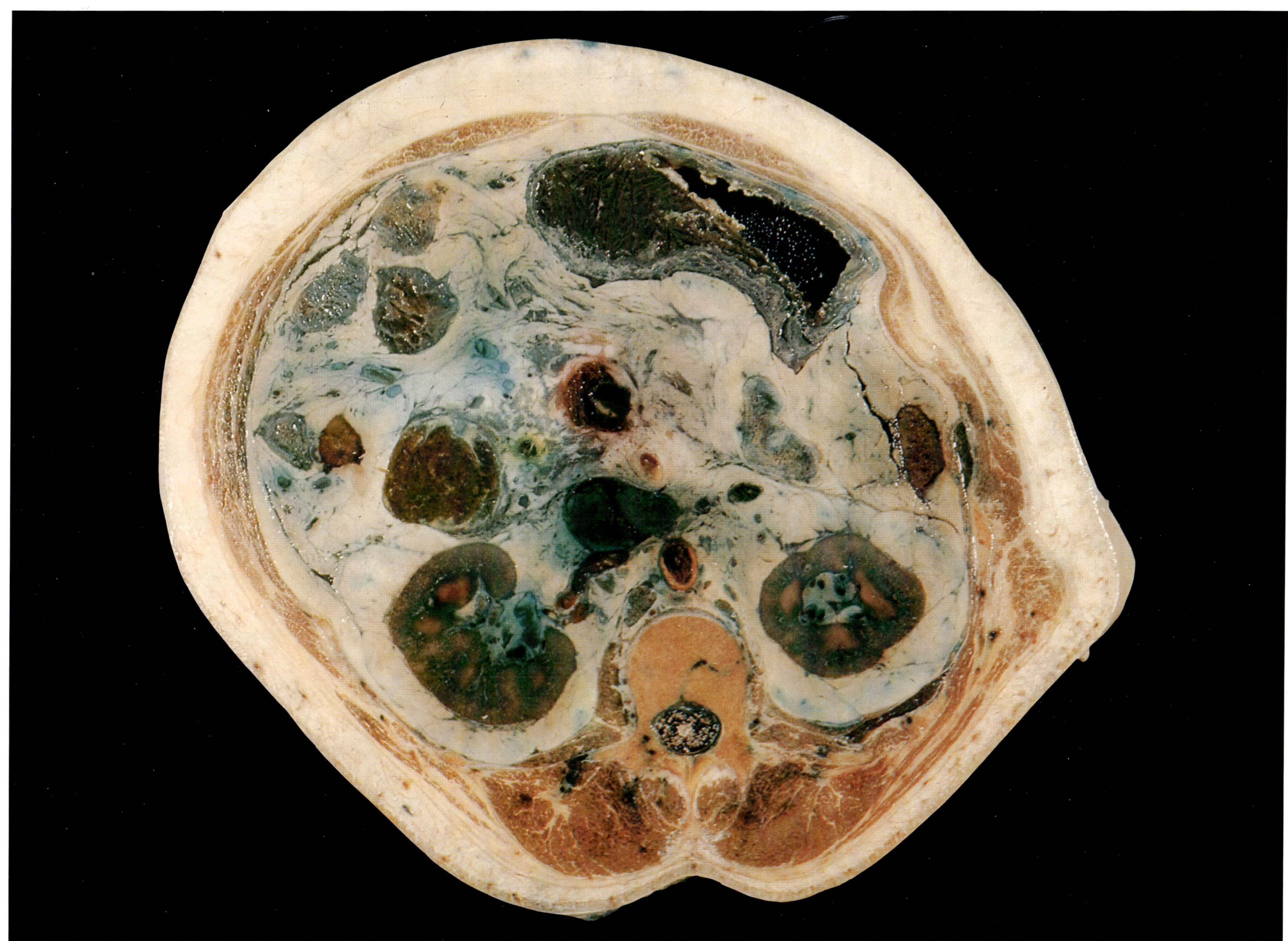

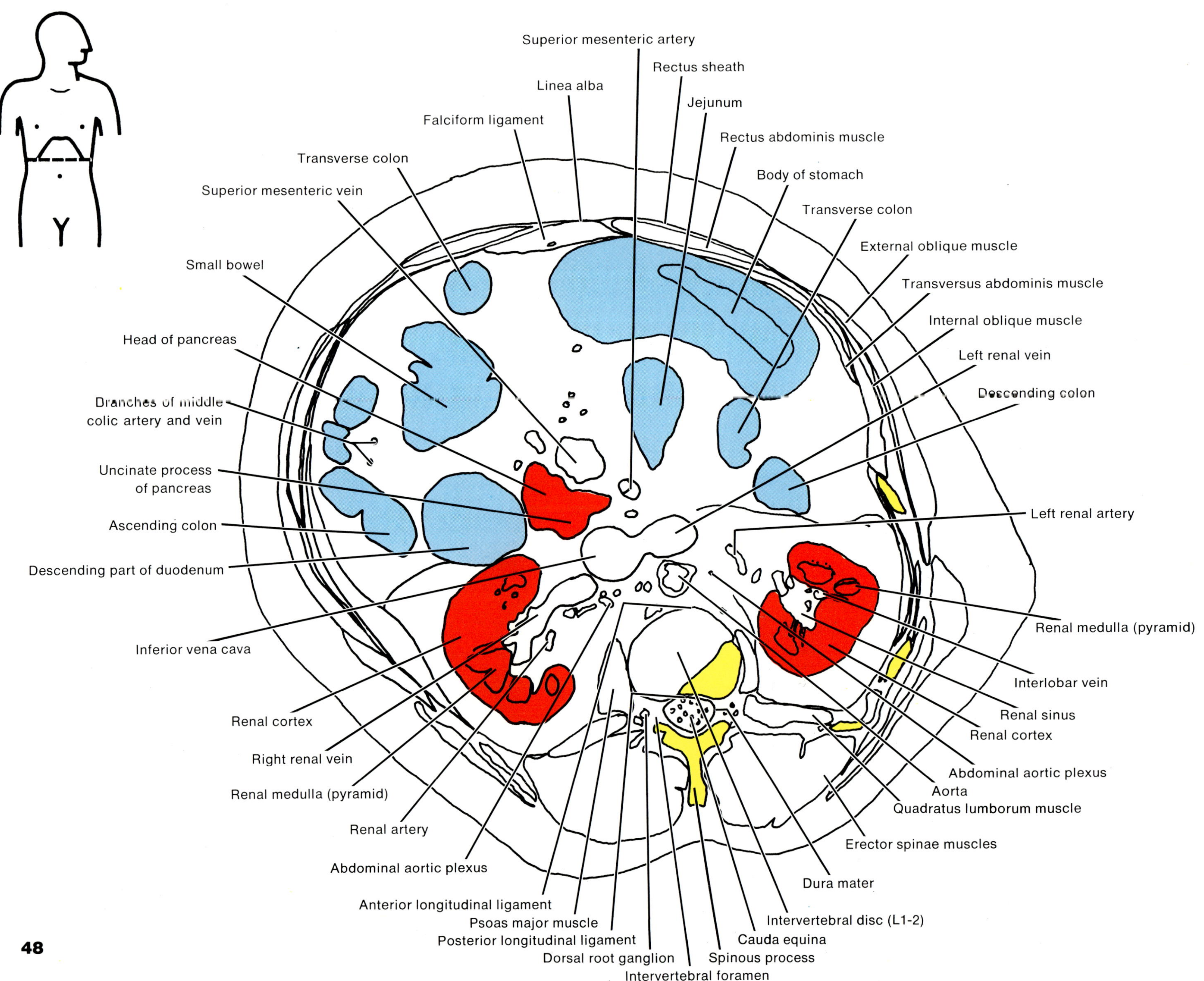

Superior mesenteric artery
Rectus sheath
Linea alba
Jejunum
Falciform ligament
Rectus abdominis muscle
Transverse colon
Body of stomach
Superior mesenteric vein
Transverse colon
Small bowel
External oblique muscle
Transversus abdominis muscle
Head of pancreas
Internal oblique muscle
Left renal vein
Branches of middle colic artery and vein
Descending colon
Uncinate process of pancreas
Left renal artery
Ascending colon
Descending part of duodenum
Renal medulla (pyramid)
Inferior vena cava
Interlobar vein
Renal sinus
Renal cortex
Renal cortex
Right renal vein
Abdominal aortic plexus
Renal medulla (pyramid)
Aorta
Quadratus lumborum muscle
Renal artery
Erector spinae muscles
Abdominal aortic plexus
Dura mater
Anterior longitudinal ligament
Intervertebral disc (L1-2)
Psoas major muscle
Cauda equina
Posterior longitudinal ligament
Spinous process
Dorsal root ganglion
Intervertebral foramen

TRANSVERSE **Abdomen**

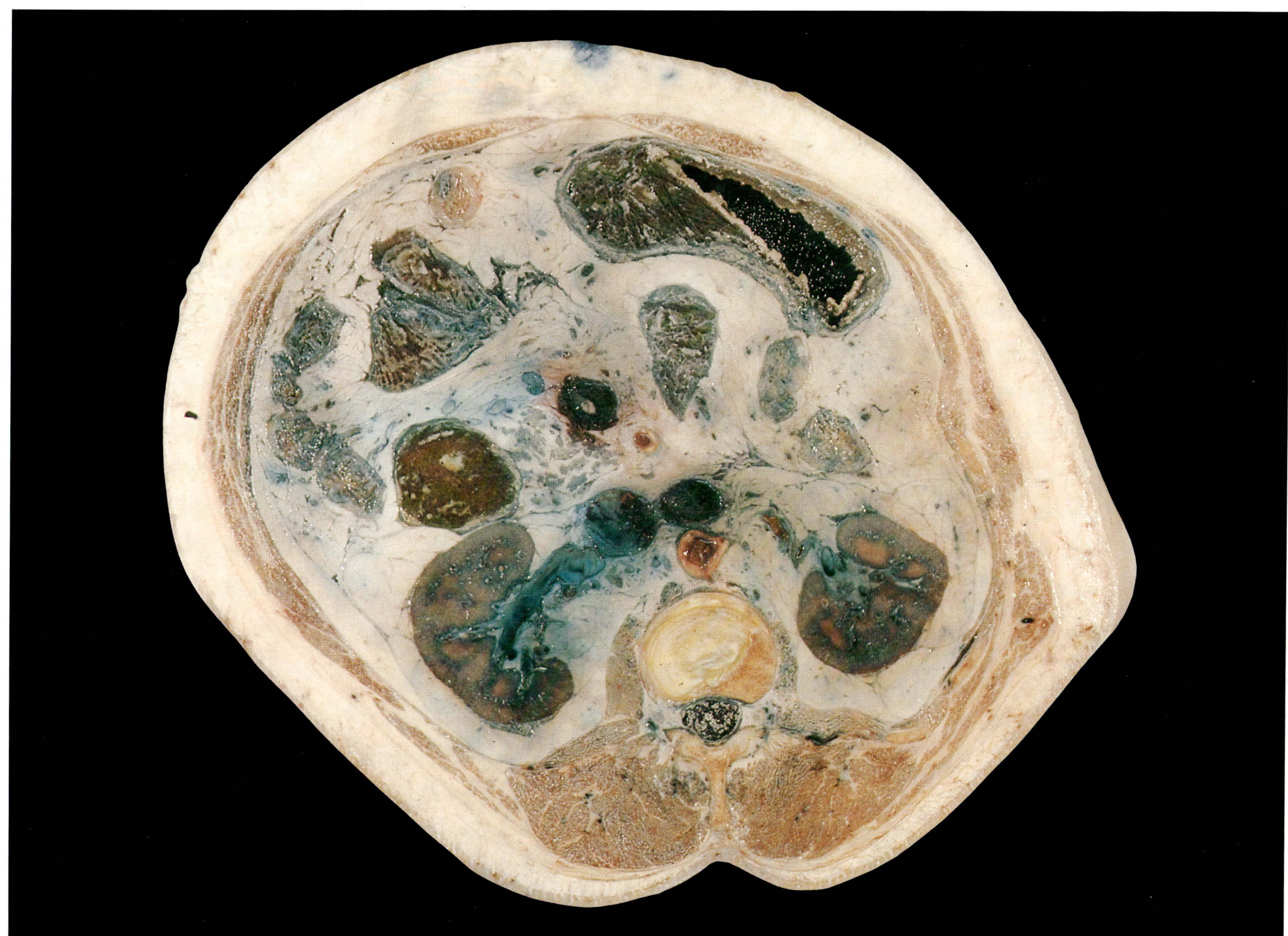

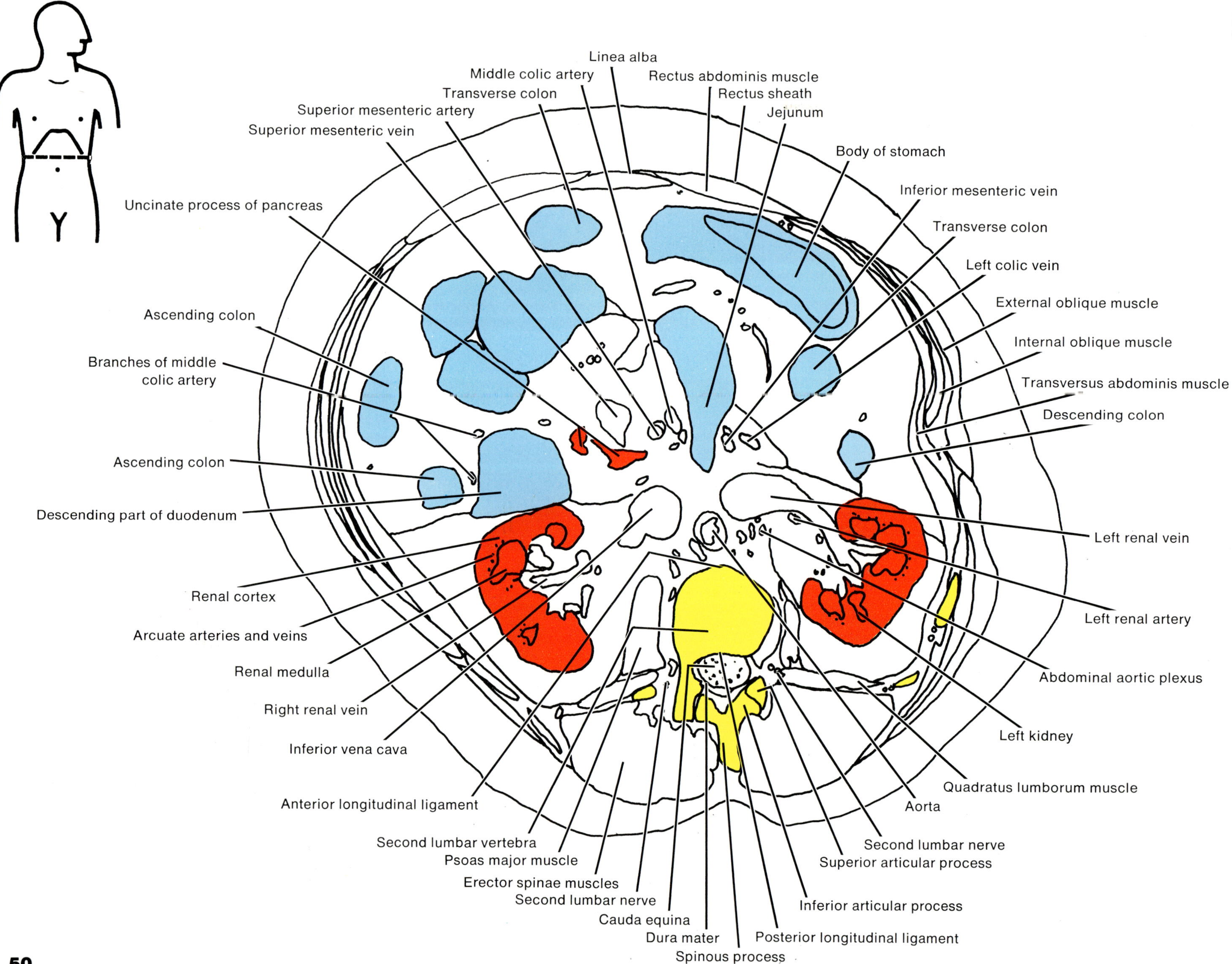

Linea alba
Middle colic artery
Transverse colon
Superior mesenteric artery
Superior mesenteric vein
Rectus abdominis muscle
Rectus sheath
Jejunum
Body of stomach
Uncinate process of pancreas
Inferior mesenteric vein
Transverse colon
Left colic vein
Ascending colon
External oblique muscle
Internal oblique muscle
Branches of middle colic artery
Transversus abdominis muscle
Descending colon
Ascending colon
Descending part of duodenum
Left renal vein
Renal cortex
Arcuate arteries and veins
Left renal artery
Renal medulla
Right renal vein
Abdominal aortic plexus
Inferior vena cava
Left kidney
Anterior longitudinal ligament
Quadratus lumborum muscle
Second lumbar vertebra
Aorta
Psoas major muscle
Second lumbar nerve
Erector spinae muscles
Superior articular process
Second lumbar nerve
Inferior articular process
Cauda equina
Dura mater
Posterior longitudinal ligament
Spinous process

TRANSVERSE **Abdomen**

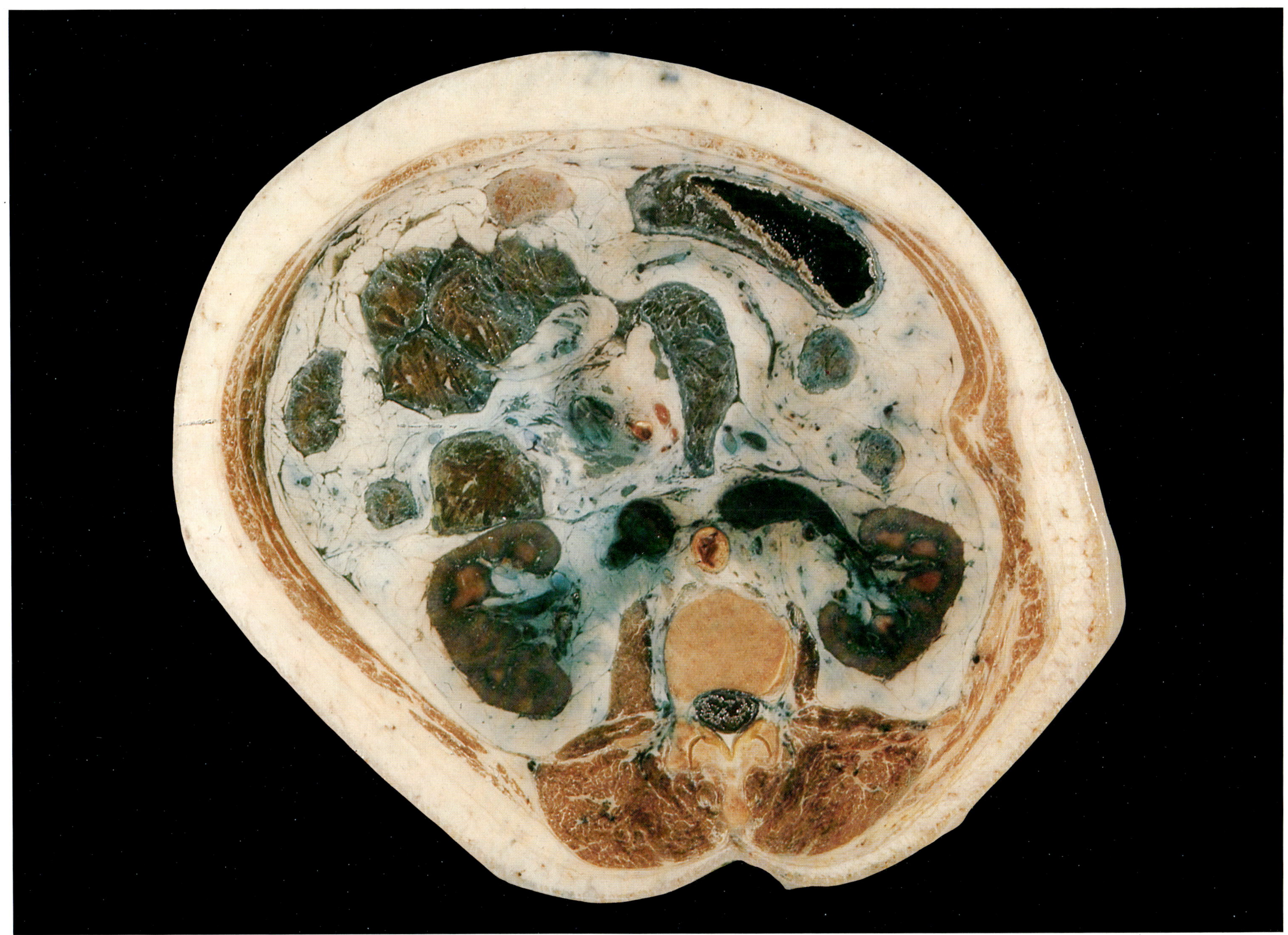

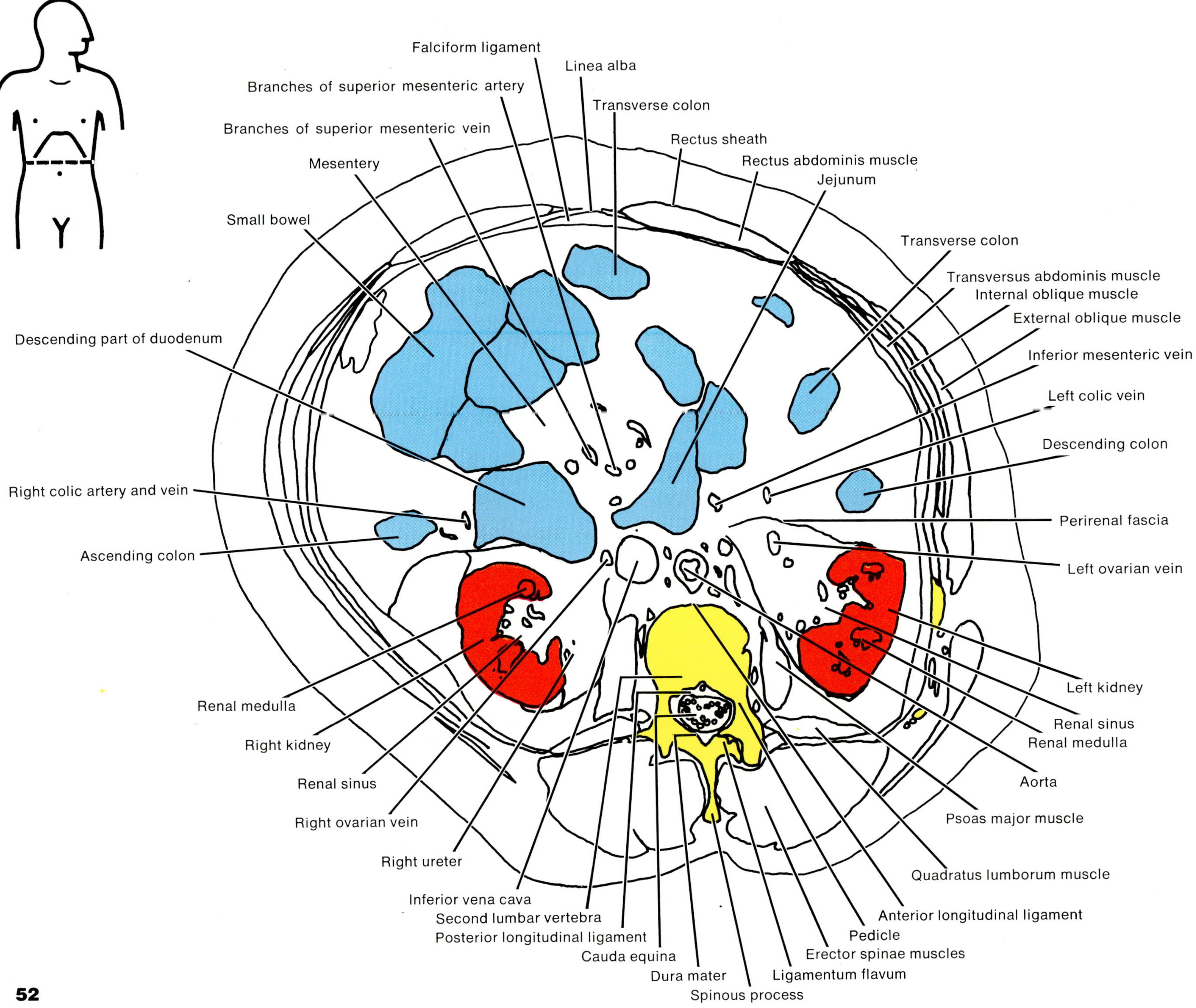

Falciform ligament
Linea alba
Branches of superior mesenteric artery
Transverse colon
Branches of superior mesenteric vein
Rectus sheath
Mesentery
Rectus abdominis muscle
Jejunum
Small bowel
Transverse colon
Transversus abdominis muscle
Internal oblique muscle
External oblique muscle
Descending part of duodenum
Inferior mesenteric vein
Left colic vein
Descending colon
Right colic artery and vein
Perirenal fascia
Ascending colon
Left ovarian vein
Left kidney
Renal sinus
Renal medulla
Renal medulla
Right kidney
Renal sinus
Aorta
Right ovarian vein
Psoas major muscle
Right ureter
Quadratus lumborum muscle
Inferior vena cava
Anterior longitudinal ligament
Second lumbar vertebra
Pedicle
Posterior longitudinal ligament
Erector spinae muscles
Cauda equina
Ligamentum flavum
Dura mater
Spinous process

TRANSVERSE **Abdomen**

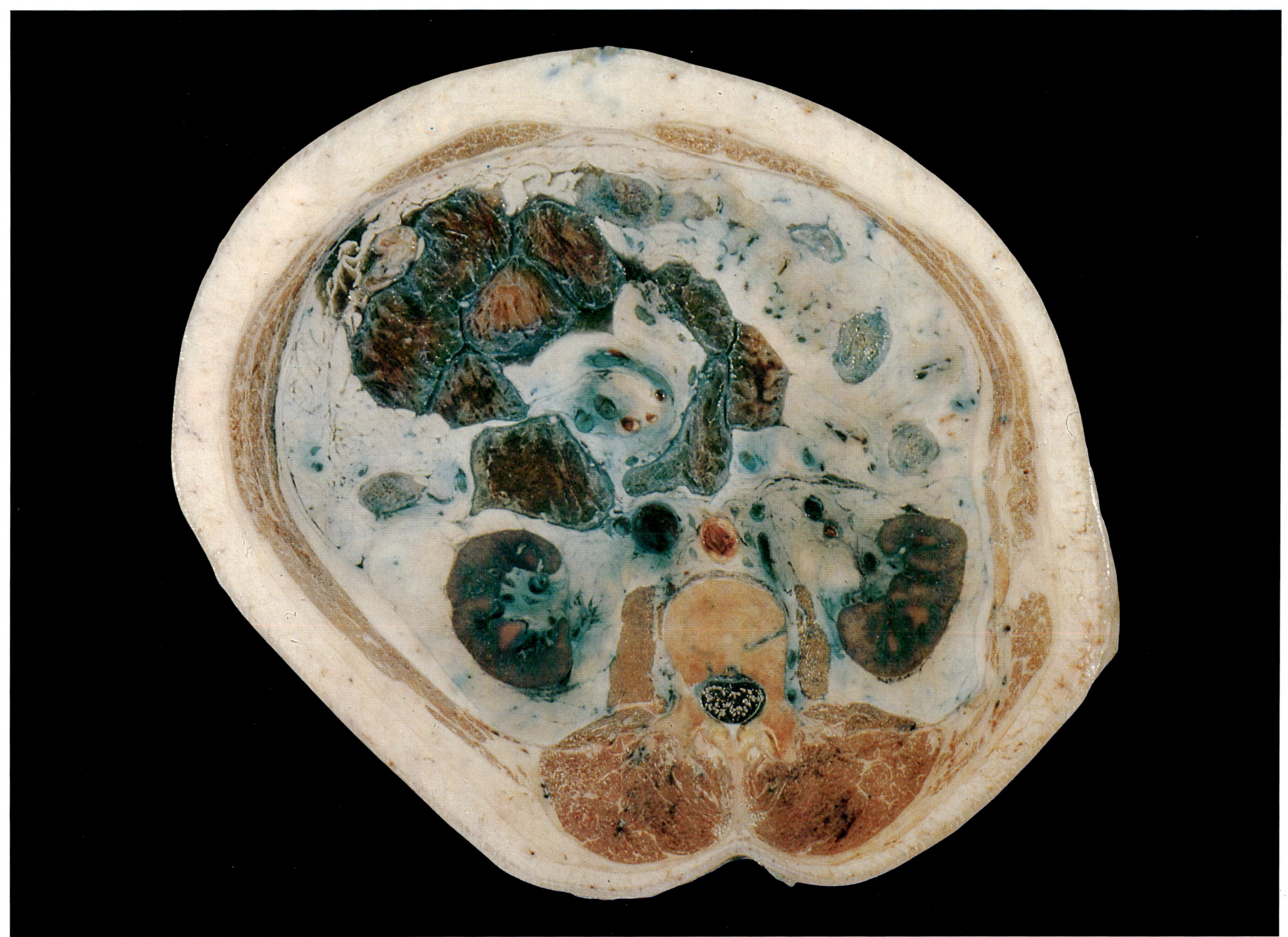

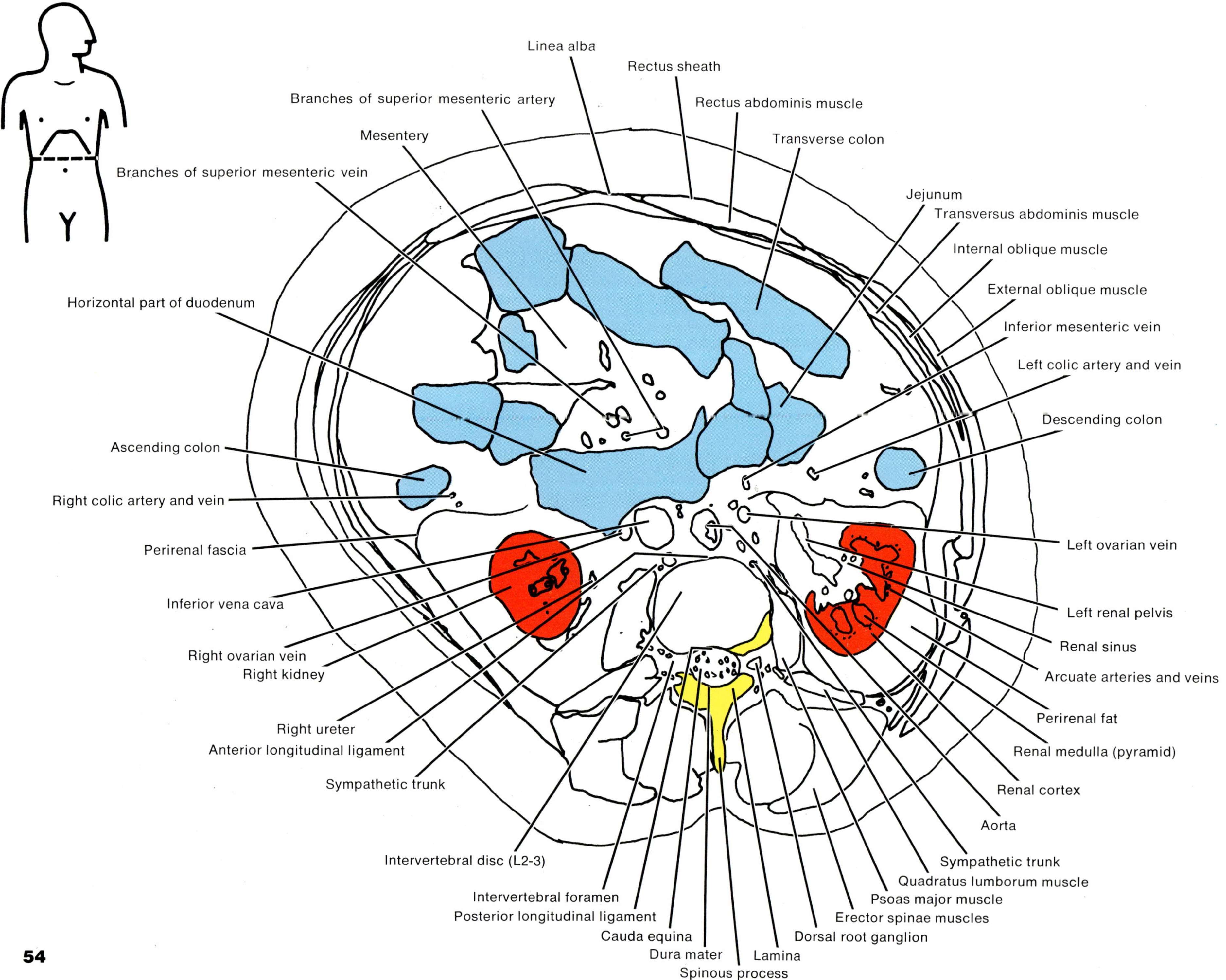

Linea alba
Rectus sheath
Branches of superior mesenteric artery
Rectus abdominis muscle
Mesentery
Transverse colon
Branches of superior mesenteric vein
Jejunum
Transversus abdominis muscle
Internal oblique muscle
Horizontal part of duodenum
External oblique muscle
Inferior mesenteric vein
Left colic artery and vein
Descending colon
Ascending colon
Right colic artery and vein
Left ovarian vein
Perirenal fascia
Left renal pelvis
Inferior vena cava
Renal sinus
Right ovarian vein
Arcuate arteries and veins
Right kidney
Perirenal fat
Right ureter
Renal medulla (pyramid)
Anterior longitudinal ligament
Renal cortex
Sympathetic trunk
Aorta
Sympathetic trunk
Quadratus lumborum muscle
Intervertebral disc (L2-3)
Psoas major muscle
Intervertebral foramen
Erector spinae muscles
Posterior longitudinal ligament
Dorsal root ganglion
Cauda equina
Dura mater
Lamina
Spinous process

TRANSVERSE **Abdomen**

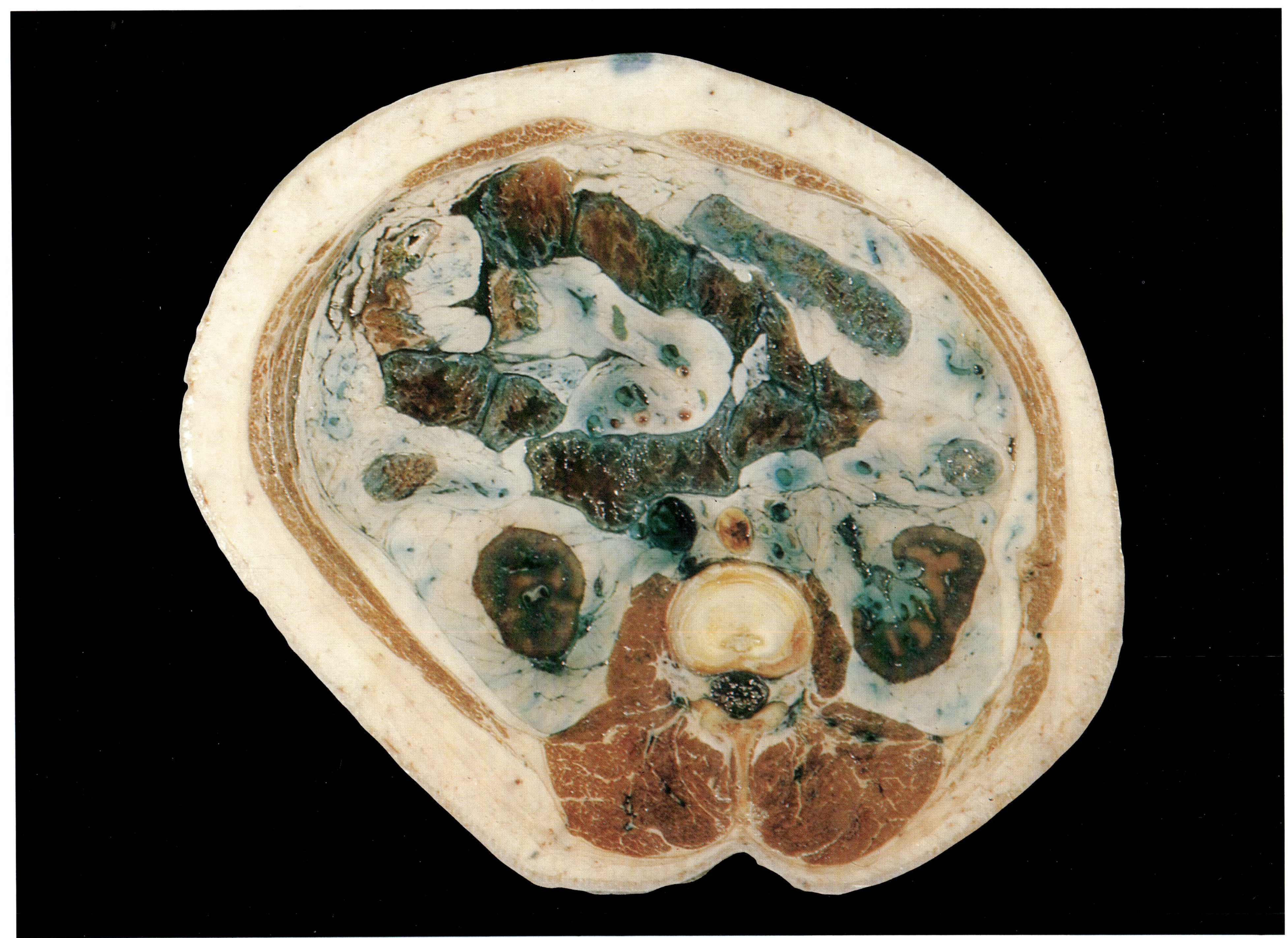

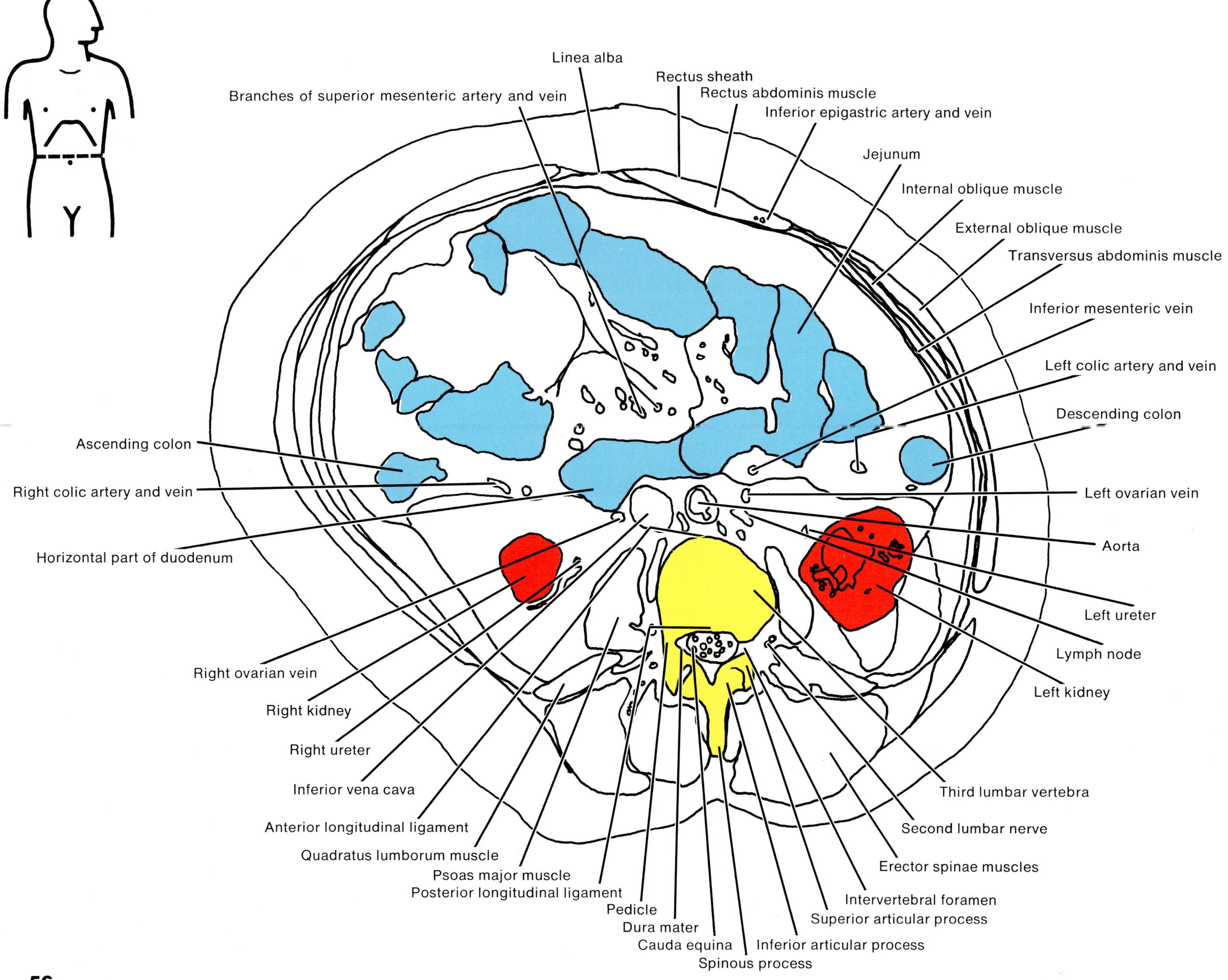

PLATE 22
Linea alba
Rectus sheath
Rectus abdominis muscle
Branches of superior mesenteric artery and vein
Inferior epigastric artery and vein
Jejunum
Internal oblique muscle
External oblique muscle
Transversus abdominis muscle
Inferior mesenteric vein
Left colic artery and vein
Descending colon
Ascending colon
Right colic artery and vein
Left ovarian vein
Horizontal part of duodenum
Aorta
Left ureter
Lymph node
Right ovarian vein
Left kidney
Right kidney
Right ureter
Inferior vena cava
Third lumbar vertebra
Anterior longitudinal ligament
Second lumbar nerve
Quadratus lumborum muscle
Erector spinae muscles
Psoas major muscle
Intervertebral foramen
Posterior longitudinal ligament
Superior articular process
Pedicle
Dura mater
Inferior articular process
Cauda equina
Spinous process

TRANSVERSE **Abdomen**

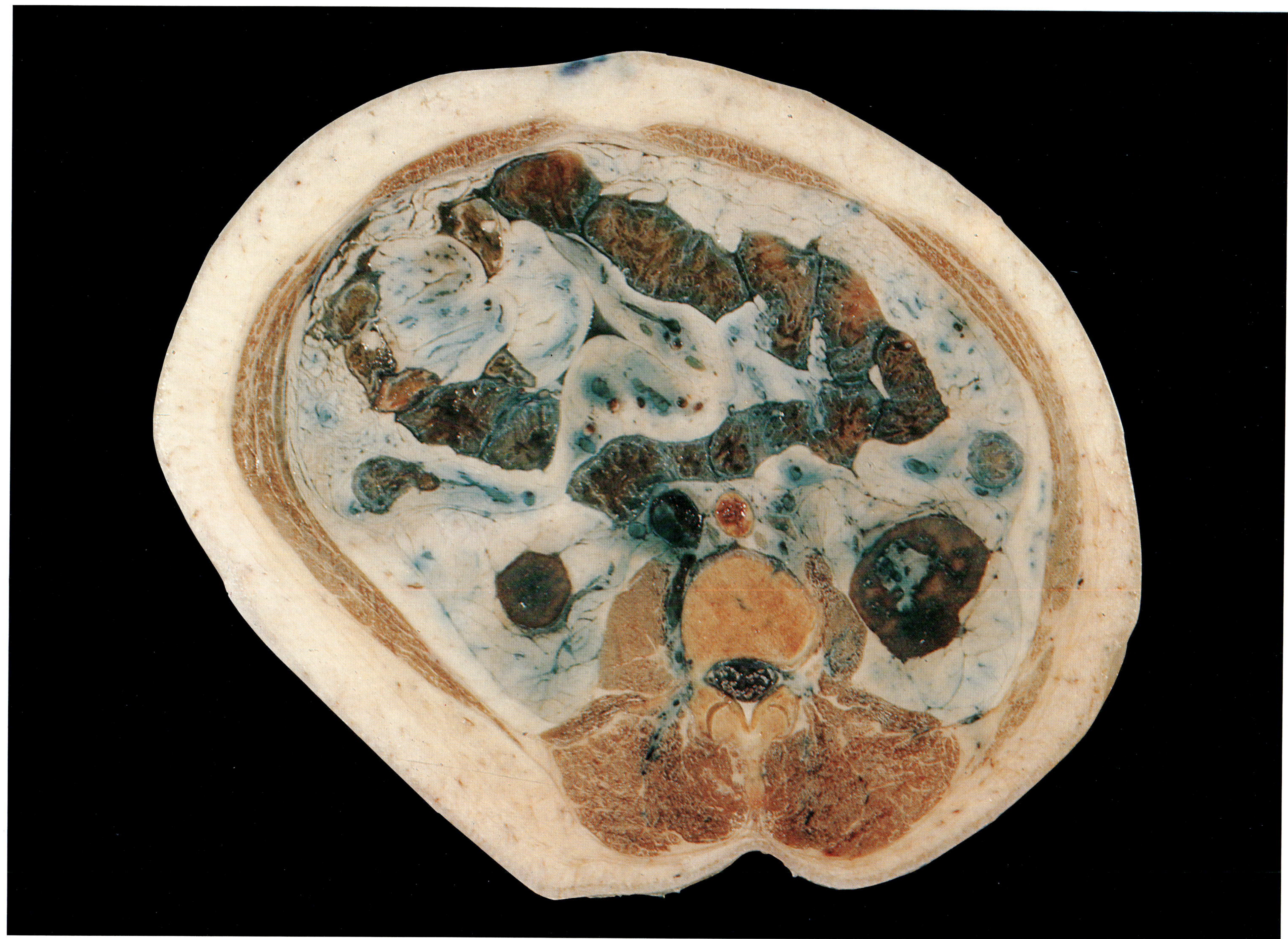

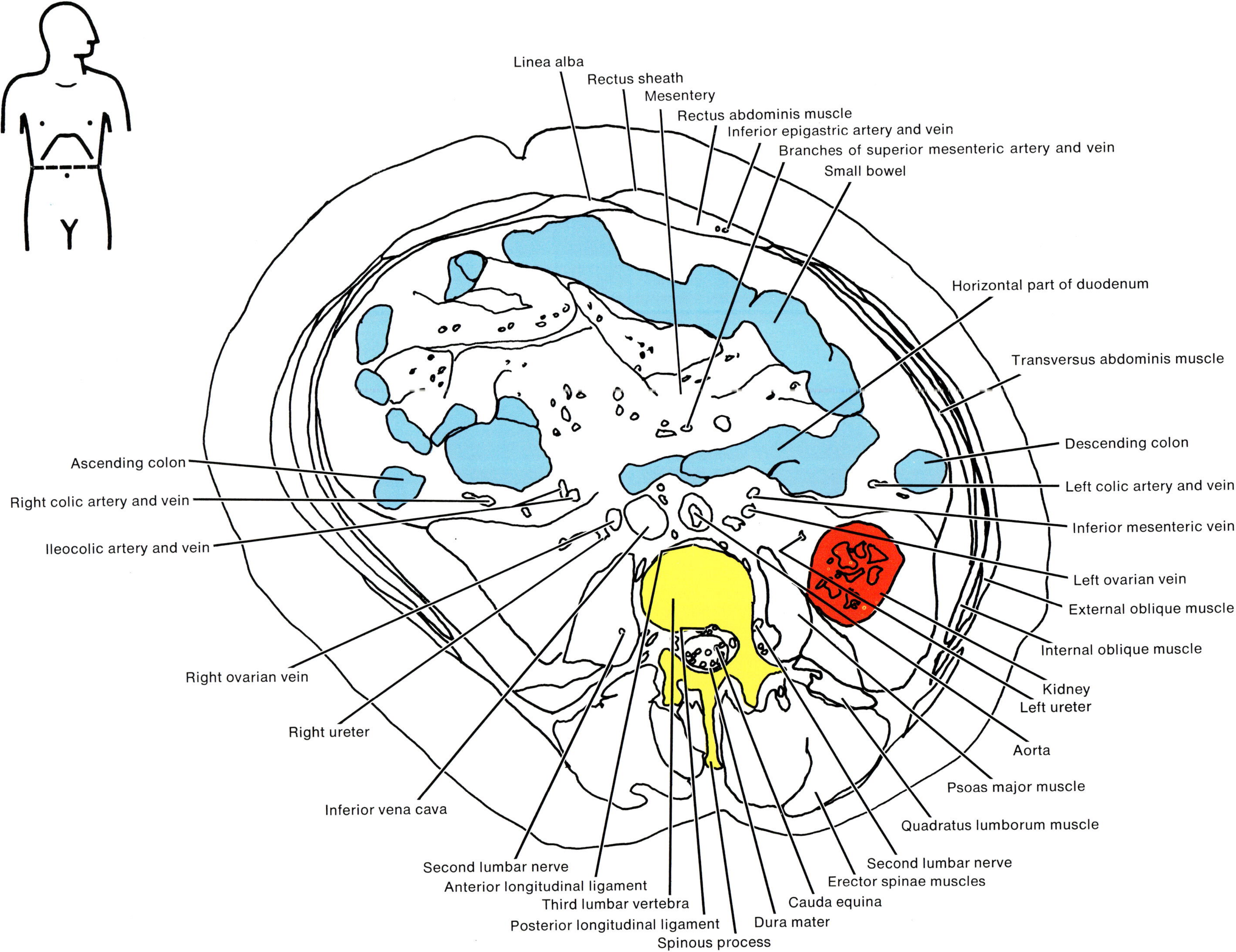

Linea alba
Rectus sheath
Mesentery
Rectus abdominis muscle
Inferior epigastric artery and vein
Branches of superior mesenteric artery and vein
Small bowel
Horizontal part of duodenum
Transversus abdominis muscle
Descending colon
Left colic artery and vein
Inferior mesenteric vein
Left ovarian vein
External oblique muscle
Internal oblique muscle
Kidney
Left ureter
Aorta
Psoas major muscle
Quadratus lumborum muscle
Second lumbar nerve
Erector spinae muscles
Cauda equina
Dura mater
Spinous process
Third lumbar vertebra
Posterior longitudinal ligament
Anterior longitudinal ligament
Second lumbar nerve
Inferior vena cava
Right ureter
Right ovarian vein
Ileocolic artery and vein
Right colic artery and vein
Ascending colon

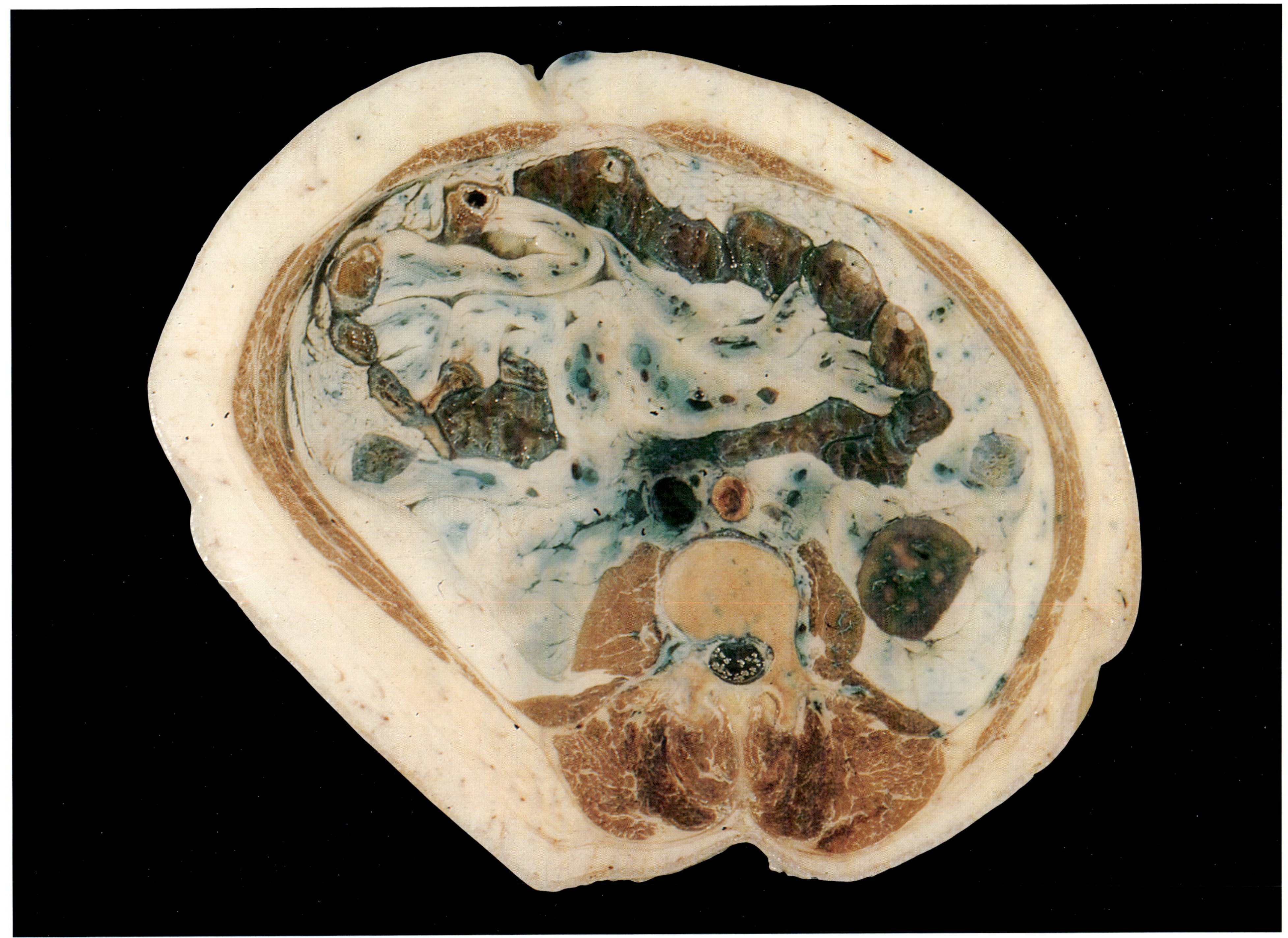

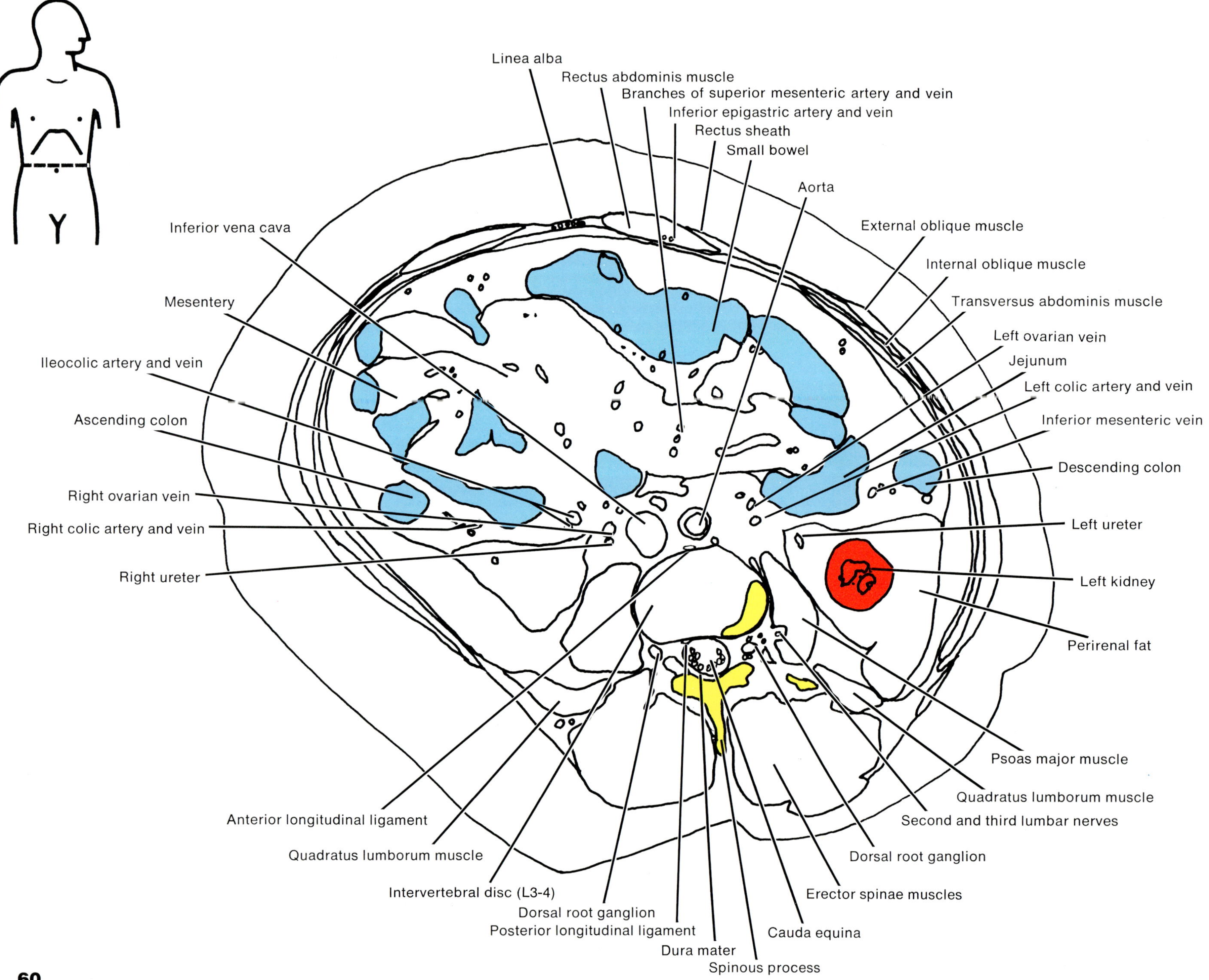

Linea alba
Rectus abdominis muscle
Branches of superior mesenteric artery and vein
Inferior epigastric artery and vein
Rectus sheath
Small bowel
Aorta
External oblique muscle
Internal oblique muscle
Transversus abdominis muscle
Left ovarian vein
Jejunum
Left colic artery and vein
Inferior mesenteric vein
Descending colon
Left ureter
Left kidney
Perirenal fat
Psoas major muscle
Quadratus lumborum muscle
Second and third lumbar nerves
Dorsal root ganglion
Erector spinae muscles
Cauda equina
Spinous process
Dura mater
Posterior longitudinal ligament
Dorsal root ganglion
Intervertebral disc (L3-4)
Quadratus lumborum muscle
Anterior longitudinal ligament
Right ureter
Right colic artery and vein
Right ovarian vein
Ascending colon
Ileocolic artery and vein
Mesentery
Inferior vena cava

TRANSVERSE **Abdomen**

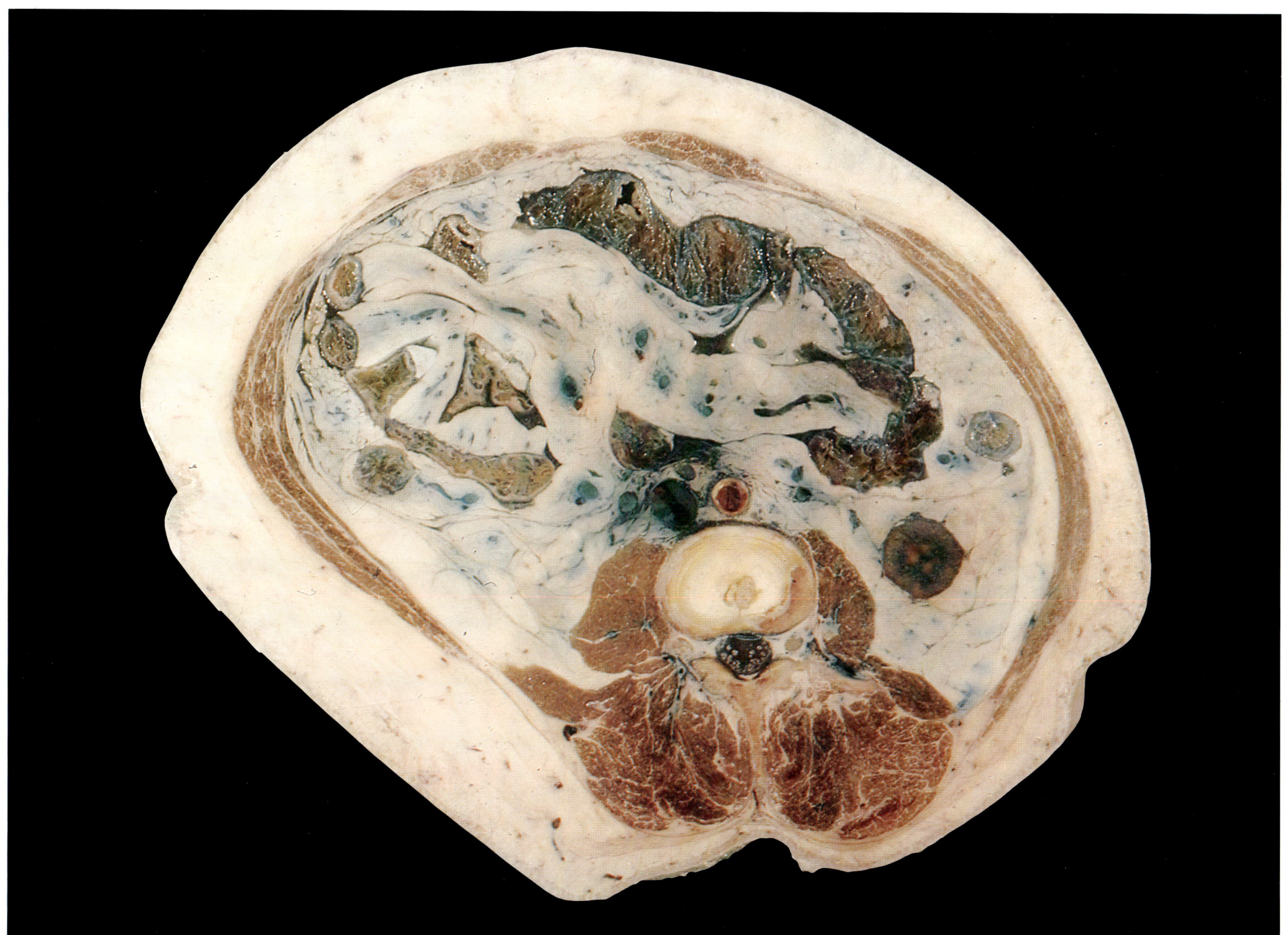

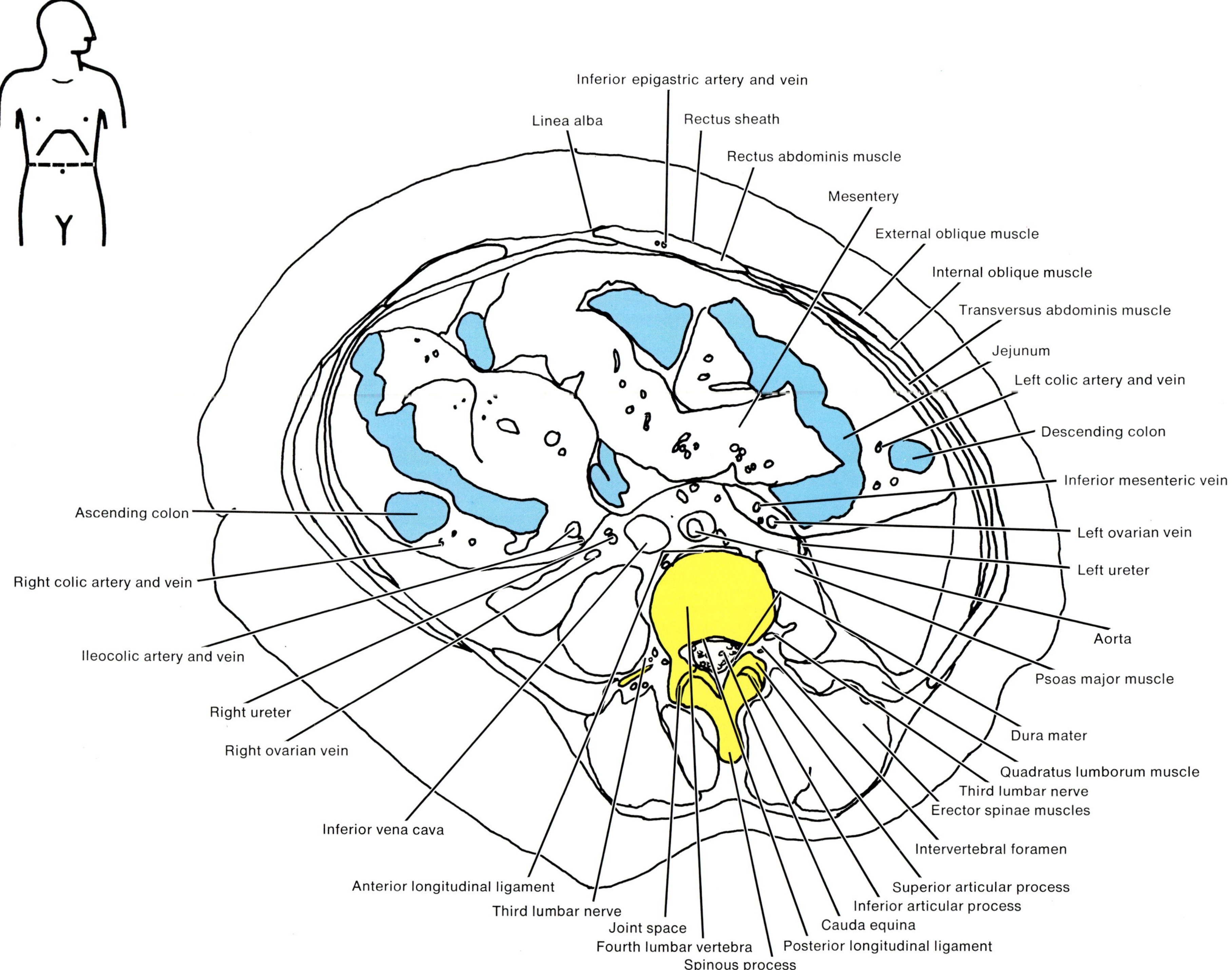

Inferior epigastric artery and vein
Linea alba
Rectus sheath
Rectus abdominis muscle
Mesentery
External oblique muscle
Internal oblique muscle
Transversus abdominis muscle
Jejunum
Left colic artery and vein
Descending colon
Inferior mesenteric vein
Left ovarian vein
Left ureter
Aorta
Psoas major muscle
Dura mater
Quadratus lumborum muscle
Third lumbar nerve
Erector spinae muscles
Intervertebral foramen
Superior articular process
Inferior articular process
Cauda equina
Posterior longitudinal ligament
Spinous process
Fourth lumbar vertebra
Joint space
Third lumbar nerve
Anterior longitudinal ligament
Inferior vena cava
Right ovarian vein
Right ureter
Ileocolic artery and vein
Right colic artery and vein
Ascending colon

TRANSVERSE **Abdomen**

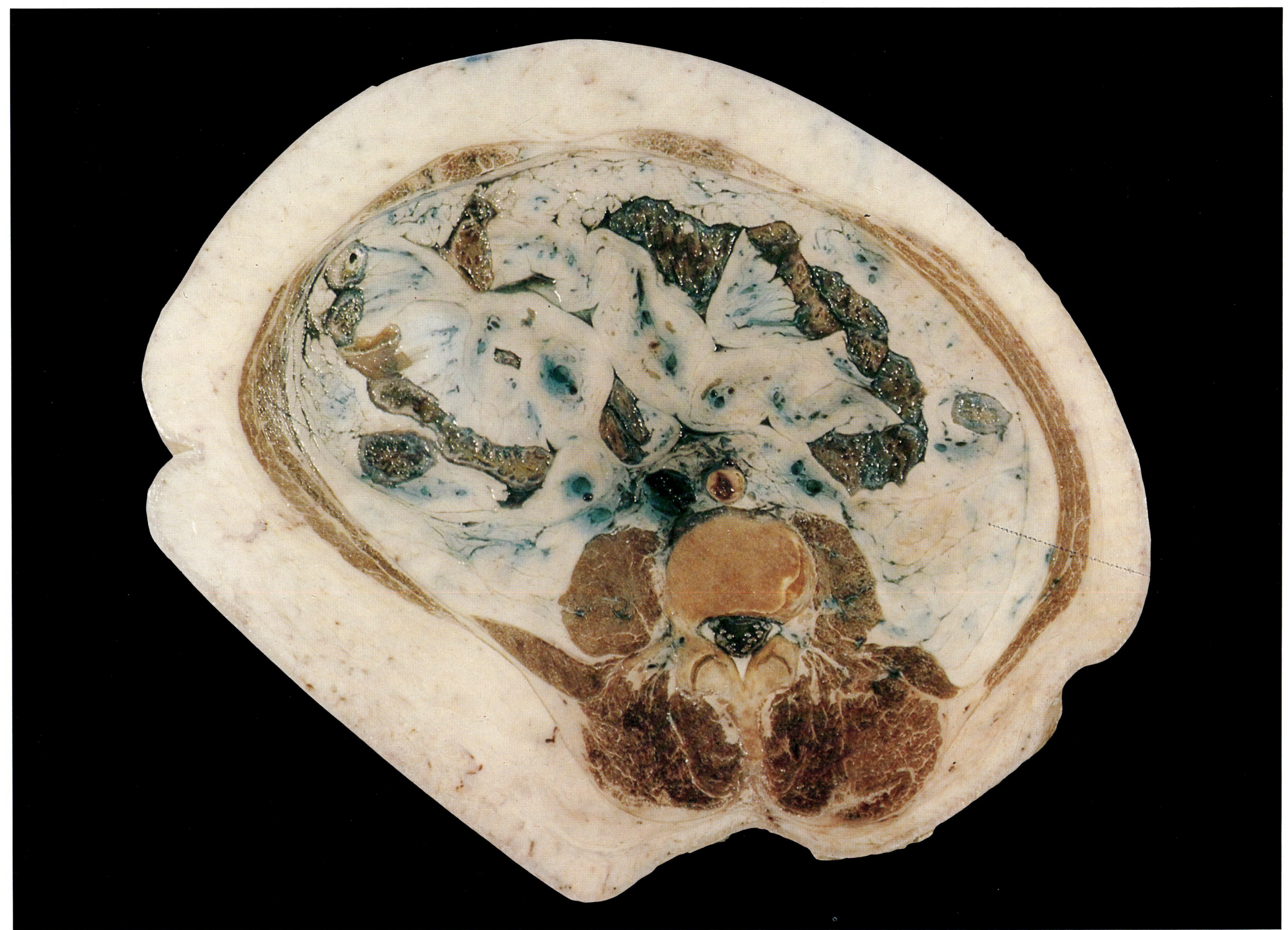

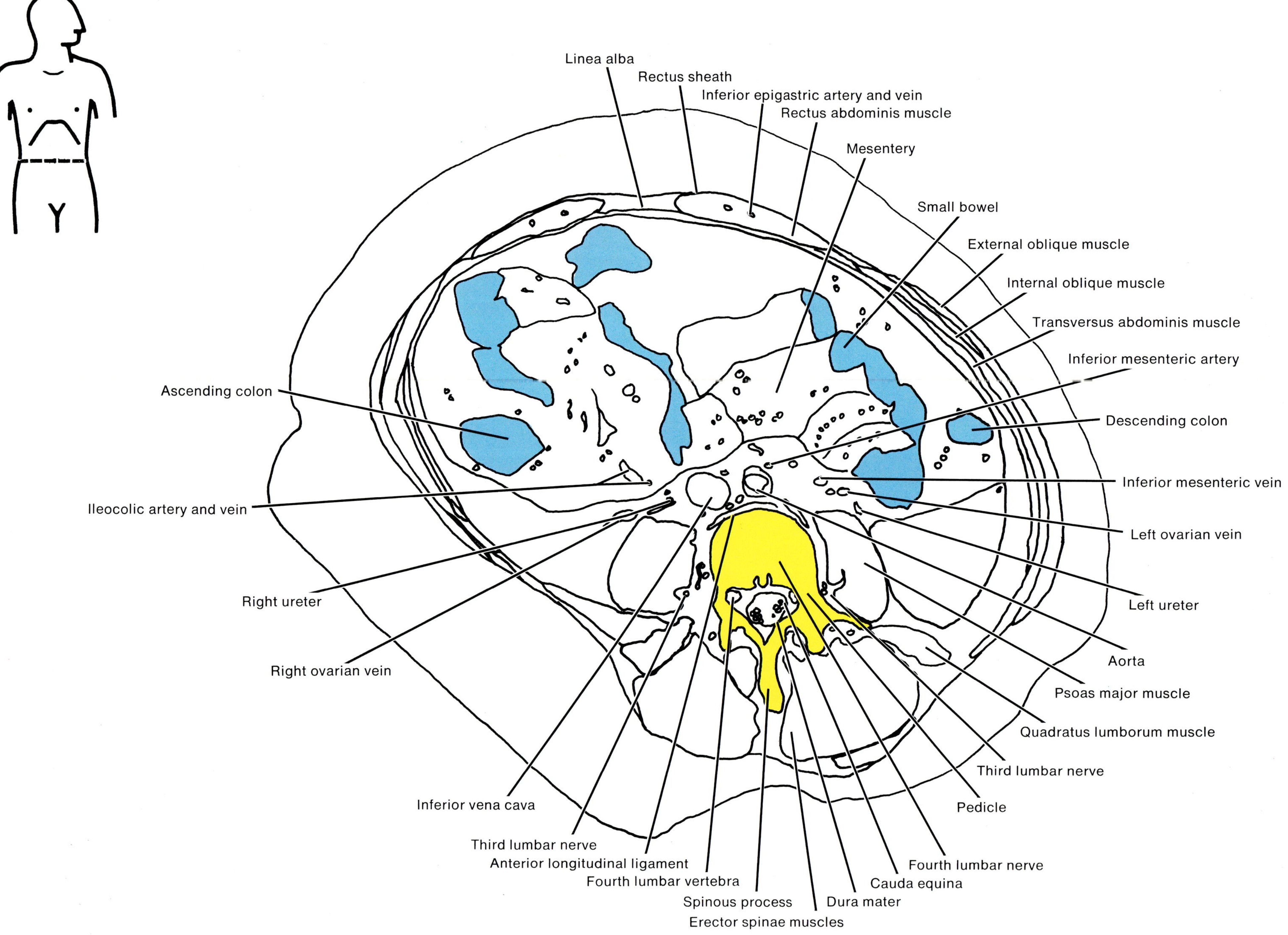
Linea alba
Rectus sheath
Inferior epigastric artery and vein
Rectus abdominis muscle
Mesentery
Small bowel
External oblique muscle
Internal oblique muscle
Transversus abdominis muscle
Inferior mesenteric artery
Descending colon
Inferior mesenteric vein
Left ovarian vein
Left ureter
Aorta
Psoas major muscle
Quadratus lumborum muscle
Third lumbar nerve
Pedicle
Fourth lumbar nerve
Cauda equina
Dura mater
Spinous process
Erector spinae muscles
Fourth lumbar vertebra
Anterior longitudinal ligament
Third lumbar nerve
Inferior vena cava
Right ovarian vein
Right ureter
Ileocolic artery and vein
Ascending colon

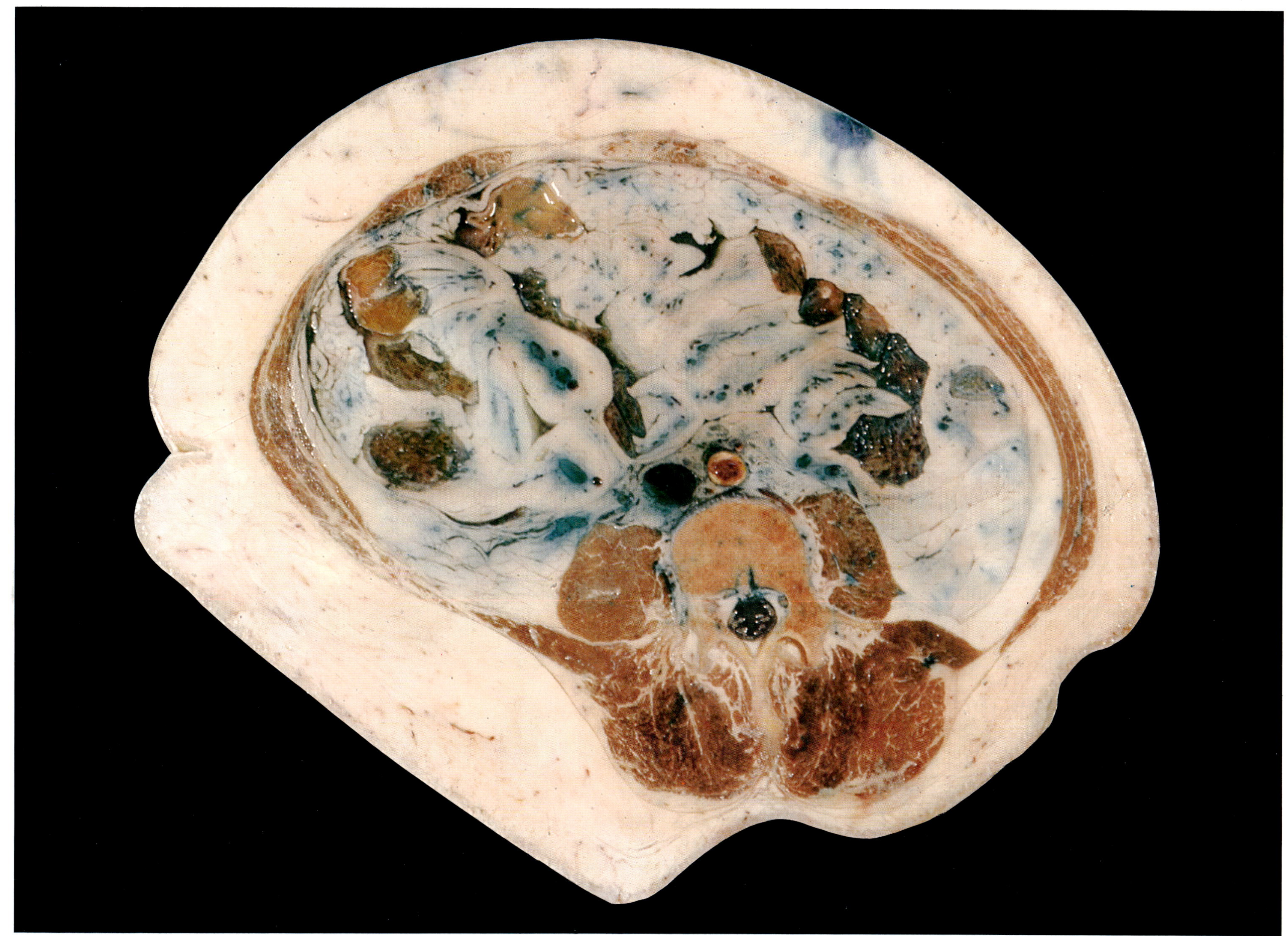

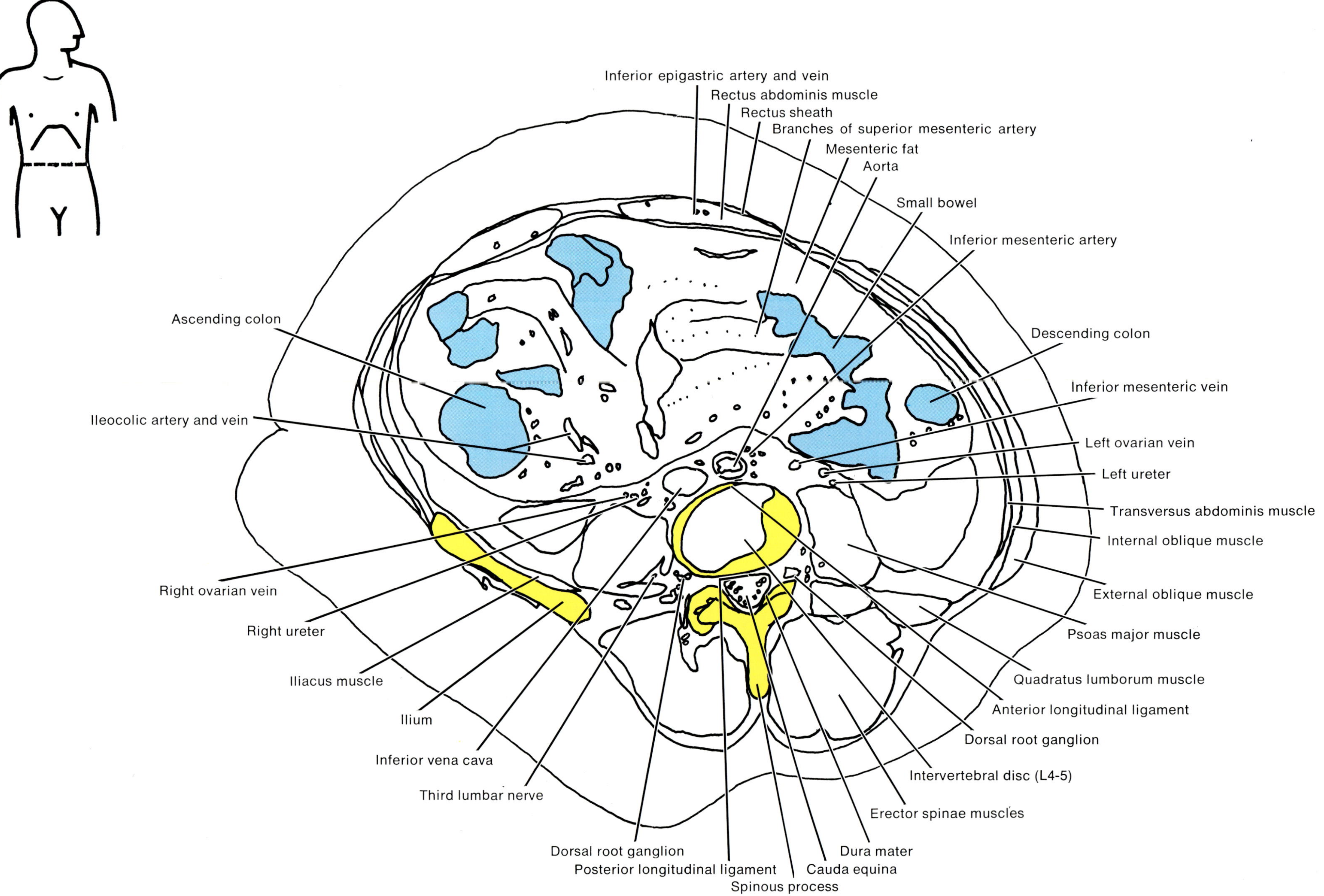

Inferior epigastric artery and vein
Rectus abdominis muscle
Rectus sheath
Branches of superior mesenteric artery
Mesenteric fat
Aorta
Small bowel
Inferior mesenteric artery
Descending colon
Inferior mesenteric vein
Left ovarian vein
Left ureter
Transversus abdominis muscle
Internal oblique muscle
External oblique muscle
Psoas major muscle
Quadratus lumborum muscle
Anterior longitudinal ligament
Dorsal root ganglion
Intervertebral disc (L4-5)
Erector spinae muscles
Dura mater
Cauda equina
Spinous process
Posterior longitudinal ligament
Dorsal root ganglion
Third lumbar nerve
Inferior vena cava
Ilium
Iliacus muscle
Right ureter
Right ovarian vein
Ileocolic artery and vein
Ascending colon

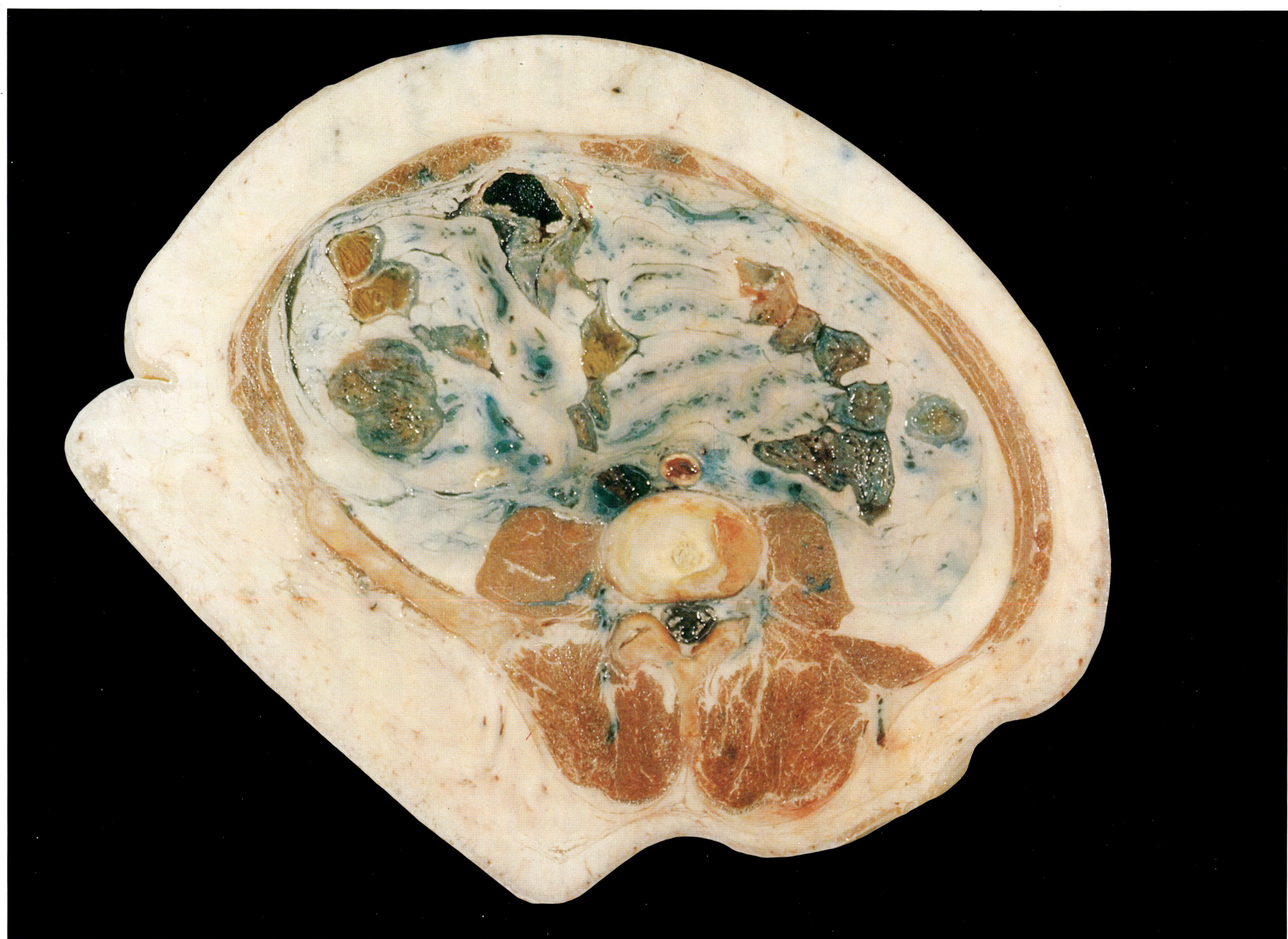

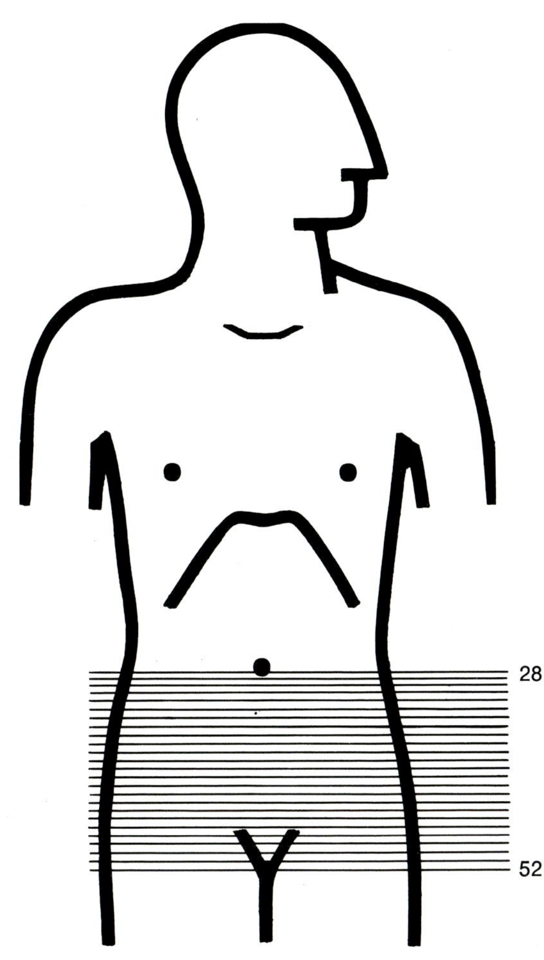

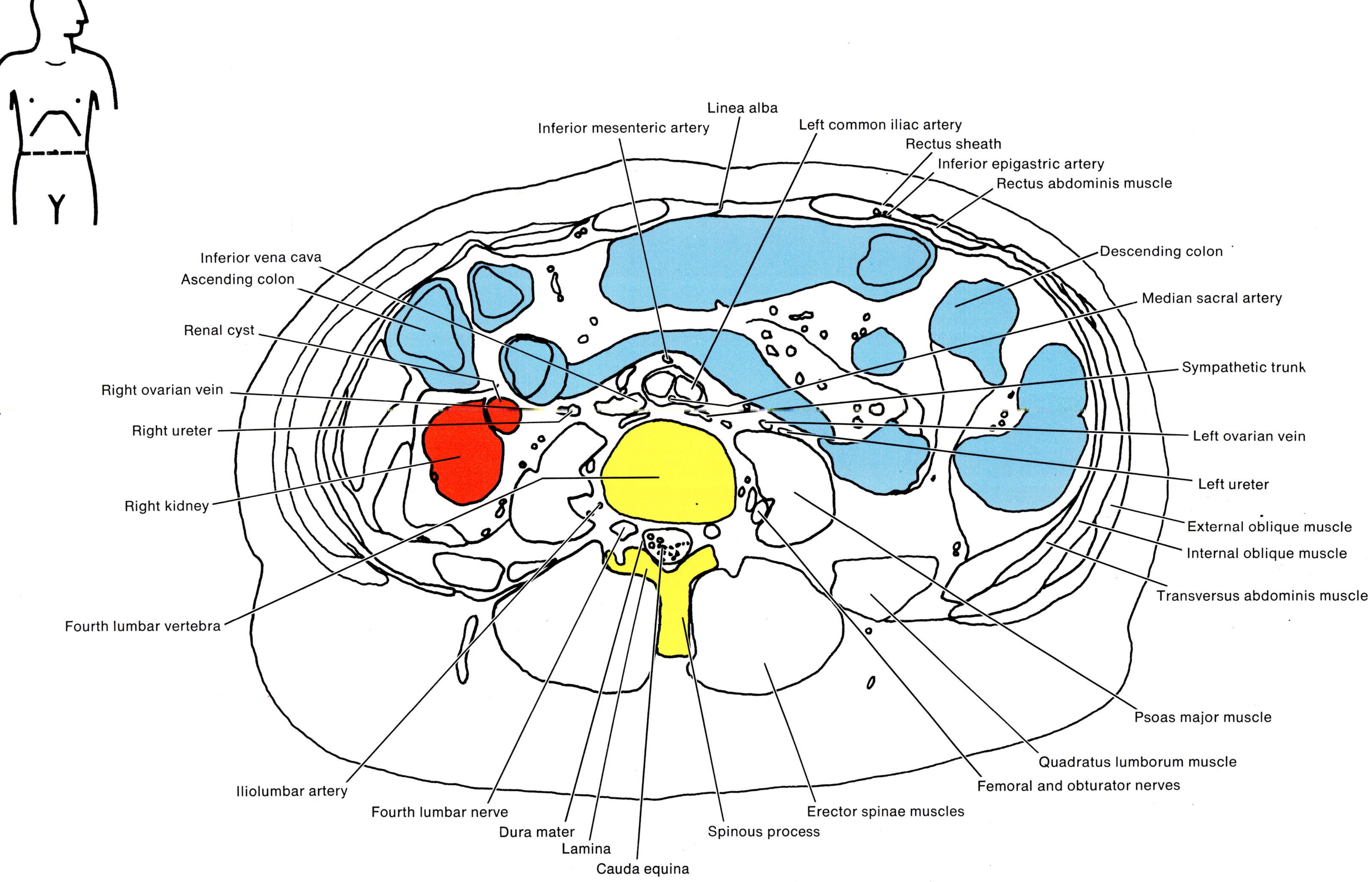

Linea alba
Inferior mesenteric artery
Left common iliac artery
Rectus sheath
Inferior epigastric artery
Rectus abdominis muscle
Inferior vena cava
Ascending colon
Descending colon
Median sacral artery
Renal cyst
Sympathetic trunk
Right ovarian vein
Right ureter
Left ovarian vein
Right kidney
Left ureter
External oblique muscle
Internal oblique muscle
Transversus abdominis muscle
Fourth lumbar vertebra
Iliolumbar artery
Psoas major muscle
Quadratus lumborum muscle
Fourth lumbar nerve
Femoral and obturator nerves
Dura mater
Erector spinae muscles
Lamina
Spinous process
Cauda equina

TRANSVERSE **Pelvis—female**

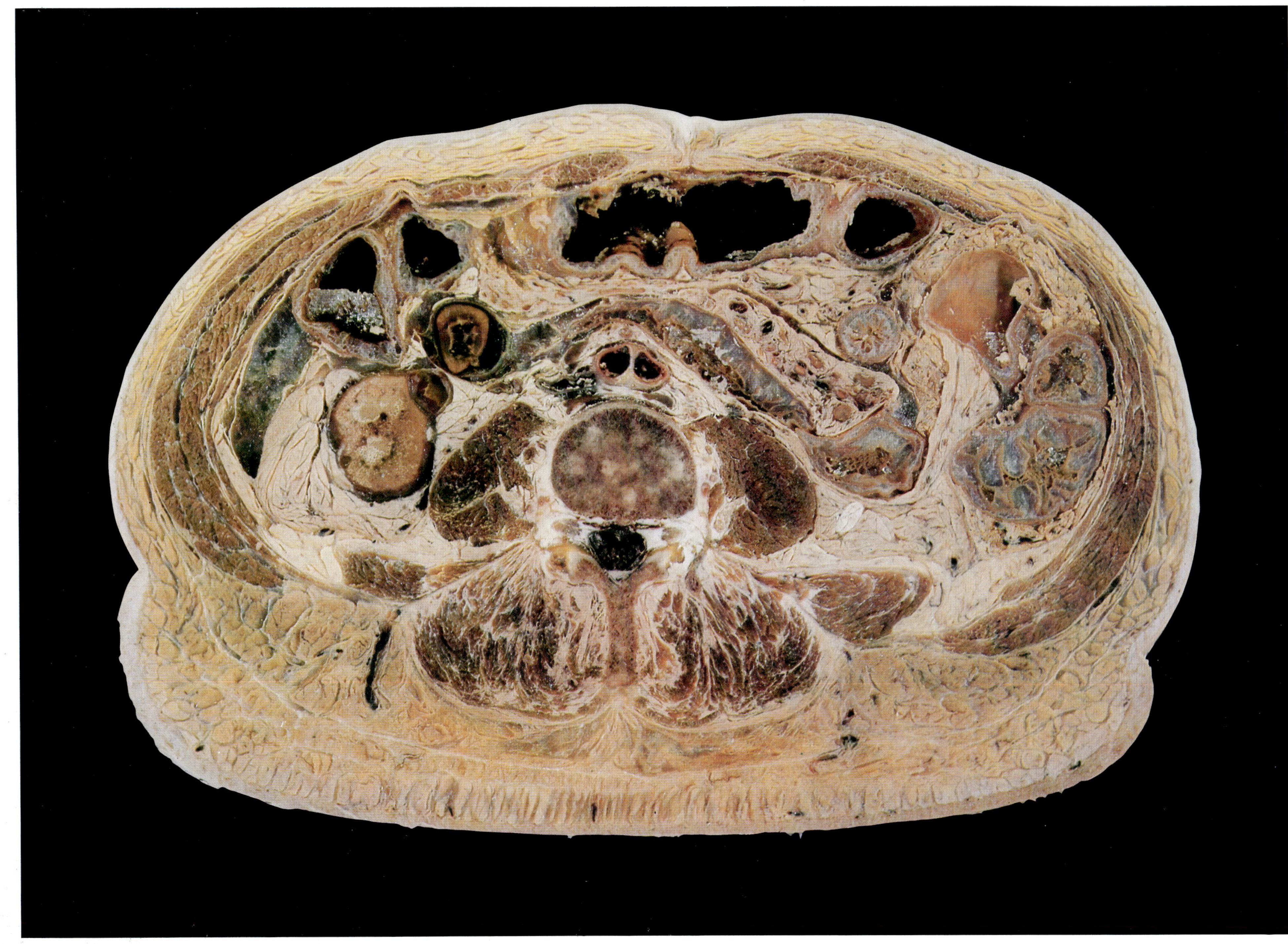

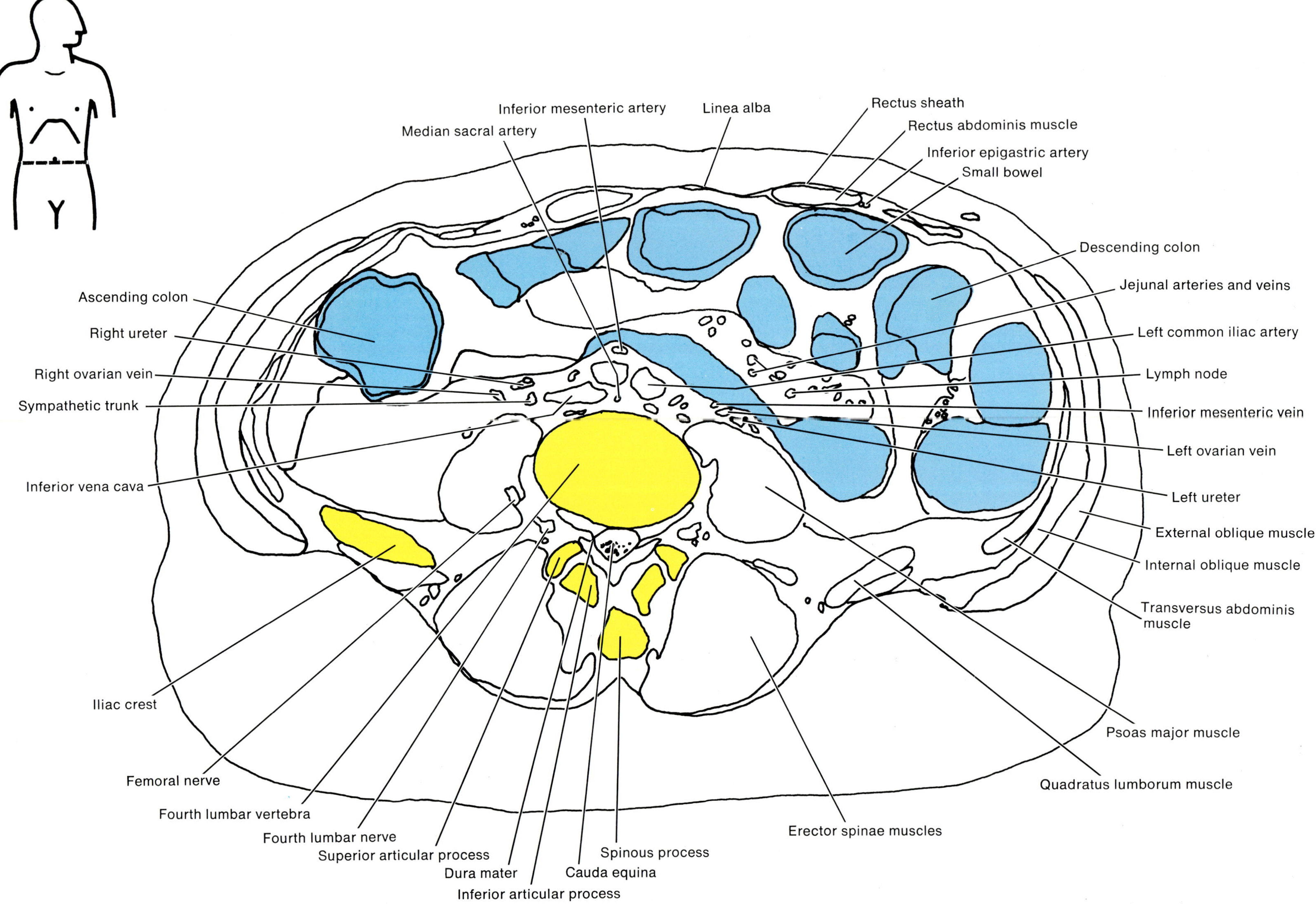

Inferior mesenteric artery
Median sacral artery
Linea alba
Rectus sheath
Rectus abdominis muscle
Inferior epigastric artery
Small bowel
Descending colon
Jejunal arteries and veins
Left common iliac artery
Lymph node
Inferior mesenteric vein
Left ovarian vein
Left ureter
External oblique muscle
Internal oblique muscle
Transversus abdominis muscle
Psoas major muscle
Quadratus lumborum muscle
Erector spinae muscles
Spinous process
Cauda equina
Dura mater
Inferior articular process
Superior articular process
Fourth lumbar nerve
Fourth lumbar vertebra
Femoral nerve
Iliac crest
Inferior vena cava
Sympathetic trunk
Right ovarian vein
Right ureter
Ascending colon

TRANSVERSE **Pelvis—female**

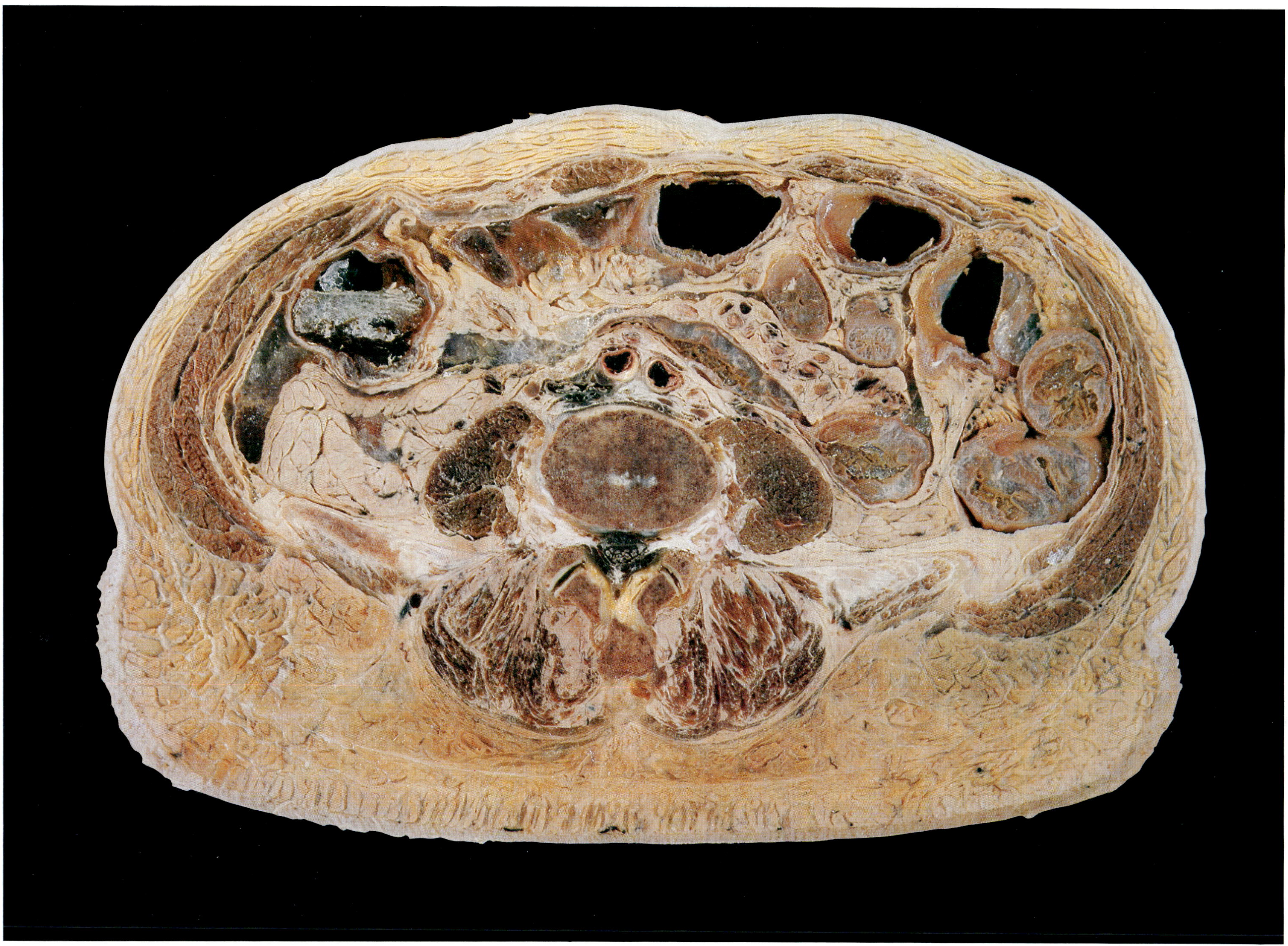

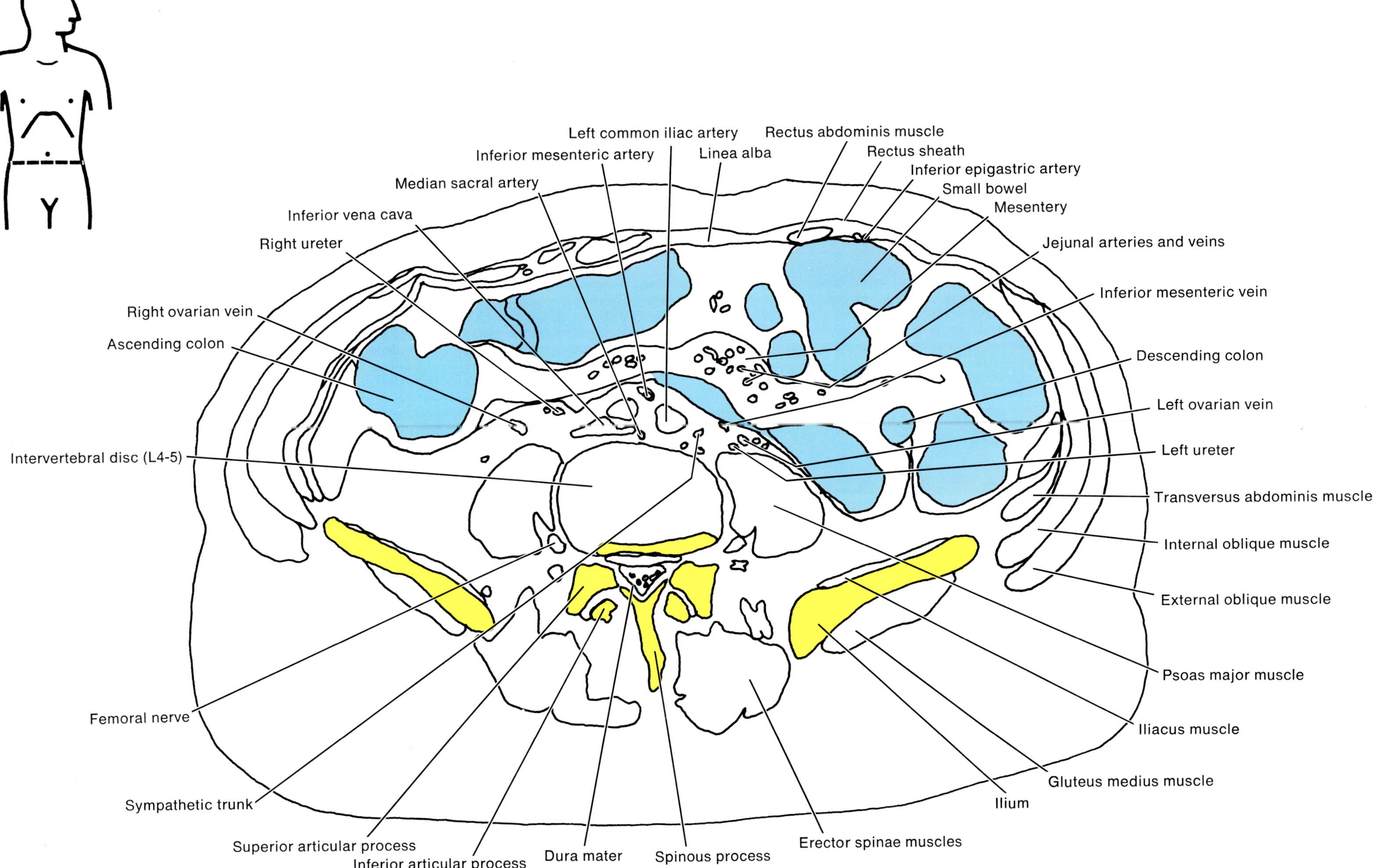

Left common iliac artery
Inferior mesenteric artery
Linea alba
Rectus abdominis muscle
Rectus sheath
Inferior epigastric artery
Small bowel
Mesentery
Median sacral artery
Inferior vena cava
Jejunal arteries and veins
Right ureter
Inferior mesenteric vein
Right ovarian vein
Ascending colon
Descending colon
Left ovarian vein
Intervertebral disc (L4-5)
Left ureter
Transversus abdominis muscle
Internal oblique muscle
External oblique muscle
Psoas major muscle
Femoral nerve
Iliacus muscle
Gluteus medius muscle
Sympathetic trunk
Ilium
Superior articular process
Inferior articular process
Dura mater
Spinous process
Erector spinae muscles

TRANSVERSE **Pelvis—female**

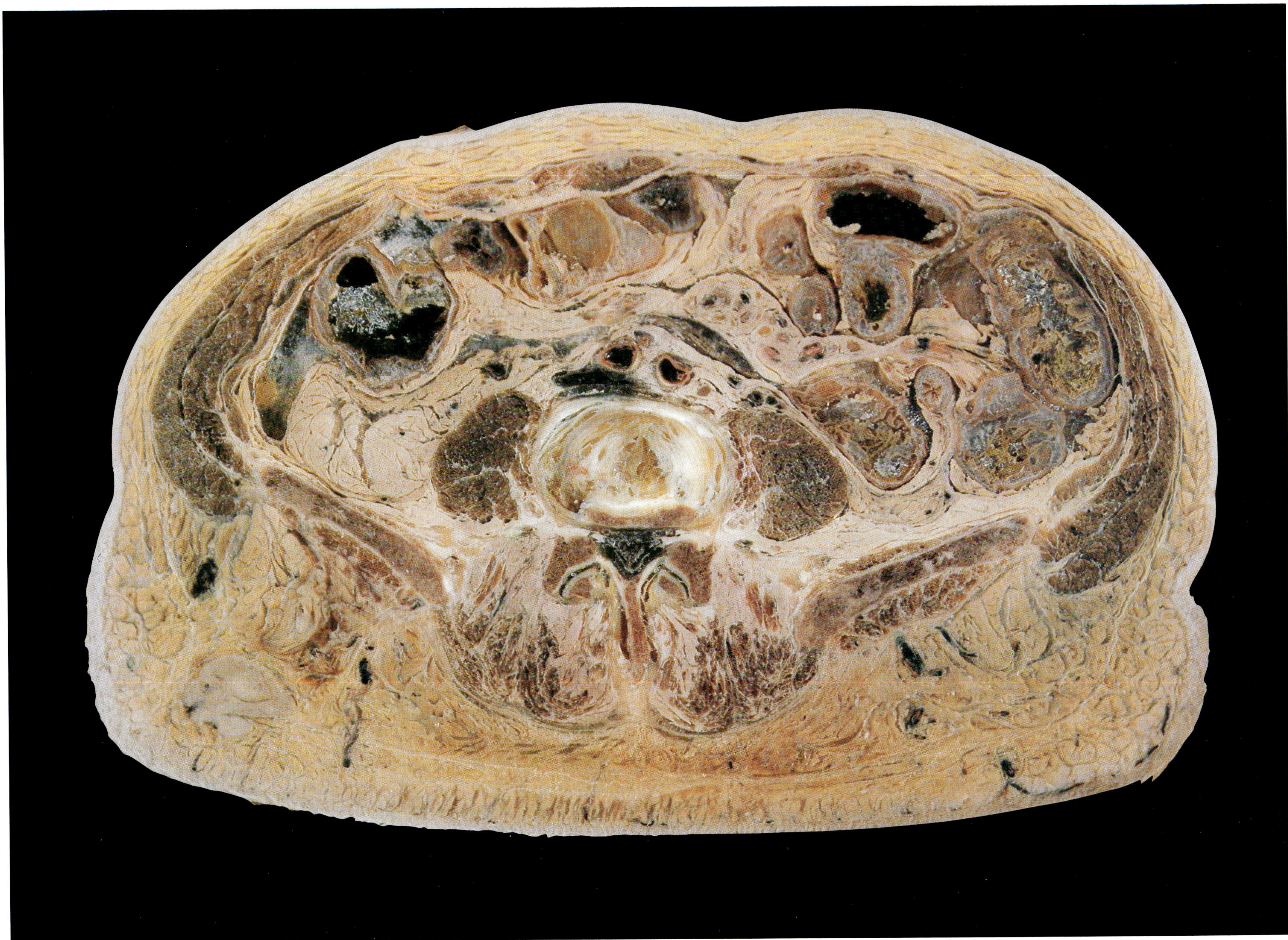

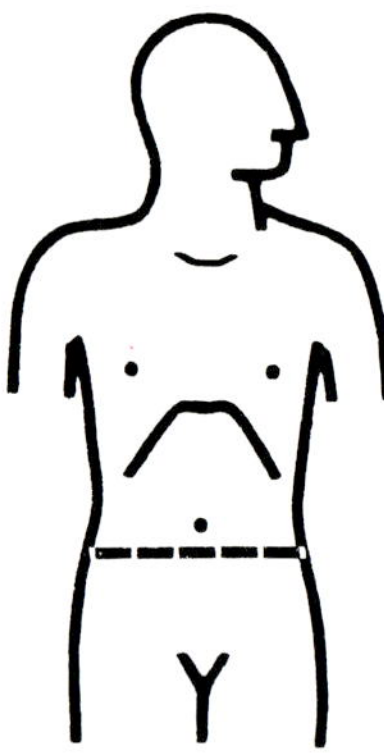

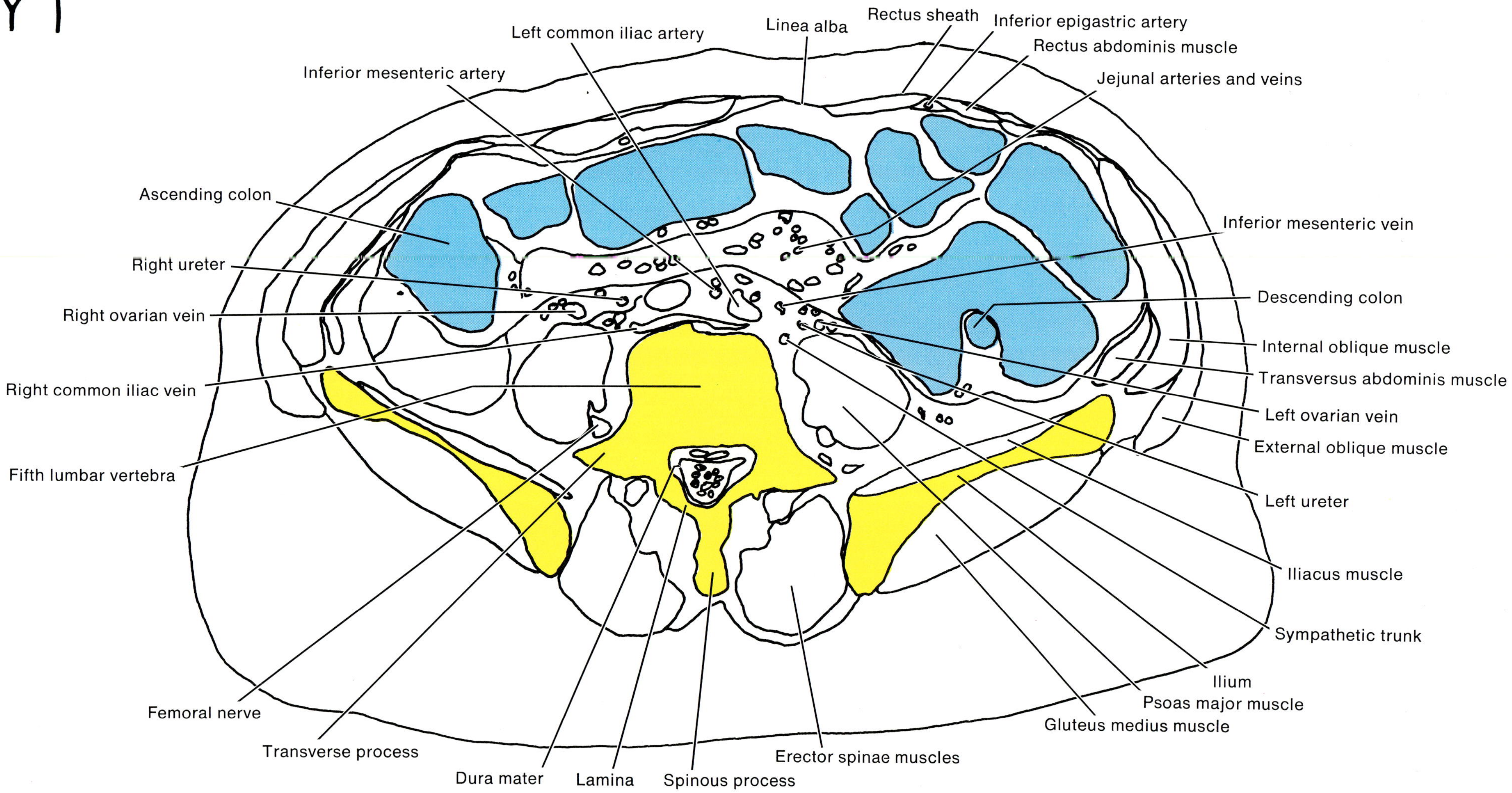

Left common iliac artery
Linea alba
Rectus sheath
Inferior epigastric artery
Rectus abdominis muscle
Inferior mesenteric artery
Jejunal arteries and veins
Ascending colon
Inferior mesenteric vein
Right ureter
Right ovarian vein
Descending colon
Internal oblique muscle
Right common iliac vein
Transversus abdominis muscle
Left ovarian vein
External oblique muscle
Fifth lumbar vertebra
Left ureter
Iliacus muscle
Sympathetic trunk
Ilium
Psoas major muscle
Femoral nerve
Gluteus medius muscle
Transverse process
Erector spinae muscles
Dura mater
Lamina
Spinous process

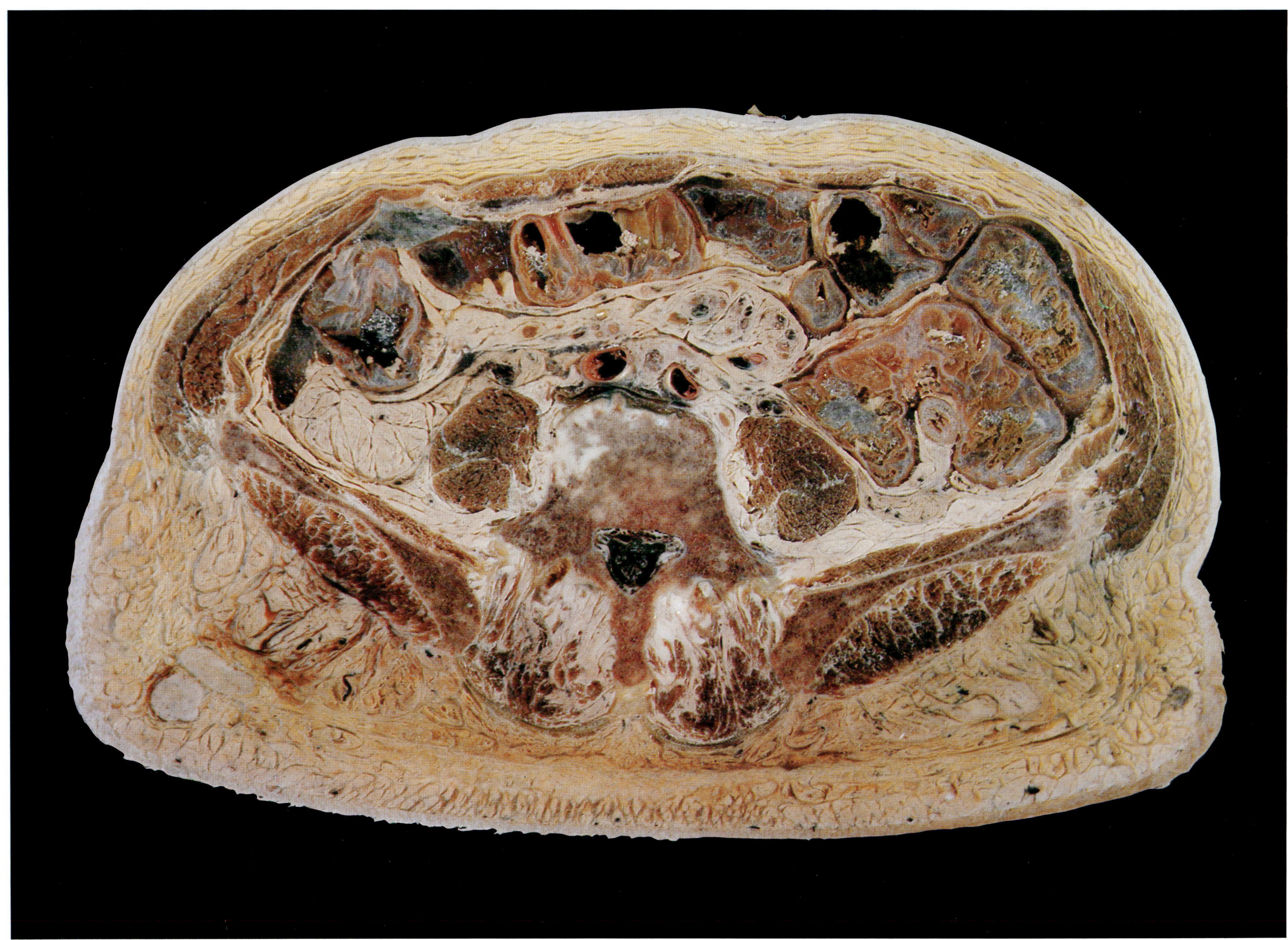

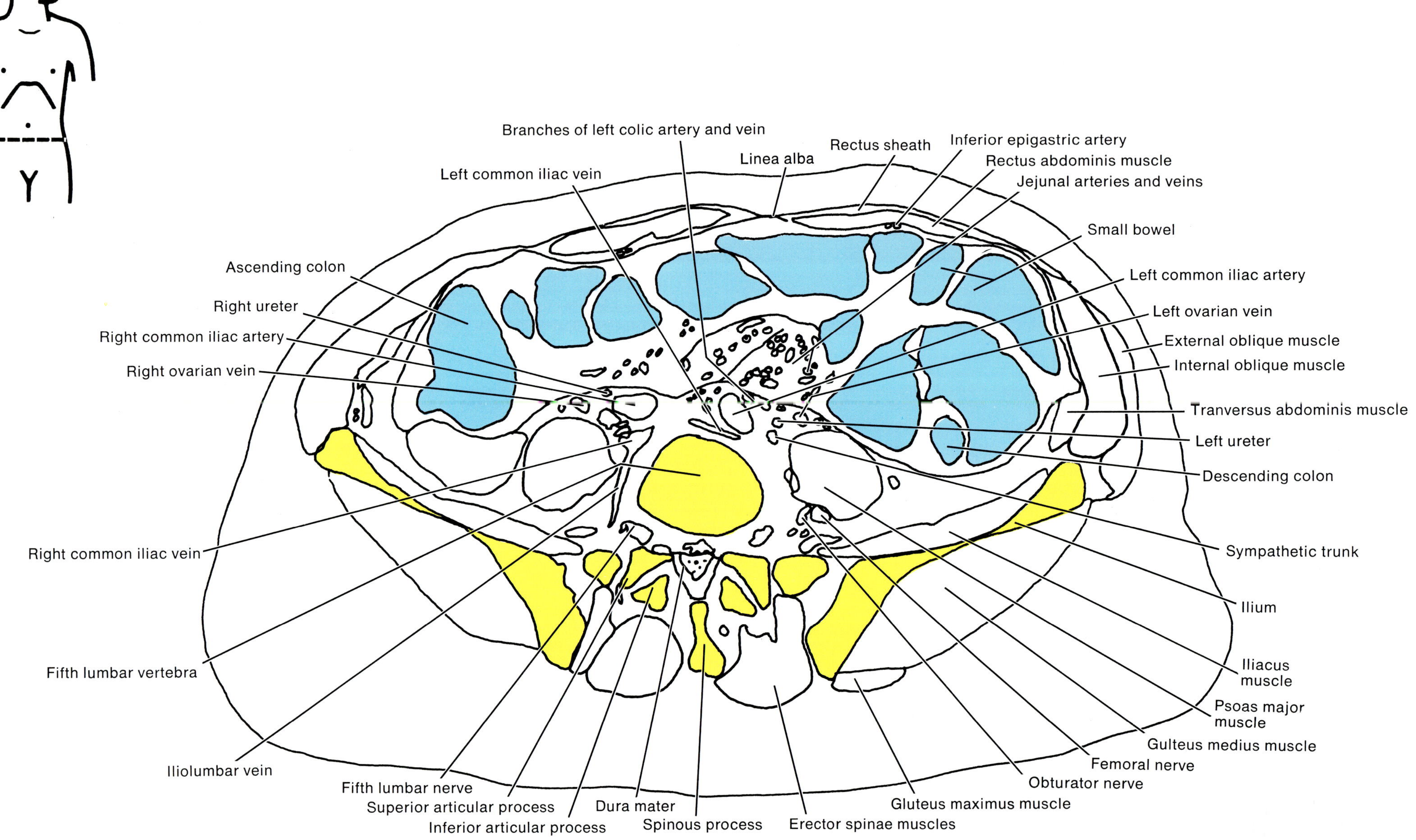
Branches of left colic artery and vein
Rectus sheath
Inferior epigastric artery
Linea alba
Rectus abdominis muscle
Jejunal arteries and veins
Left common iliac vein
Small bowel
Ascending colon
Left common iliac artery
Right ureter
Left ovarian vein
Right common iliac artery
External oblique muscle
Right ovarian vein
Internal oblique muscle
Tranversus abdominis muscle
Left ureter
Descending colon
Right common iliac vein
Sympathetic trunk
Ilium
Fifth lumbar vertebra
Iliacus muscle
Psoas major muscle
Gulteus medius muscle
Iliolumbar vein
Femoral nerve
Fifth lumbar nerve
Obturator nerve
Superior articular process
Dura mater
Gluteus maximus muscle
Inferior articular process
Spinous process
Erector spinae muscles

TRANSVERSE **Pelvis—female**

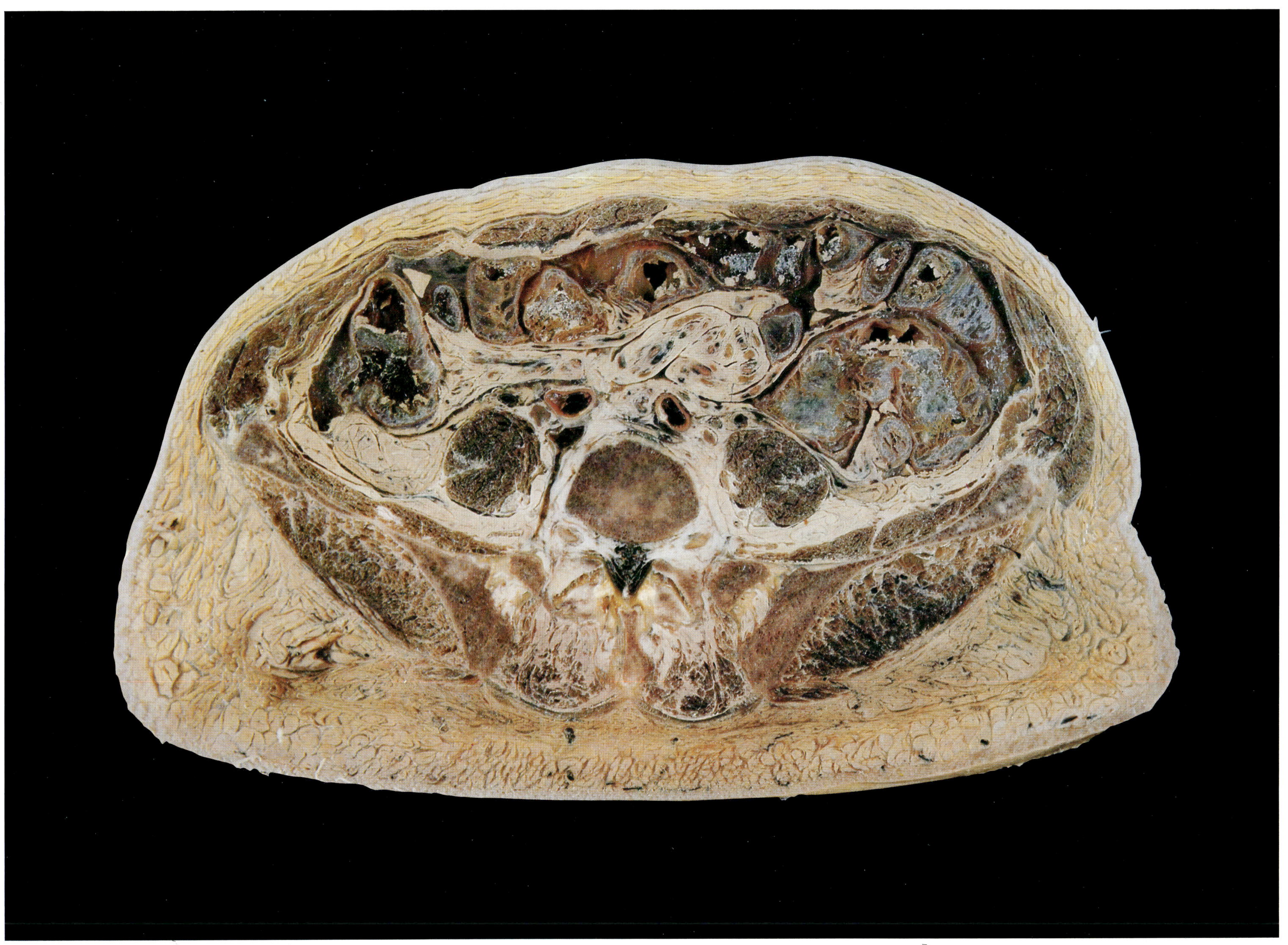

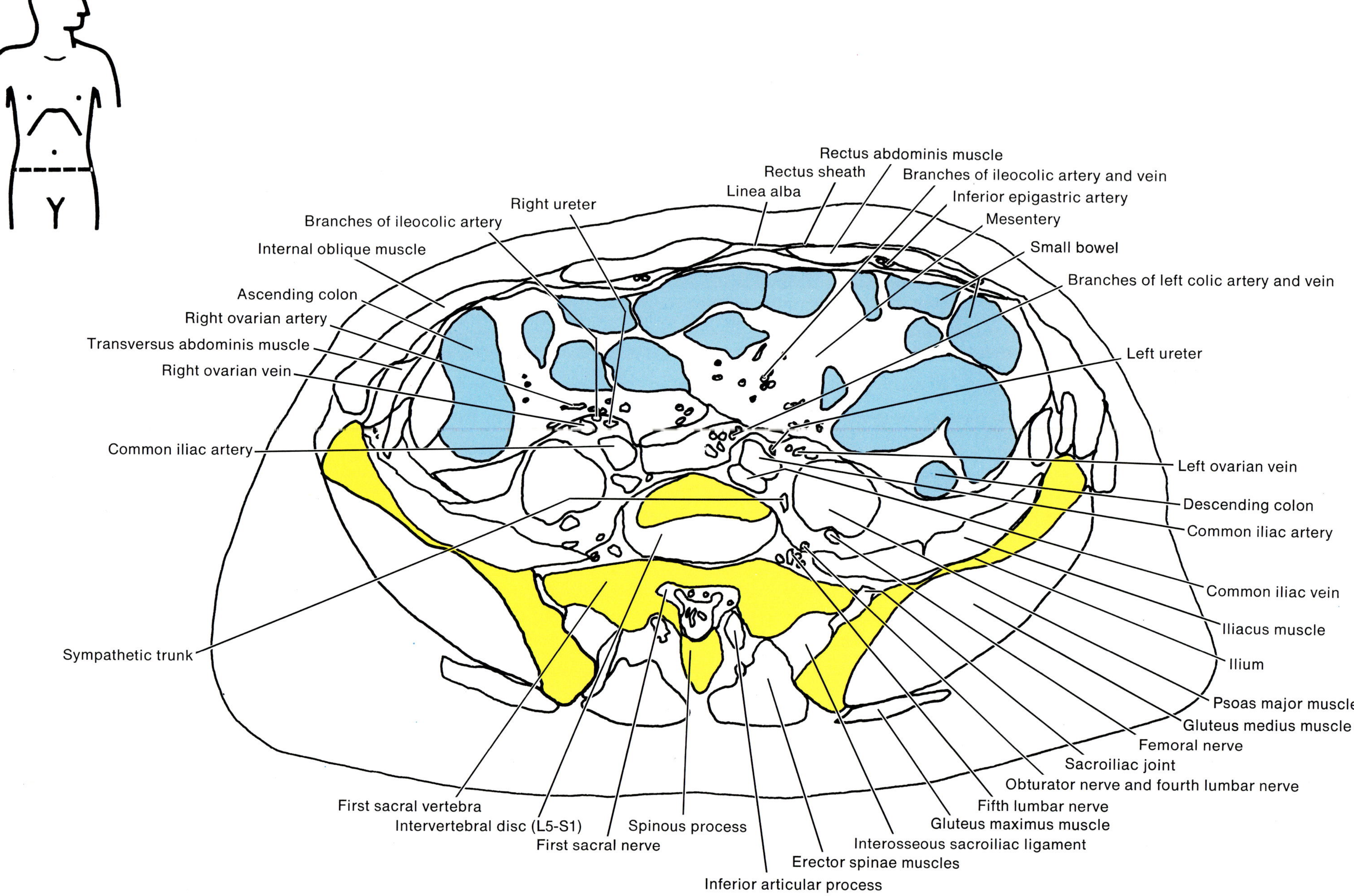

Rectus abdominis muscle
Rectus sheath
Linea alba
Branches of ileocolic artery and vein
Inferior epigastric artery
Mesentery
Small bowel
Branches of left colic artery and vein
Right ureter
Branches of ileocolic artery
Internal oblique muscle
Ascending colon
Right ovarian artery
Transversus abdominis muscle
Right ovarian vein
Left ureter
Common iliac artery
Left ovarian vein
Descending colon
Common iliac artery
Common iliac vein
Iliacus muscle
Ilium
Psoas major muscle
Sympathetic trunk
Gluteus medius muscle
Femoral nerve
Sacroiliac joint
Obturator nerve and fourth lumbar nerve
Fifth lumbar nerve
Gluteus maximus muscle
Interosseous sacroiliac ligament
First sacral vertebra
Intervertebral disc (L5-S1)
Spinous process
First sacral nerve
Erector spinae muscles
Inferior articular process

TRANSVERSE **Pelvis—female**

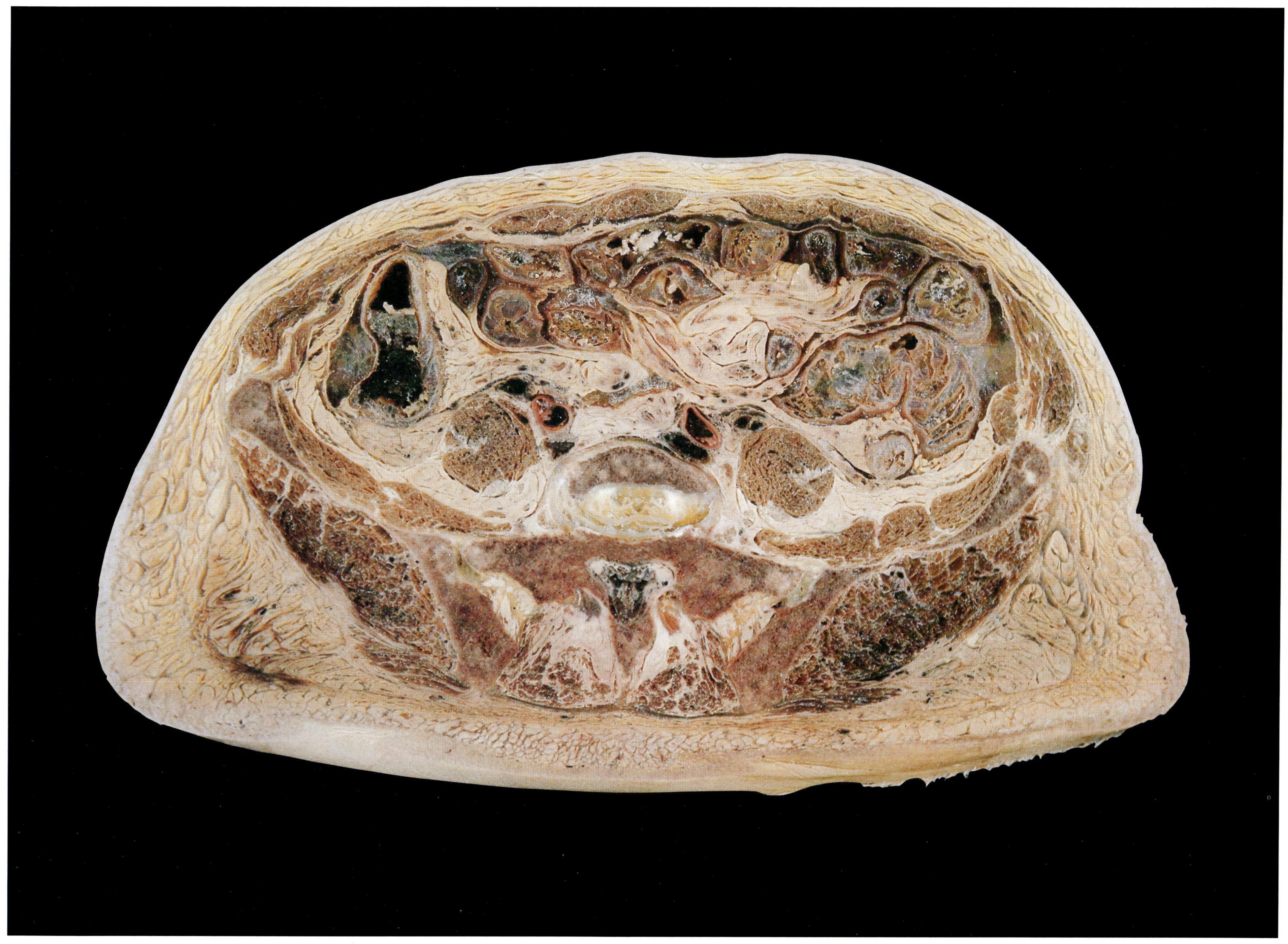

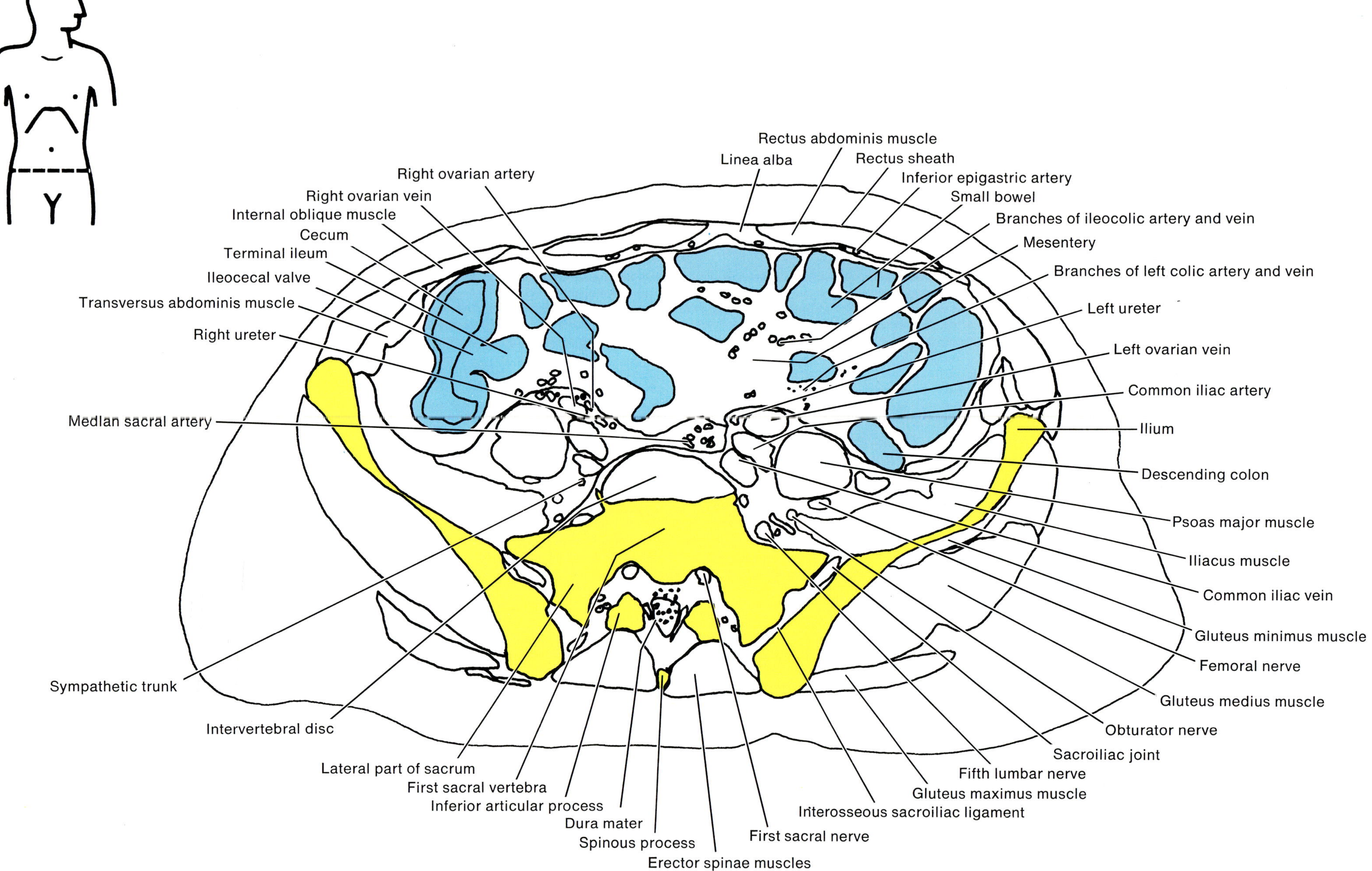

Rectus abdominis muscle
Linea alba
Rectus sheath
Inferior epigastric artery
Small bowel
Branches of ileocolic artery and vein
Right ovarian artery
Mesentery
Right ovarian vein
Branches of left colic artery and vein
Internal oblique muscle
Cecum
Left ureter
Terminal ileum
Ileocecal valve
Left ovarian vein
Transversus abdominis muscle
Common iliac artery
Right ureter
Ilium
Median sacral artery
Descending colon
Psoas major muscle
Iliacus muscle
Common iliac vein
Gluteus minimus muscle
Femoral nerve
Sympathetic trunk
Gluteus medius muscle
Obturator nerve
Intervertebral disc
Sacroiliac joint
Lateral part of sacrum
Fifth lumbar nerve
First sacral vertebra
Gluteus maximus muscle
Inferior articular process
Interosseous sacroiliac ligament
Dura mater
Spinous process
First sacral nerve
Erector spinae muscles

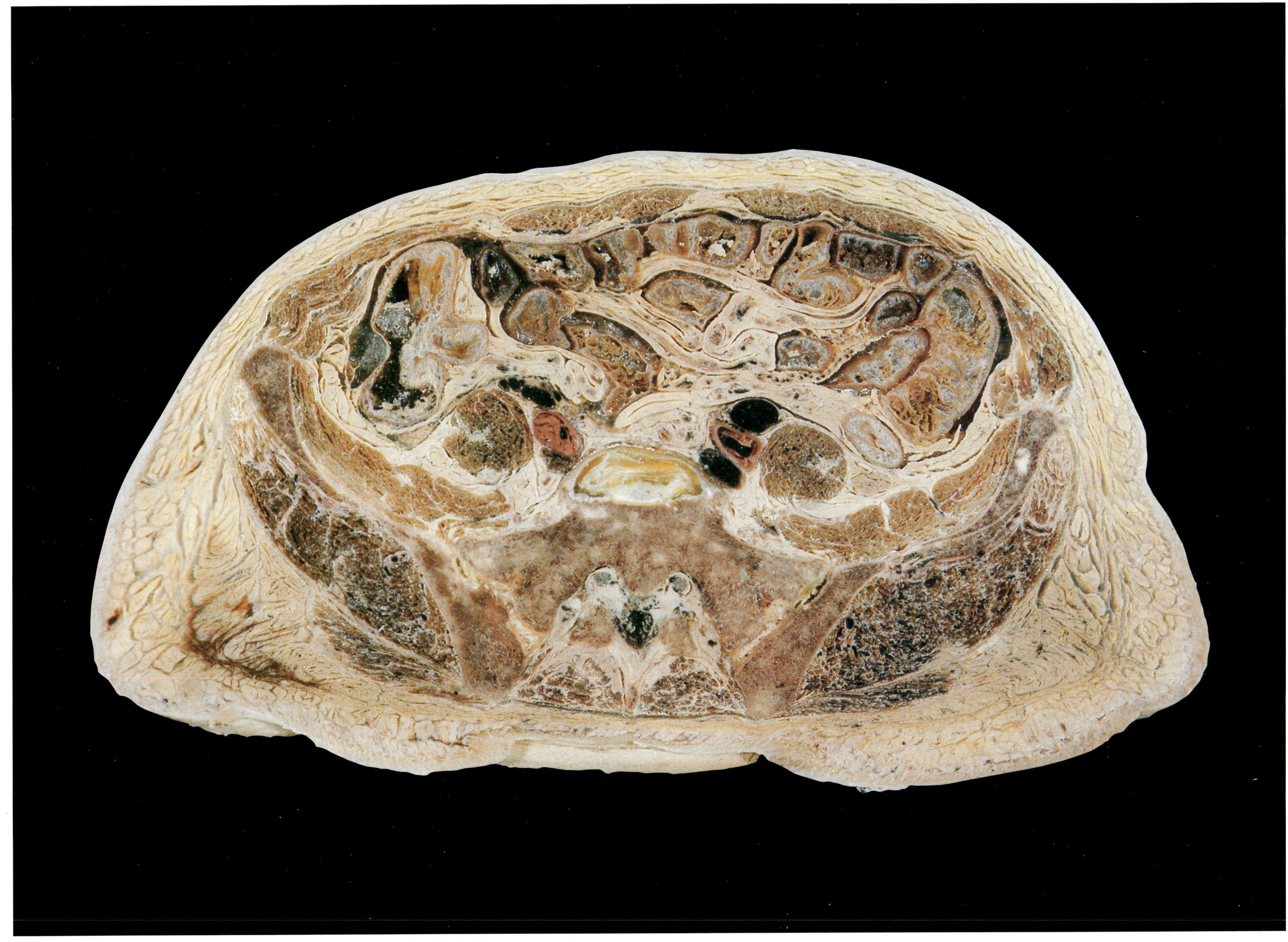

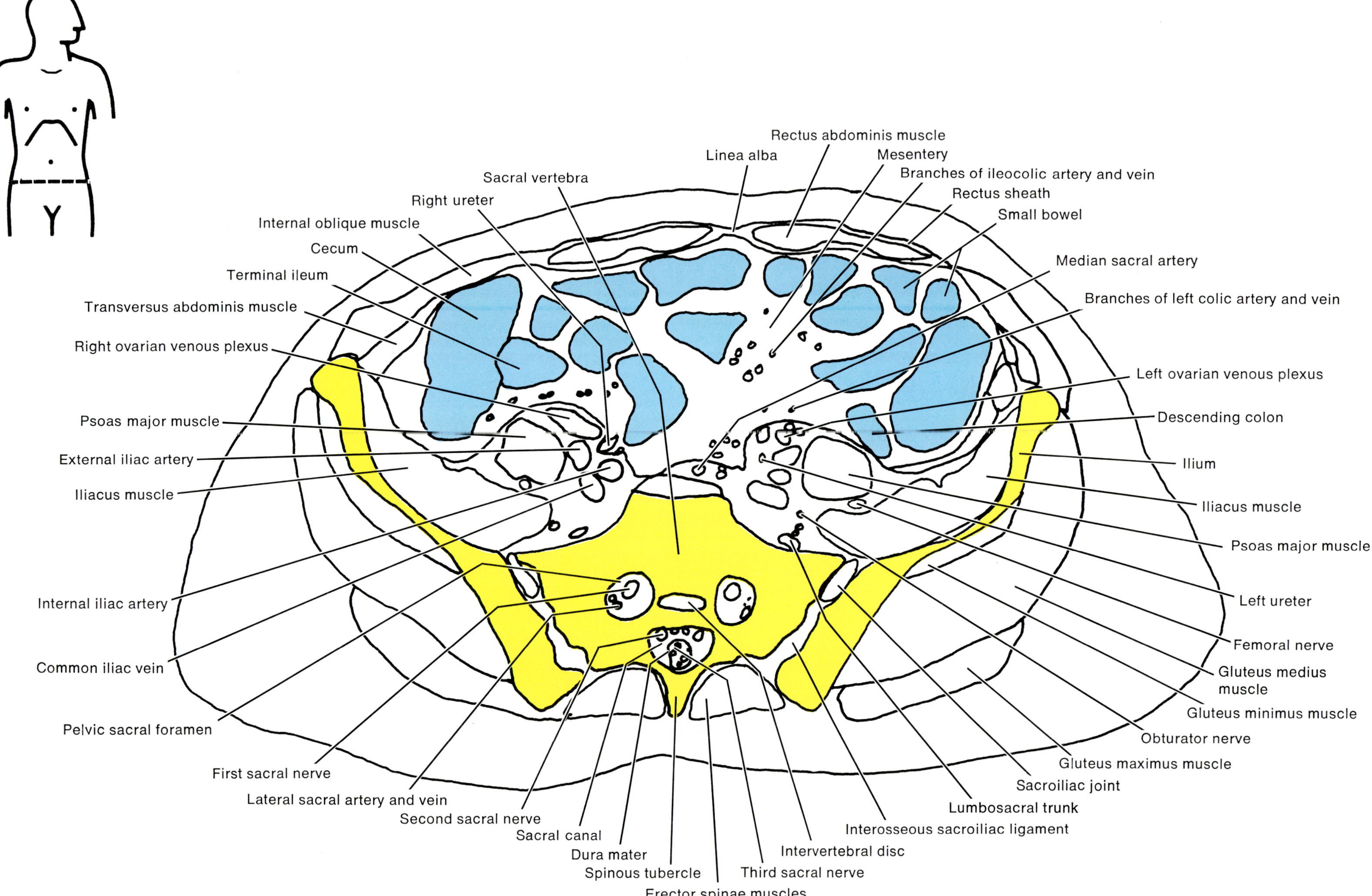
Rectus abdominis muscle
Linea alba
Mesentery
Branches of ileocolic artery and vein
Rectus sheath
Small bowel
Sacral vertebra
Right ureter
Internal oblique muscle
Cecum
Terminal ileum
Transversus abdominis muscle
Right ovarian venous plexus
Median sacral artery
Branches of left colic artery and vein
Psoas major muscle
External iliac artery
Iliacus muscle
Left ovarian venous plexus
Descending colon
Ilium
Iliacus muscle
Psoas major muscle
Internal iliac artery
Common iliac vein
Pelvic sacral foramen
Left ureter
Femoral nerve
Gluteus medius muscle
Gluteus minimus muscle
Obturator nerve
Gluteus maximus muscle
Sacroiliac joint
Lumbosacral trunk
Interosseous sacroiliac ligament
First sacral nerve
Lateral sacral artery and vein
Second sacral nerve
Sacral canal
Dura mater
Spinous tubercle
Erector spinae muscles
Third sacral nerve
Intervertebral disc

TRANSVERSE **Pelvis—female**

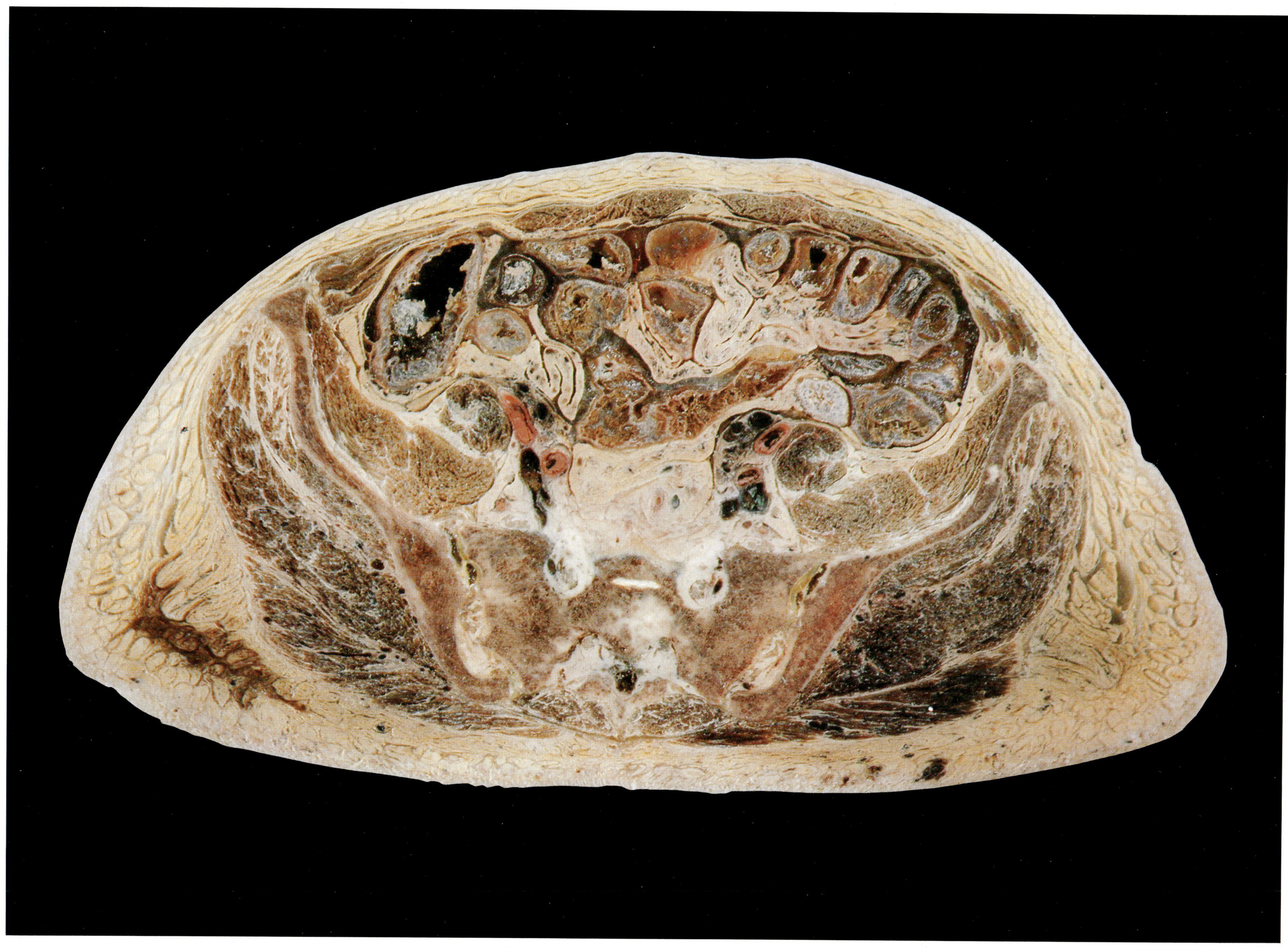

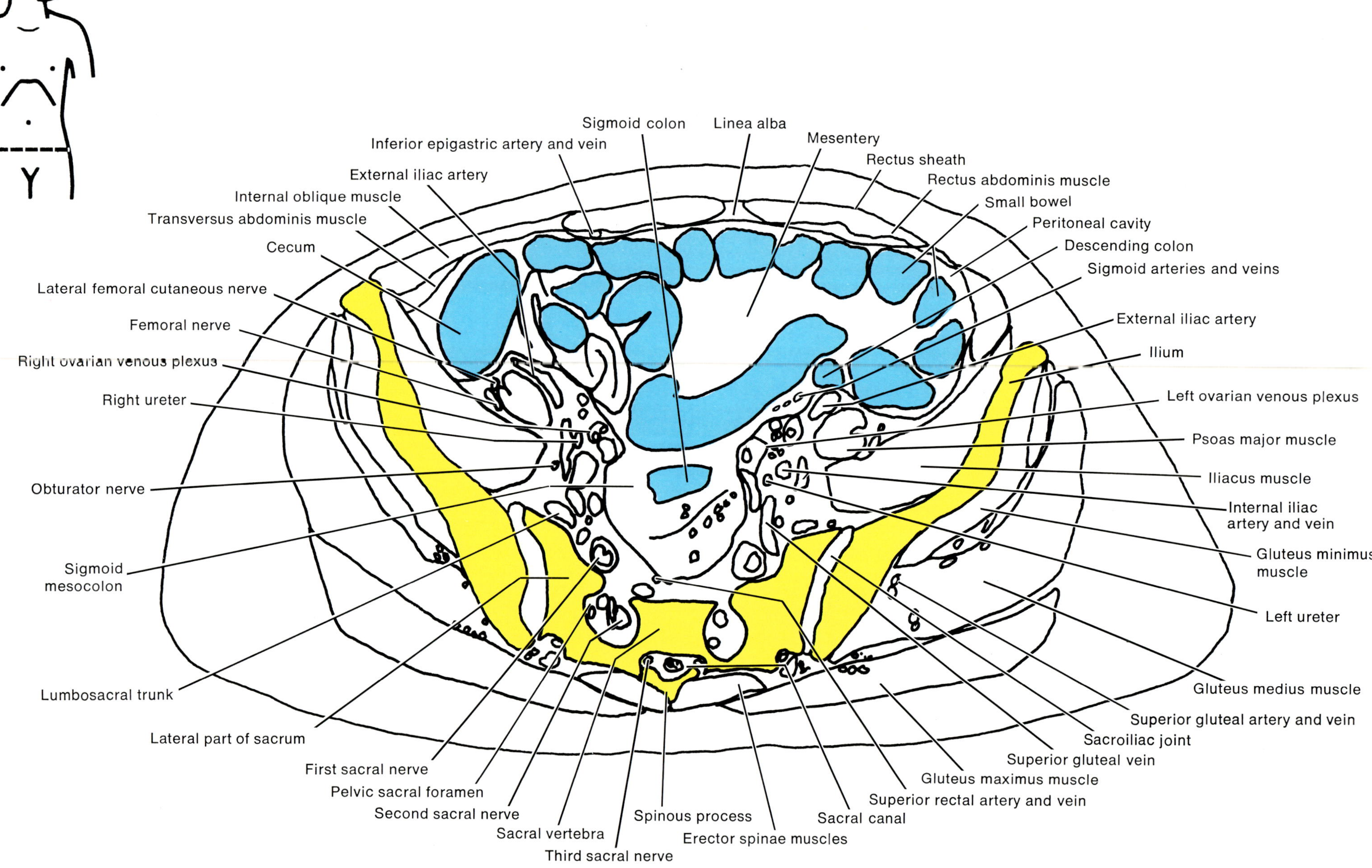

Sigmoid colon
Linea alba
Mesentery
Inferior epigastric artery and vein
Rectus sheath
External iliac artery
Rectus abdominis muscle
Internal oblique muscle
Small bowel
Transversus abdominis muscle
Peritoneal cavity
Cecum
Descending colon
Sigmoid arteries and veins
Lateral femoral cutaneous nerve
External iliac artery
Femoral nerve
Ilium
Right ovarian venous plexus
Left ovarian venous plexus
Right ureter
Psoas major muscle
Iliacus muscle
Obturator nerve
Internal iliac artery and vein
Sigmoid mesocolon
Gluteus minimus muscle
Left ureter
Lumbosacral trunk
Gluteus medius muscle
Lateral part of sacrum
Superior gluteal artery and vein
Sacroiliac joint
First sacral nerve
Superior gluteal vein
Pelvic sacral foramen
Gluteus maximus muscle
Second sacral nerve
Superior rectal artery and vein
Sacral vertebra
Sacral canal
Spinous process
Third sacral nerve
Erector spinae muscles

TRANSVERSE **Pelvis—female**

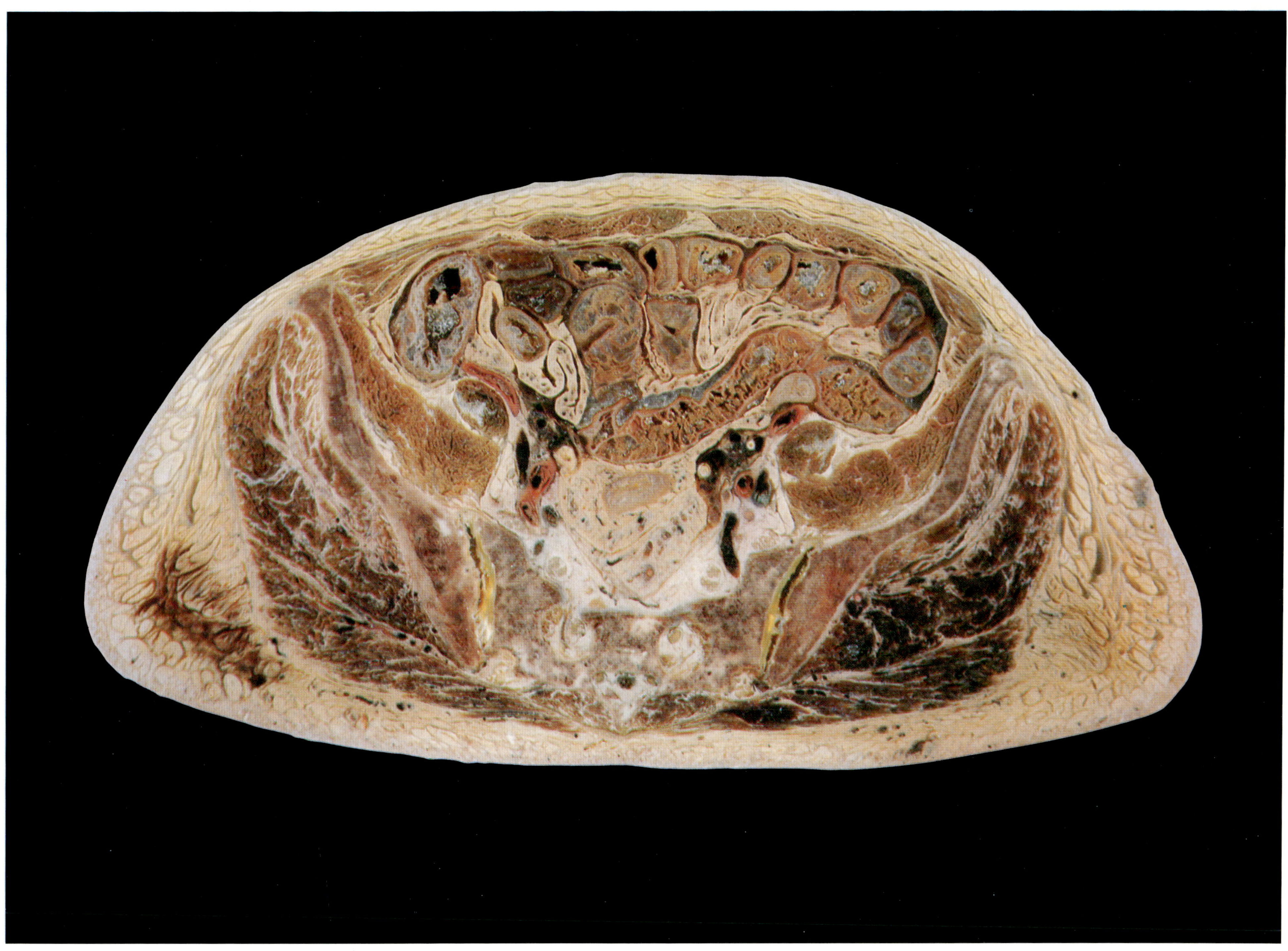

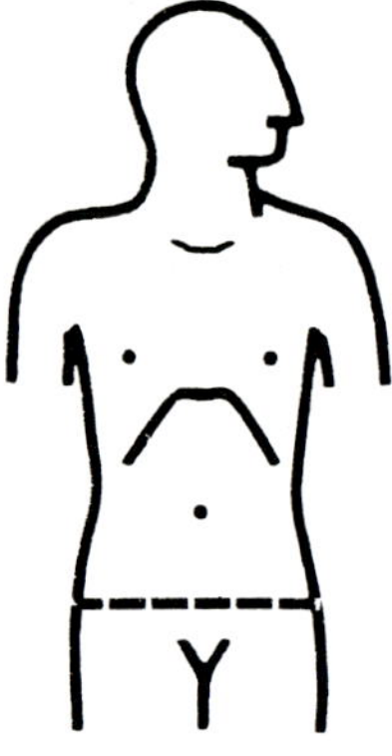

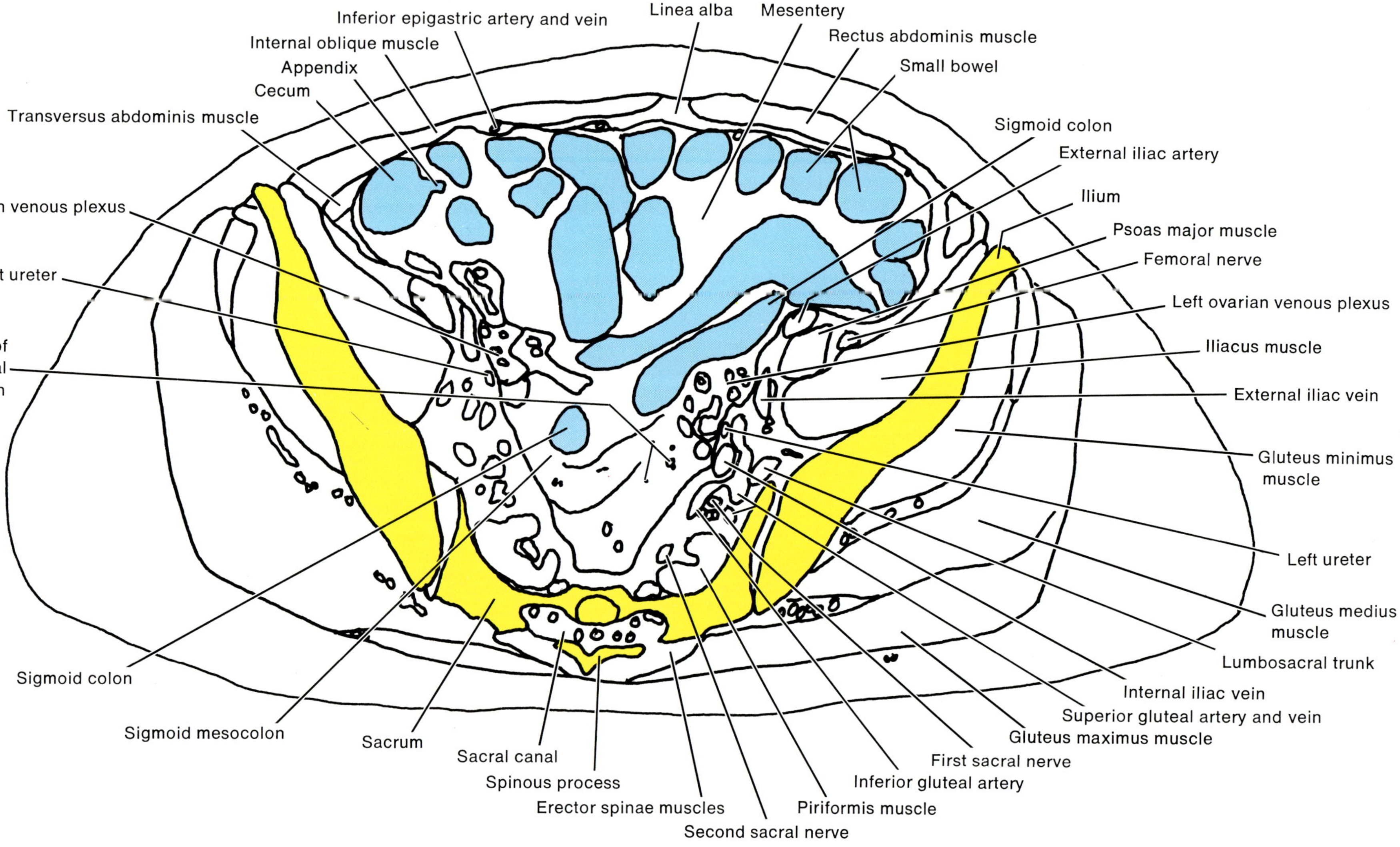

Inferior epigastric artery and vein
Internal oblique muscle
Appendix
Cecum
Transversus abdominis muscle
Linea alba
Mesentery
Rectus abdominis muscle
Small bowel
Right ovarian venous plexus
Sigmoid colon
External iliac artery
Ilium
Psoas major muscle
Femoral nerve
Right ureter
Left ovarian venous plexus
Iliacus muscle
Branches of superior rectal artery and vein
External iliac vein
Gluteus minimus muscle
Left ureter
Gluteus medius muscle
Sigmoid colon
Lumbosacral trunk
Internal iliac vein
Superior gluteal artery and vein
Gluteus maximus muscle
Sigmoid mesocolon
Sacrum
Sacral canal
First sacral nerve
Inferior gluteal artery
Spinous process
Piriformis muscle
Erector spinae muscles
Second sacral nerve

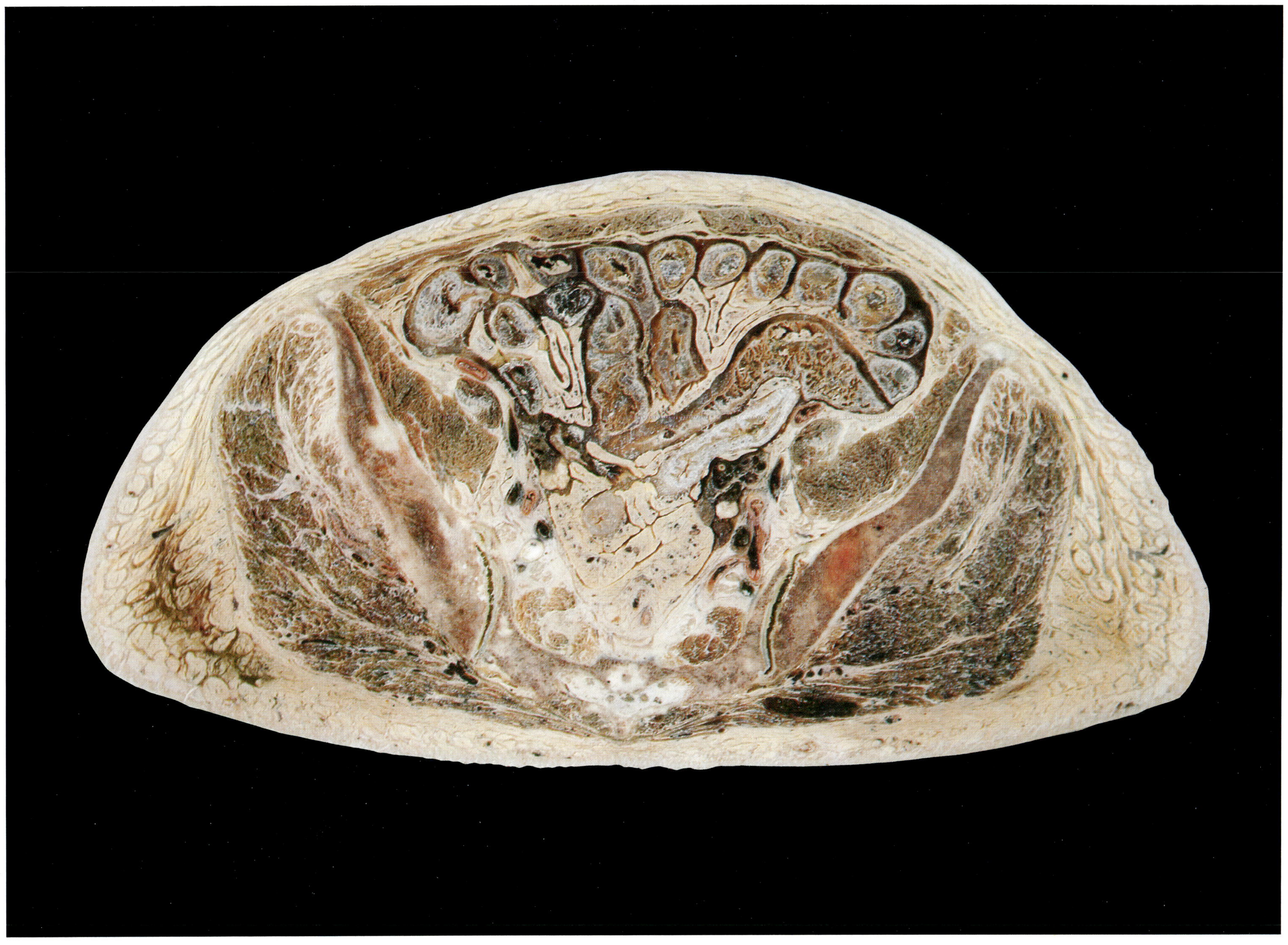

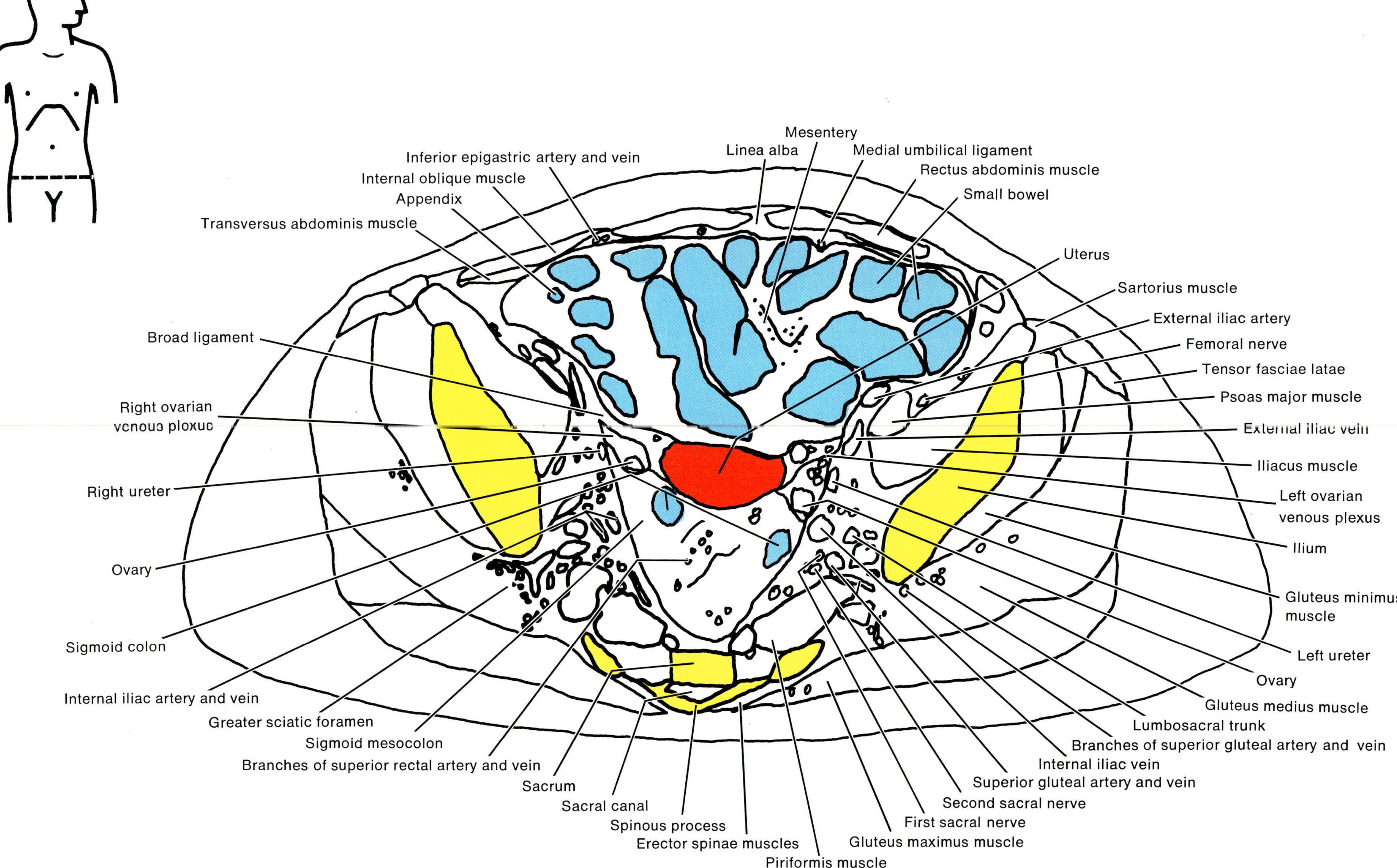

Mesentery
Linea alba
Inferior epigastric artery and vein
Medial umbilical ligament
Internal oblique muscle
Rectus abdominis muscle
Appendix
Small bowel
Transversus abdominis muscle
Uterus
Sartorius muscle
External iliac artery
Broad ligament
Femoral nerve
Tensor fasciae latae
Psoas major muscle
Right ovarian venous plexus
External iliac vein
Iliacus muscle
Right ureter
Left ovarian venous plexus
Ilium
Ovary
Gluteus minimus muscle
Sigmoid colon
Left ureter
Internal iliac artery and vein
Ovary
Greater sciatic foramen
Gluteus medius muscle
Sigmoid mesocolon
Lumbosacral trunk
Branches of superior rectal artery and vein
Branches of superior gluteal artery and vein
Sacrum
Internal iliac vein
Sacral canal
Superior gluteal artery and vein
Spinous process
Second sacral nerve
Erector spinae muscles
First sacral nerve
Piriformis muscle
Gluteus maximus muscle

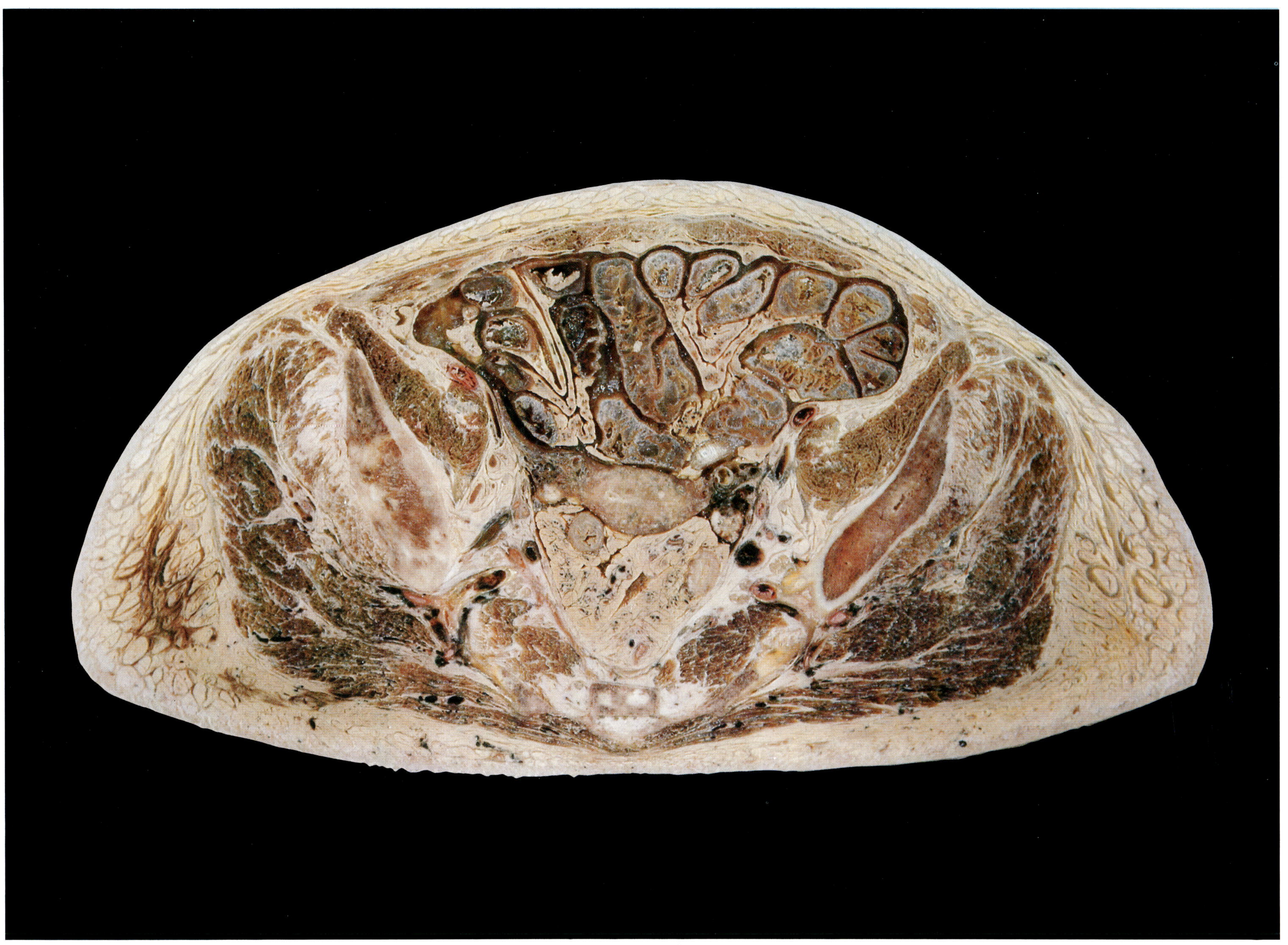

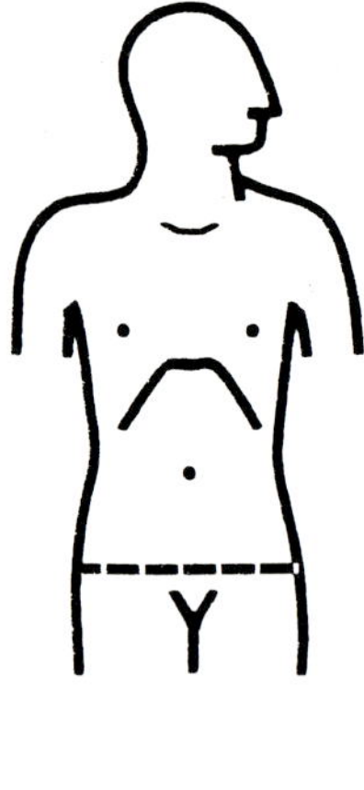

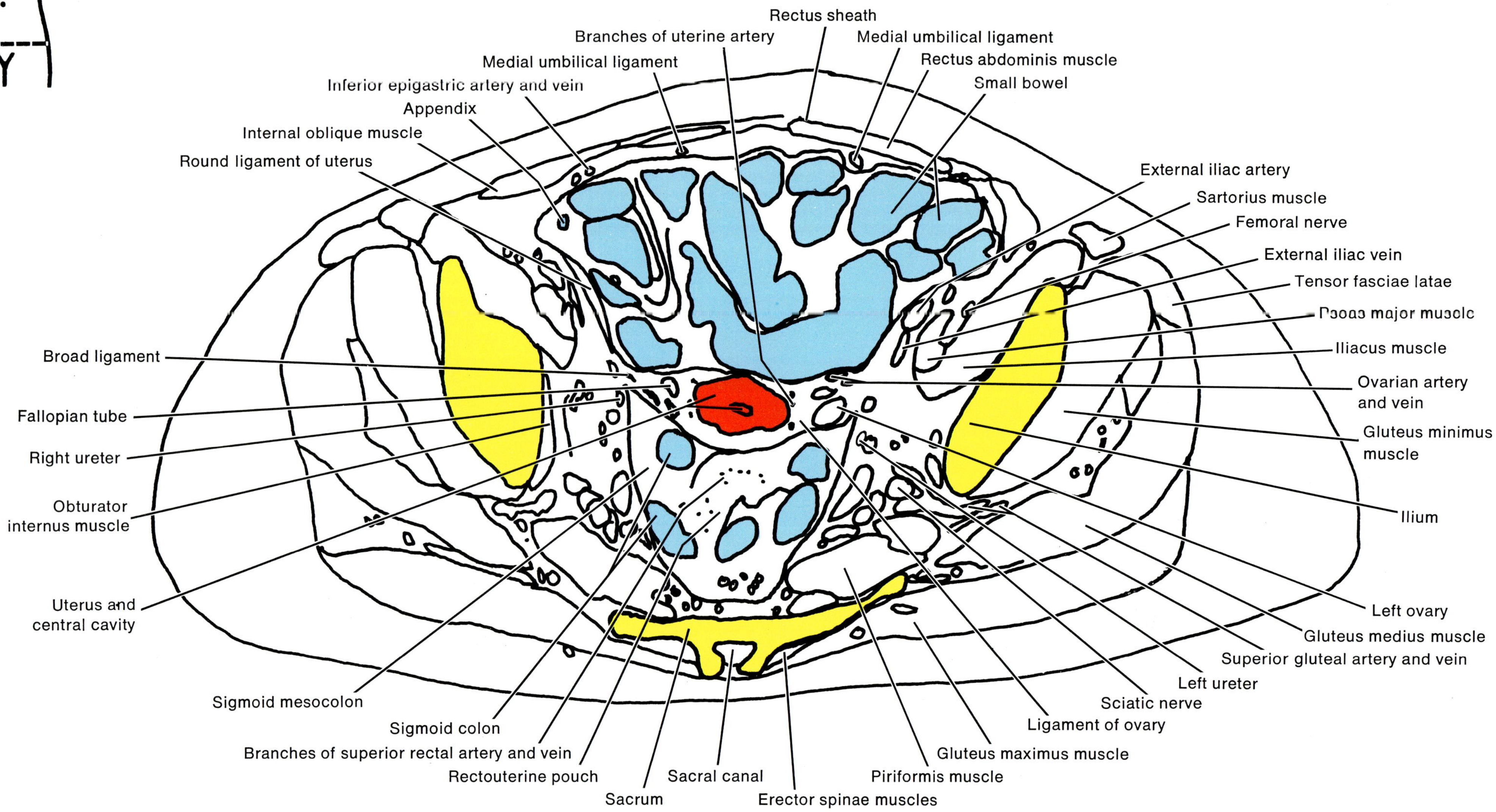

Rectus sheath
Branches of uterine artery
Medial umbilical ligament
Rectus abdominis muscle
Medial umbilical ligament
Small bowel
Inferior epigastric artery and vein
Appendix
Internal oblique muscle
Round ligament of uterus
External iliac artery
Sartorius muscle
Femoral nerve
External iliac vein
Tensor fasciae latae
Psoas major muscle
Broad ligament
Iliacus muscle
Ovarian artery and vein
Fallopian tube
Gluteus minimus muscle
Right ureter
Obturator internus muscle
Ilium
Uterus and central cavity
Left ovary
Gluteus medius muscle
Superior gluteal artery and vein
Left ureter
Sciatic nerve
Sigmoid mesocolon
Ligament of ovary
Sigmoid colon
Gluteus maximus muscle
Branches of superior rectal artery and vein
Rectouterine pouch
Sacral canal
Piriformis muscle
Sacrum
Erector spinae muscles

TRANSVERSE **Pelvis—female**

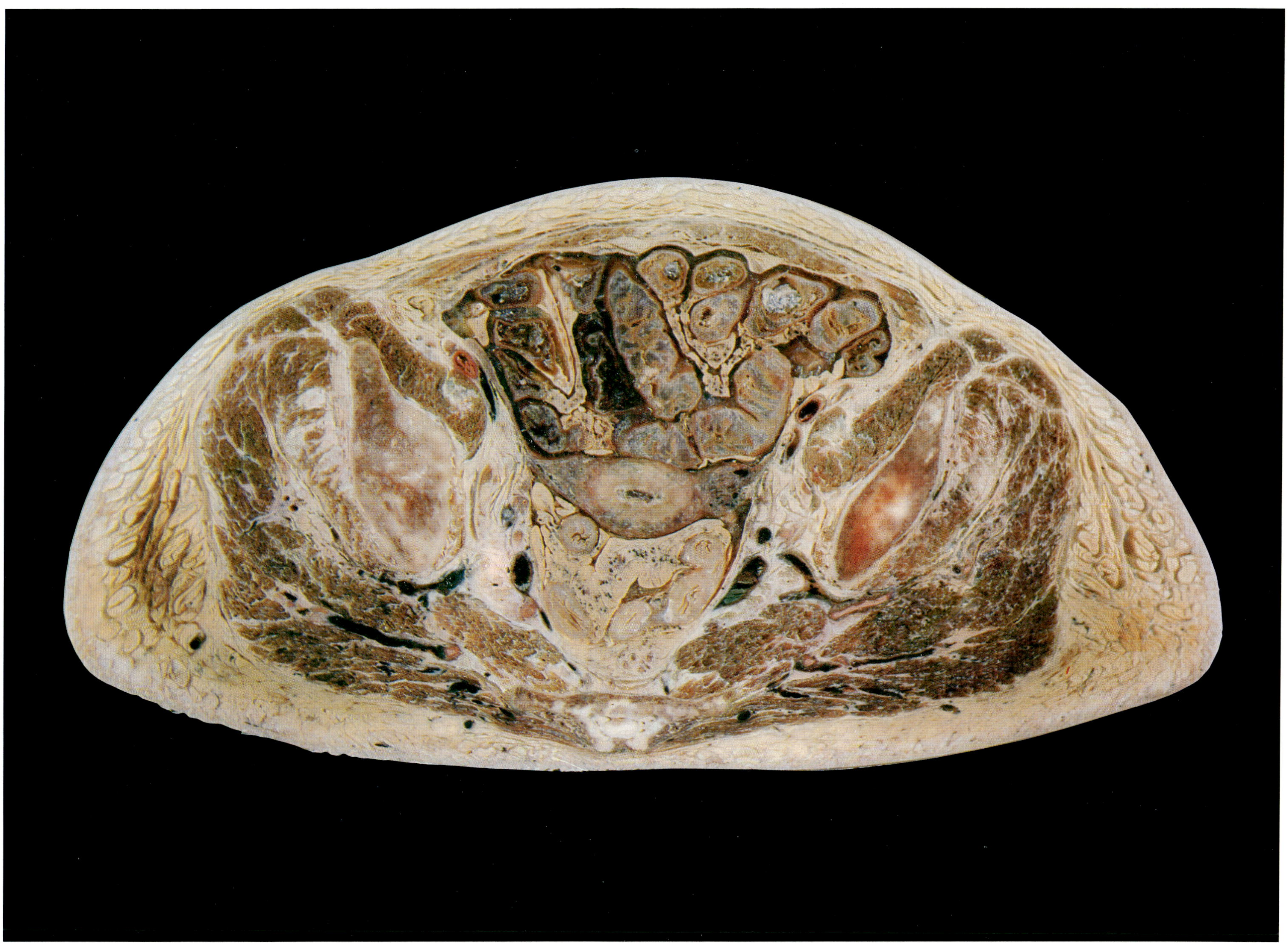

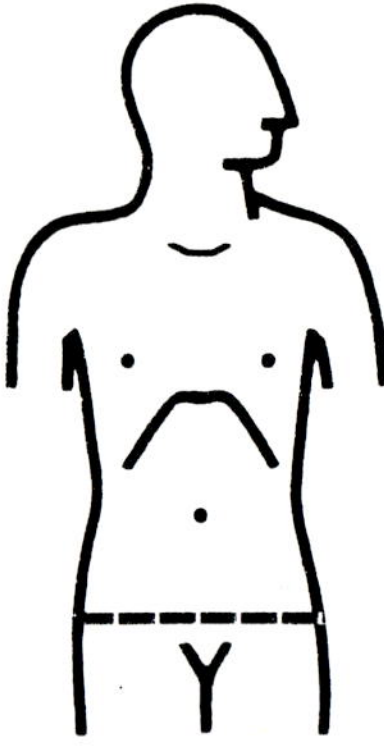

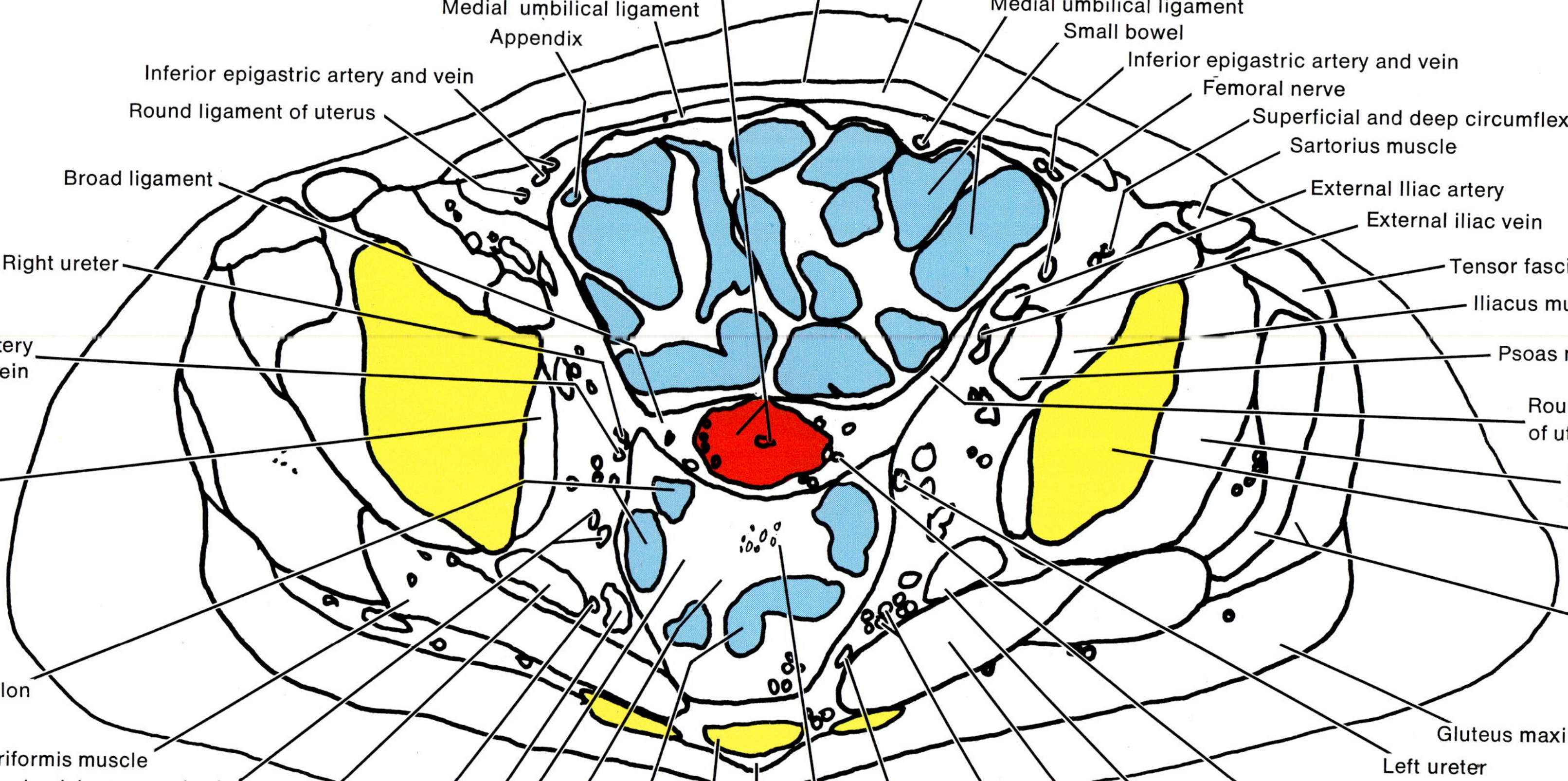

Uterus and central cavity
Rectus sheath
Rectus abdominis muscle
Medial umbilical ligament
Medial umbilical ligament
Appendix
Small bowel
Inferior epigastric artery and vein
Inferior epigastric artery and vein
Femoral nerve
Round ligament of uterus
Superficial and deep circumflex iliac arteries
Sartorius muscle
Broad ligament
External Iliac artery
External iliac vein
Right ureter
Tensor fasciae latae
Iliacus muscle
Uterine artery and vein
Psoas major muscle
Round ligament of uterus
Obturator internus muscle
Gluteus minimus muscle
Ilium
Sigmoid colon
Gluteus medius muscle
Piriformis muscle
Internal pudendal artery and vein
Sciatic nerve
Inferior gluteal artery
Inferior gluteal vein
Sigmoid mesocolon
Rectouterine pouch
Rectum
Sacrum
Sacral canal
Pudendal nerve
Piriformis muscle
Inferior gluteal artery and vein
Branches of superior rectal artery and vein
Sciatic nerve
Branches of uterine artery
Left ureter
Gluteus maximus muscle

TRANSVERSE **Pelvis—female**

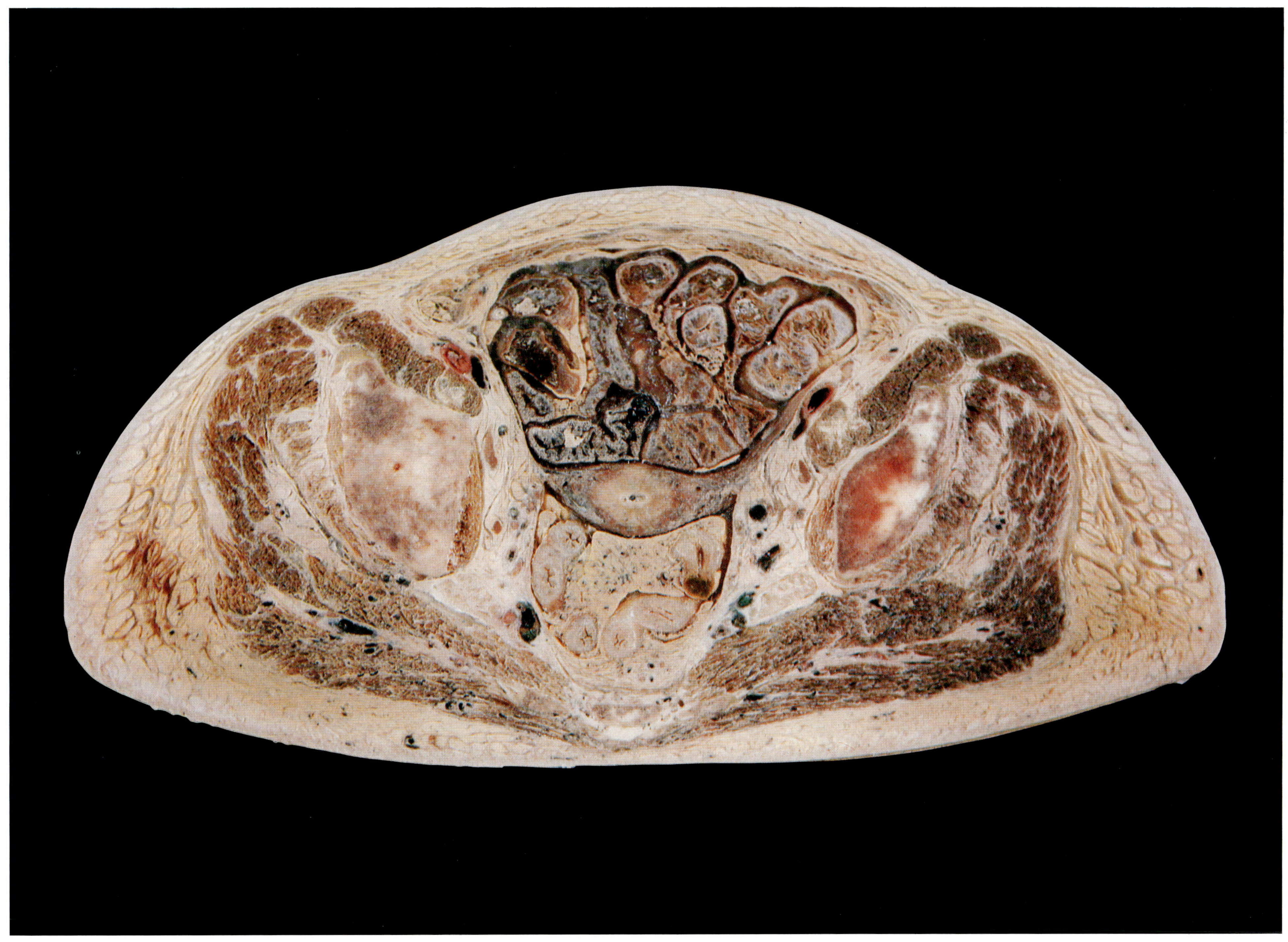

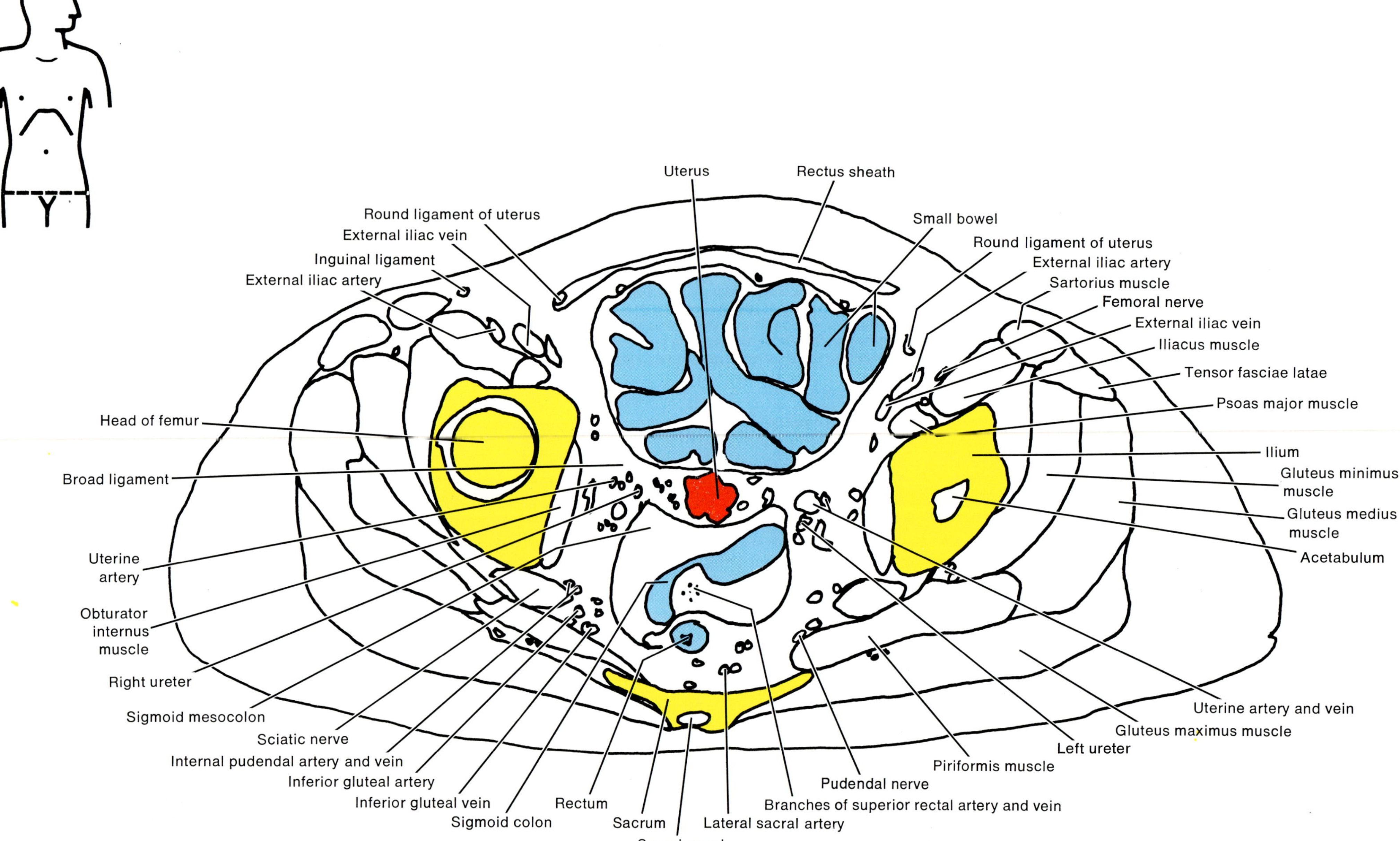
Uterus
Rectus sheath
Round ligament of uterus
External iliac vein
Inguinal ligament
External iliac artery
Small bowel
Round ligament of uterus
External iliac artery
Sartorius muscle
Femoral nerve
External iliac vein
Iliacus muscle
Tensor fasciae latae
Psoas major muscle
Head of femur
Ilium
Gluteus minimus muscle
Broad ligament
Gluteus medius muscle
Acetabulum
Uterine artery
Obturator internus muscle
Right ureter
Sigmoid mesocolon
Sciatic nerve
Internal pudendal artery and vein
Inferior gluteal artery
Inferior gluteal vein
Sigmoid colon
Rectum
Sacrum
Sacral canal
Lateral sacral artery
Branches of superior rectal artery and vein
Pudendal nerve
Piriformis muscle
Left ureter
Gluteus maximus muscle
Uterine artery and vein

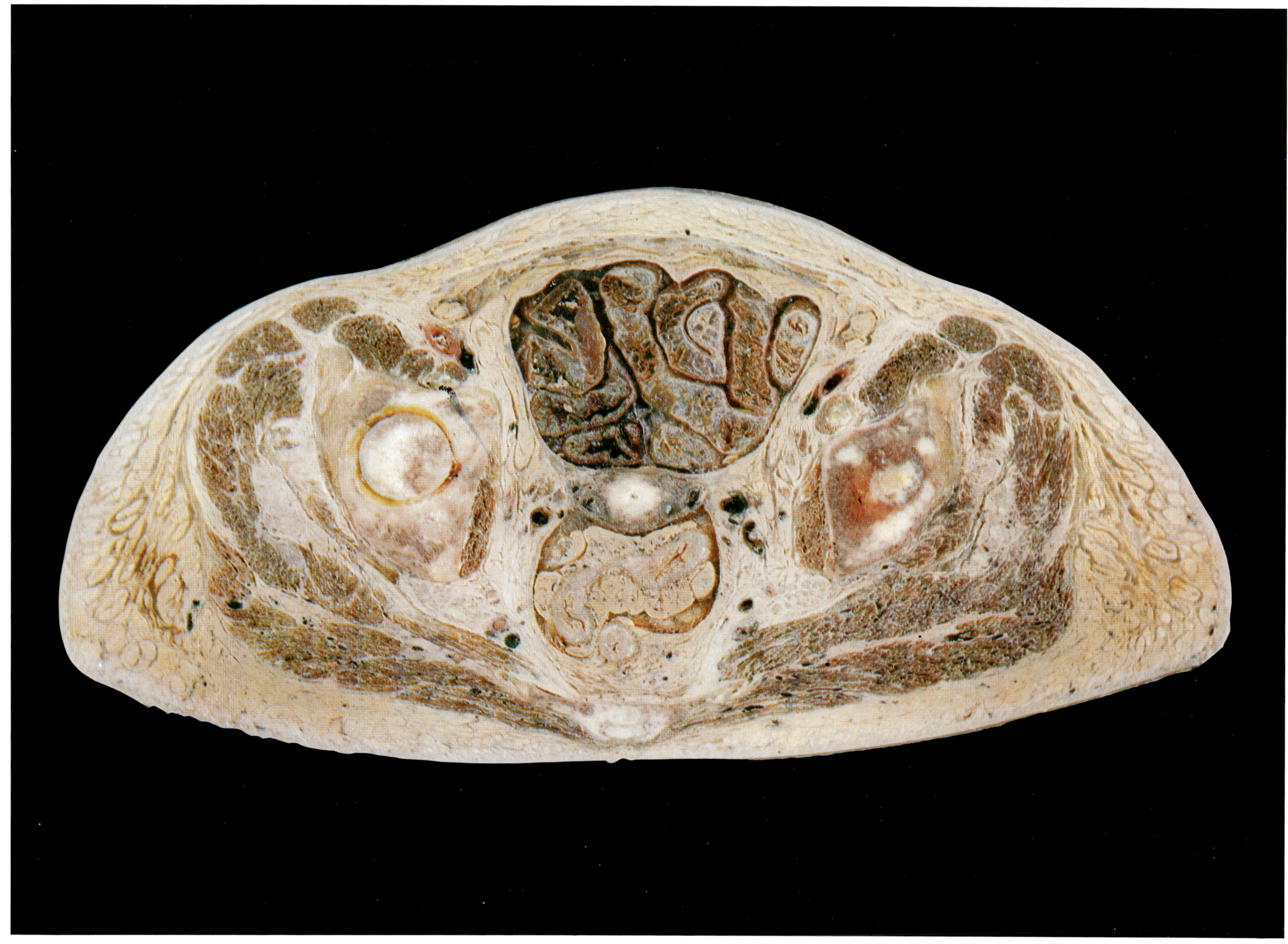

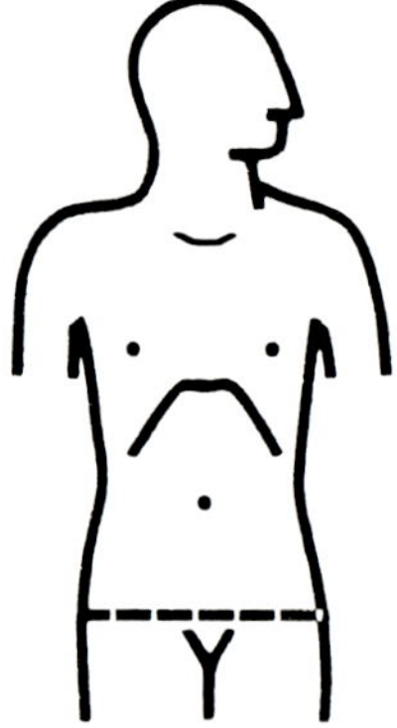

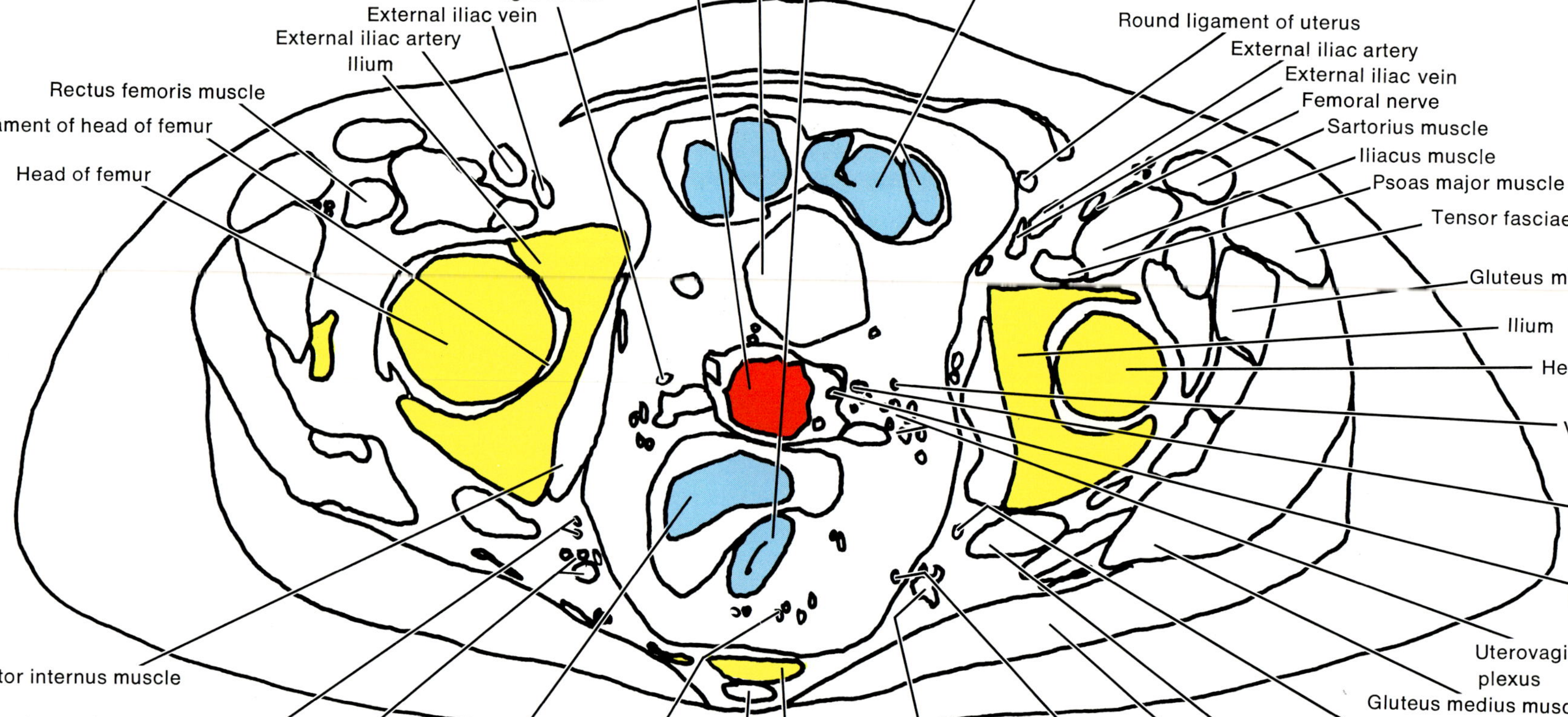

Urinary bladder
Cervix
Rectum
Right ureter
Small bowel
External iliac vein
External iliac artery
Ilium
Round ligament of uterus
External iliac artery
External iliac vein
Femoral nerve
Rectus femoris muscle
Sartorius muscle
Ligament of head of femur
Iliacus muscle
Head of femur
Psoas major muscle
Tensor fasciae latae
Gluteus minimus muscle
Ilium
Head of femur
Vaginal artery
Left ureter
Uterine artery
Uterovaginal venous plexus
Obturator internus muscle
Gluteus medius muscle
Internal pudendal artery and vein
Internal pudendal artery
Inferior gluteal artery and vein
Sciatic nerve
Lateral sacral artery
Sacrum
Pudendal nerve
Sigmoid colon
Sacral canal
Inferior gluteal artery and vein
Gluteus maximus muscle

TRANSVERSE **Pelvis—female**

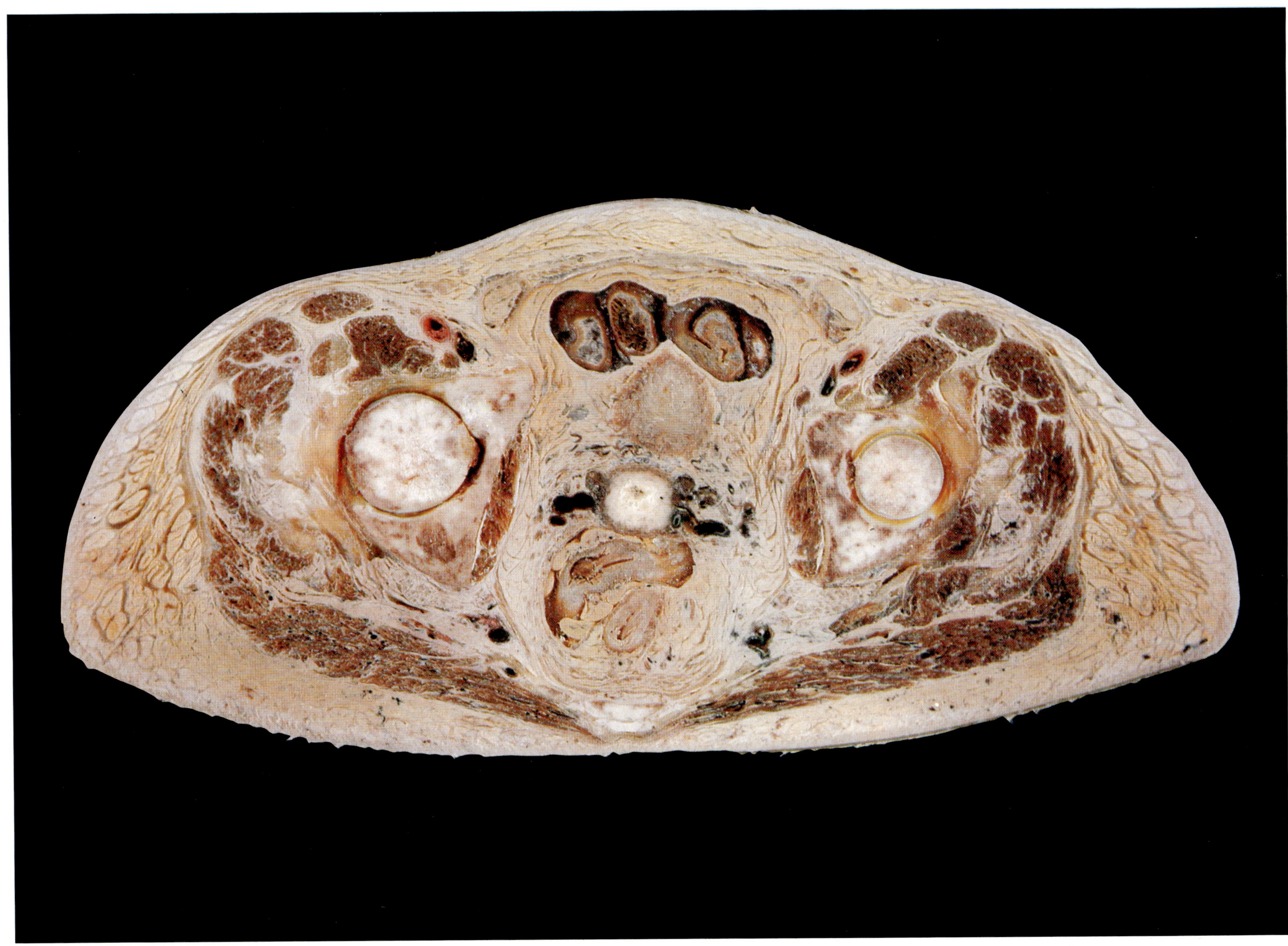

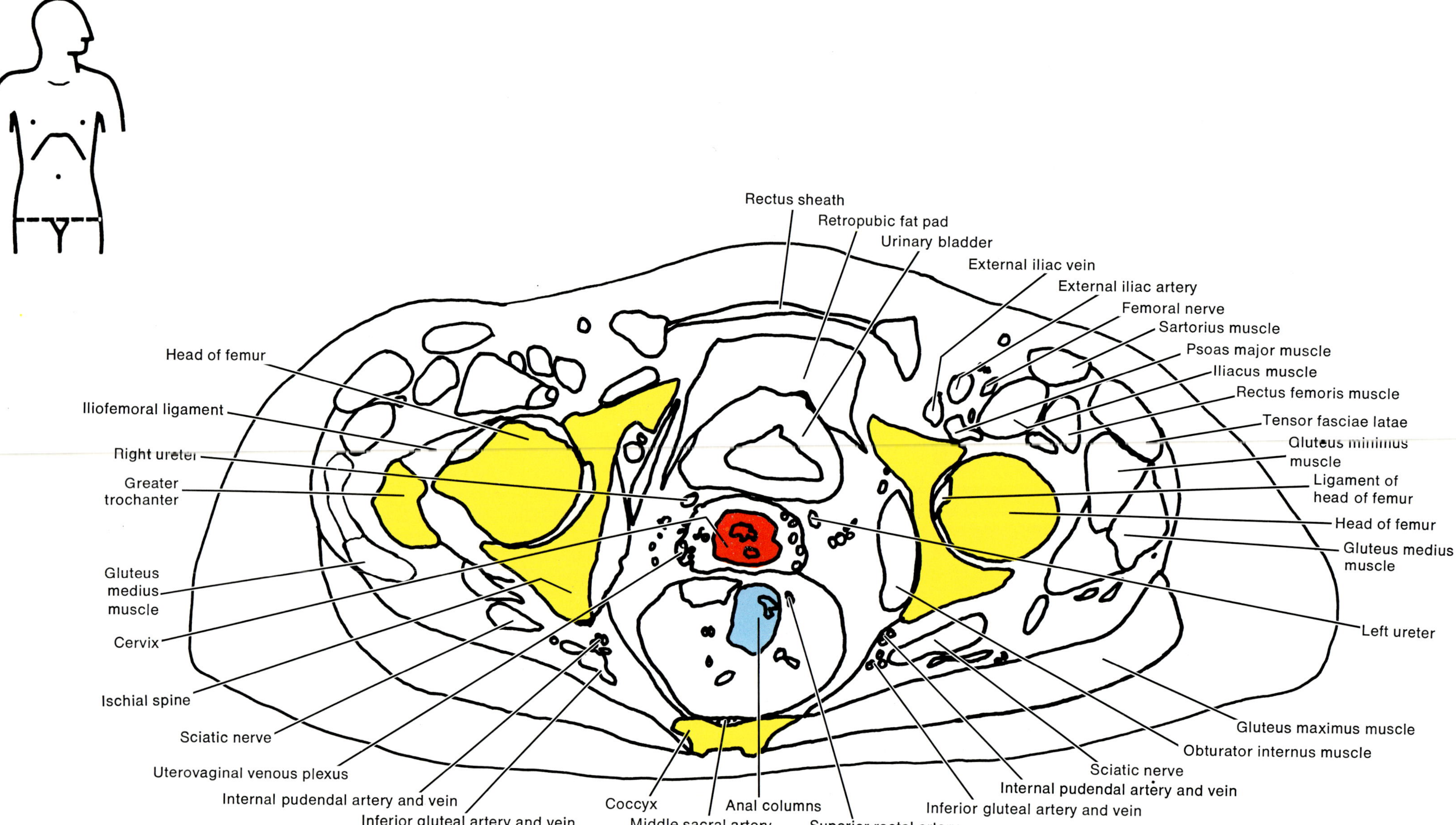

Rectus sheath
Retropubic fat pad
Urinary bladder
External iliac vein
External iliac artery
Femoral nerve
Sartorius muscle
Psoas major muscle
Iliacus muscle
Rectus femoris muscle
Tensor fasciae latae
Gluteus minimus muscle
Ligament of head of femur
Head of femur
Gluteus medius muscle
Head of femur
Iliofemoral ligament
Right ureter
Greater trochanter
Gluteus medius muscle
Cervix
Ischial spine
Sciatic nerve
Uterovaginal venous plexus
Internal pudendal artery and vein
Inferior gluteal artery and vein
Coccyx
Middle sacral artery
Anal columns
Superior rectal artery
Inferior gluteal artery and vein
Internal pudendal artery and vein
Sciatic nerve
Left ureter
Gluteus maximus muscle
Obturator internus muscle

TRANSVERSE **Pelvis—female**

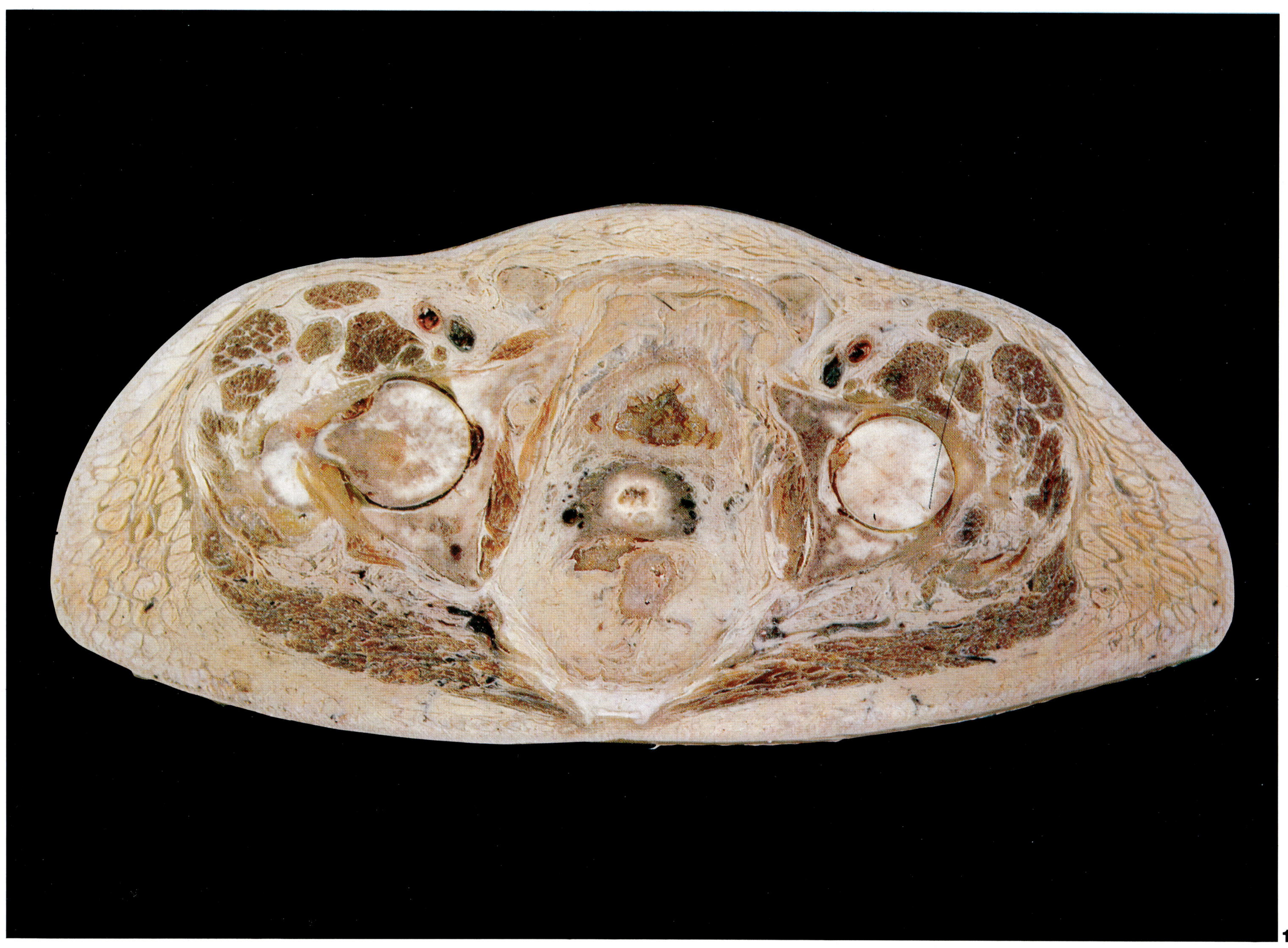

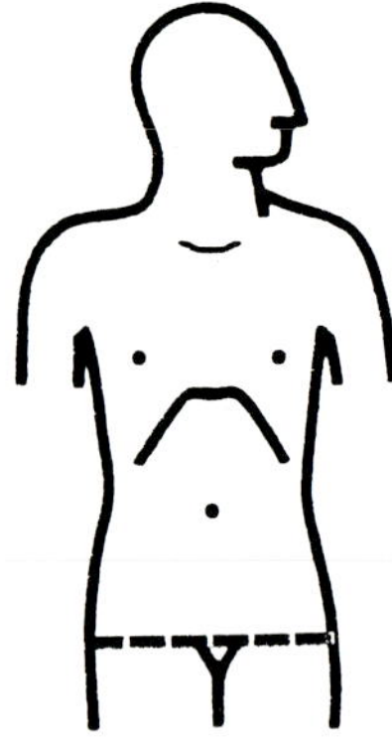

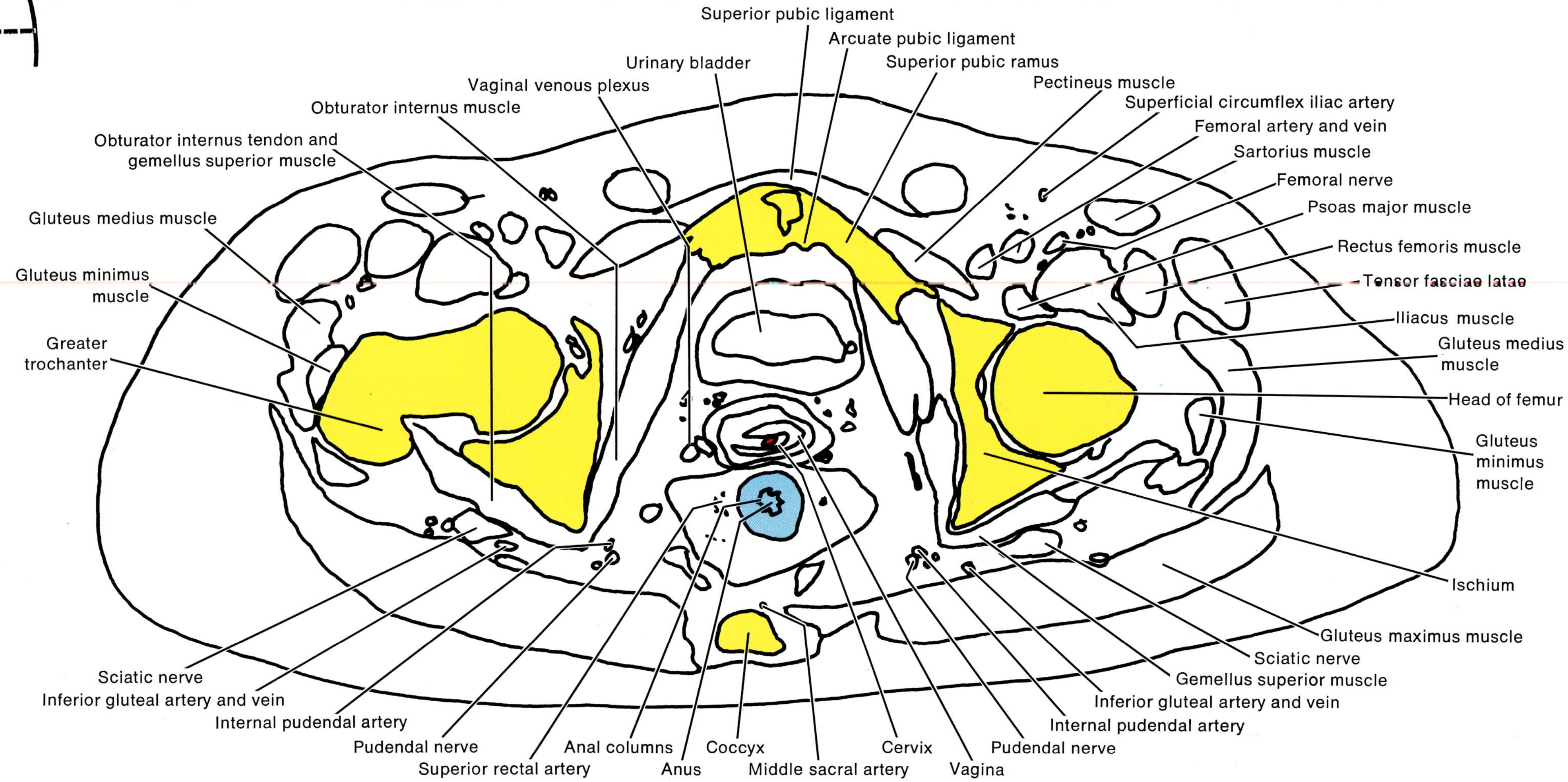

Superior pubic ligament
Arcuate pubic ligament
Superior pubic ramus
Urinary bladder
Vaginal venous plexus
Pectineus muscle
Superficial circumflex iliac artery
Obturator internus muscle
Femoral artery and vein
Obturator internus tendon and gemellus superior muscle
Sartorius muscle
Femoral nerve
Gluteus medius muscle
Psoas major muscle
Rectus femoris muscle
Gluteus minimus muscle
Tensor fasciae latae
Iliacus muscle
Gluteus medius muscle
Greater trochanter
Head of femur
Gluteus minimus muscle
Ischium
Gluteus maximus muscle
Sciatic nerve
Gemellus superior muscle
Sciatic nerve
Inferior gluteal artery and vein
Inferior gluteal artery and vein
Internal pudendal artery
Internal pudendal artery
Pudendal nerve
Pudendal nerve
Anal columns
Coccyx
Cervix
Vagina
Superior rectal artery
Anus
Middle sacral artery

TRANSVERSE **Pelvis—female**

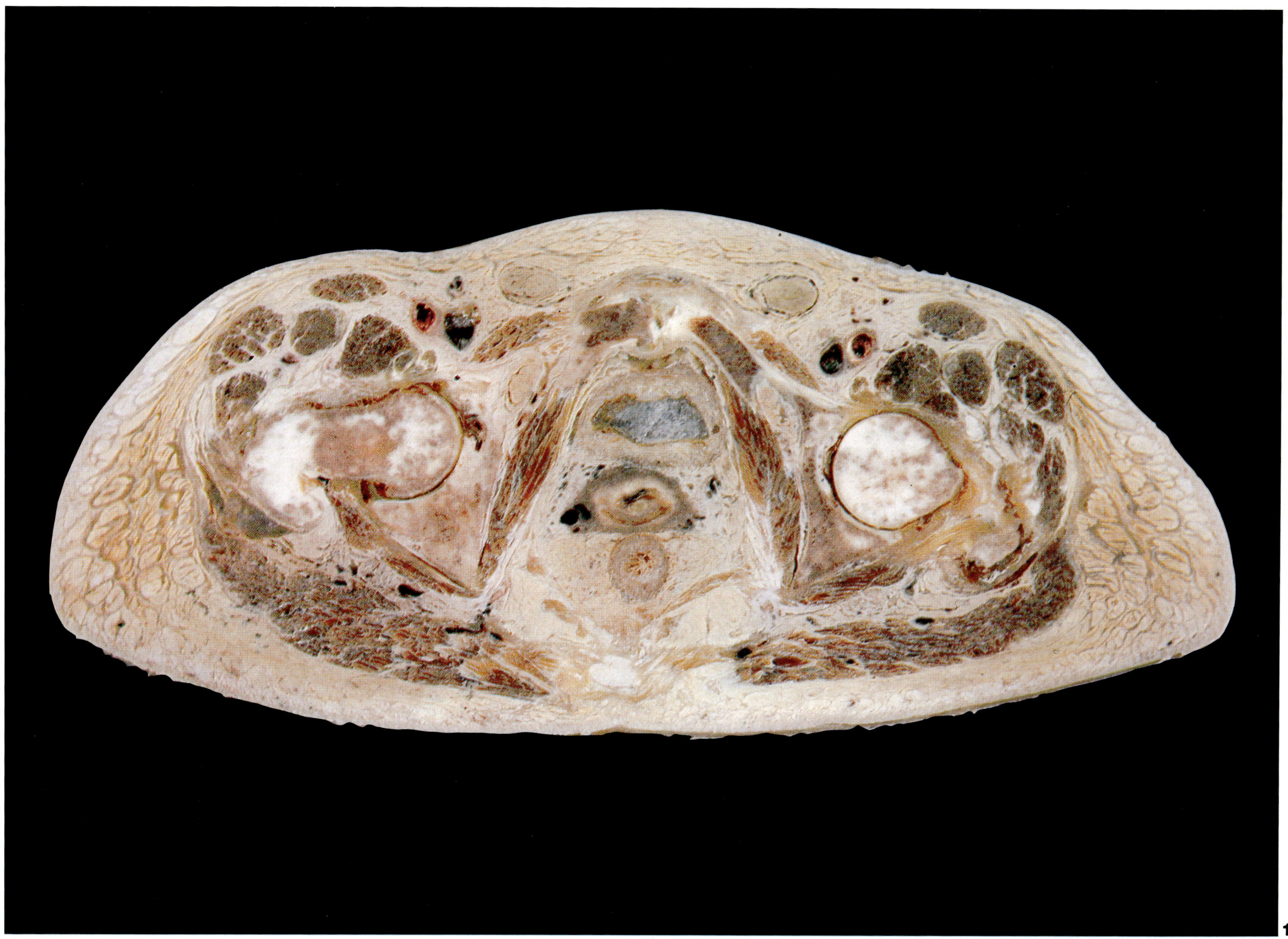

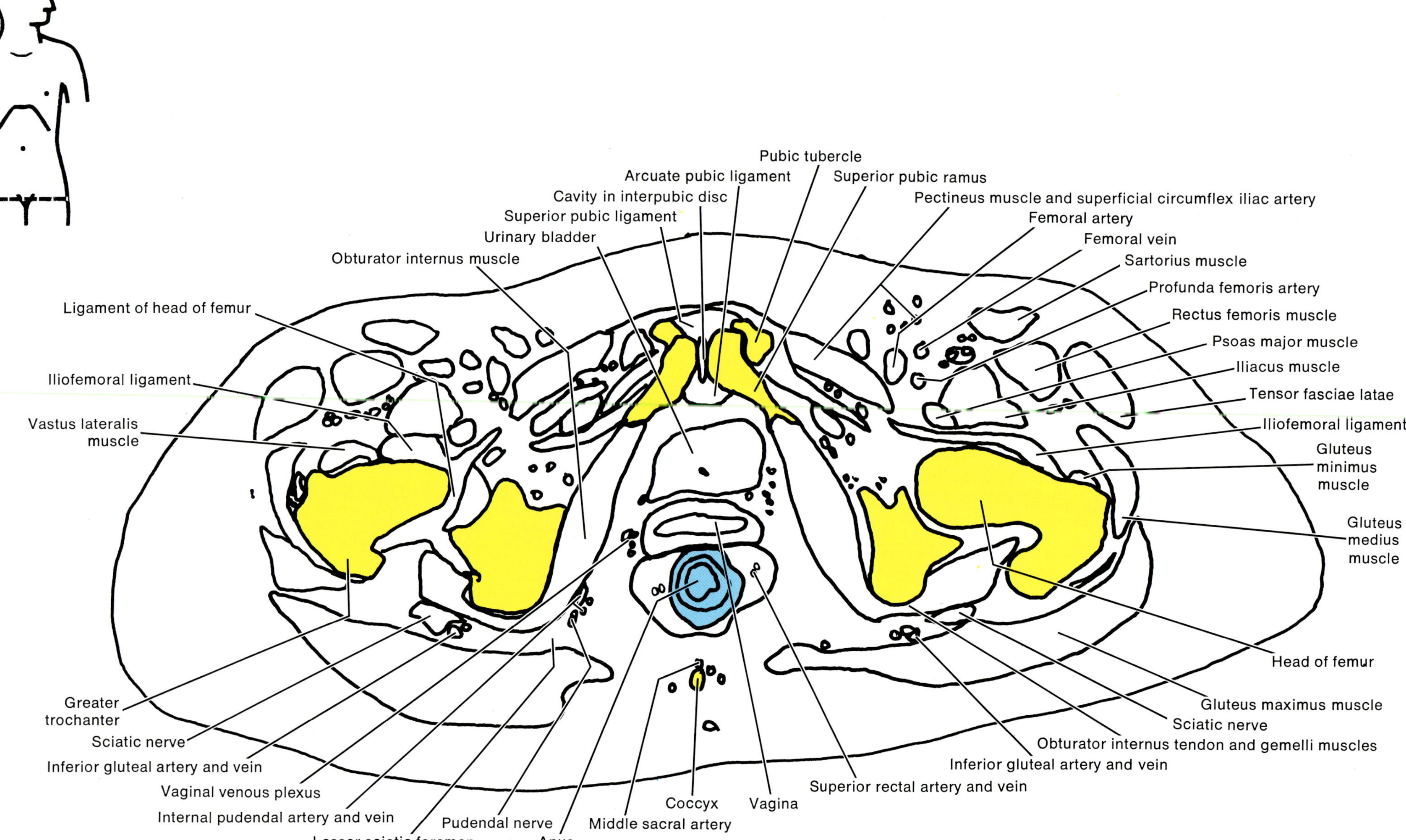

Pubic tubercle
Arcuate pubic ligament
Superior pubic ramus
Cavity in interpubic disc
Pectineus muscle and superficial circumflex iliac artery
Superior pubic ligament
Femoral artery
Urinary bladder
Femoral vein
Obturator internus muscle
Sartorius muscle
Profunda femoris artery
Ligament of head of femur
Rectus femoris muscle
Psoas major muscle
Iliofemoral ligament
Iliacus muscle
Tensor fasciae latae
Vastus lateralis muscle
Iliofemoral ligament
Gluteus minimus muscle
Gluteus medius muscle
Head of femur
Greater trochanter
Gluteus maximus muscle
Sciatic nerve
Sciatic nerve
Inferior gluteal artery and vein
Obturator internus tendon and gemelli muscles
Vaginal venous plexus
Inferior gluteal artery and vein
Internal pudendal artery and vein
Superior rectal artery and vein
Lesser sciatic foramen
Pudendal nerve
Coccyx
Vagina
Anus
Middle sacral artery

TRANSVERSE **Pelvis—female**

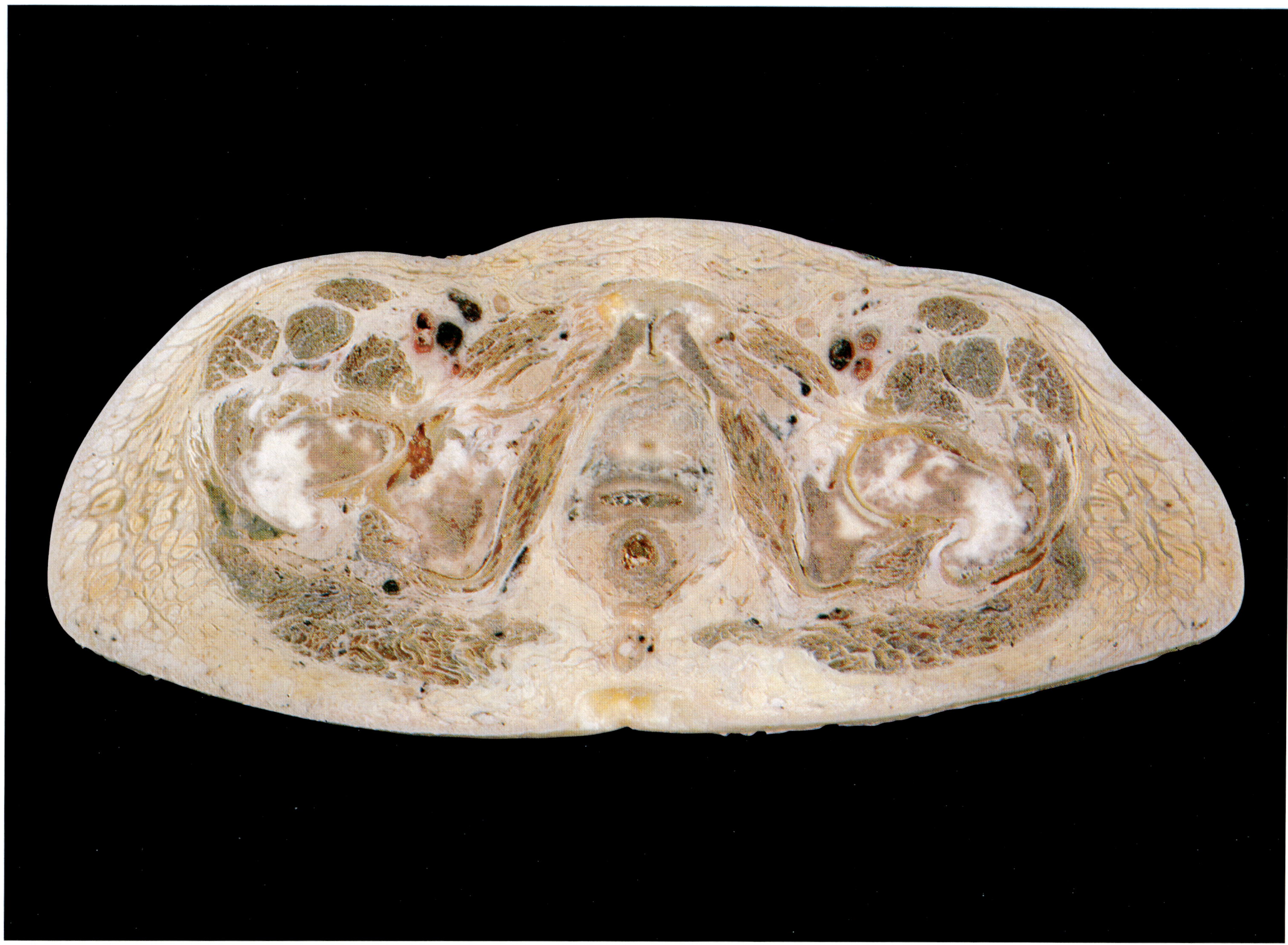

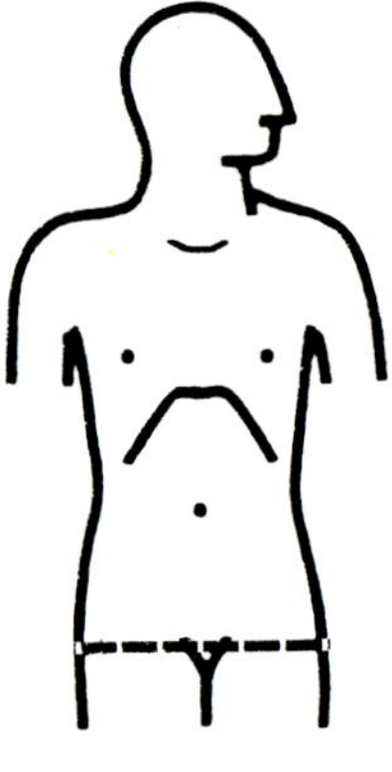

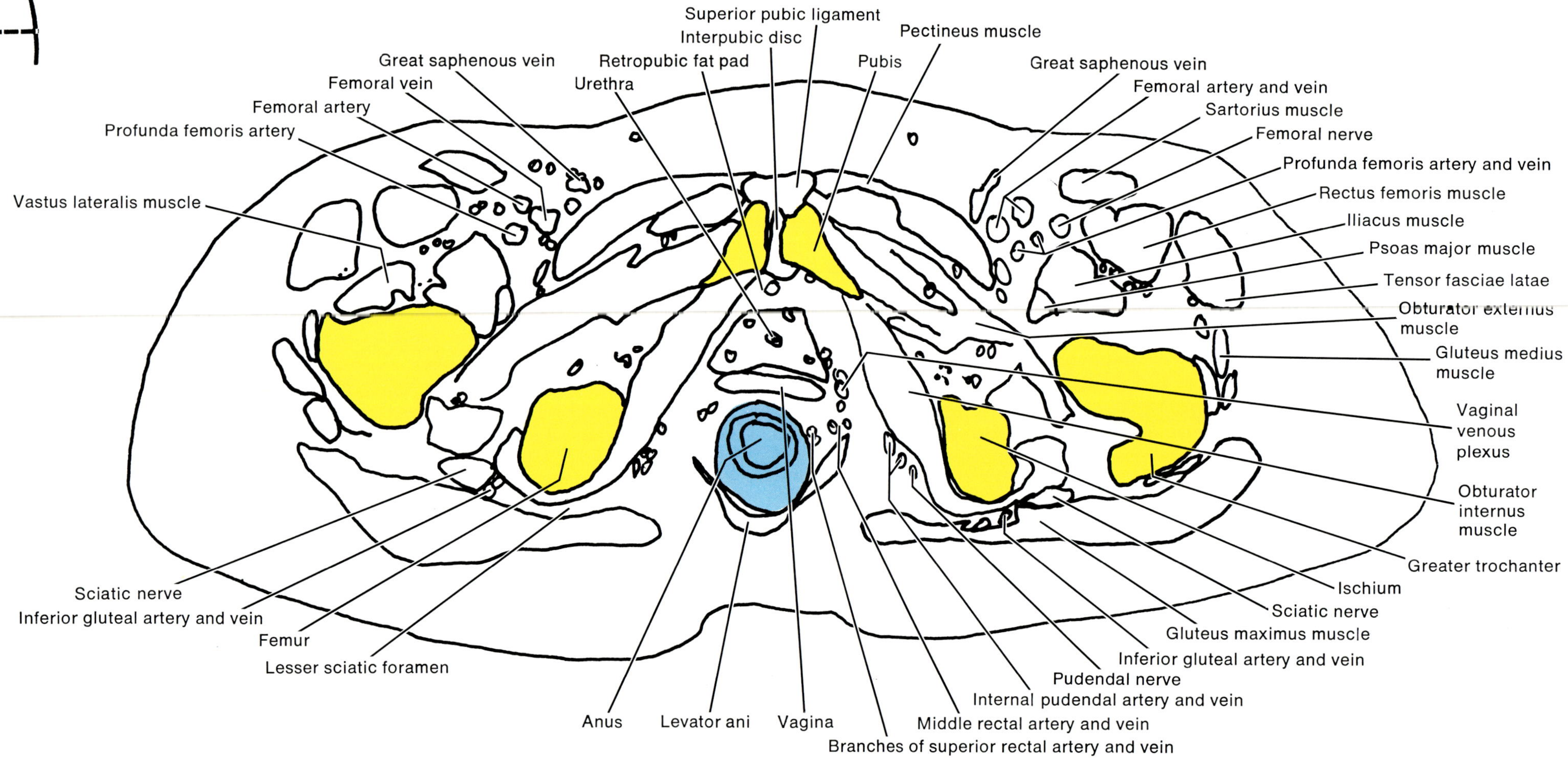

Superior pubic ligament
Interpubic disc
Retropubic fat pad
Urethra
Pectineus muscle
Pubis
Great saphenous vein
Great saphenous vein
Femoral vein
Femoral artery
Profunda femoris artery
Vastus lateralis muscle
Femoral artery and vein
Sartorius muscle
Femoral nerve
Profunda femoris artery and vein
Rectus femoris muscle
Iliacus muscle
Psoas major muscle
Tensor fasciae latae
Obturator externus muscle
Gluteus medius muscle
Vaginal venous plexus
Obturator internus muscle
Greater trochanter
Ischium
Sciatic nerve
Gluteus maximus muscle
Inferior gluteal artery and vein
Pudendal nerve
Internal pudendal artery and vein
Middle rectal artery and vein
Branches of superior rectal artery and vein
Anus
Levator ani
Vagina
Sciatic nerve
Inferior gluteal artery and vein
Femur
Lesser sciatic foramen

TRANSVERSE **Pelvis—female**

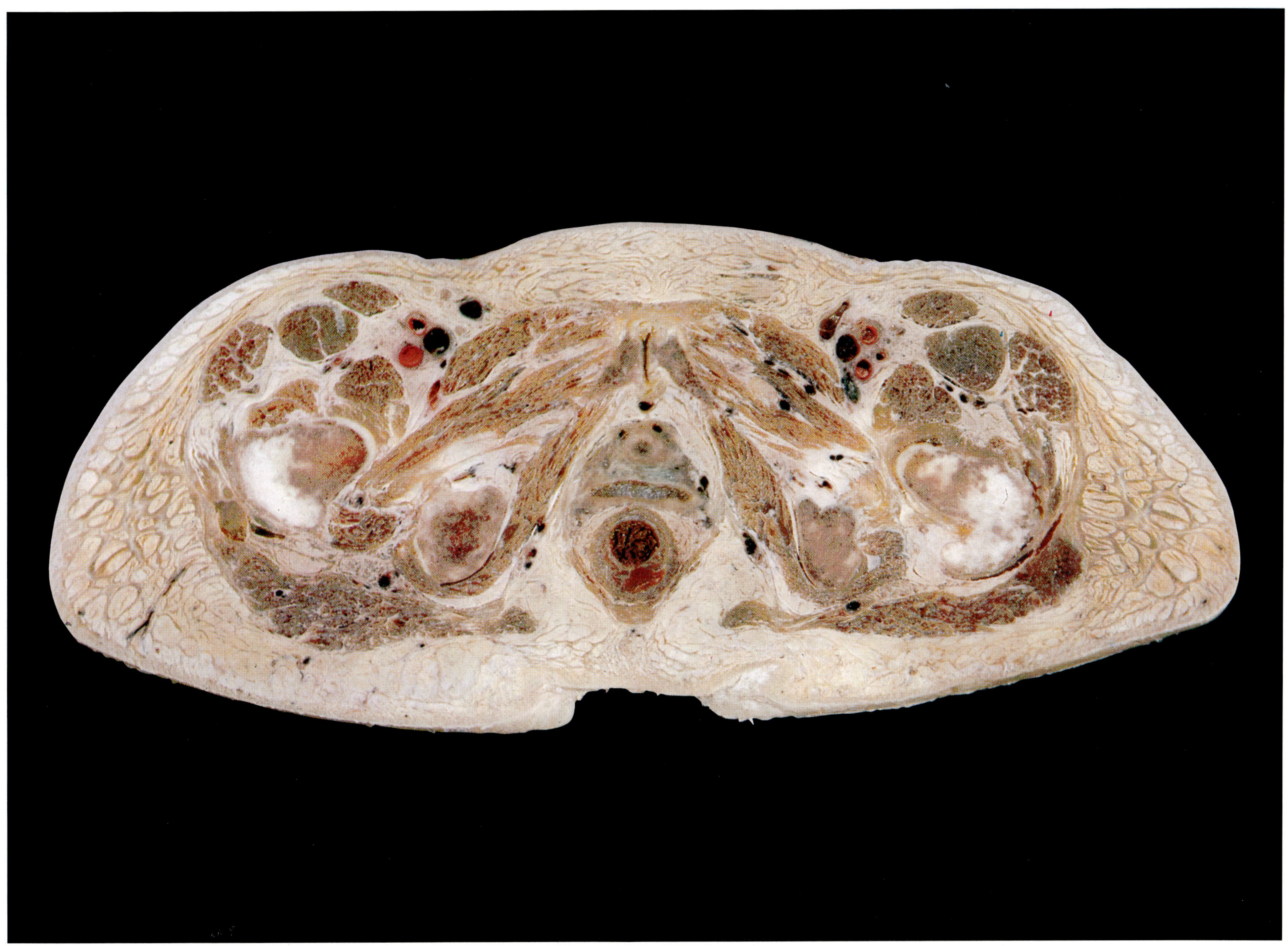

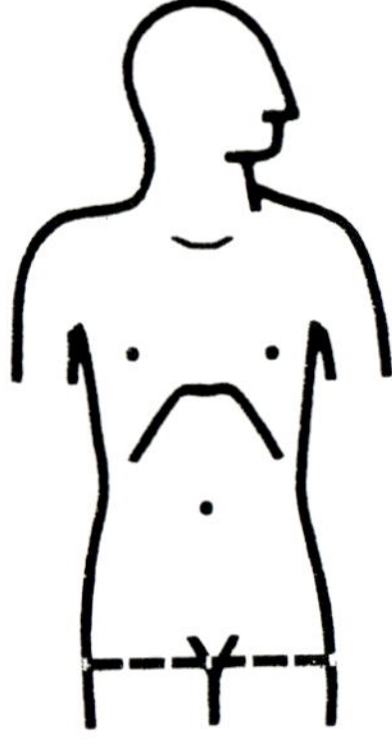

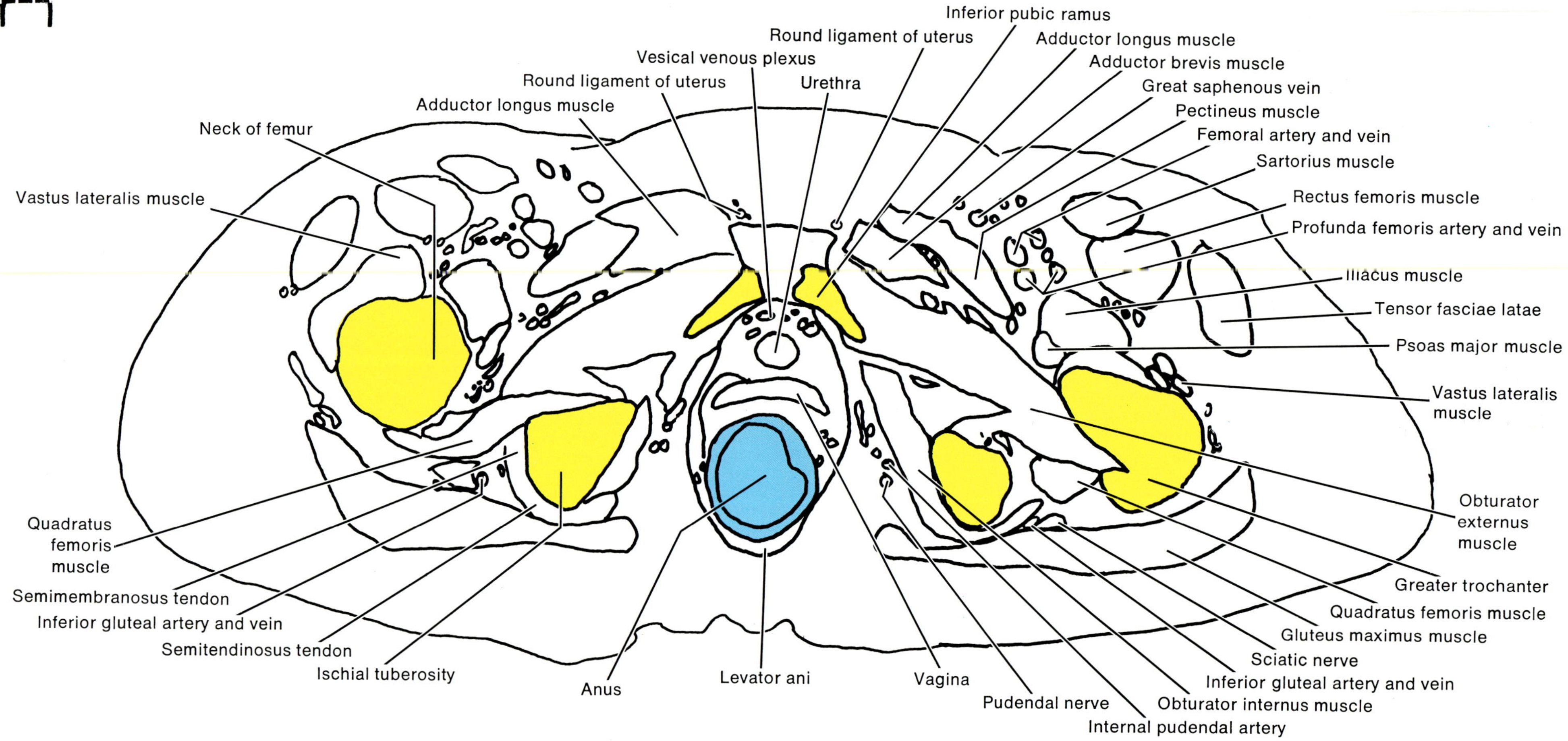

Inferior pubic ramus
Round ligament of uterus
Vesical venous plexus
Adductor longus muscle
Adductor brevis muscle
Great saphenous vein
Pectineus muscle
Femoral artery and vein
Sartorius muscle
Round ligament of uterus
Urethra
Adductor longus muscle
Neck of femur
Rectus femoris muscle
Profunda femoris artery and vein
Vastus lateralis muscle
Iliacus muscle
Tensor fasciae latae
Psoas major muscle
Vastus lateralis muscle
Obturator externus muscle
Quadratus femoris muscle
Greater trochanter
Quadratus femoris muscle
Semimembranosus tendon
Gluteus maximus muscle
Inferior gluteal artery and vein
Sciatic nerve
Semitendinosus tendon
Inferior gluteal artery and vein
Ischial tuberosity
Obturator internus muscle
Anus
Internal pudendal artery
Levator ani
Vagina
Pudendal nerve

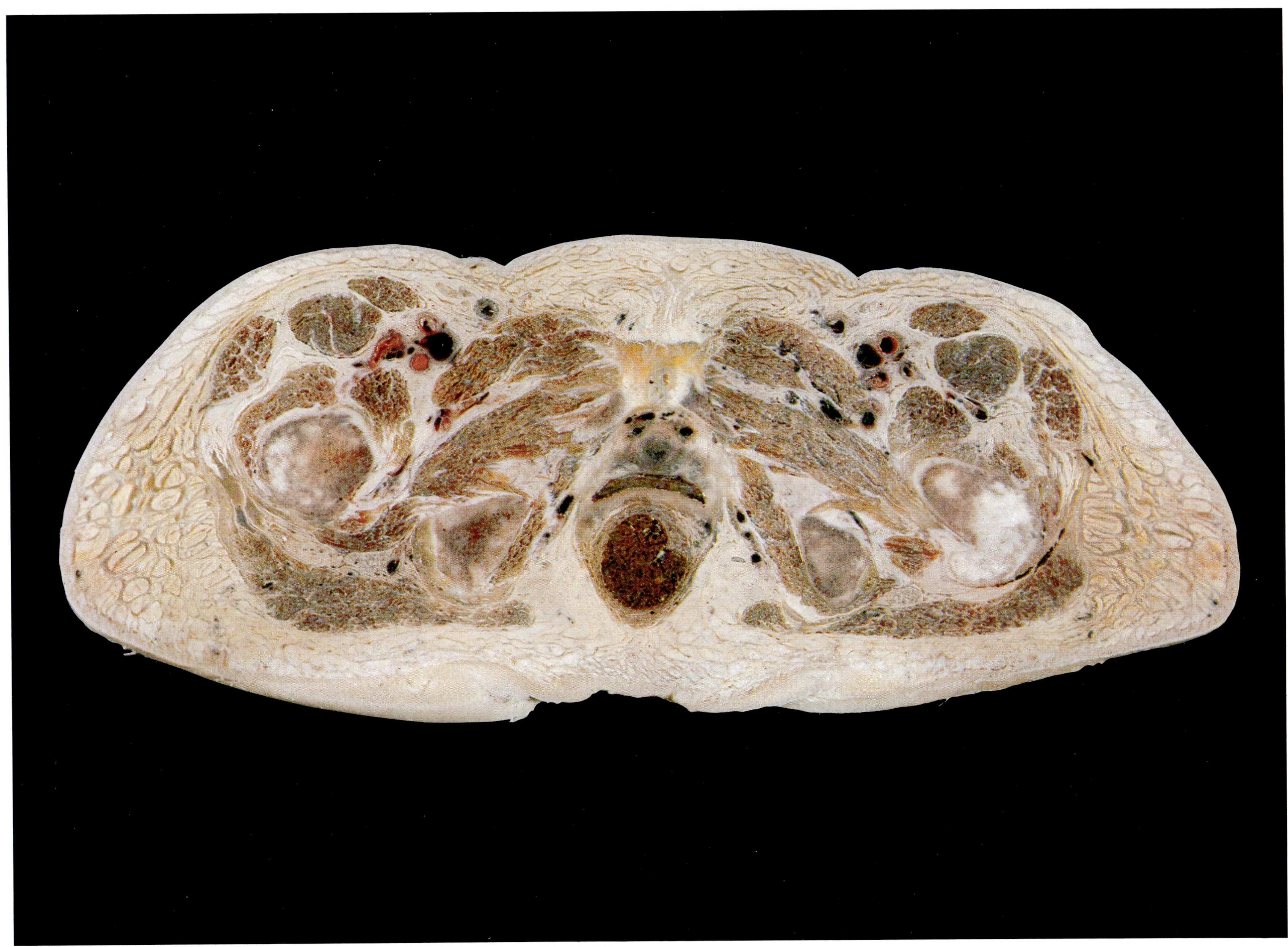

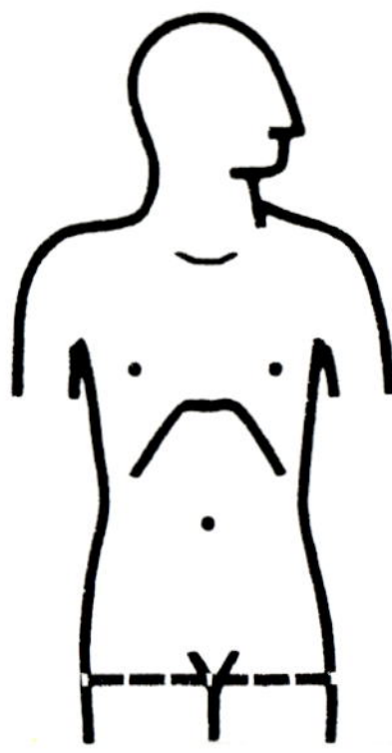

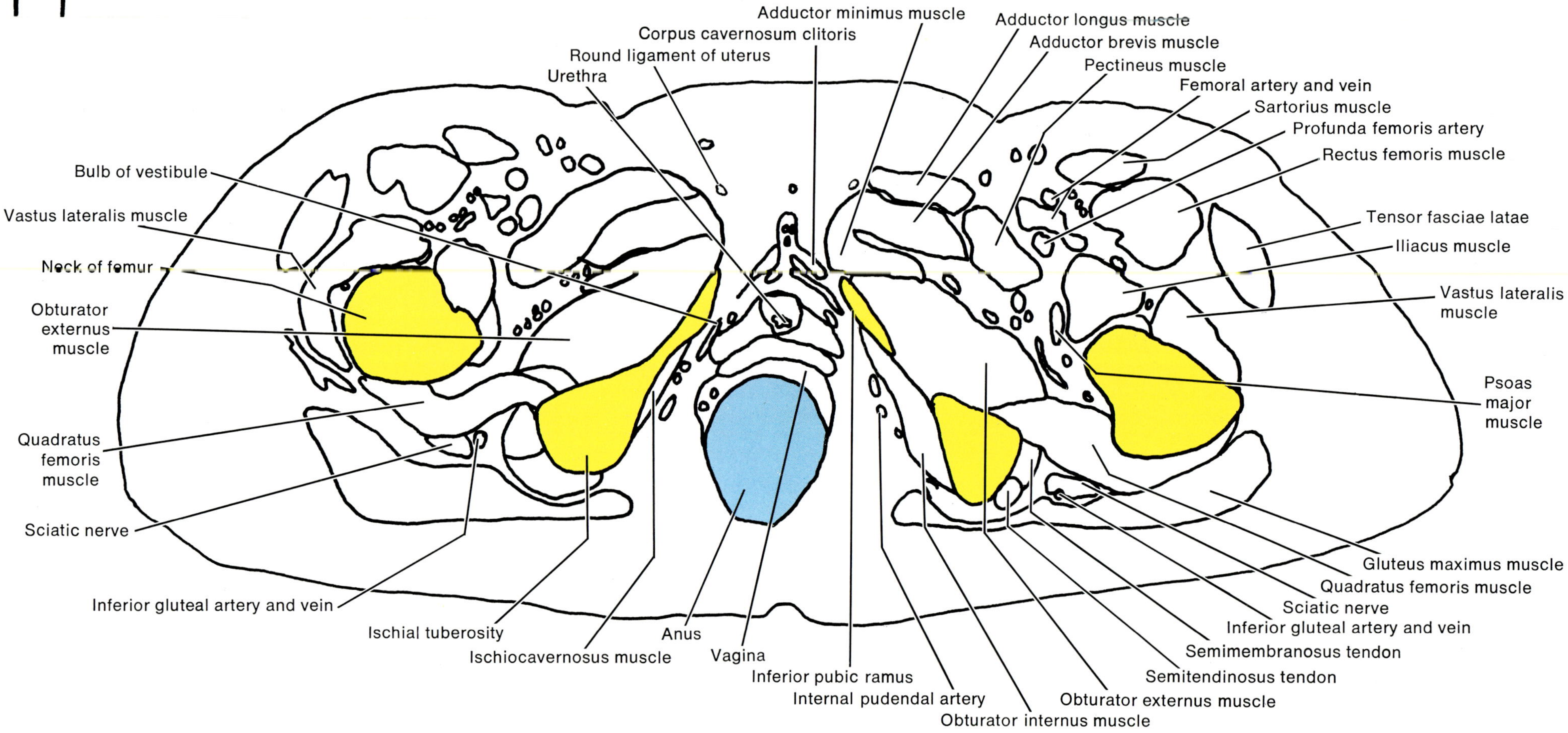

Adductor minimus muscle
Corpus cavernosum clitoris
Round ligament of uterus
Urethra
Adductor longus muscle
Adductor brevis muscle
Pectineus muscle
Femoral artery and vein
Sartorius muscle
Profunda femoris artery
Rectus femoris muscle

Bulb of vestibule
Vastus lateralis muscle
Neck of femur
Obturator externus muscle
Quadratus femoris muscle
Sciatic nerve

Tensor fasciae latae
Iliacus muscle
Vastus lateralis muscle
Psoas major muscle

Inferior gluteal artery and vein
Ischial tuberosity
Ischiocavernosus muscle
Anus
Vagina
Inferior pubic ramus
Internal pudendal artery
Obturator internus muscle

Gluteus maximus muscle
Quadratus femoris muscle
Sciatic nerve
Inferior gluteal artery and vein
Semimembranosus tendon
Semitendinosus tendon
Obturator externus muscle

TRANSVERSE **Pelvis—female**

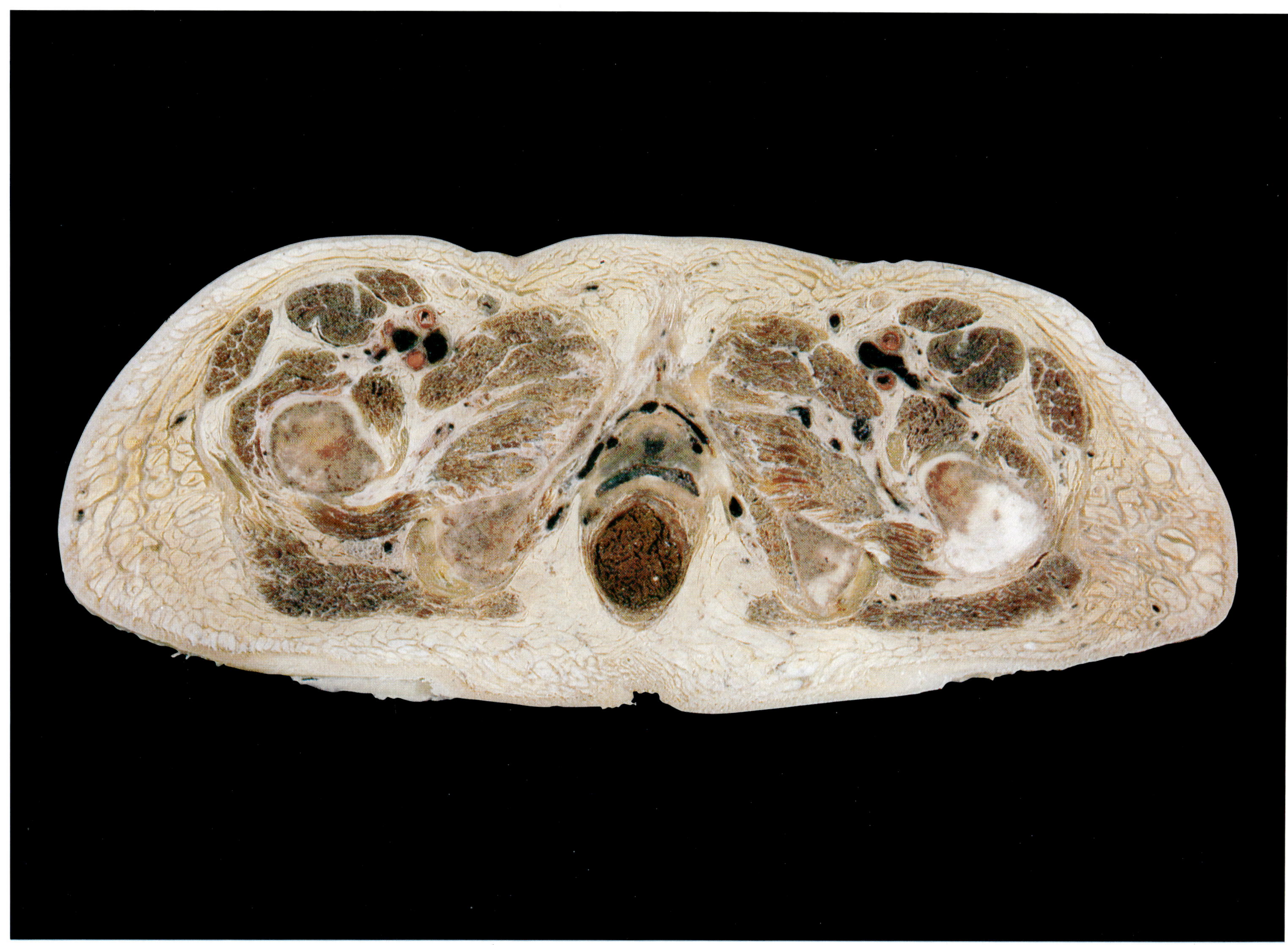

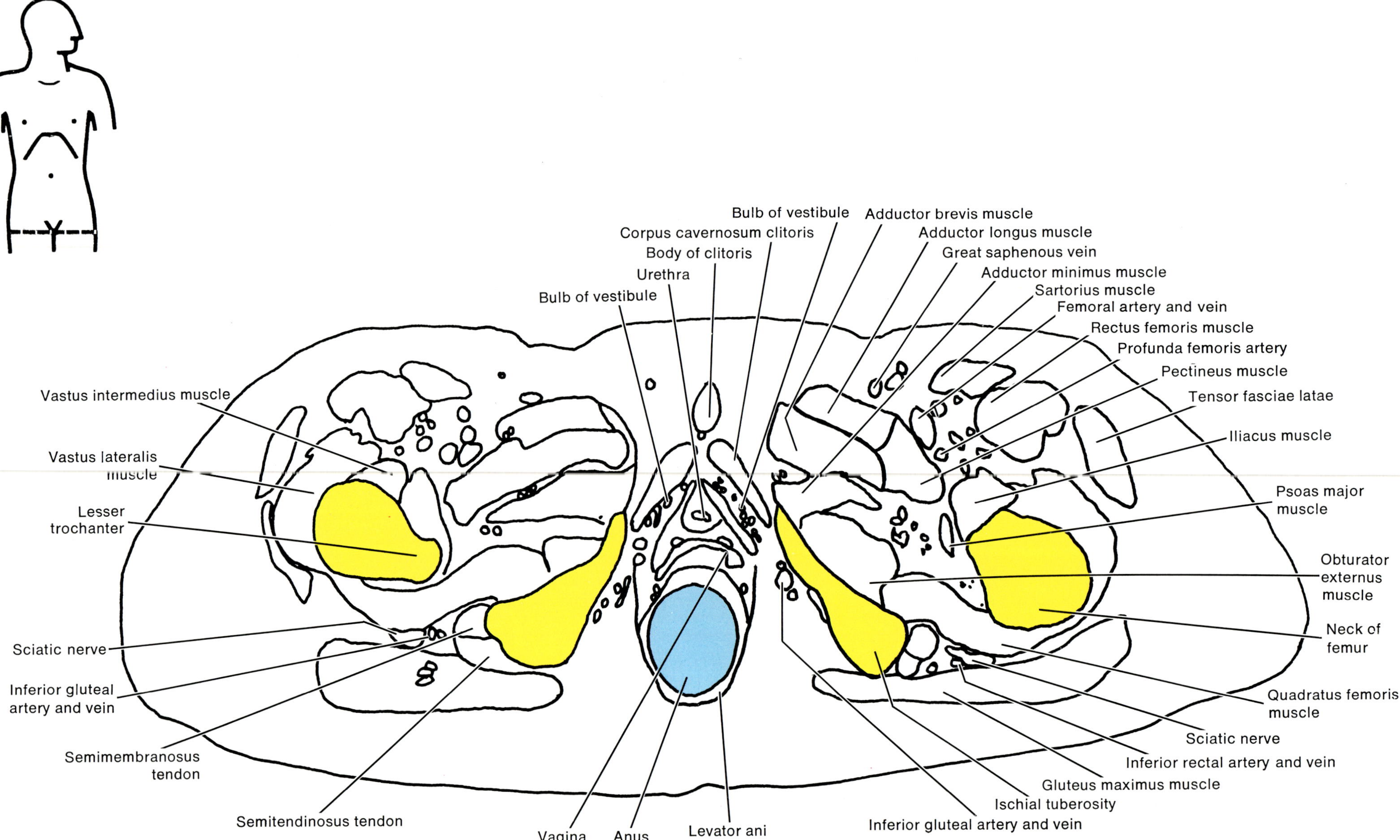
Bulb of vestibule
Corpus cavernosum clitoris
Body of clitoris
Urethra
Bulb of vestibule
Adductor brevis muscle
Adductor longus muscle
Great saphenous vein
Adductor minimus muscle
Sartorius muscle
Femoral artery and vein
Rectus femoris muscle
Profunda femoris artery
Pectineus muscle
Tensor fasciae latae
Iliacus muscle
Psoas major muscle
Vastus intermedius muscle
Vastus lateralis muscle
Lesser trochanter
Obturator externus muscle
Neck of femur
Sciatic nerve
Inferior gluteal artery and vein
Quadratus femoris muscle
Semimembranosus tendon
Sciatic nerve
Inferior rectal artery and vein
Semitendinosus tendon
Gluteus maximus muscle
Ischial tuberosity
Inferior gluteal artery and vein
Vagina
Anus
Levator ani

TRANSVERSE **Pelvis—female**

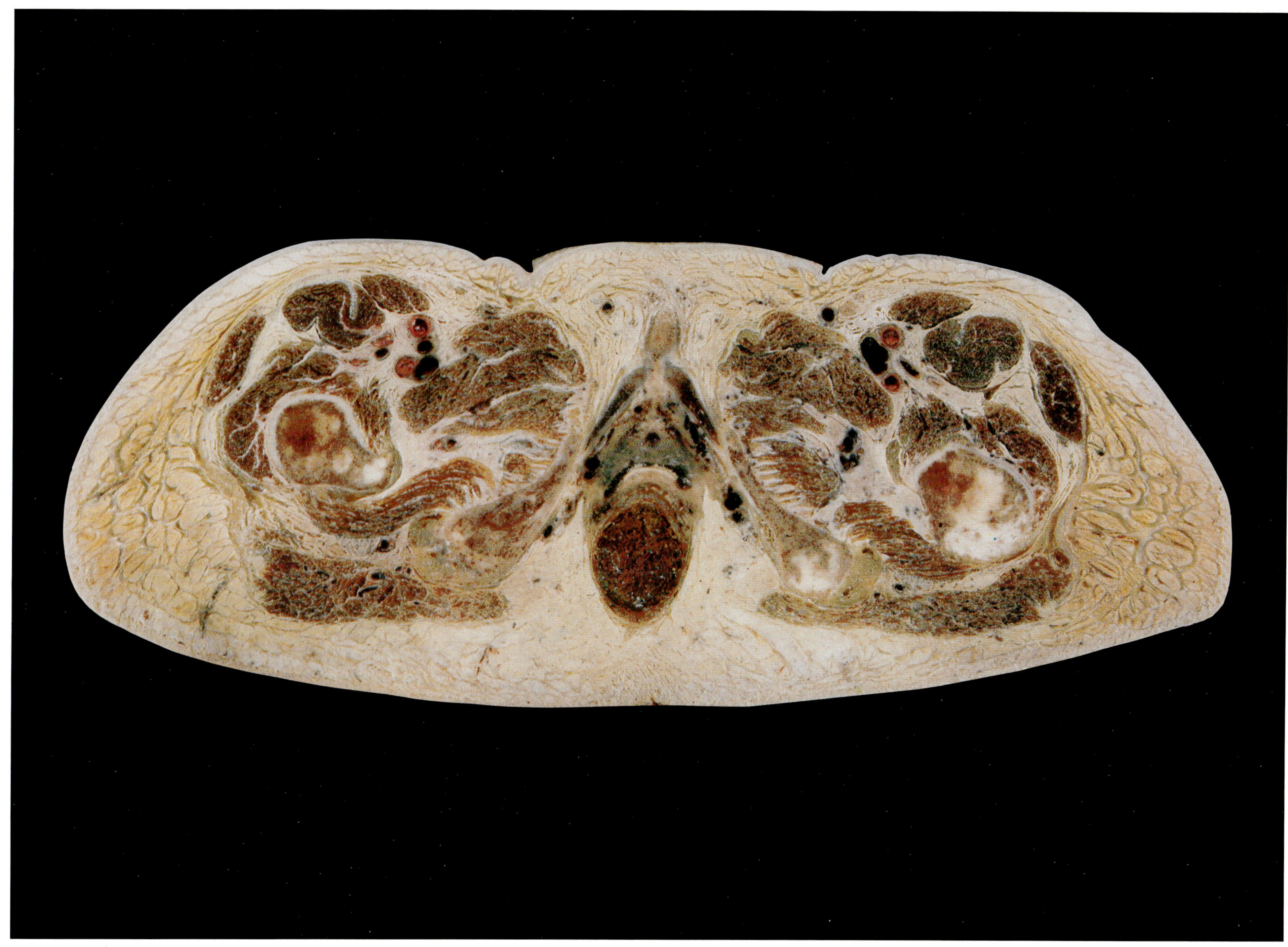

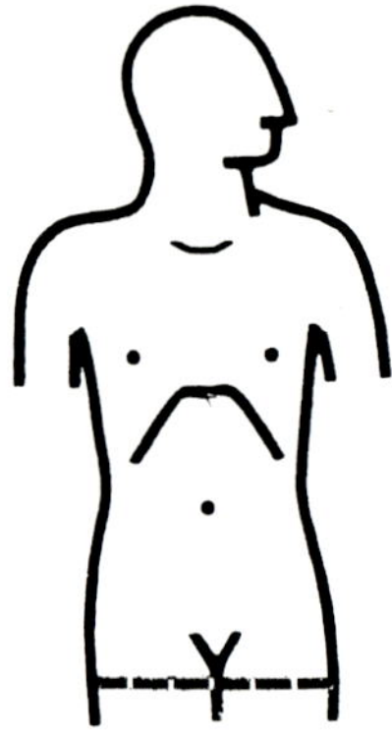

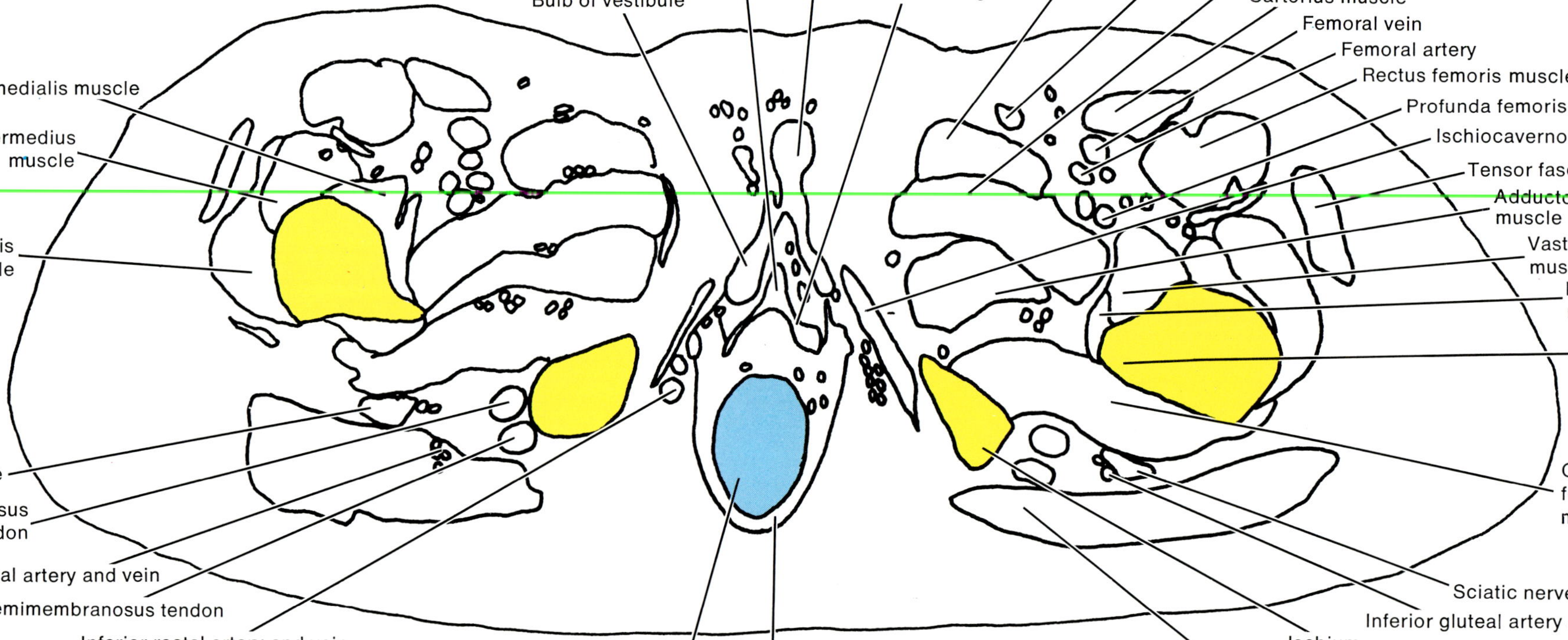

Great saphenous vein
Glans clitoridis
Adductor longus muscle
Adductor brevis muscle
Urethra
Vestibule of vagina
Sartorius muscle
Bulb of vestibule
Femoral vein
Femoral artery
Rectus femoris muscle
Vastus medialis muscle
Profunda femoris artery
Vastus intermedius muscle
Ischiocavernosus muscle
Tensor fasciae latae
Adductor minimus muscle
Vastus lateralis muscle
Vastus medialis muscle
Psoas major muscle
Lesser trochanter
Sciatic nerve
Semitendinosus tendon
Quadratus femoris muscle
Inferior gluteal artery and vein
Semimembranosus tendon
Sciatic nerve
Inferior rectal artery and vein
Inferior gluteal artery and vein
Anus
Levator ani
Ischium
Gluteus maximus muscle

TRANSVERSE **Pelvis—female**

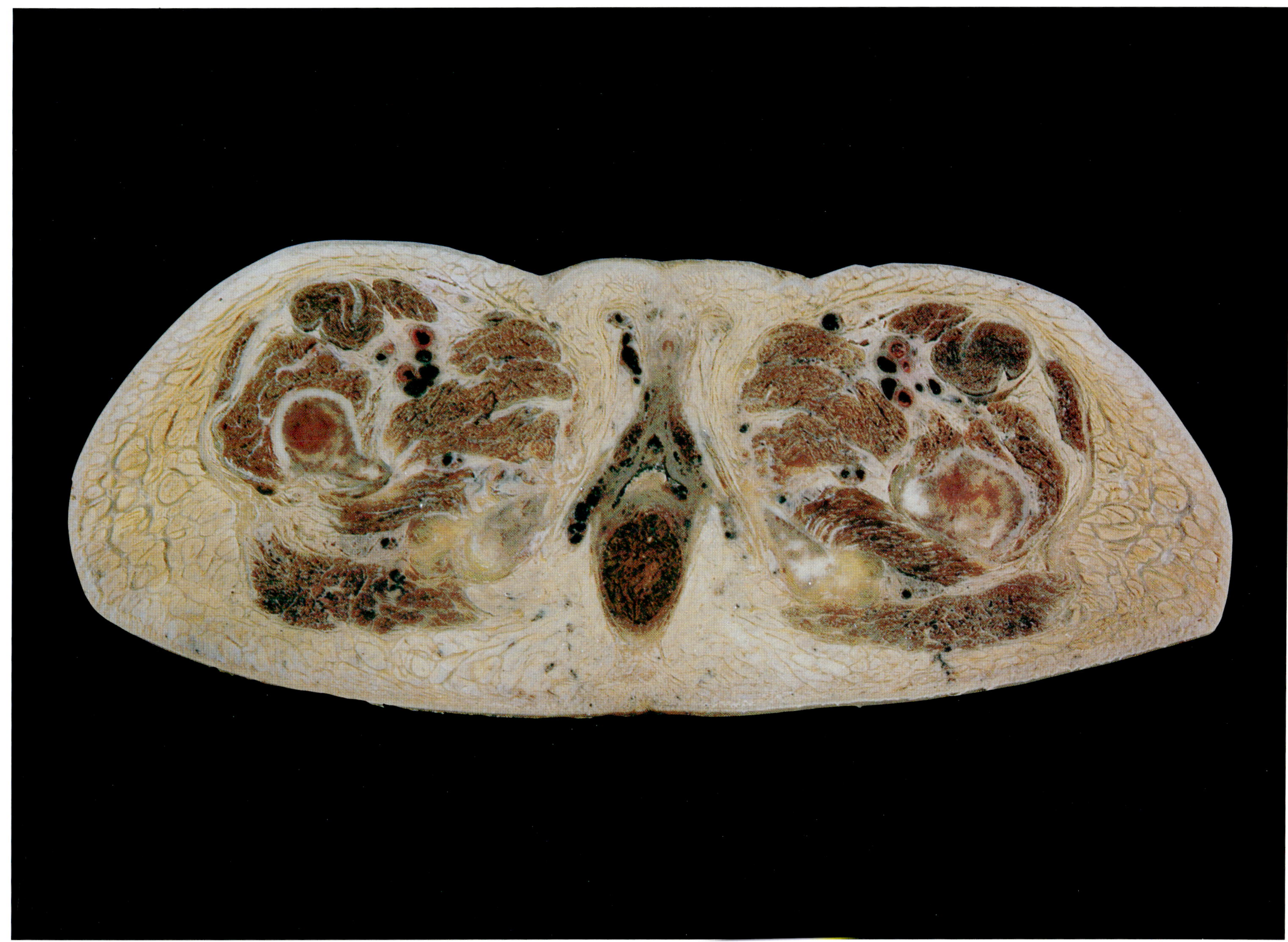

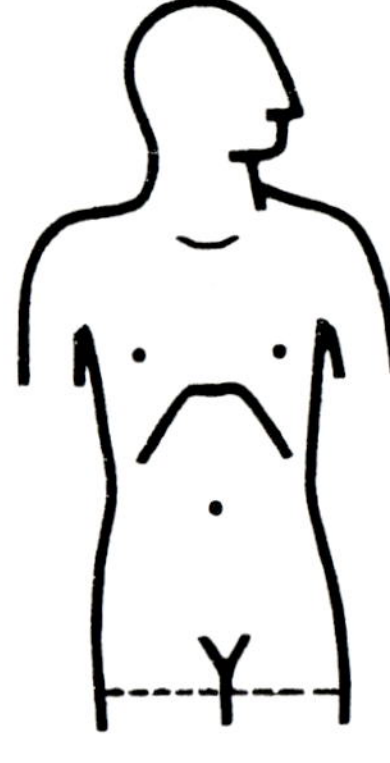

Semimembranosus tendon
Bulb of vestibule
Glans clitoridis
Vestibule of vagina
Gracilis muscle
Adductor longus muscle
Sartorius muscle
Femoral artery
Femoral vein
Vastus medialis muscle
Vastus intermedius muscle
Femur
Vastus lateralis muscle
Rectus femoris muscle
Deep femoral artery
Psoas major muscle
Tensor fasciae latae
Vastus medialis muscle
Pectineus muscle
Adductor brevis muscle
Adductor minimus muscle
Vastus lateralis muscle
Biceps femoris muscle (long head)
Semitendinosus muscle
Semimembranosus tendon
Sciatic nerve
Sphincter ani externus
Anus with feces
Sphincter ani internus
Inferior gluteal artery and vein
Gluteus maximus muscle

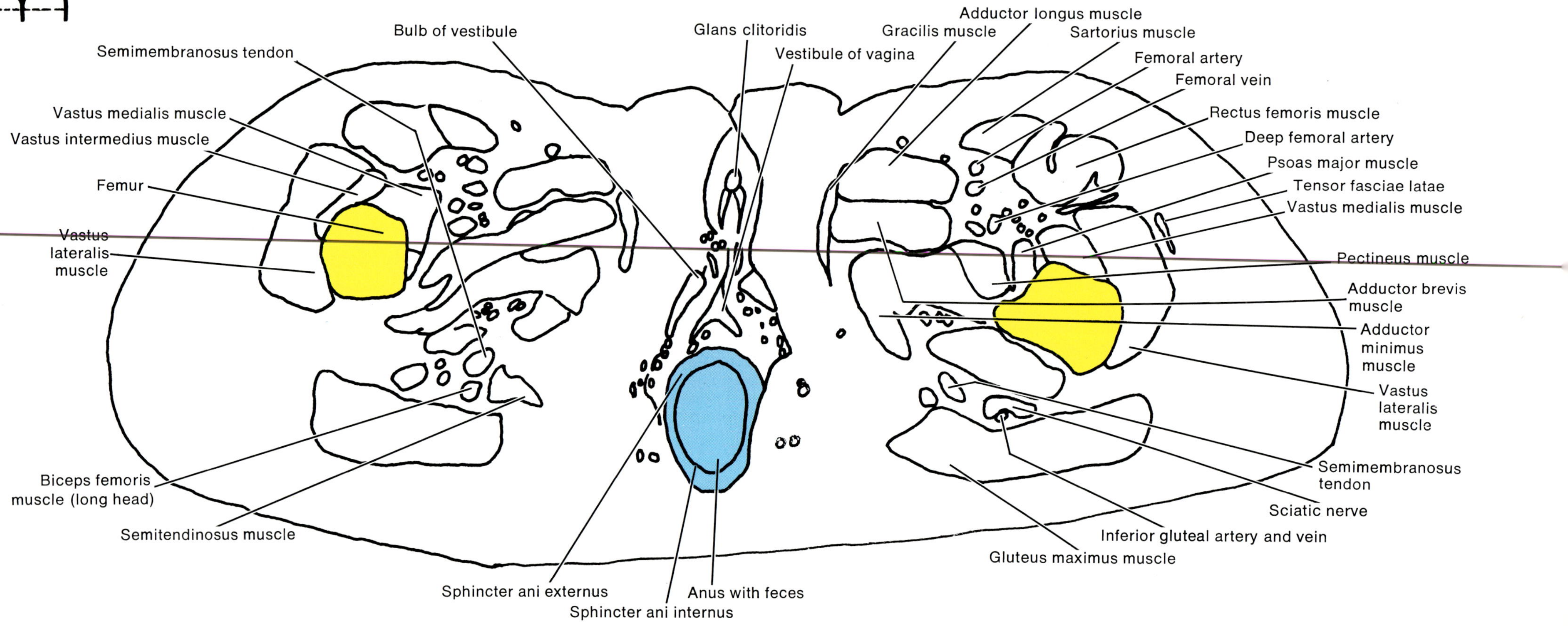

TRANSVERSE **Pelvis—female**

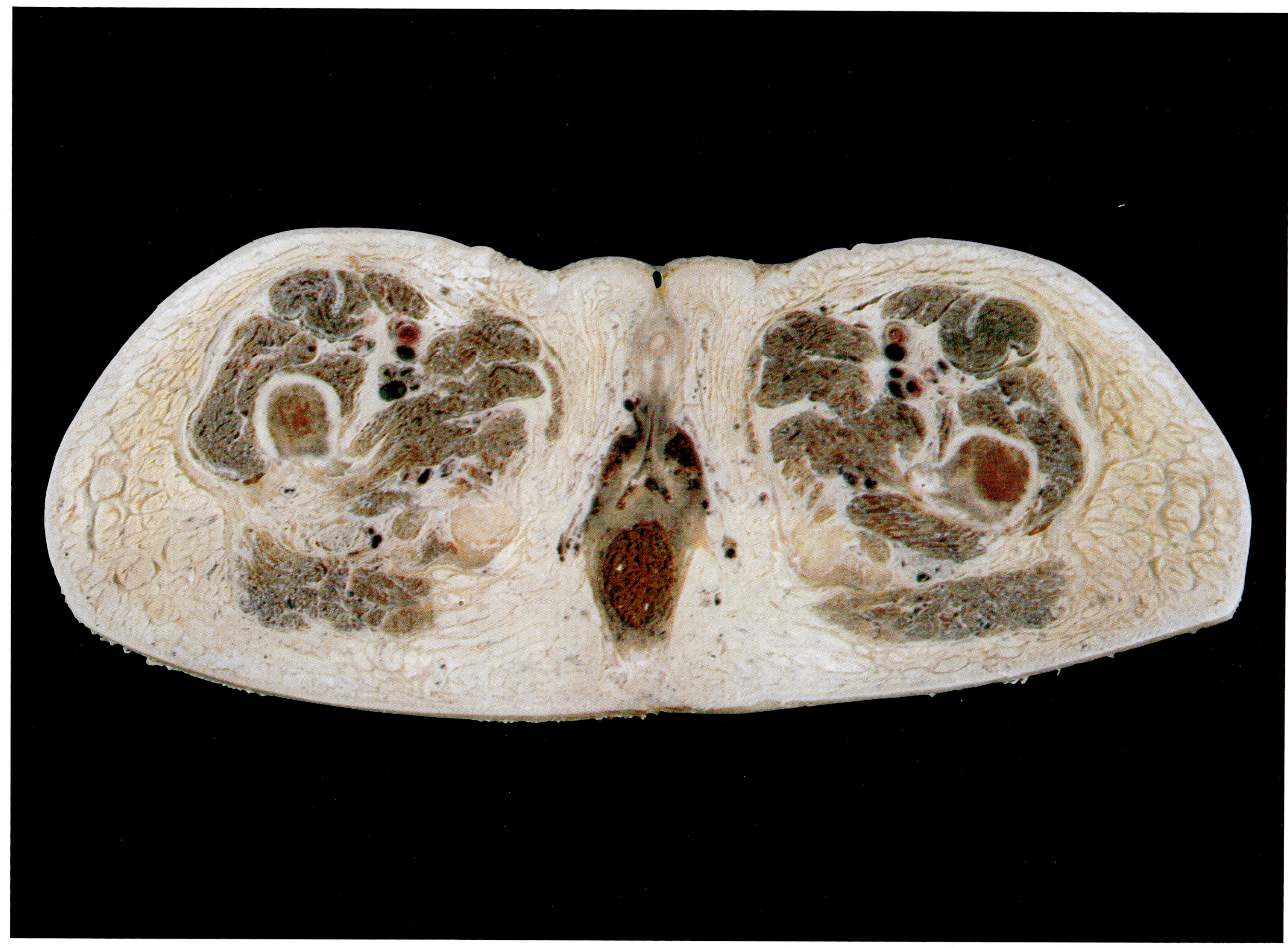

Pelvis—male

PLATES 53-64

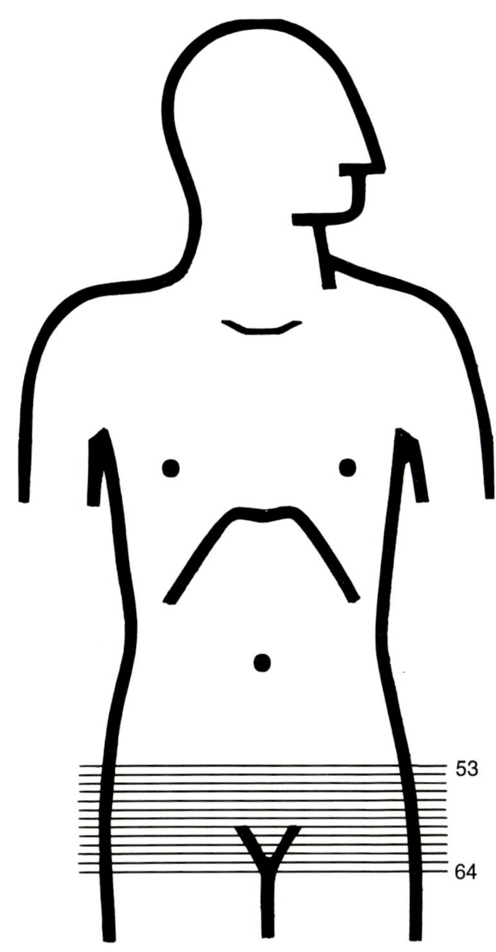

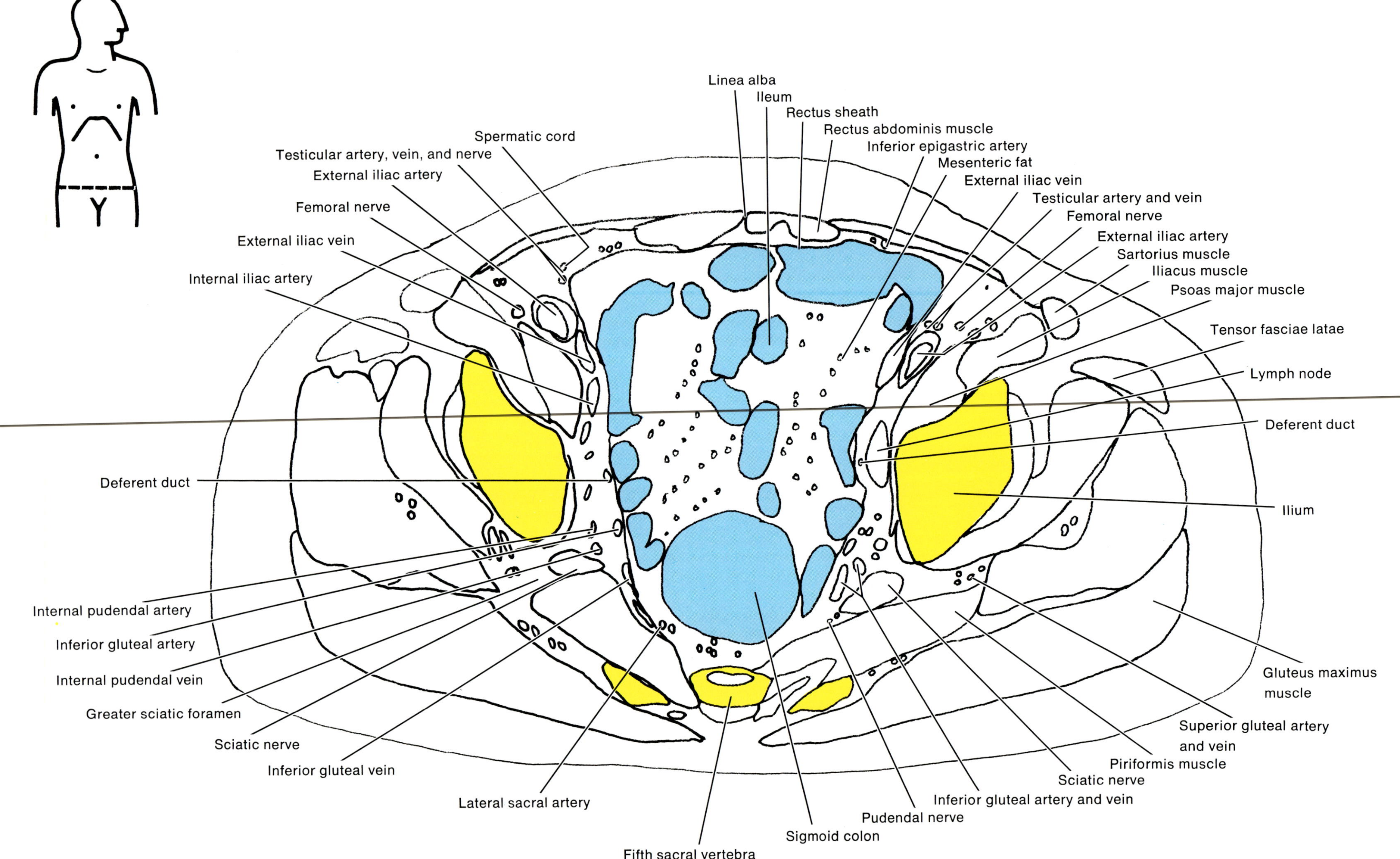

Linea alba
Ileum
Rectus sheath
Rectus abdominis muscle
Inferior epigastric artery
Mesenteric fat
External iliac vein
Testicular artery and vein
Femoral nerve
External iliac artery
Sartorius muscle
Iliacus muscle
Psoas major muscle
Tensor fasciae latae
Lymph node
Deferent duct
Ilium
Gluteus maximus muscle
Superior gluteal artery and vein
Piriformis muscle
Sciatic nerve
Inferior gluteal artery and vein
Pudendal nerve
Sigmoid colon
Fifth sacral vertebra
Lateral sacral artery
Inferior gluteal vein
Sciatic nerve
Greater sciatic foramen
Internal pudendal vein
Inferior gluteal artery
Internal pudendal artery
Deferent duct
Internal iliac artery
External iliac vein
Femoral nerve
External iliac artery
Testicular artery, vein, and nerve
Spermatic cord

TRANSVERSE **Pelvis—male**

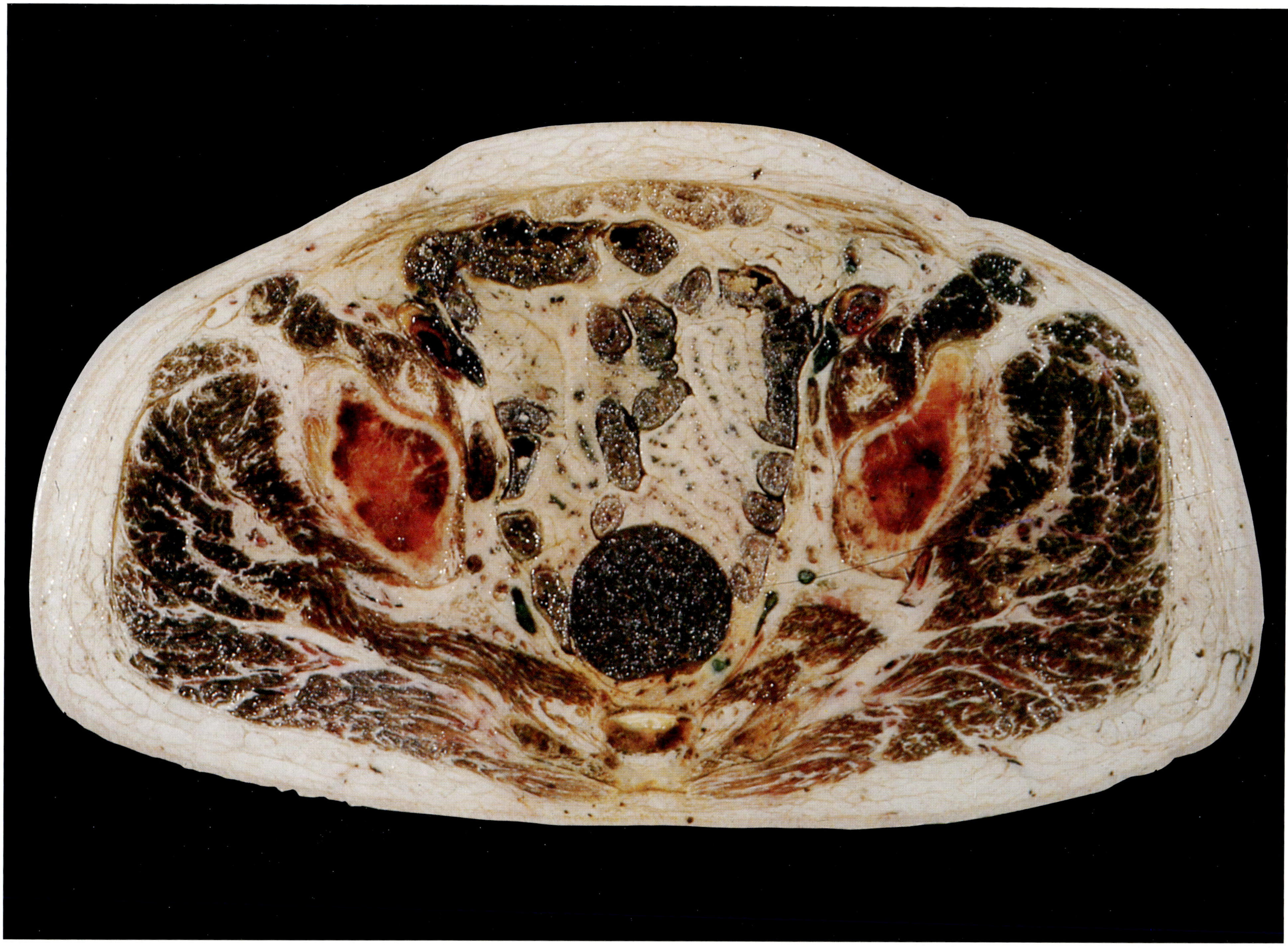

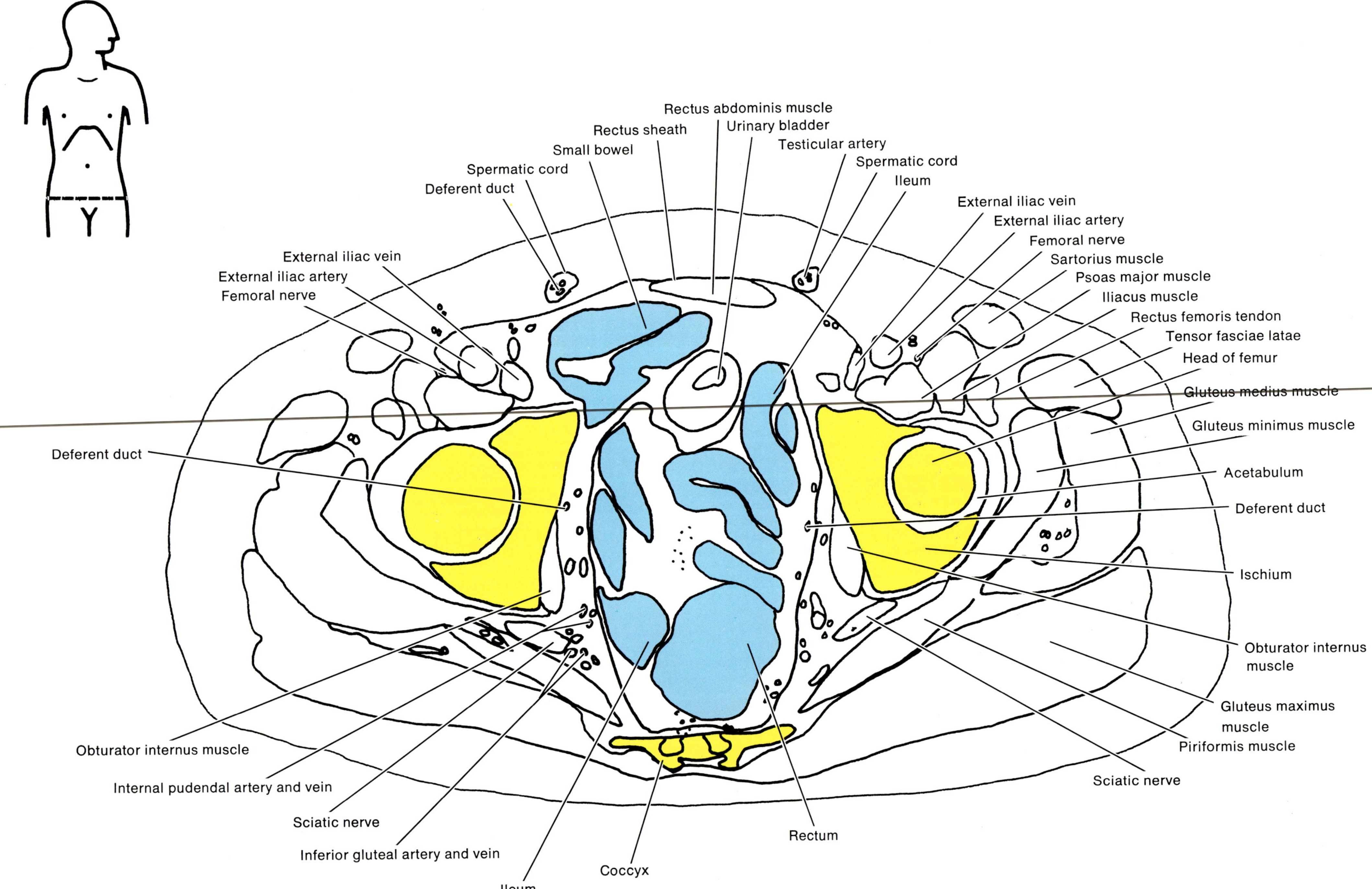

Rectus abdominis muscle
Rectus sheath
Urinary bladder
Small bowel
Testicular artery
Spermatic cord
Spermatic cord
Ileum
Deferent duct
External iliac vein
External iliac artery
Femoral nerve
Sartorius muscle
External iliac vein
Psoas major muscle
External iliac artery
Iliacus muscle
Femoral nerve
Rectus femoris tendon
Tensor fasciae latae
Head of femur
Gluteus medius muscle
Deferent duct
Gluteus minimus muscle
Acetabulum
Deferent duct
Ischium
Obturator internus
muscle
Gluteus maximus
muscle
Obturator internus muscle
Piriformis muscle
Internal pudendal artery and vein
Sciatic nerve
Sciatic nerve
Inferior gluteal artery and vein
Rectum
Coccyx
Ileum

TRANSVERSE **Pelvis—male**

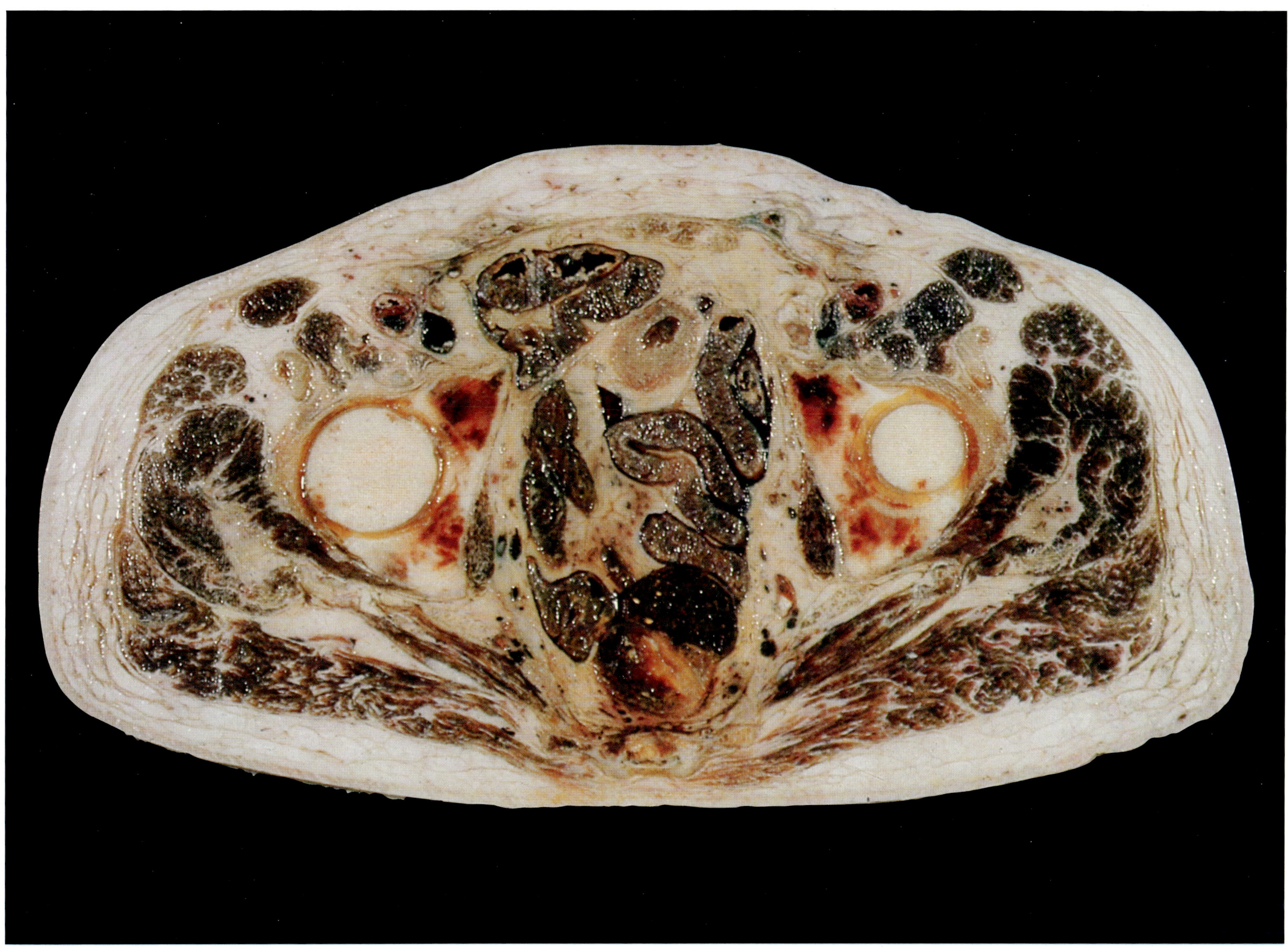

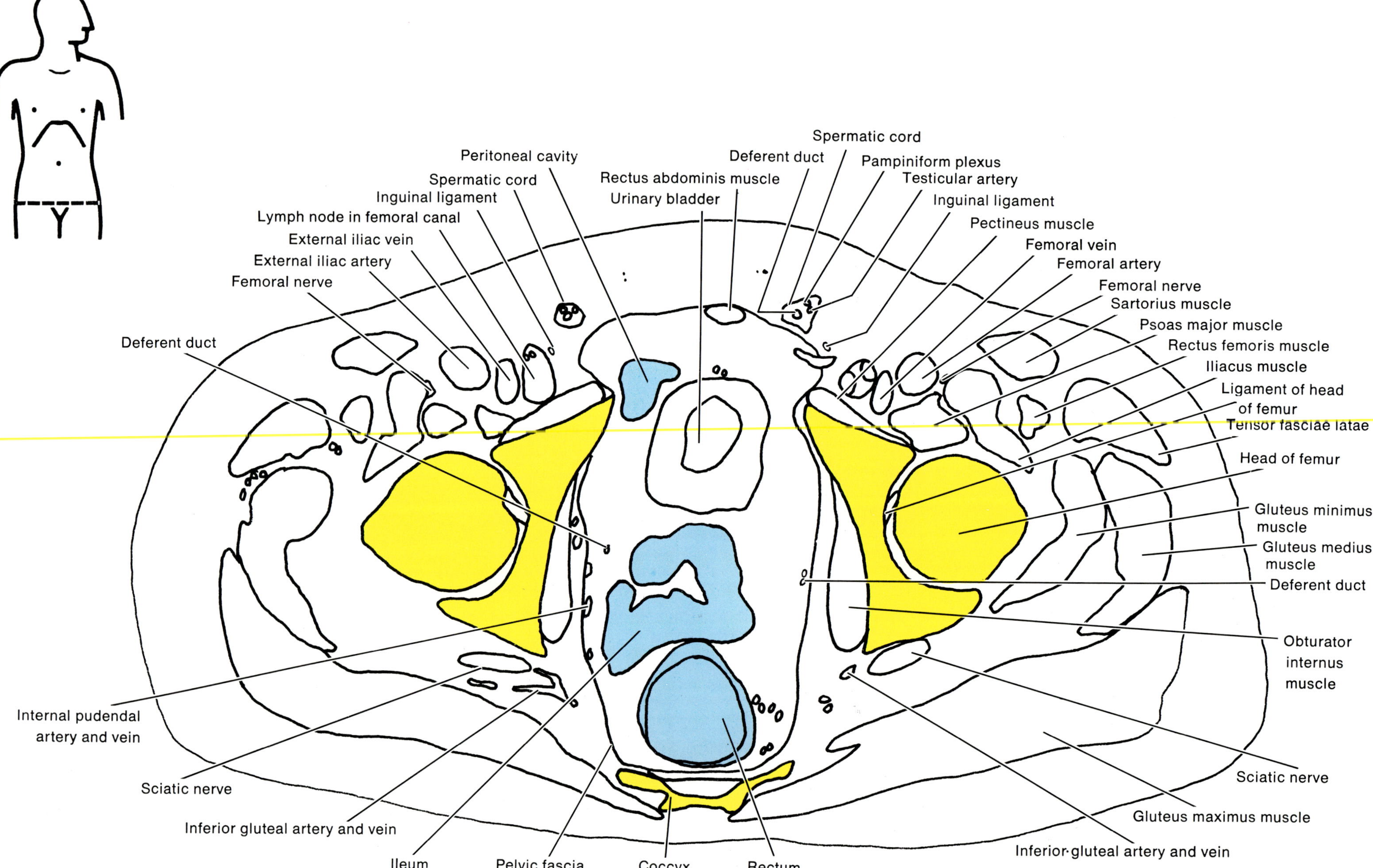
Peritoneal cavity
Spermatic cord
Inguinal ligament
Lymph node in femoral canal
External iliac vein
External iliac artery
Femoral nerve
Deferent duct
Rectus abdominis muscle
Urinary bladder
Spermatic cord
Deferent duct
Pampiniform plexus
Testicular artery
Inguinal ligament
Pectineus muscle
Femoral vein
Femoral artery
Femoral nerve
Sartorius muscle
Psoas major muscle
Rectus femoris muscle
Iliacus muscle
Ligament of head of femur
Tensor fasciae latae
Head of femur
Gluteus minimus muscle
Gluteus medius muscle
Deferent duct
Obturator internus muscle
Internal pudendal artery and vein
Sciatic nerve
Inferior gluteal artery and vein
Ileum
Pelvic fascia
Coccyx
Rectum
Sciatic nerve
Gluteus maximus muscle
Inferior gluteal artery and vein

TRANSVERSE **Pelvis—male**

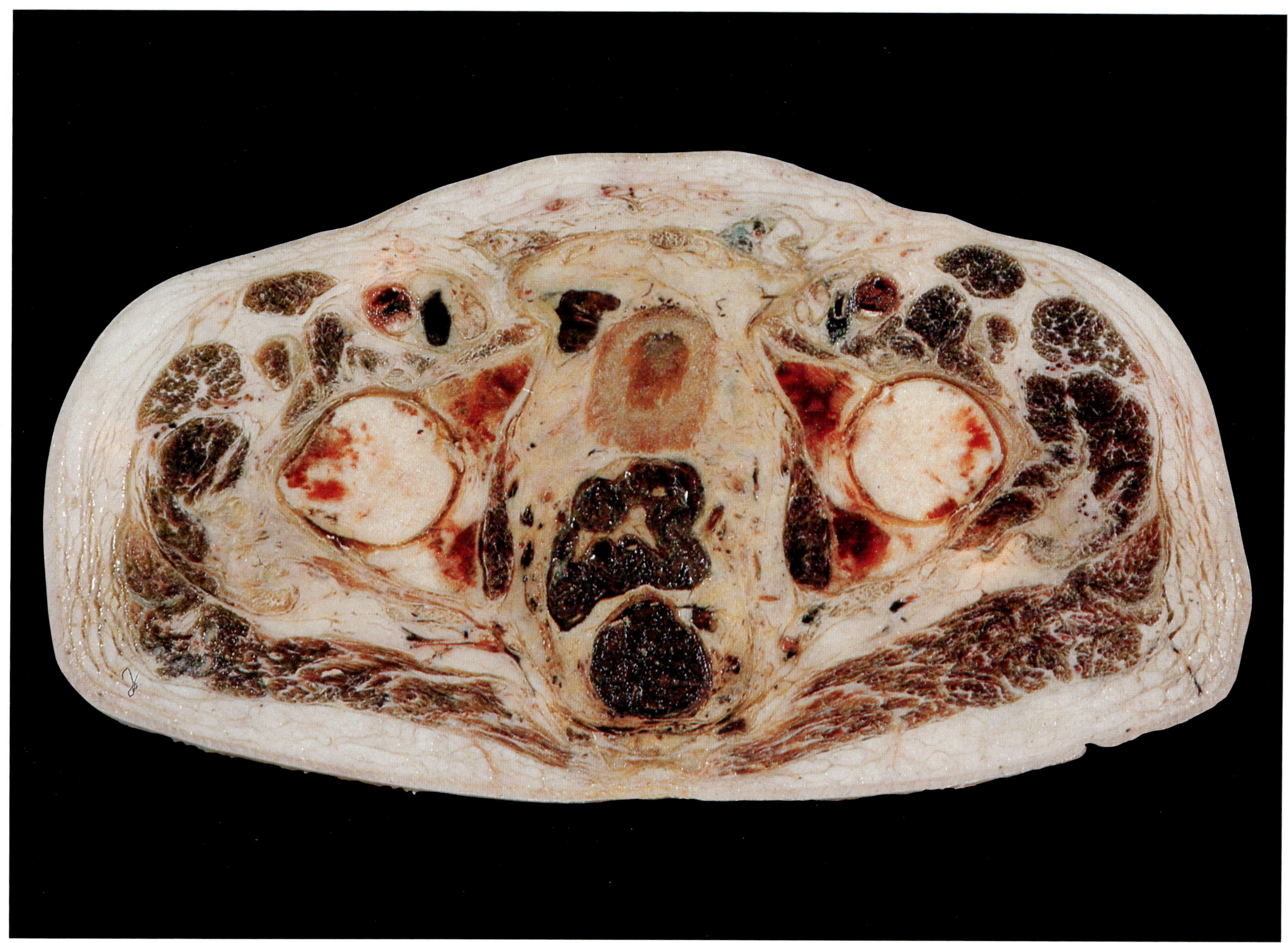

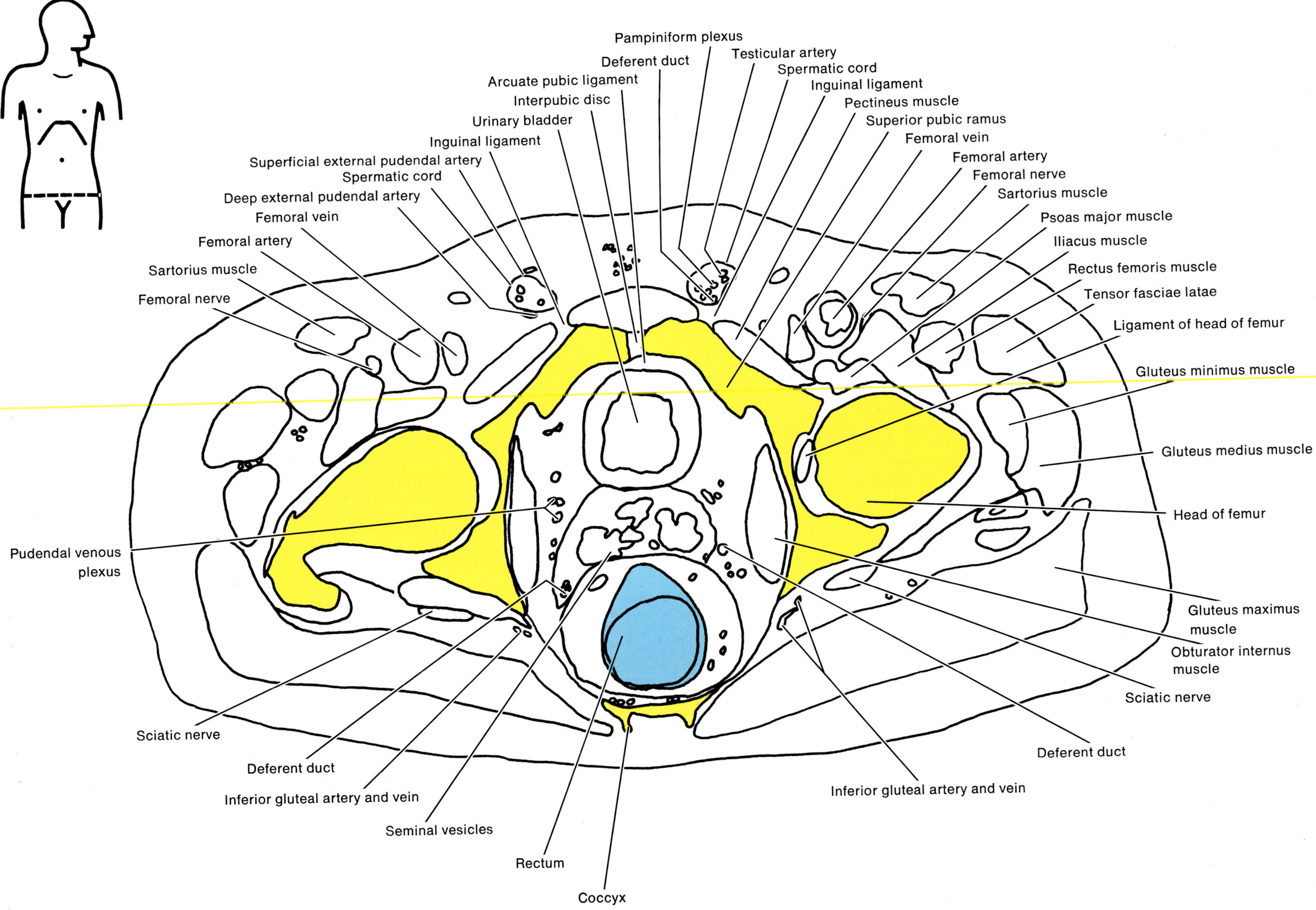
Pampiniform plexus
Deferent duct
Testicular artery
Arcuate pubic ligament
Spermatic cord
Interpubic disc
Inguinal ligament
Urinary bladder
Pectineus muscle
Superior pubic ramus
Inguinal ligament
Femoral vein
Superficial external pudendal artery
Femoral artery
Spermatic cord
Femoral nerve
Deep external pudendal artery
Sartorius muscle
Femoral vein
Psoas major muscle
Femoral artery
Iliacus muscle
Sartorius muscle
Rectus femoris muscle
Femoral nerve
Tensor fasciae latae
Ligament of head of femur
Gluteus minimus muscle
Gluteus medius muscle
Head of femur
Pudendal venous plexus
Gluteus maximus muscle
Obturator internus muscle
Sciatic nerve
Sciatic nerve
Deferent duct
Deferent duct
Inferior gluteal artery and vein
Inferior gluteal artery and vein
Seminal vesicles
Rectum
Coccyx

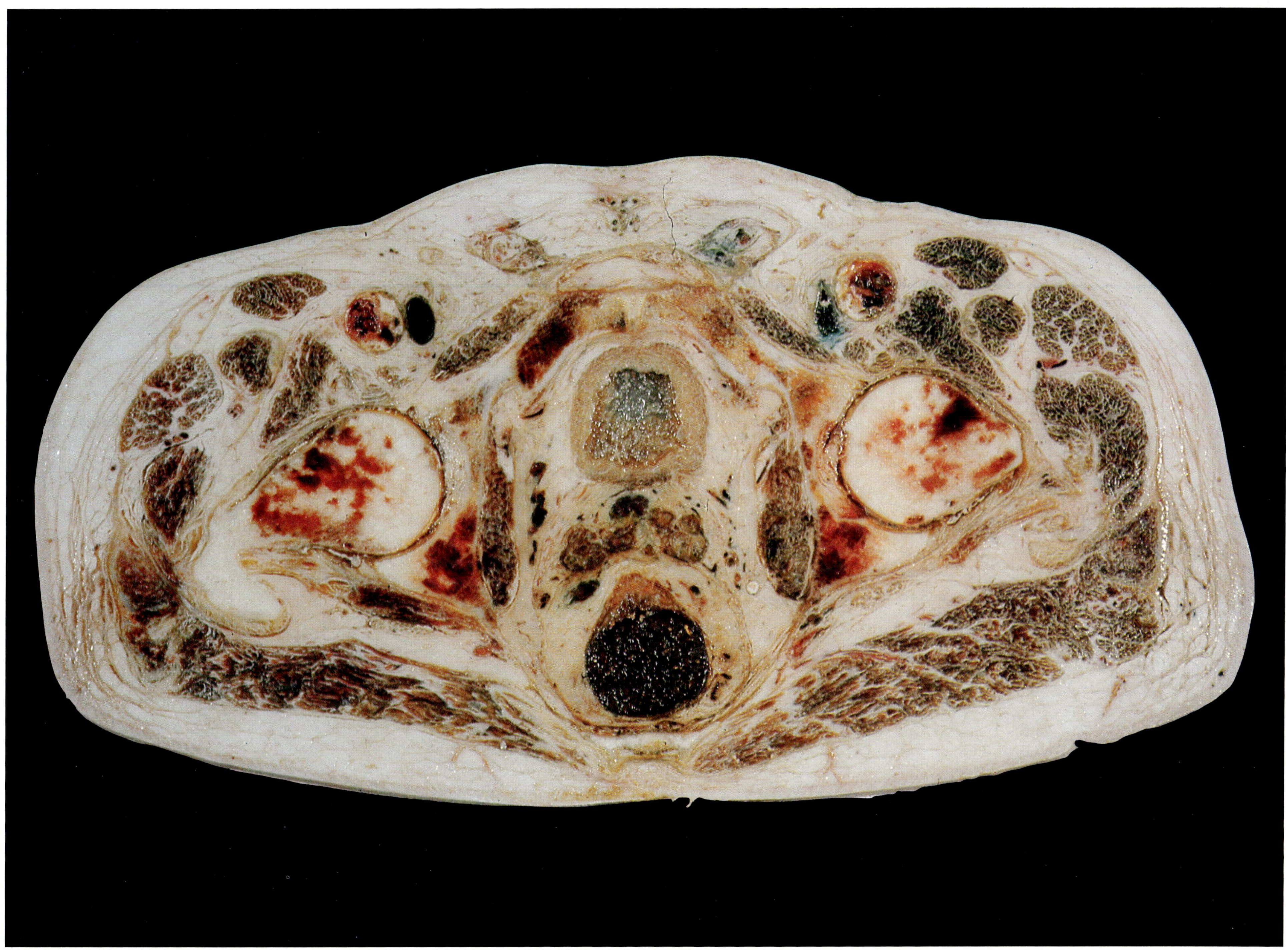

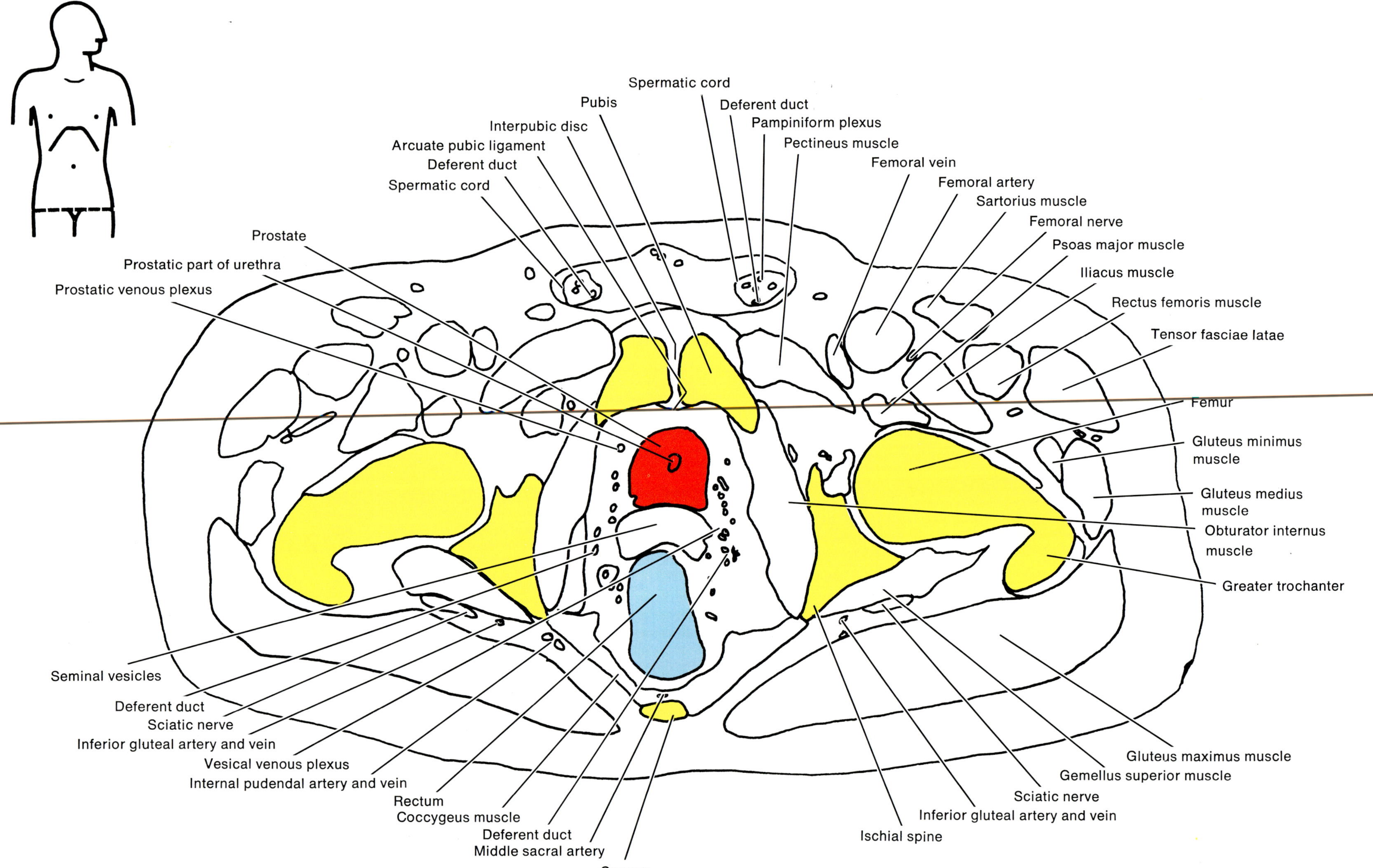

Spermatic cord
Pubis
Deferent duct
Interpubic disc
Pampiniform plexus
Arcuate pubic ligament
Pectineus muscle
Deferent duct
Femoral vein
Spermatic cord
Femoral artery
Sartorius muscle
Femoral nerve
Prostate
Psoas major muscle
Prostatic part of urethra
Iliacus muscle
Prostatic venous plexus
Rectus femoris muscle
Tensor fasciae latae
Femur
Gluteus minimus muscle
Gluteus medius muscle
Obturator internus muscle
Greater trochanter
Seminal vesicles
Deferent duct
Sciatic nerve
Inferior gluteal artery and vein
Vesical venous plexus
Internal pudendal artery and vein
Gluteus maximus muscle
Gemellus superior muscle
Rectum
Coccygeus muscle
Sciatic nerve
Deferent duct
Inferior gluteal artery and vein
Middle sacral artery
Ischial spine
Coccyx

TRANSVERSE **Pelvis—male**

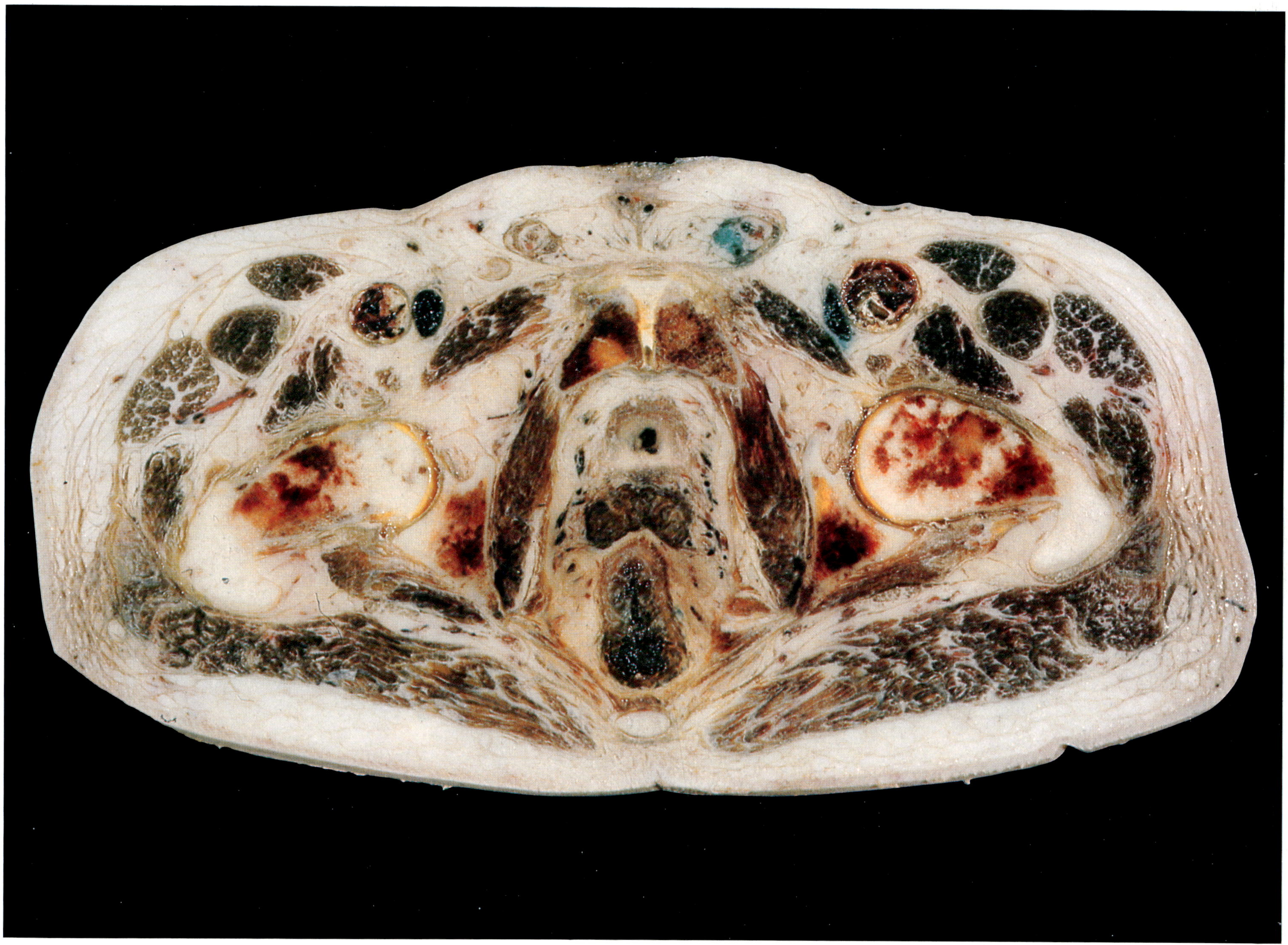

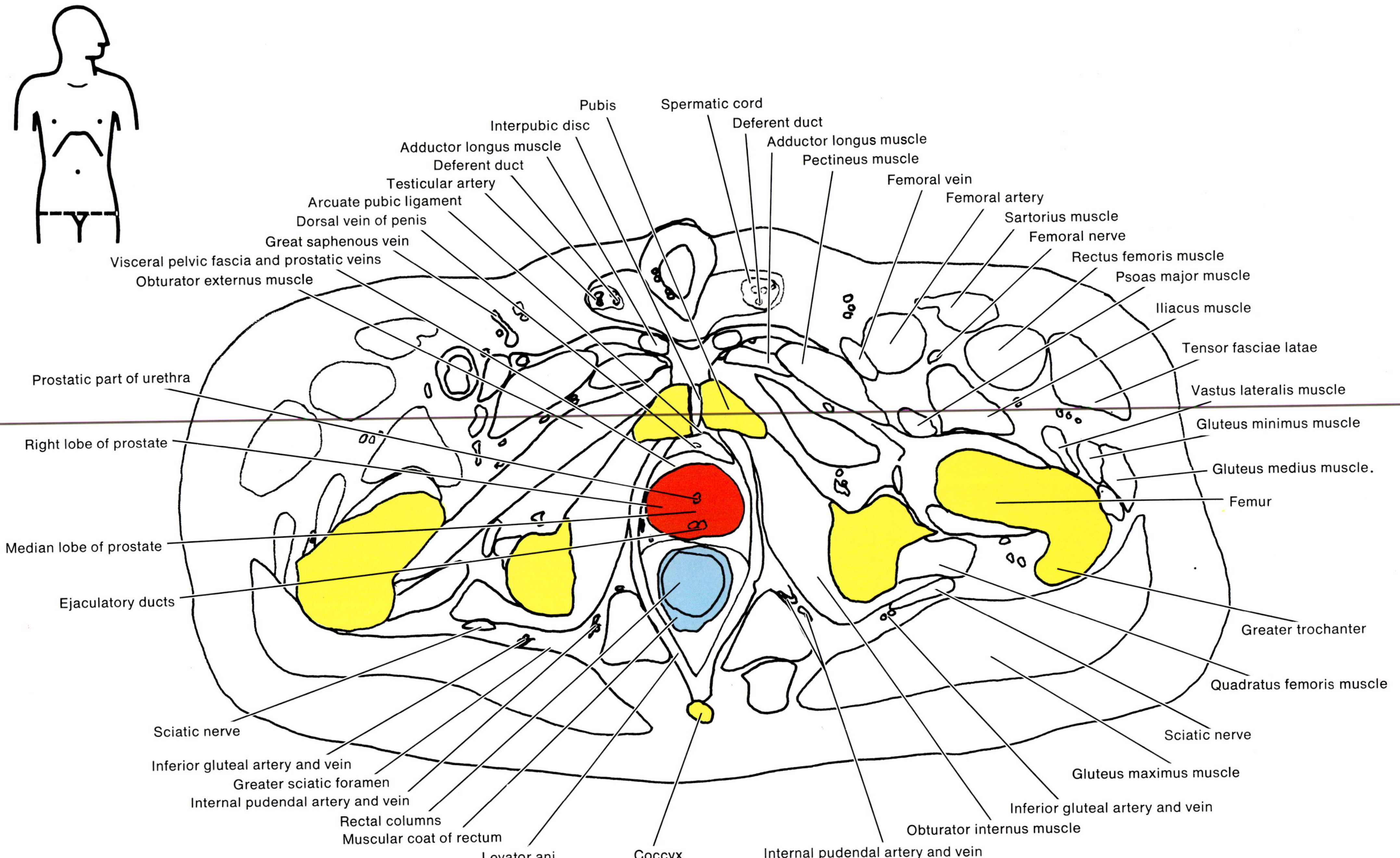

Pubis
Spermatic cord
Interpubic disc
Deferent duct
Adductor longus muscle
Adductor longus muscle
Deferent duct
Pectineus muscle
Testicular artery
Femoral vein
Arcuate pubic ligament
Femoral artery
Dorsal vein of penis
Sartorius muscle
Great saphenous vein
Femoral nerve
Visceral pelvic fascia and prostatic veins
Rectus femoris muscle
Obturator externus muscle
Psoas major muscle
Iliacus muscle
Prostatic part of urethra
Tensor fasciae latae
Vastus lateralis muscle
Right lobe of prostate
Gluteus minimus muscle
Gluteus medius muscle.
Median lobe of prostate
Femur
Ejaculatory ducts
Greater trochanter
Quadratus femoris muscle
Sciatic nerve
Sciatic nerve
Inferior gluteal artery and vein
Greater sciatic foramen
Gluteus maximus muscle
Internal pudendal artery and vein
Inferior gluteal artery and vein
Rectal columns
Obturator internus muscle
Muscular coat of rectum
Levator ani
Coccyx
Internal pudendal artery and vein

TRANSVERSE **Pelvis—male**

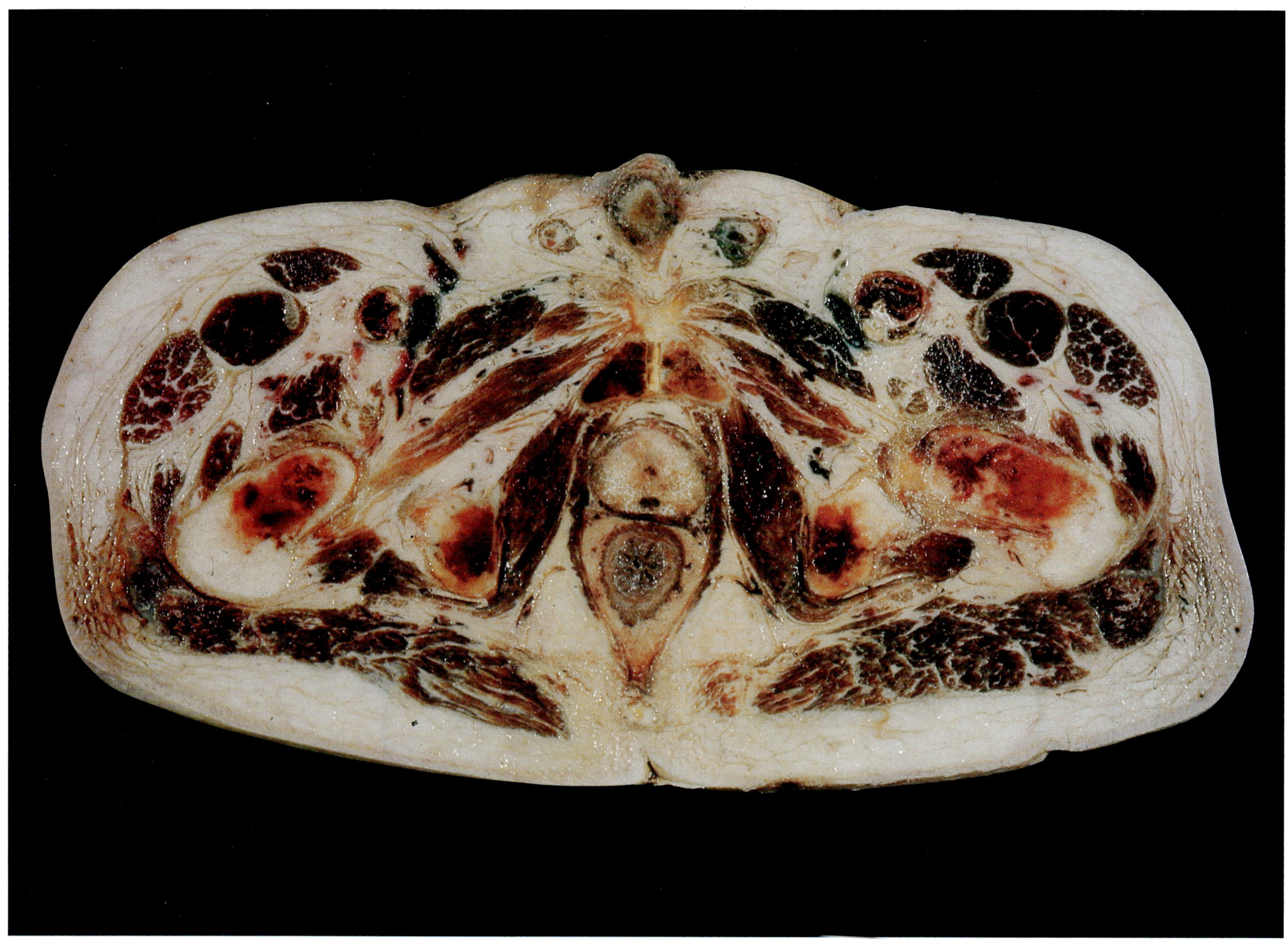

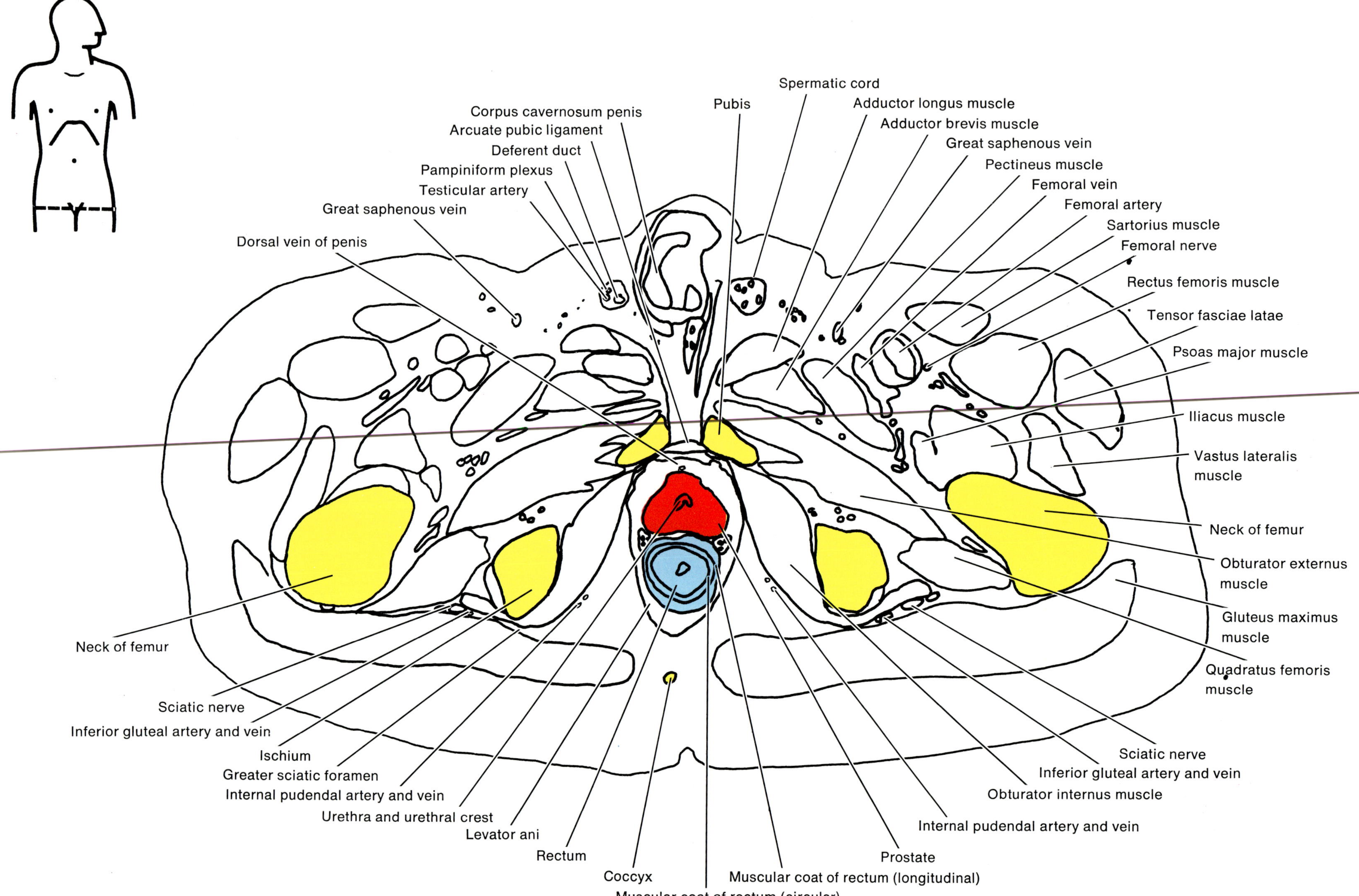

Corpus cavernosum penis
Arcuate pubic ligament
Deferent duct
Pampiniform plexus
Testicular artery
Great saphenous vein
Dorsal vein of penis
Pubis
Spermatic cord
Adductor longus muscle
Adductor brevis muscle
Great saphenous vein
Pectineus muscle
Femoral vein
Femoral artery
Sartorius muscle
Femoral nerve
Rectus femoris muscle
Tensor fasciae latae
Psoas major muscle
Iliacus muscle
Vastus lateralis muscle
Neck of femur
Obturator externus muscle
Gluteus maximus muscle
Quadratus femoris muscle
Sciatic nerve
Inferior gluteal artery and vein
Obturator internus muscle
Internal pudendal artery and vein
Prostate
Muscular coat of rectum (longitudinal)
Muscular coat of rectum (circular)
Coccyx
Rectum
Levator ani
Urethra and urethral crest
Internal pudendal artery and vein
Greater sciatic foramen
Ischium
Inferior gluteal artery and vein
Sciatic nerve
Neck of femur

TRANSVERSE **Pelvis—male**

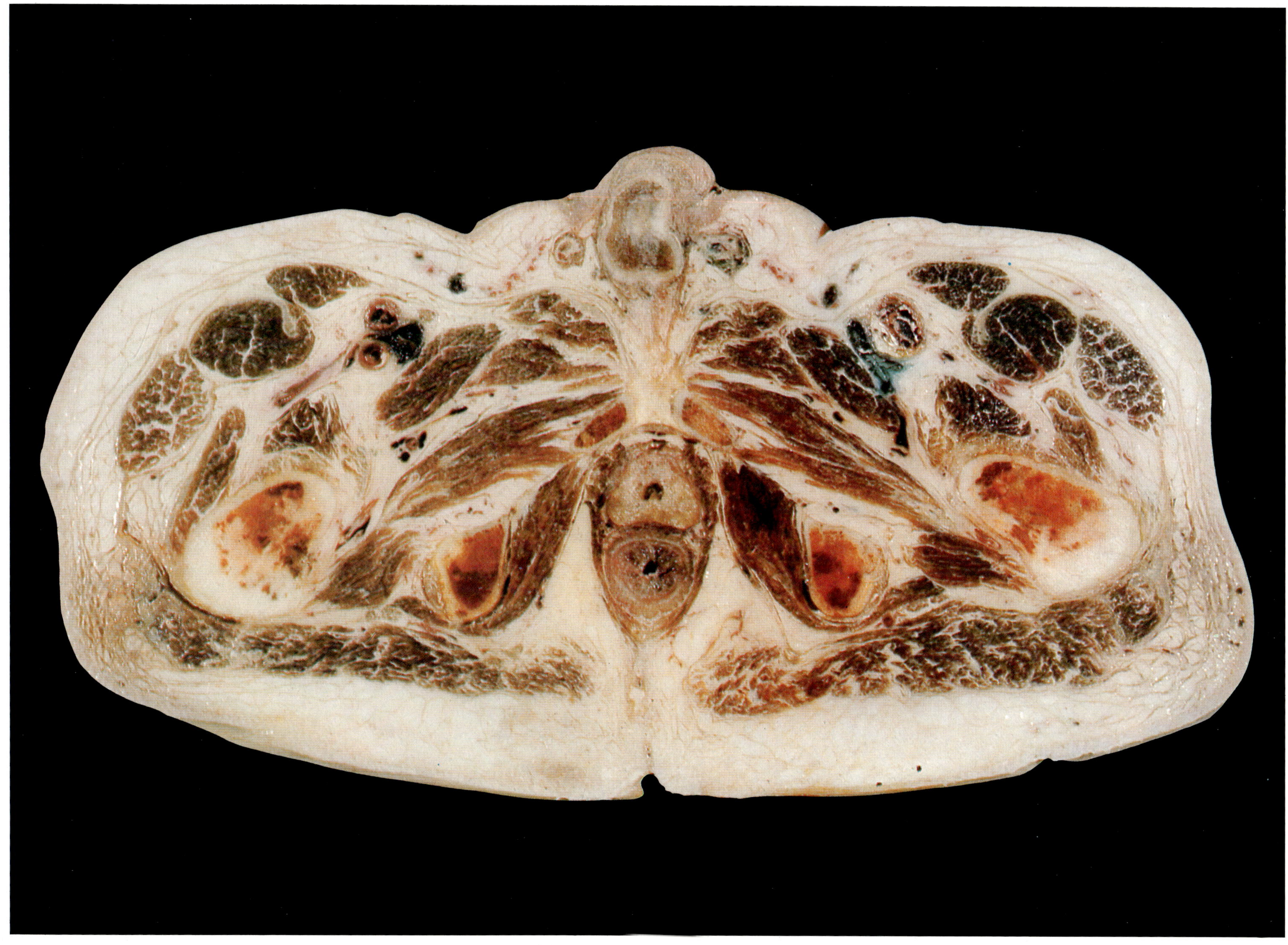

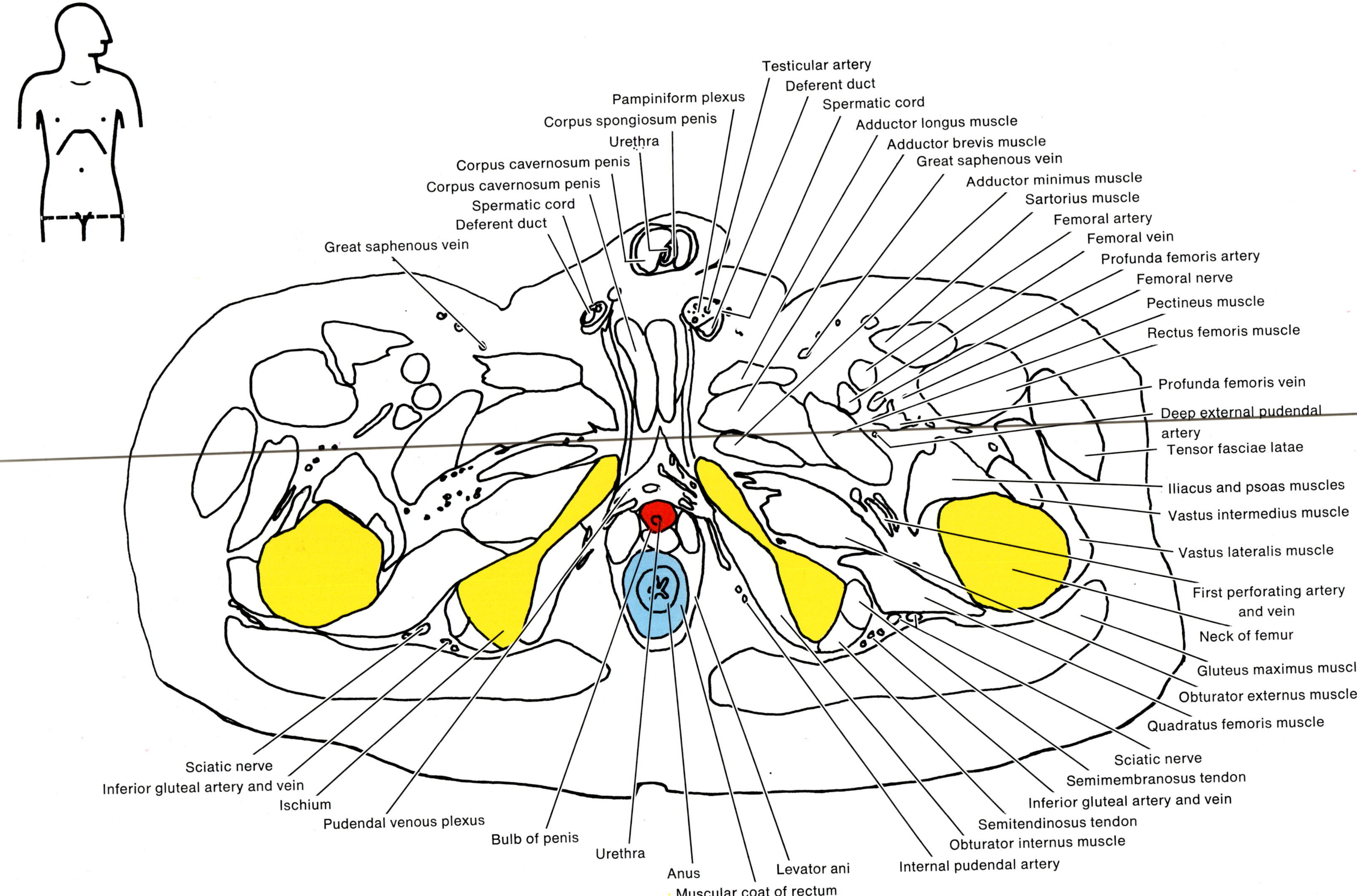

Testicular artery
Deferent duct
Spermatic cord
Adductor longus muscle
Adductor brevis muscle
Great saphenous vein
Adductor minimus muscle
Sartorius muscle
Femoral artery
Femoral vein
Profunda femoris artery
Femoral nerve
Pectineus muscle
Rectus femoris muscle
Profunda femoris vein
Deep external pudendal artery
Tensor fasciae latae
Iliacus and psoas muscles
Vastus intermedius muscle
Vastus lateralis muscle
First perforating artery and vein
Neck of femur
Gluteus maximus muscle
Obturator externus muscle
Quadratus femoris muscle
Sciatic nerve
Semimembranosus tendon
Inferior gluteal artery and vein
Semitendinosus tendon
Obturator internus muscle
Internal pudendal artery
Pampiniform plexus
Corpus spongiosum penis
Urethra
Corpus cavernosum penis
Corpus cavernosum penis
Spermatic cord
Deferent duct
Great saphenous vein
Sciatic nerve
Inferior gluteal artery and vein
Ischium
Pudendal venous plexus
Bulb of penis
Urethra
Anus
Muscular coat of rectum
Levator ani

TRANSVERSE **Pelvis—male**

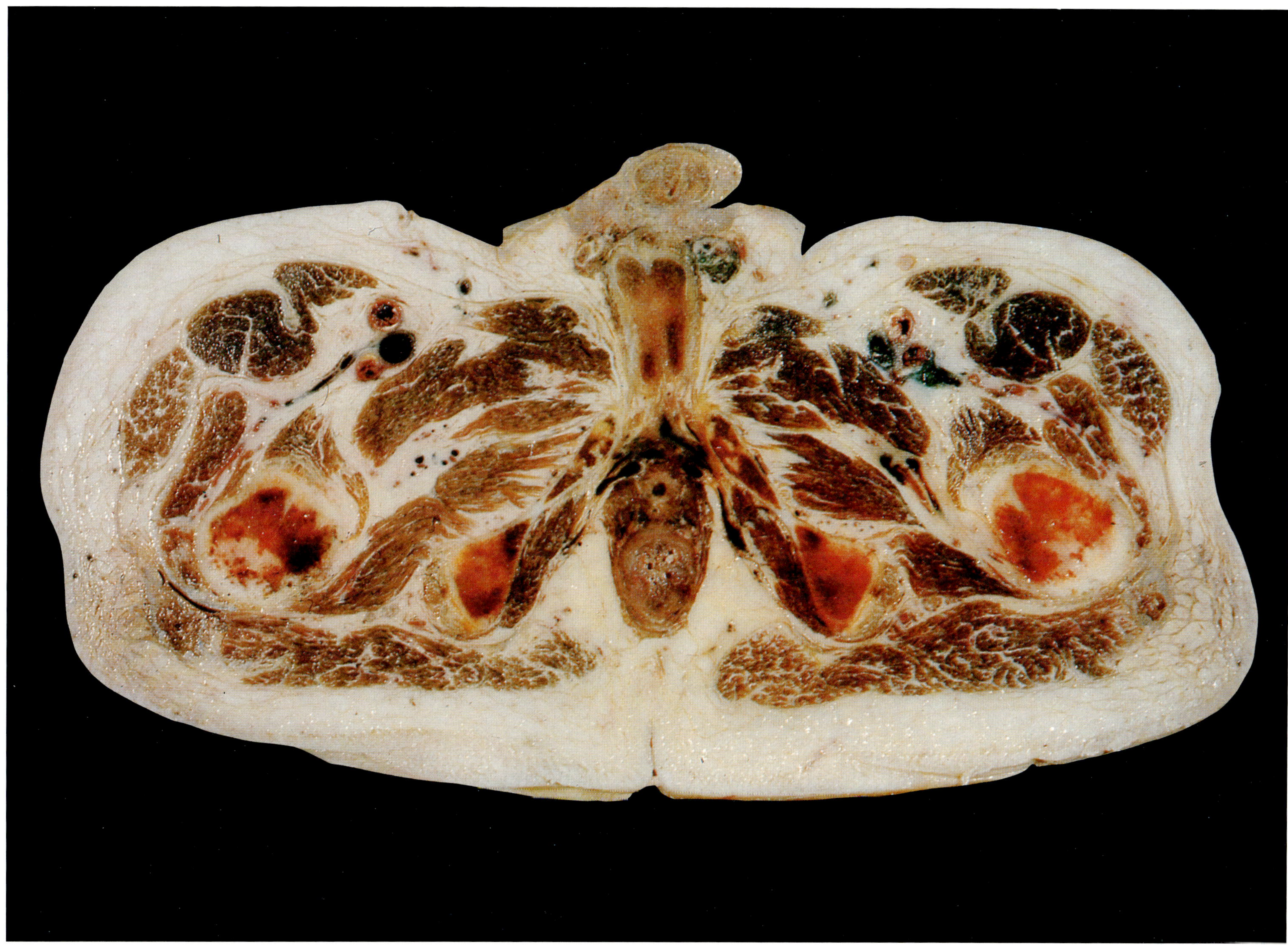

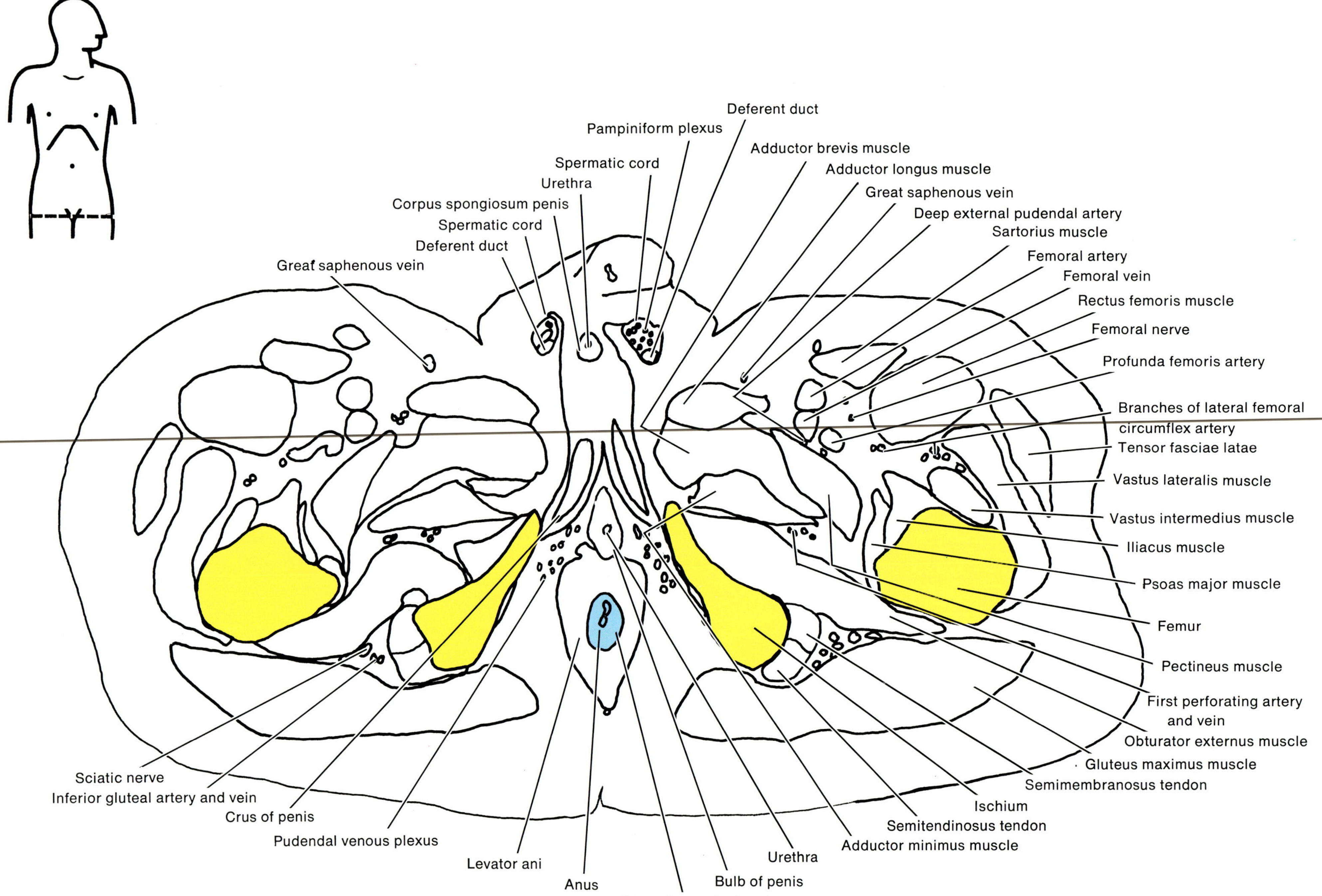
Deferent duct
Pampiniform plexus
Spermatic cord
Urethra
Corpus spongiosum penis
Spermatic cord
Deferent duct
Great saphenous vein
Adductor brevis muscle
Adductor longus muscle
Great saphenous vein
Deep external pudendal artery
Sartorius muscle
Femoral artery
Femoral vein
Rectus femoris muscle
Femoral nerve
Profunda femoris artery
Branches of lateral femoral circumflex artery
Tensor fasciae latae
Vastus lateralis muscle
Vastus intermedius muscle
Iliacus muscle
Psoas major muscle
Femur
Pectineus muscle
First perforating artery and vein
Obturator externus muscle
Gluteus maximus muscle
Semimembranosus tendon
Ischium
Semitendinosus tendon
Adductor minimus muscle
Urethra
Bulb of penis
Muscular coat of rectum
Anus
Levator ani
Pudendal venous plexus
Crus of penis
Inferior gluteal artery and vein
Sciatic nerve

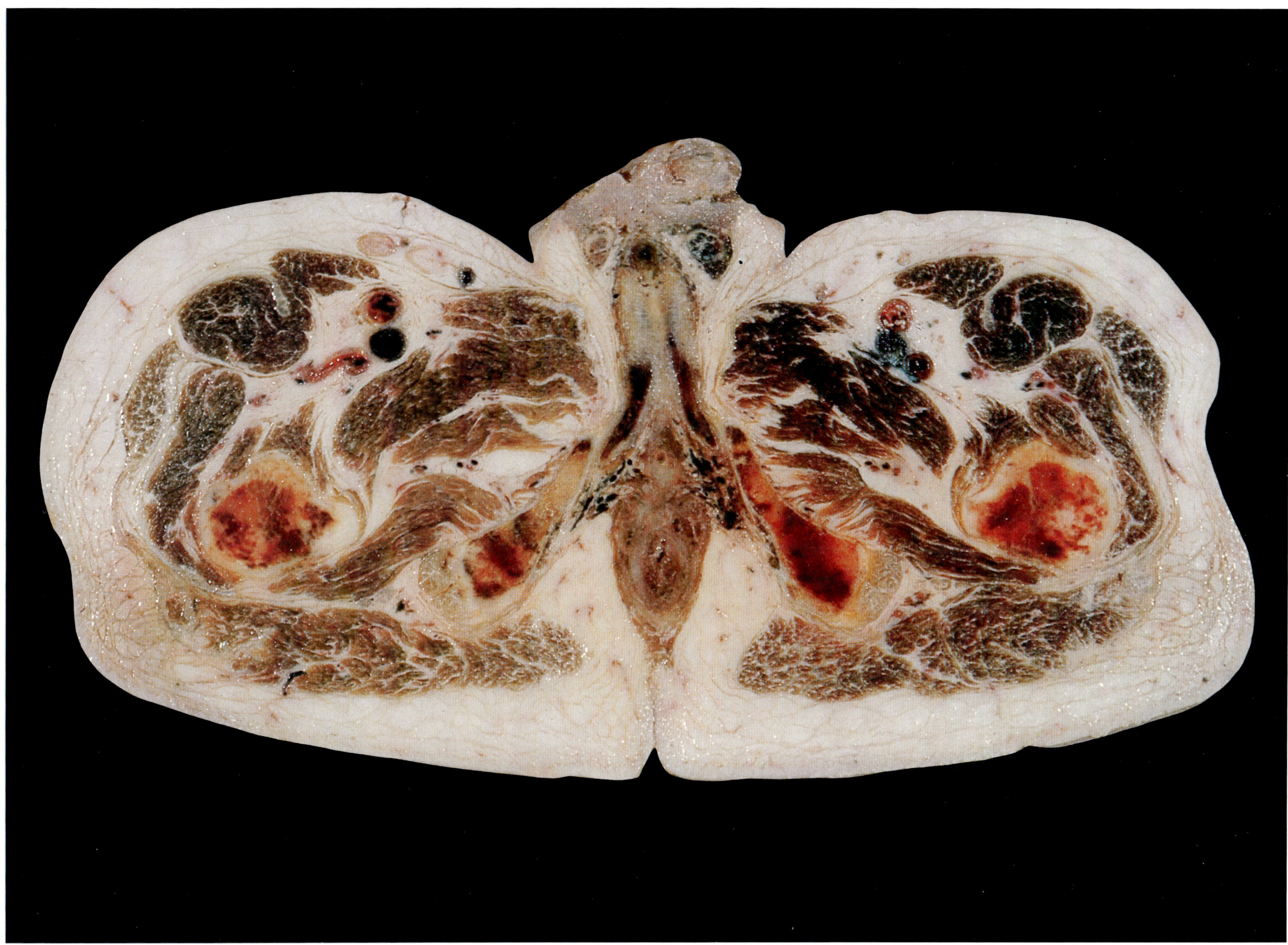

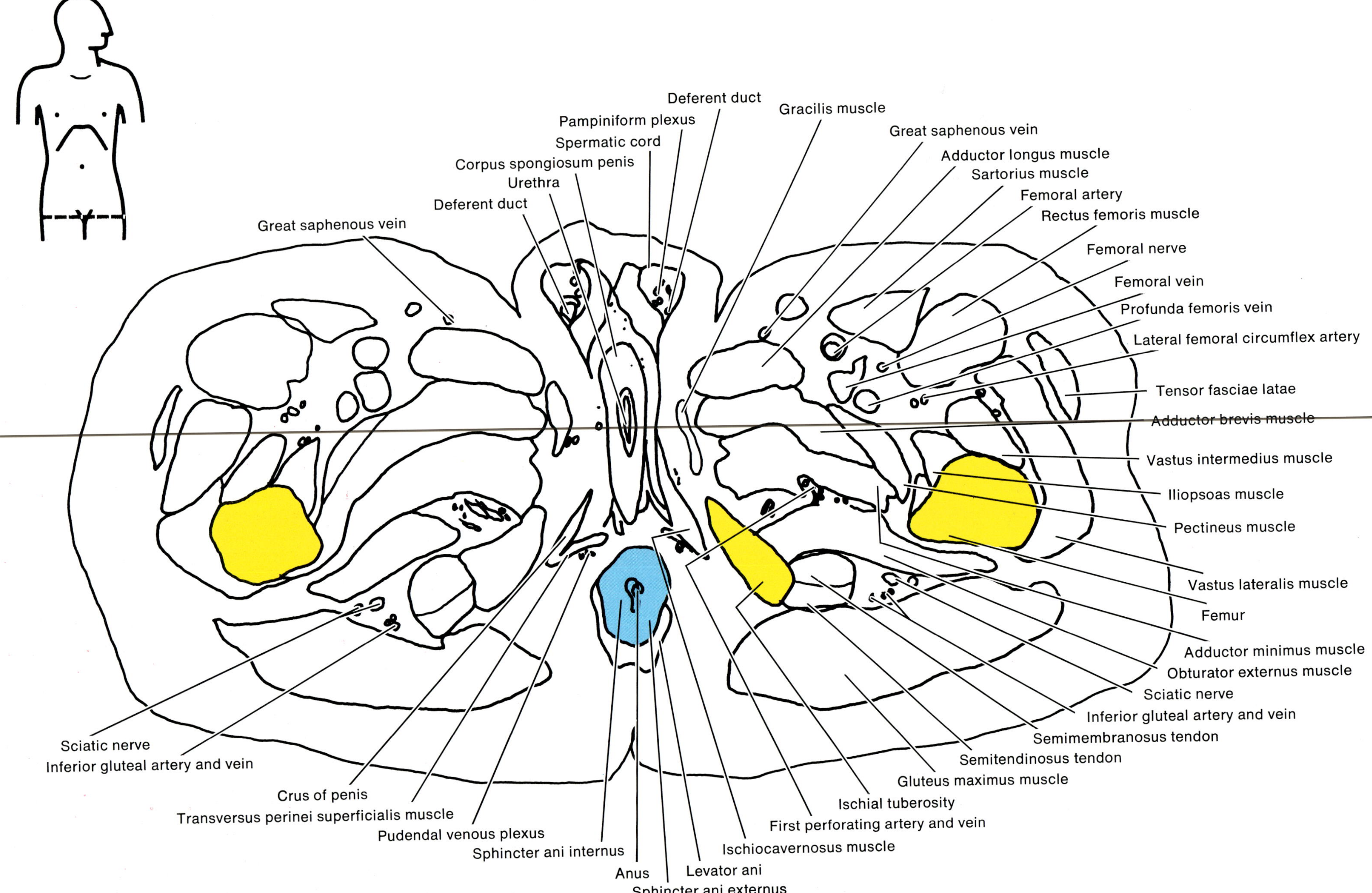

PLATE 62
Deferent duct
Pampiniform plexus
Gracilis muscle
Spermatic cord
Great saphenous vein
Corpus spongiosum penis
Adductor longus muscle
Urethra
Sartorius muscle
Deferent duct
Femoral artery
Rectus femoris muscle
Great saphenous vein
Femoral nerve
Femoral vein
Profunda femoris vein
Lateral femoral circumflex artery
Tensor fasciae latae
Adductor brevis muscle
Vastus intermedius muscle
Iliopsoas muscle
Pectineus muscle
Vastus lateralis muscle
Femur
Adductor minimus muscle
Obturator externus muscle
Sciatic nerve
Inferior gluteal artery and vein
Semimembranosus tendon
Semitendinosus tendon
Gluteus maximus muscle
Sciatic nerve
Inferior gluteal artery and vein
Ischial tuberosity
First perforating artery and vein
Crus of penis
Ischiocavernosus muscle
Transversus perinei superficialis muscle
Pudendal venous plexus
Sphincter ani internus
Levator ani
Anus
Sphincter ani externus

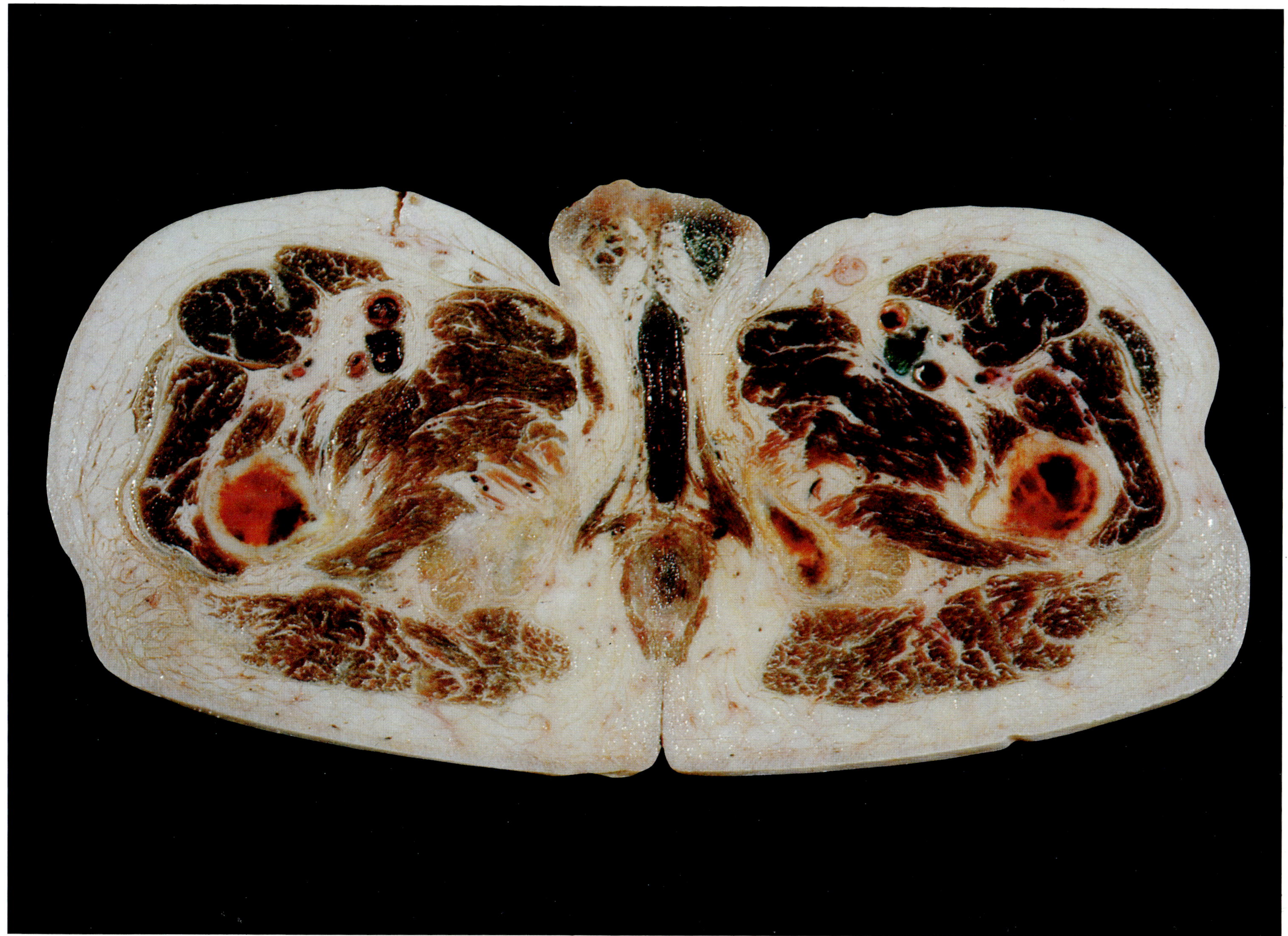

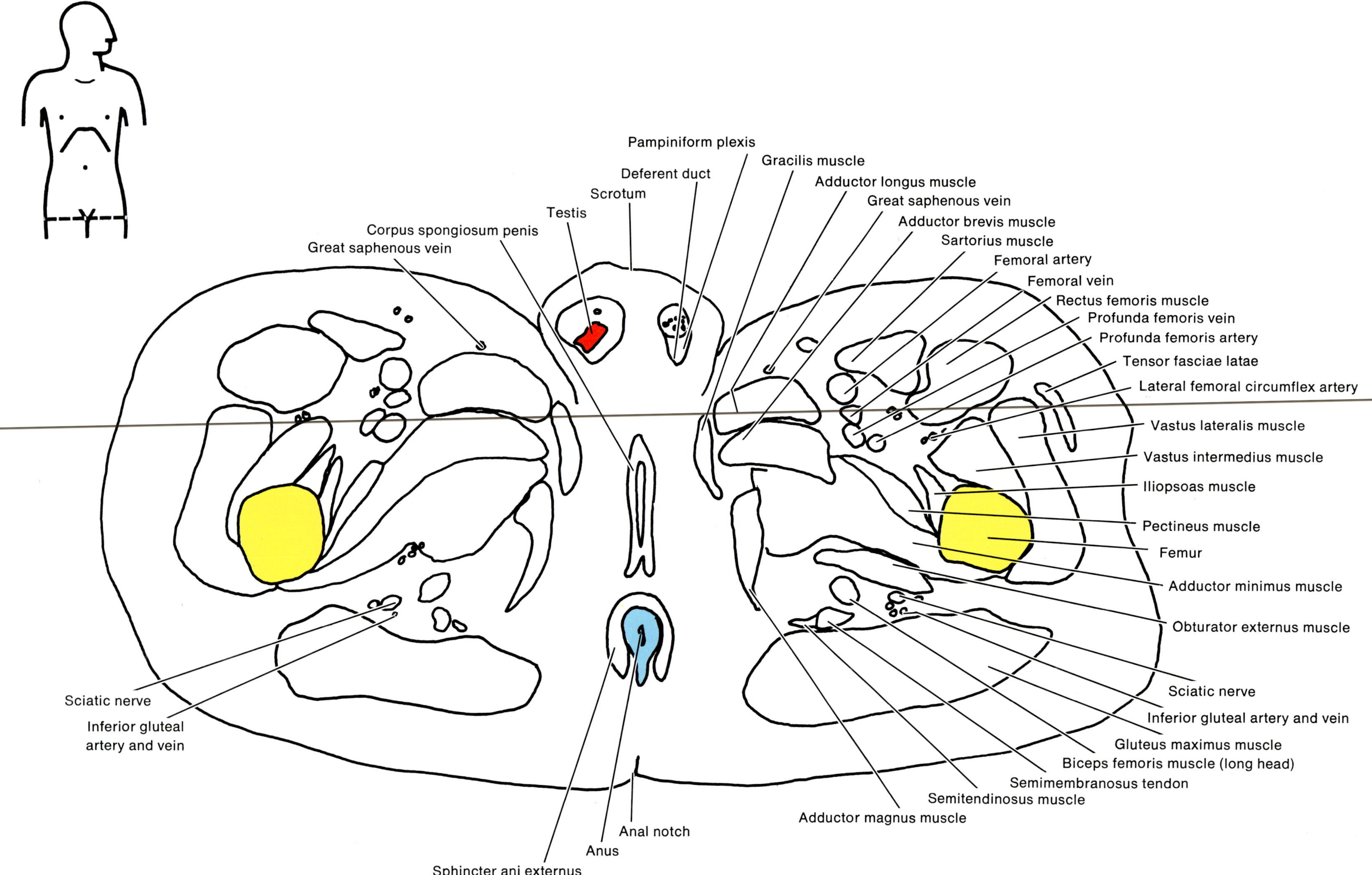

Pampiniform plexis
Deferent duct
Gracilis muscle
Adductor longus muscle
Great saphenous vein
Adductor brevis muscle
Sartorius muscle
Scrotum
Testis
Femoral artery
Corpus spongiosum penis
Femoral vein
Great saphenous vein
Rectus femoris muscle
Profunda femoris vein
Profunda femoris artery
Tensor fasciae latae
Lateral femoral circumflex artery
Vastus lateralis muscle
Vastus intermedius muscle
Iliopsoas muscle
Pectineus muscle
Femur
Adductor minimus muscle
Obturator externus muscle
Sciatic nerve
Inferior gluteal artery and vein
Sciatic nerve
Inferior gluteal
artery and vein
Gluteus maximus muscle
Biceps femoris muscle (long head)
Semimembranosus tendon
Semitendinosus muscle
Adductor magnus muscle
Anal notch
Anus
Sphincter ani externus

TRANSVERSE **Pelvis—male**

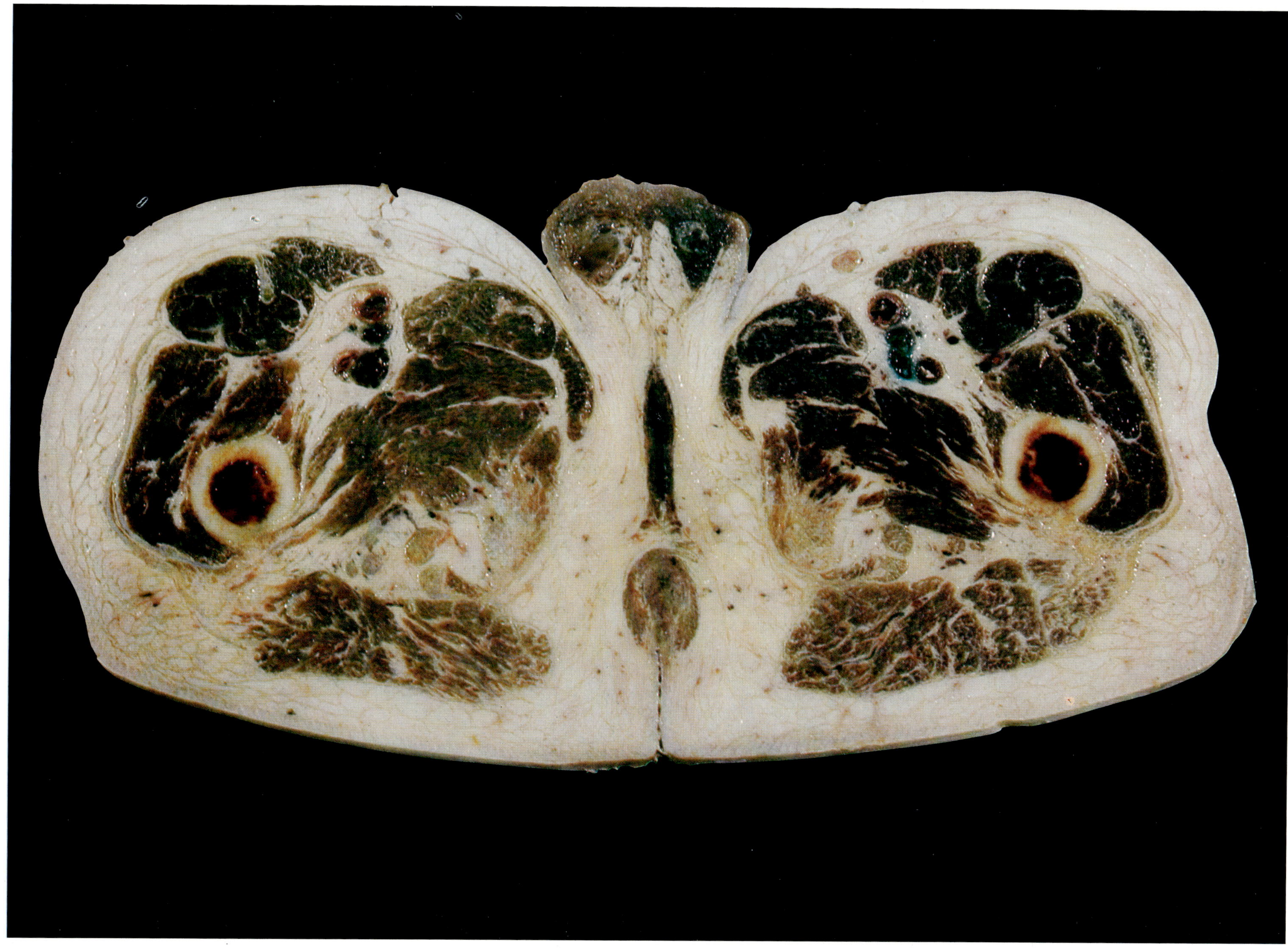

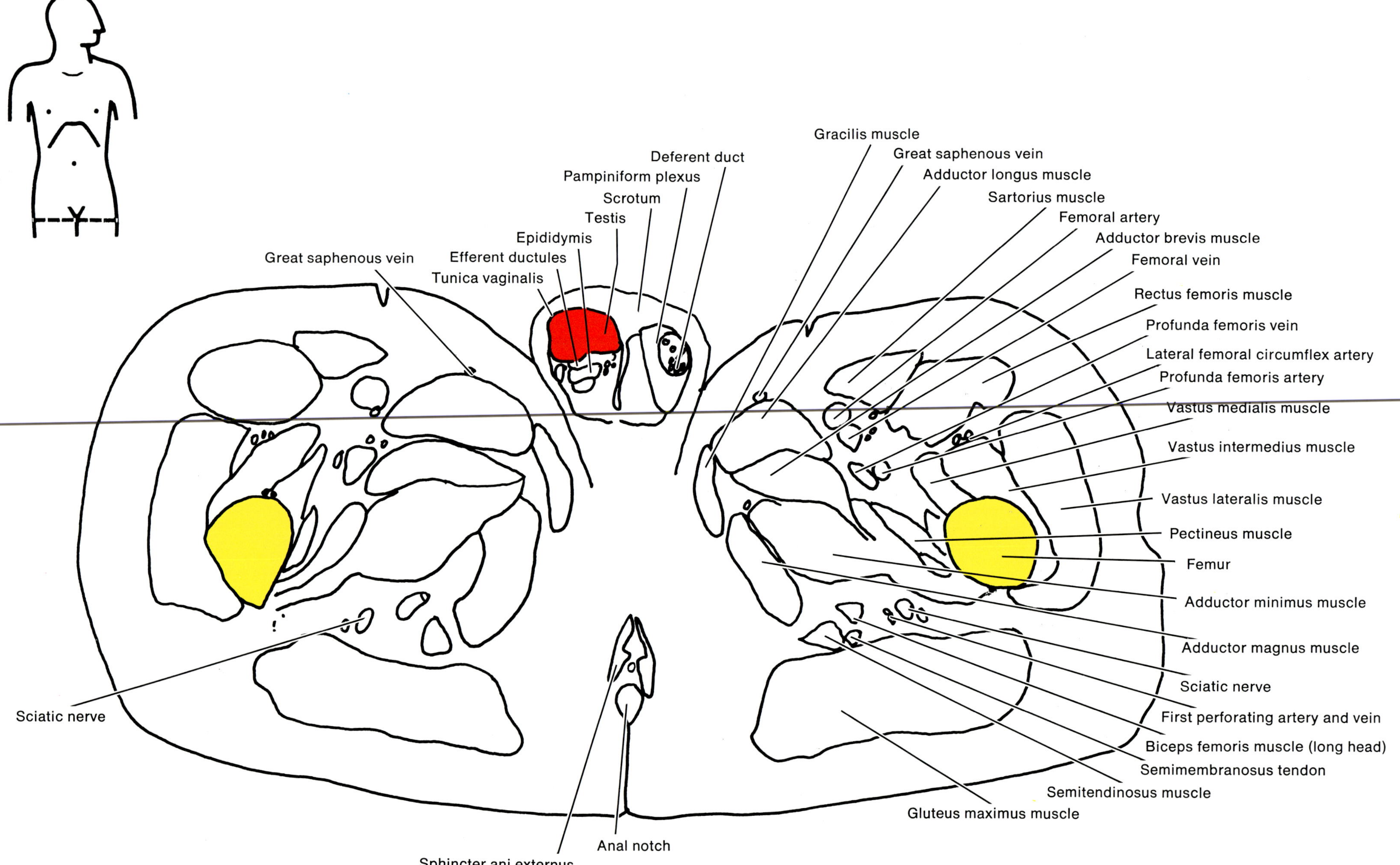

Gracilis muscle
Deferent duct
Great saphenous vein
Pampiniform plexus
Adductor longus muscle
Scrotum
Sartorius muscle
Testis
Femoral artery
Epididymis
Adductor brevis muscle
Efferent ductules
Femoral vein
Great saphenous vein
Tunica vaginalis
Rectus femoris muscle
Profunda femoris vein
Lateral femoral circumflex artery
Profunda femoris artery
Vastus medialis muscle
Vastus intermedius muscle
Vastus lateralis muscle
Pectineus muscle
Femur
Adductor minimus muscle
Adductor magnus muscle
Sciatic nerve
First perforating artery and vein
Biceps femoris muscle (long head)
Semimembranosus tendon
Semitendinosus muscle
Gluteus maximus muscle
Sciatic nerve
Anal notch
Sphincter ani externus

TRANSVERSE **Pelvis—male**

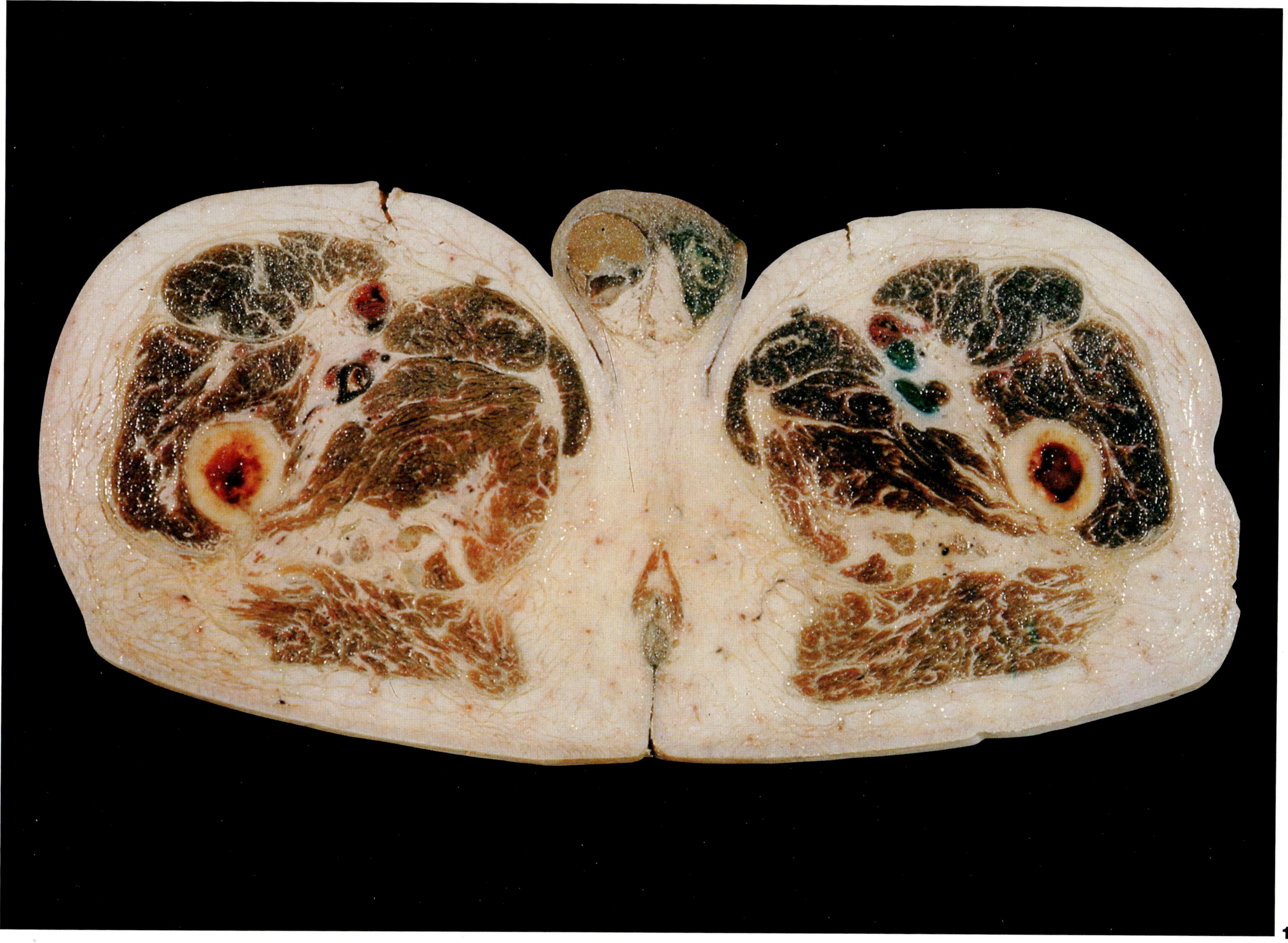

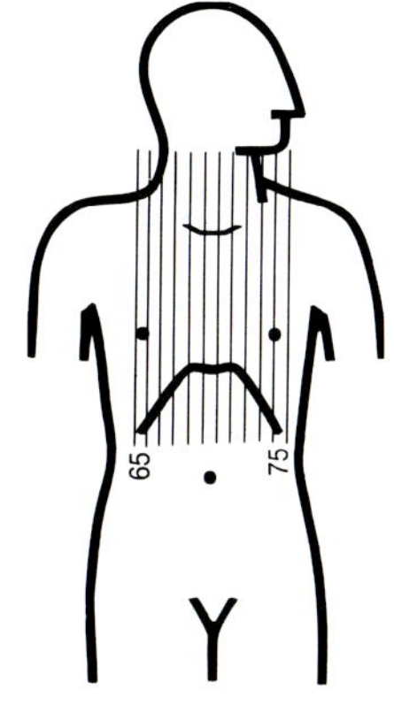

Chest

PLATES 65-75

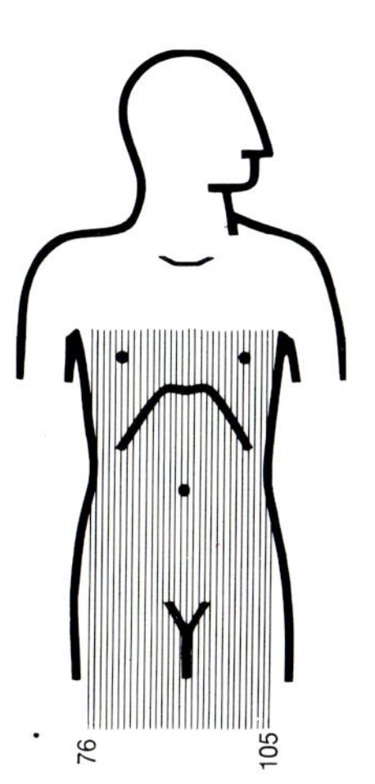

**Abdomen
and pelvis—
male**

PLATES 76-105

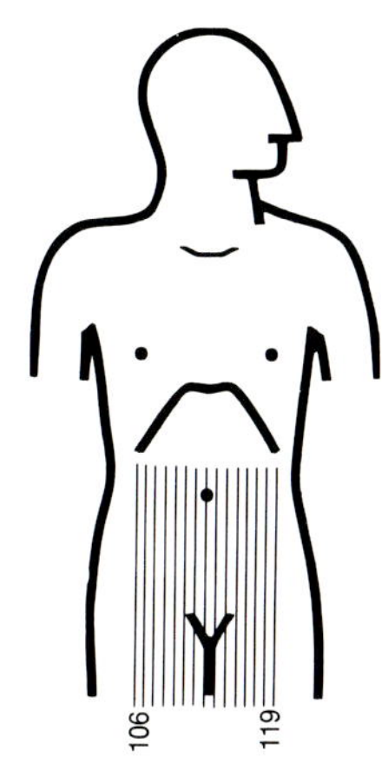

**Pelvis—
female**

PLATES 106-119

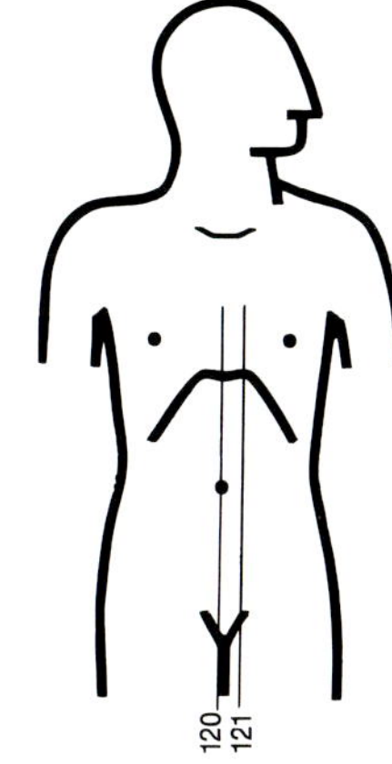

**Abdominal
aortic
aneurysm**

PLATES 120-121

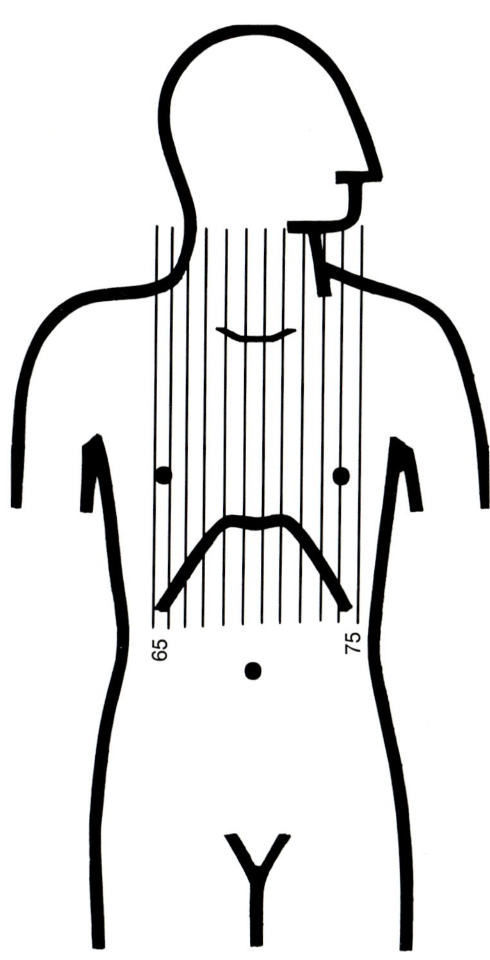
65
75

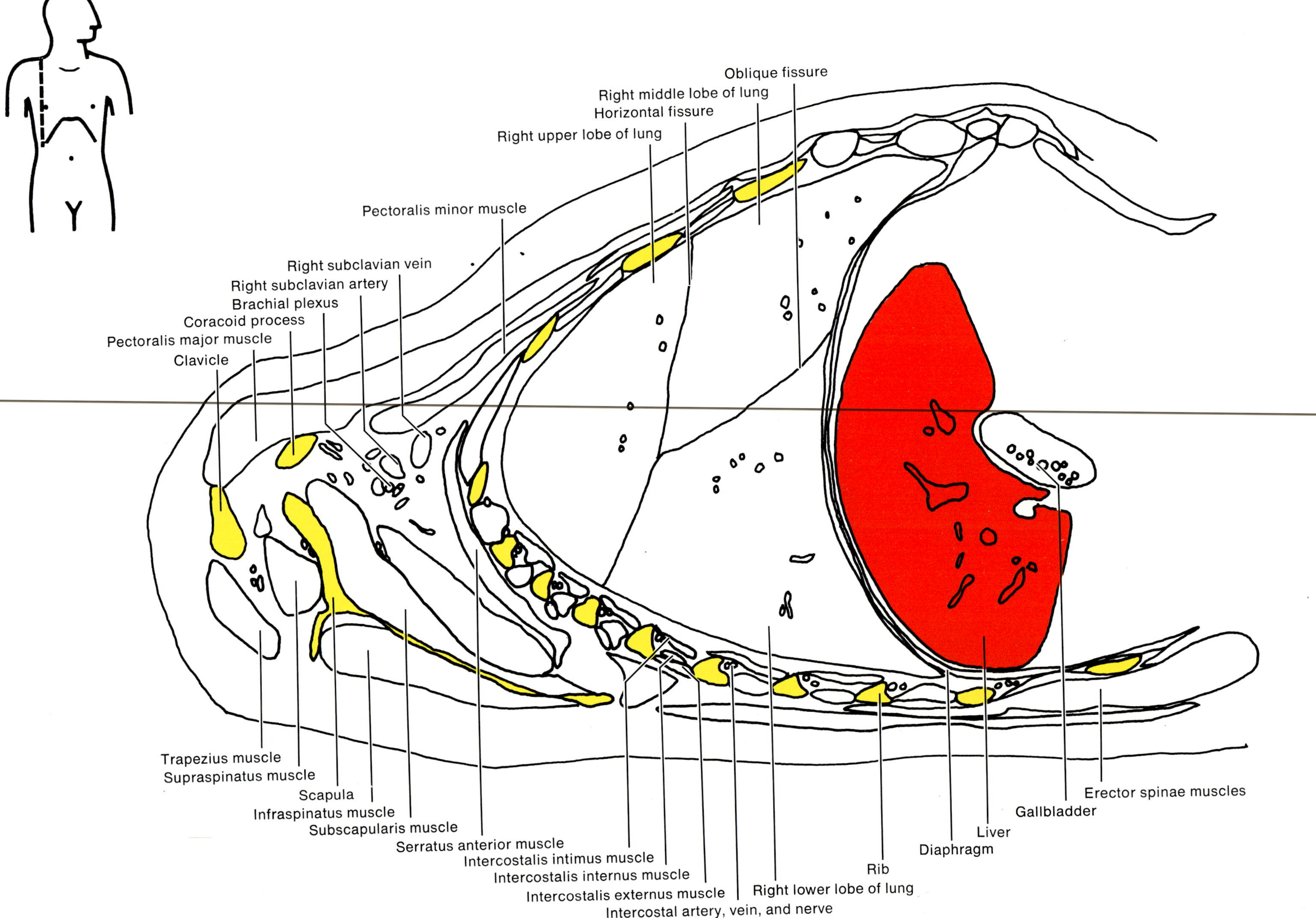
Oblique fissure
Right middle lobe of lung
Horizontal fissure
Right upper lobe of lung
Pectoralis minor muscle
Right subclavian vein
Right subclavian artery
Brachial plexus
Coracoid process
Pectoralis major muscle
Clavicle
Trapezius muscle
Supraspinatus muscle
Scapula
Infraspinatus muscle
Subscapularis muscle
Serratus anterior muscle
Intercostalis intimus muscle
Intercostalis internus muscle
Intercostalis externus muscle
Intercostal artery, vein, and nerve
Right lower lobe of lung
Rib
Diaphragm
Liver
Gallbladder
Erector spinae muscles

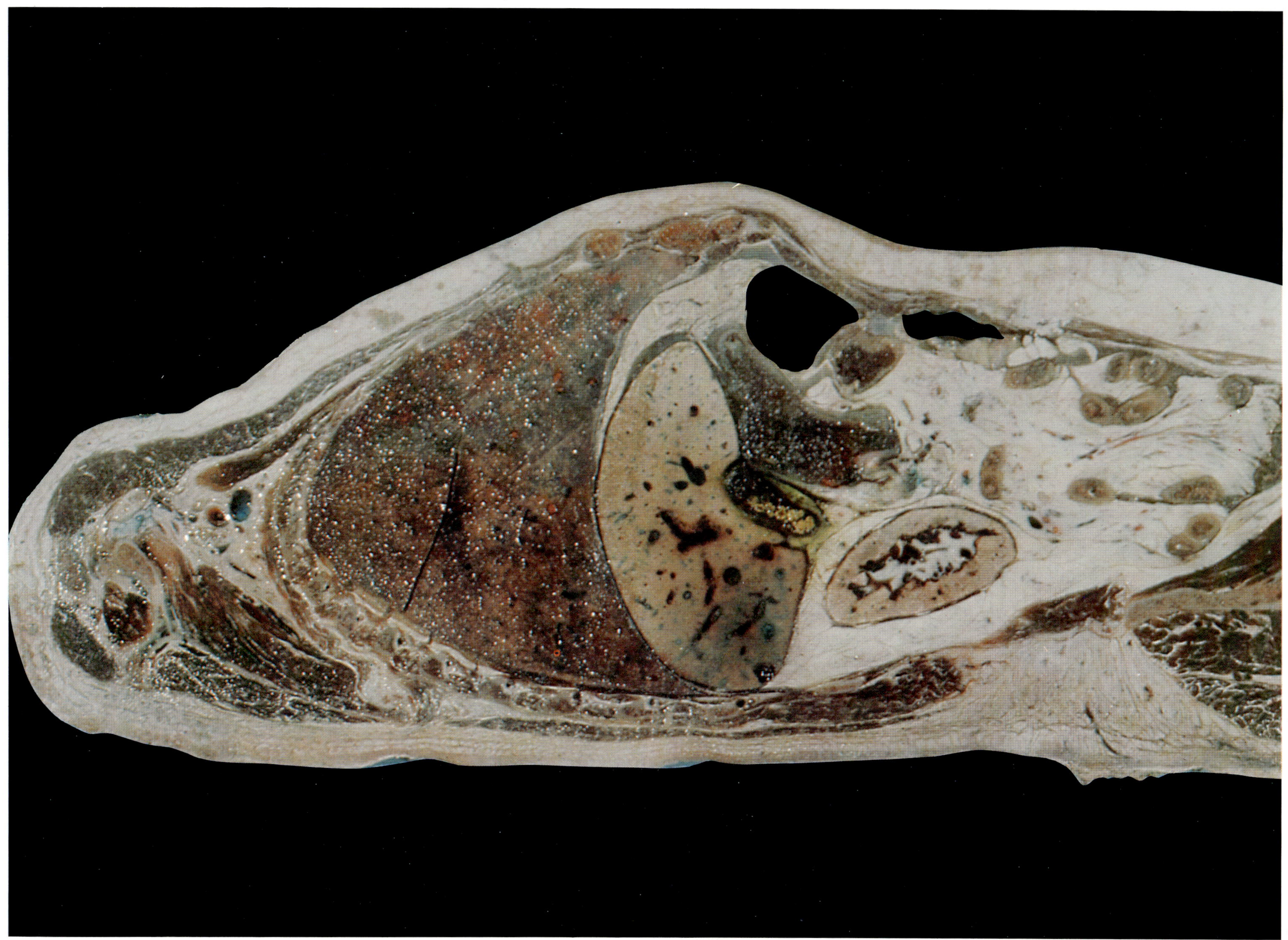

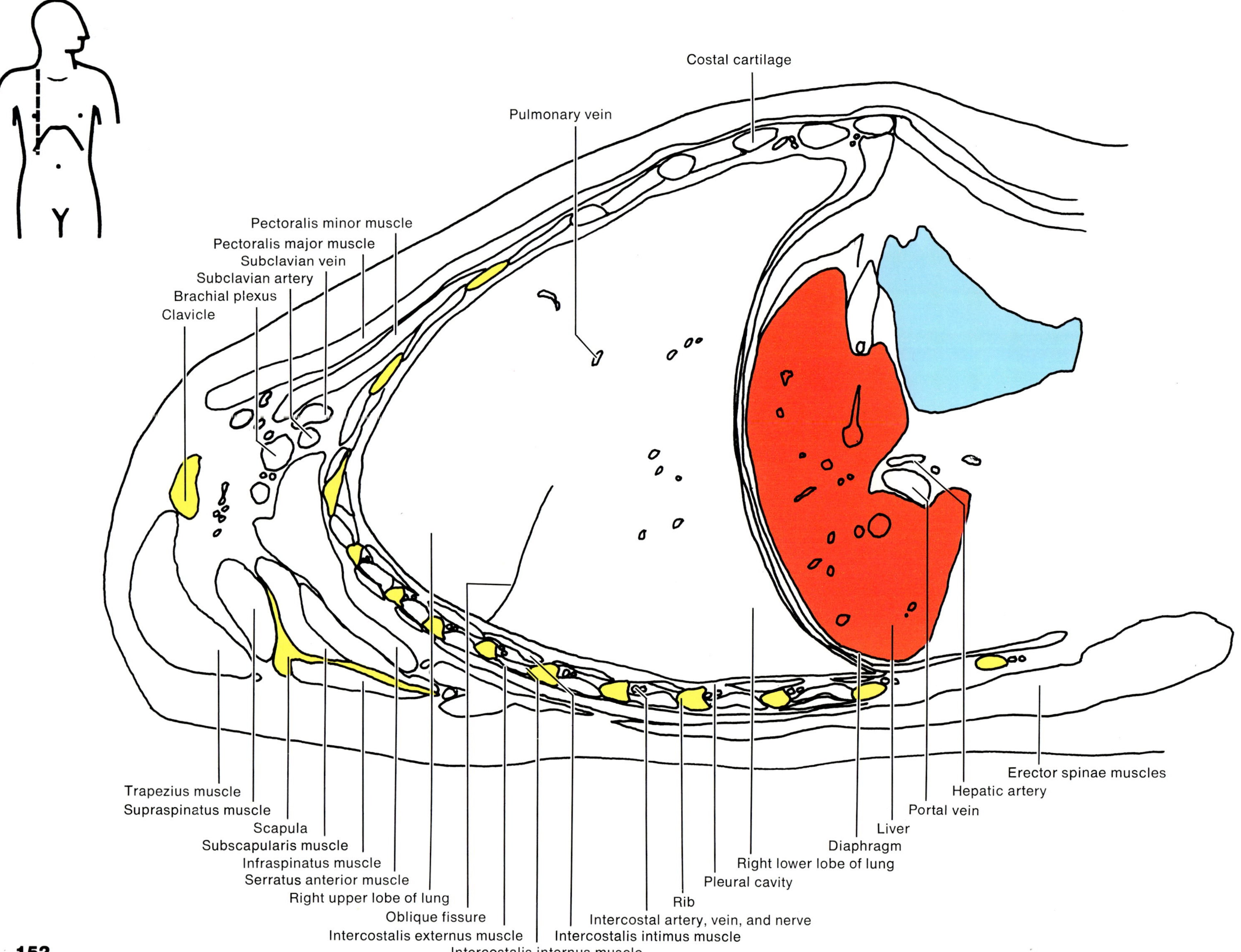
Costal cartilage
Pulmonary vein
Pectoralis minor muscle
Pectoralis major muscle
Subclavian vein
Subclavian artery
Brachial plexus
Clavicle
Erector spinae muscles
Hepatic artery
Portal vein
Liver
Diaphragm
Right lower lobe of lung
Pleural cavity
Rib
Intercostal artery, vein, and nerve
Intercostalis intimus muscle
Intercostalis internus muscle
Intercostalis externus muscle
Oblique fissure
Right upper lobe of lung
Serratus anterior muscle
Infraspinatus muscle
Subscapularis muscle
Scapula
Supraspinatus muscle
Trapezius muscle

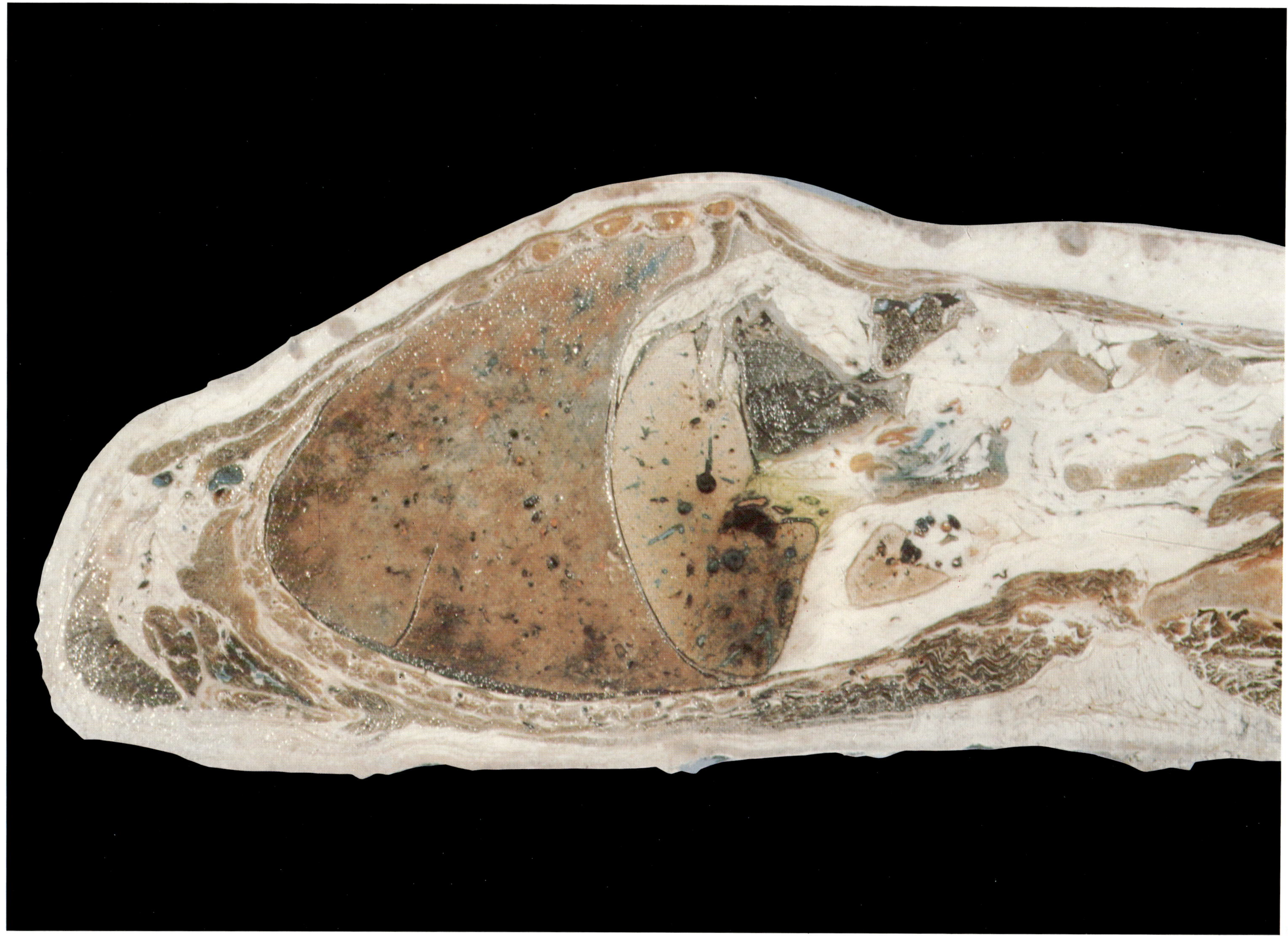

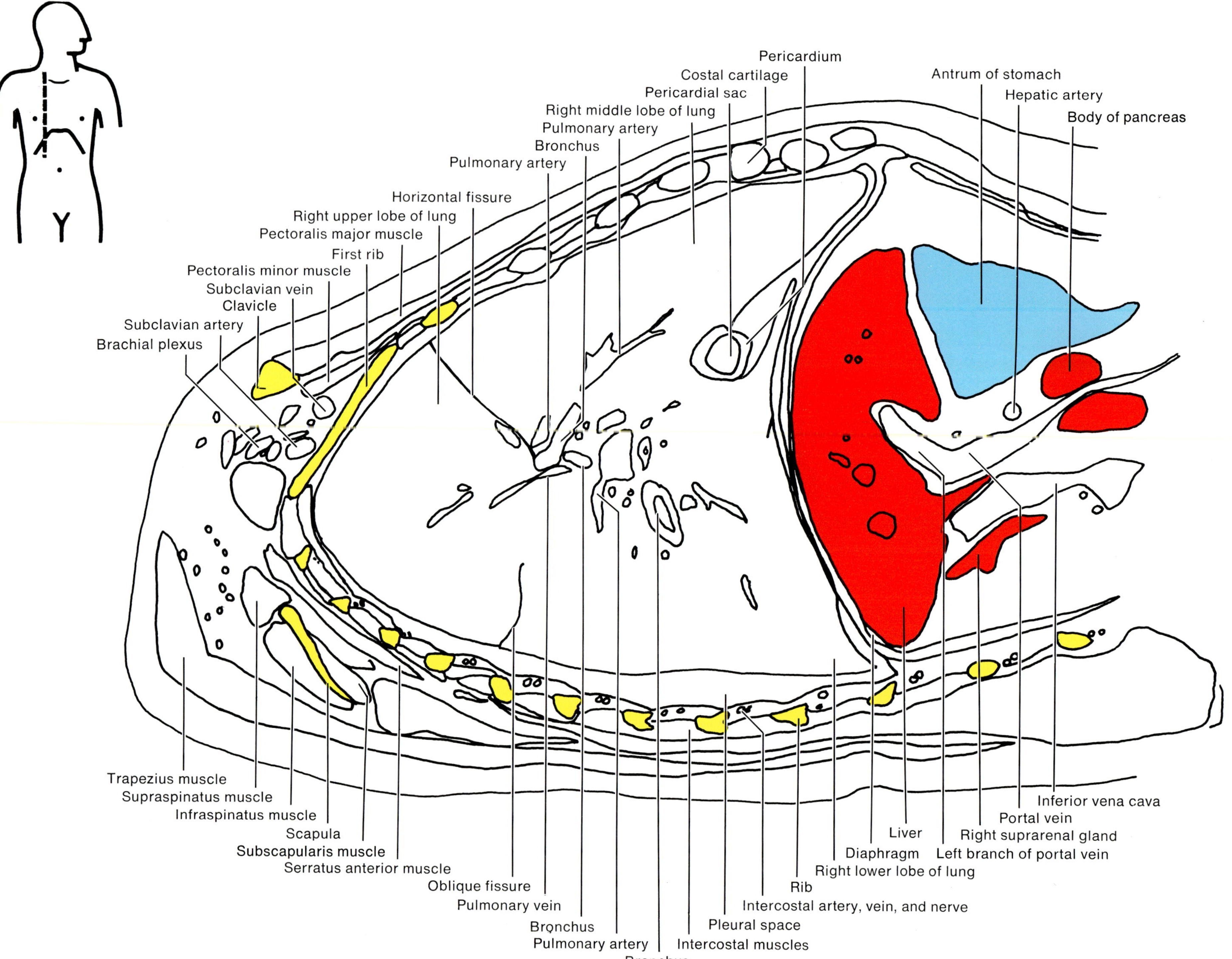
Pericardium
Costal cartilage
Pericardial sac
Right middle lobe of lung
Pulmonary artery
Bronchus
Pulmonary artery
Horizontal fissure
Right upper lobe of lung
Pectoralis major muscle
First rib
Pectoralis minor muscle
Subclavian vein
Clavicle
Subclavian artery
Brachial plexus
Antrum of stomach
Hepatic artery
Body of pancreas
Trapezius muscle
Supraspinatus muscle
Infraspinatus muscle
Scapula
Subscapularis muscle
Serratus anterior muscle
Oblique fissure
Pulmonary vein
Bronchus
Pulmonary artery
Bronchus
Intercostal muscles
Pleural space
Intercostal artery, vein, and nerve
Rib
Right lower lobe of lung
Diaphragm
Liver
Left branch of portal vein
Right suprarenal gland
Portal vein
Inferior vena cava

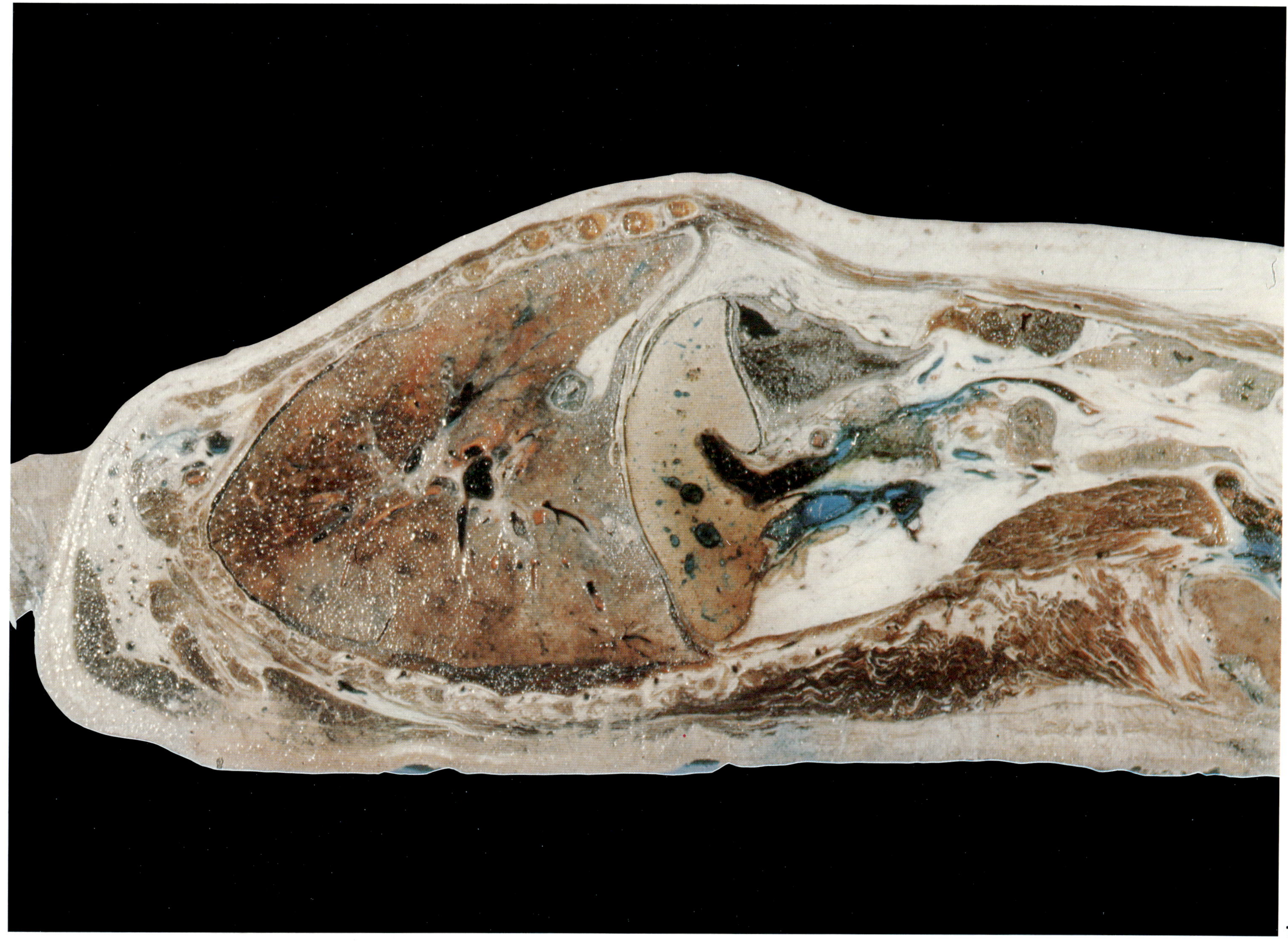

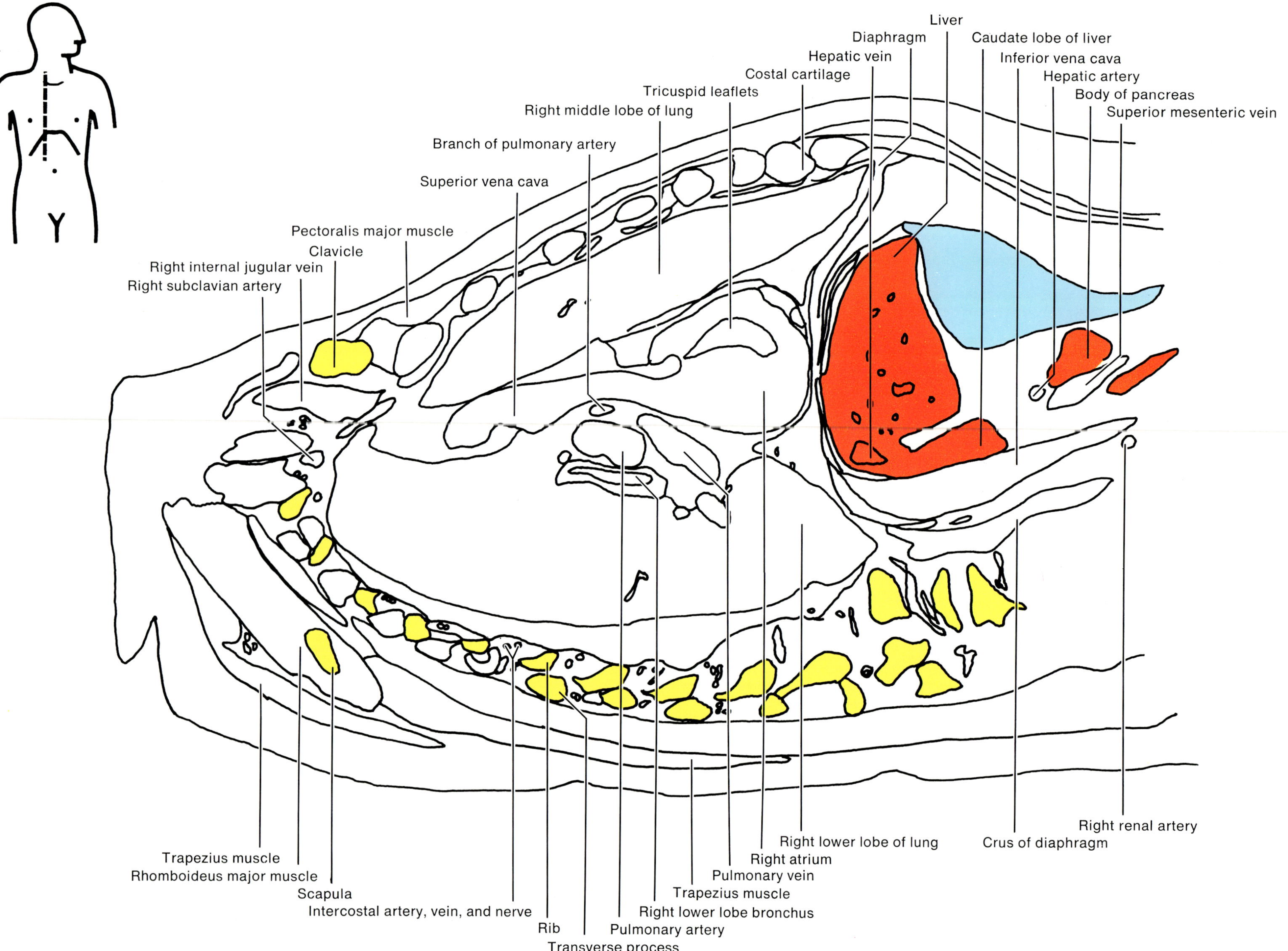

Liver
Diaphragm
Caudate lobe of liver
Hepatic vein
Inferior vena cava
Costal cartilage
Hepatic artery
Tricuspid leaflets
Body of pancreas
Right middle lobe of lung
Superior mesenteric vein
Branch of pulmonary artery
Superior vena cava
Pectoralis major muscle
Clavicle
Right internal jugular vein
Right subclavian artery
Right renal artery
Crus of diaphragm
Right lower lobe of lung
Right atrium
Pulmonary vein
Trapezius muscle
Right lower lobe bronchus
Trapezius muscle
Rhomboideus major muscle
Scapula
Intercostal artery, vein, and nerve
Rib
Pulmonary artery
Transverse process

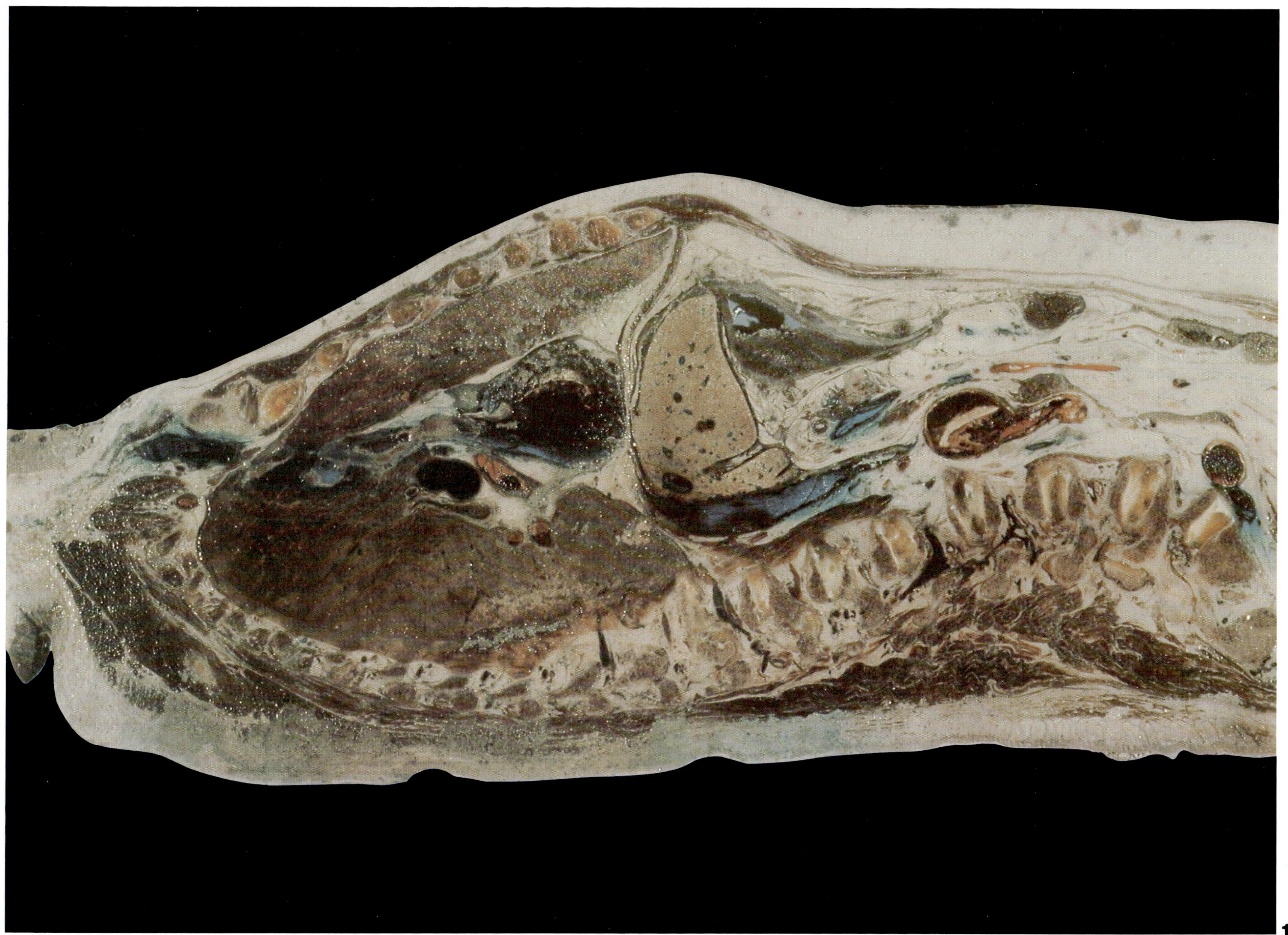

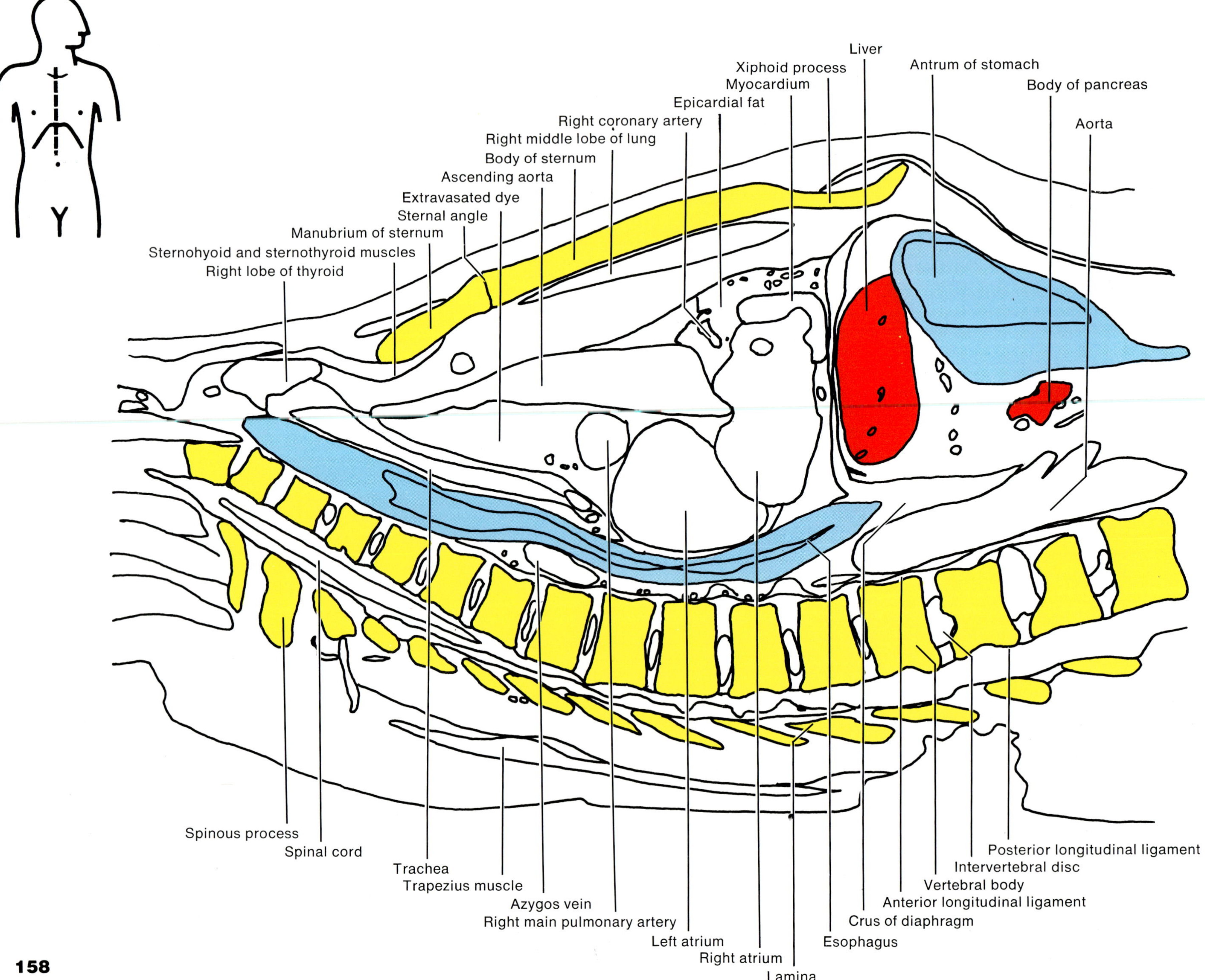

Liver
Xiphoid process
Antrum of stomach
Myocardium
Body of pancreas
Epicardial fat
Aorta
Right coronary artery
Right middle lobe of lung
Body of sternum
Ascending aorta
Extravasated dye
Sternal angle
Manubrium of sternum
Sternohyoid and sternothyroid muscles
Right lobe of thyroid
Spinous process
Spinal cord
Trachea
Trapezius muscle
Azygos vein
Right main pulmonary artery
Left atrium
Right atrium
Lamina
Esophagus
Crus of diaphragm
Anterior longitudinal ligament
Vertebral body
Intervertebral disc
Posterior longitudinal ligament

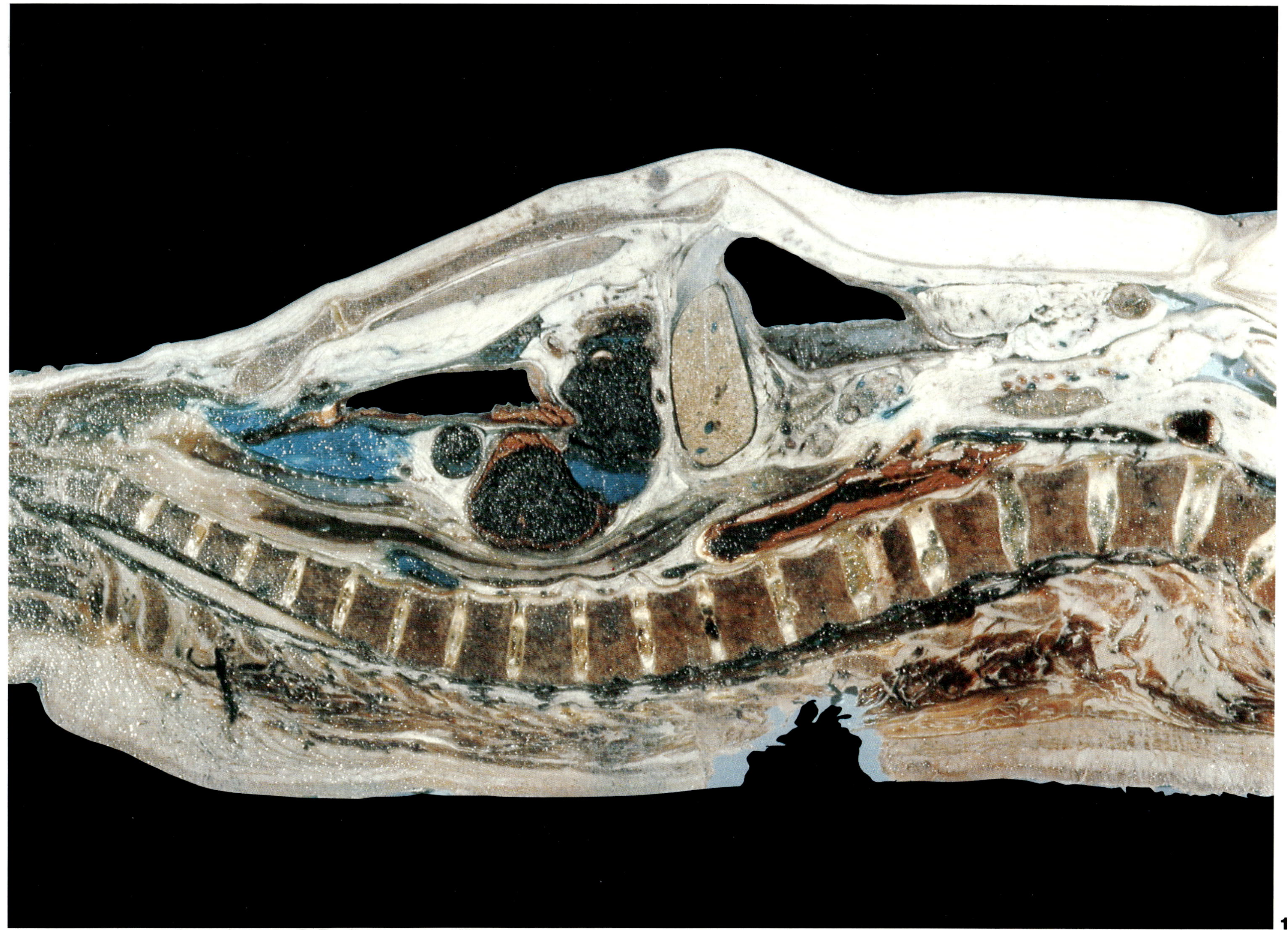

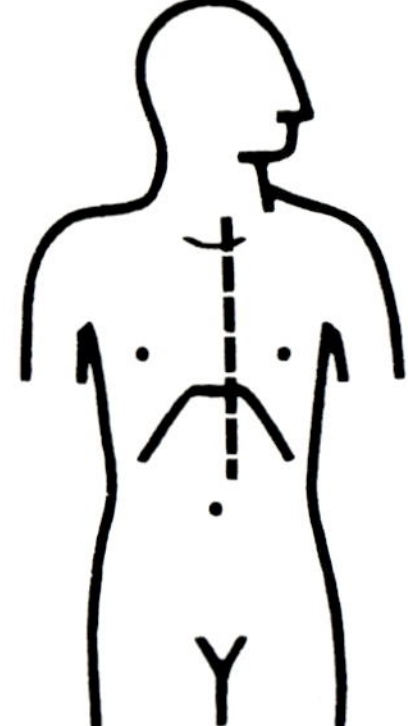

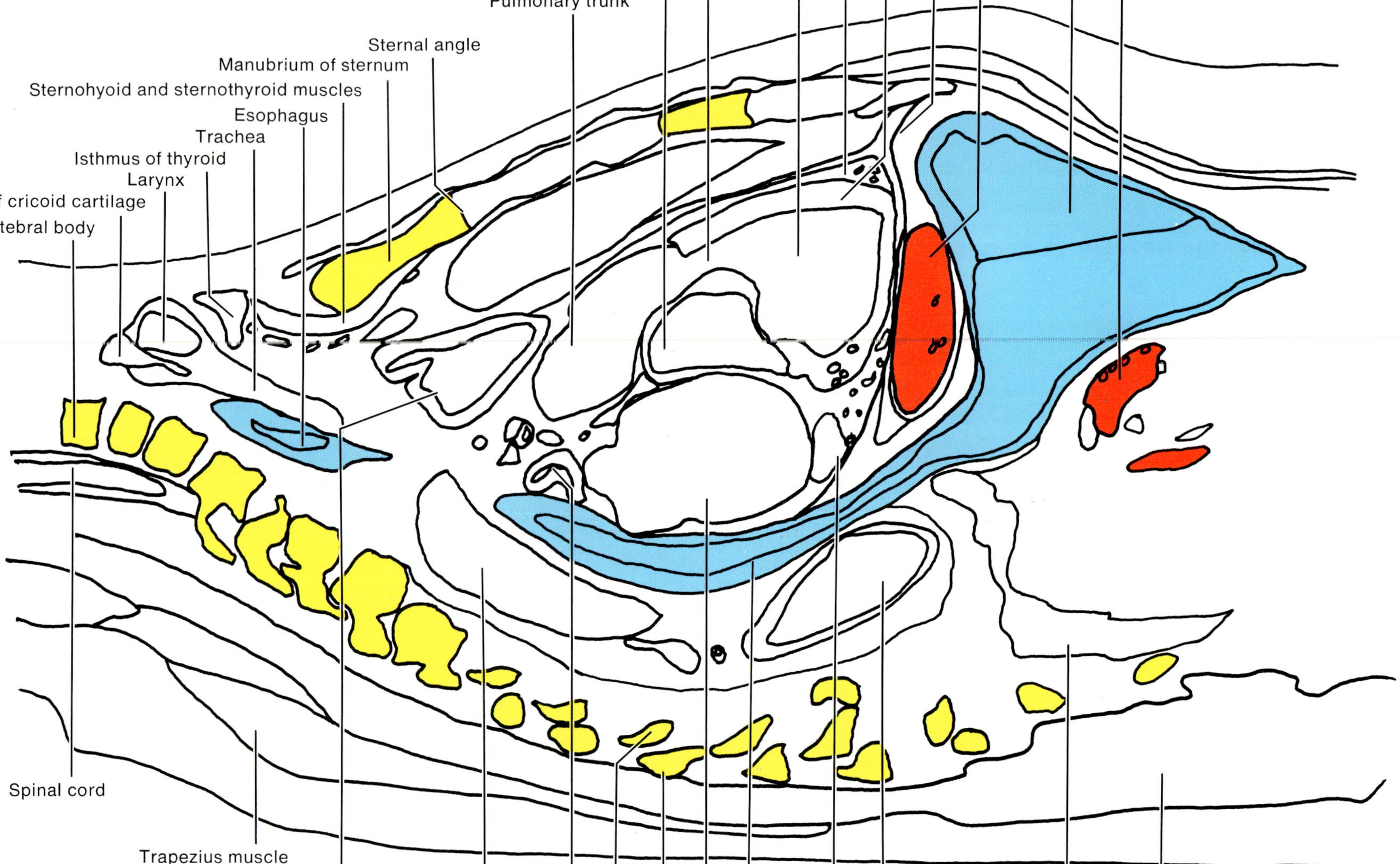

Diaphragm
Myocardium
Left lobe of liver
Epicardial fat
Fundus of stomach
Right ventricle
Body of pancreas
Pulmonary outflow tract
Ascending aorta
Pulmonary trunk
Sternal angle
Manubrium of sternum
Sternohyoid and sternothyroid muscles
Esophagus
Trachea
Isthmus of thyroid
Larynx
Lamina of cricoid cartilage
Vertebral body
Spinal cord
Trapezius muscle
Aortic arch
Aorta
Left principal bronchus
Rib
Transverse process
Left atrium
Esophagus
Coronary sinus
Aorta
Diaphragm
Erector spinae muscles

PARASAGITTAL **Chest**

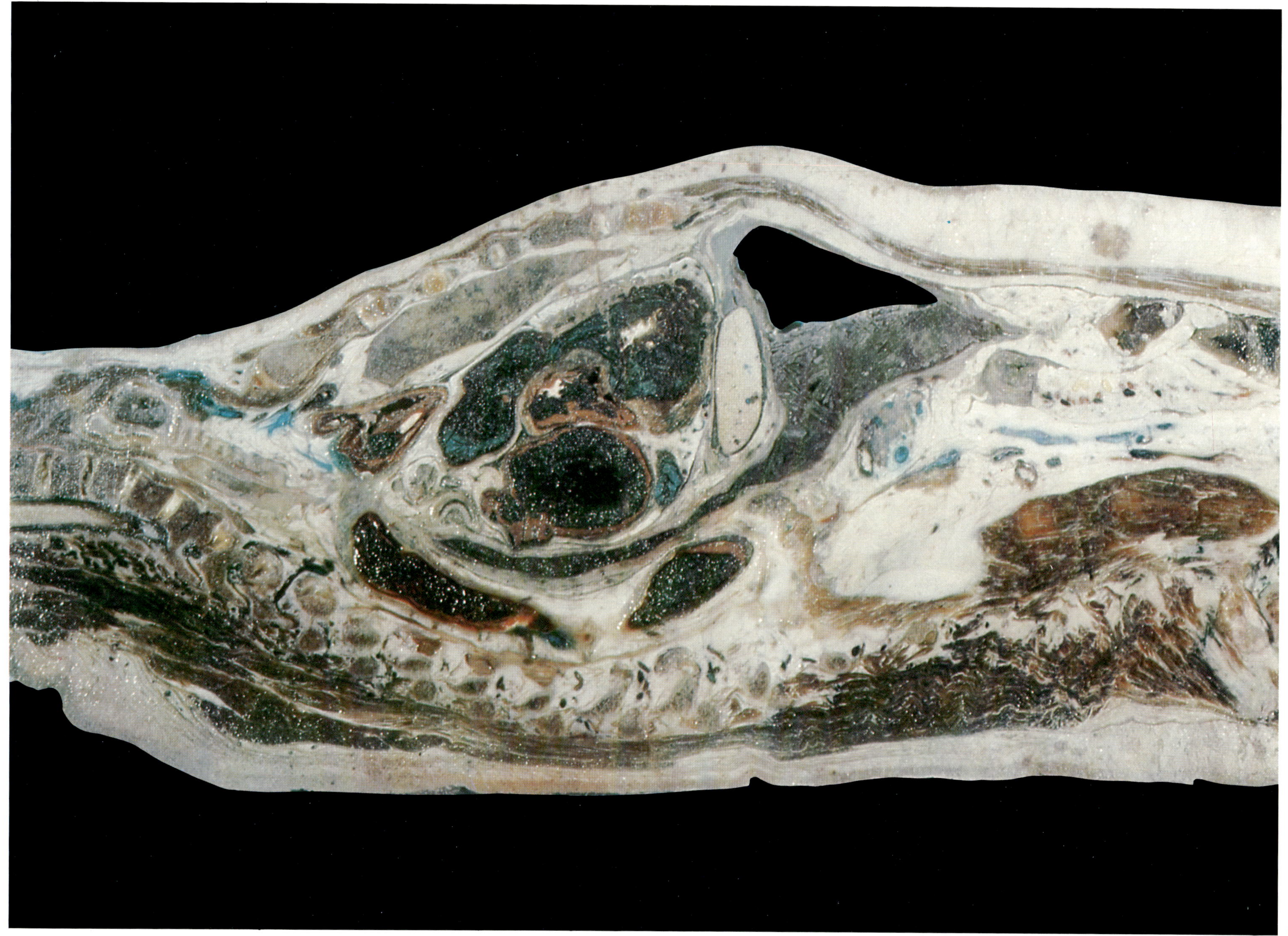

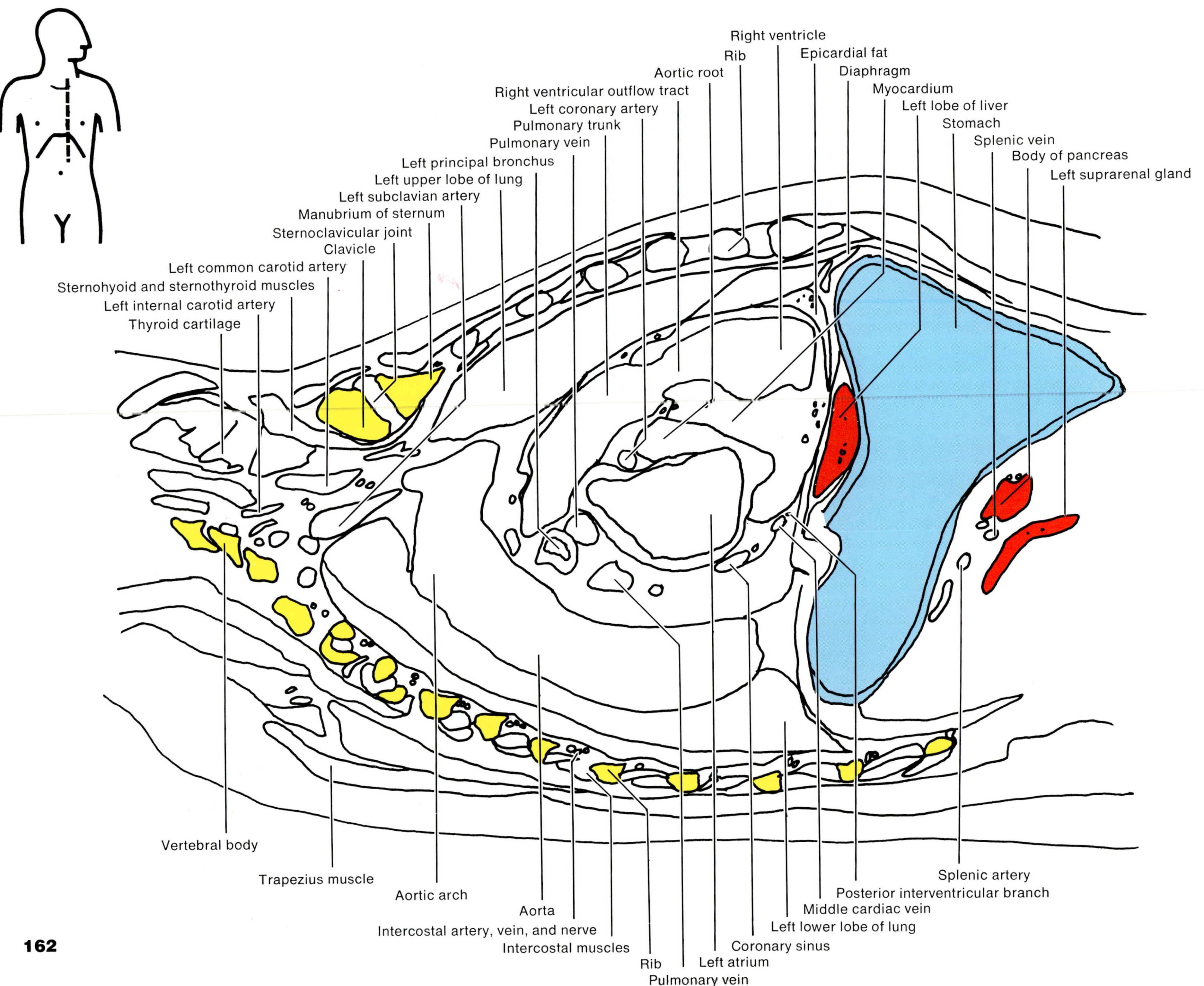

Right ventricle
Rib
Epicardial fat
Aortic root
Diaphragm
Right ventricular outflow tract
Myocardium
Left coronary artery
Left lobe of liver
Pulmonary trunk
Stomach
Pulmonary vein
Splenic vein
Left principal bronchus
Body of pancreas
Left upper lobe of lung
Left suprarenal gland
Left subclavian artery
Manubrium of sternum
Sternoclavicular joint
Clavicle
Left common carotid artery
Sternohyoid and sternothyroid muscles
Left internal carotid artery
Thyroid cartilage
Vertebral body
Trapezius muscle
Aortic arch
Aorta
Intercostal artery, vein, and nerve
Intercostal muscles
Rib
Pulmonary vein
Left atrium
Coronary sinus
Left lower lobe of lung
Middle cardiac vein
Posterior interventricular branch
Splenic artery

PARASAGITTAL **Chest**

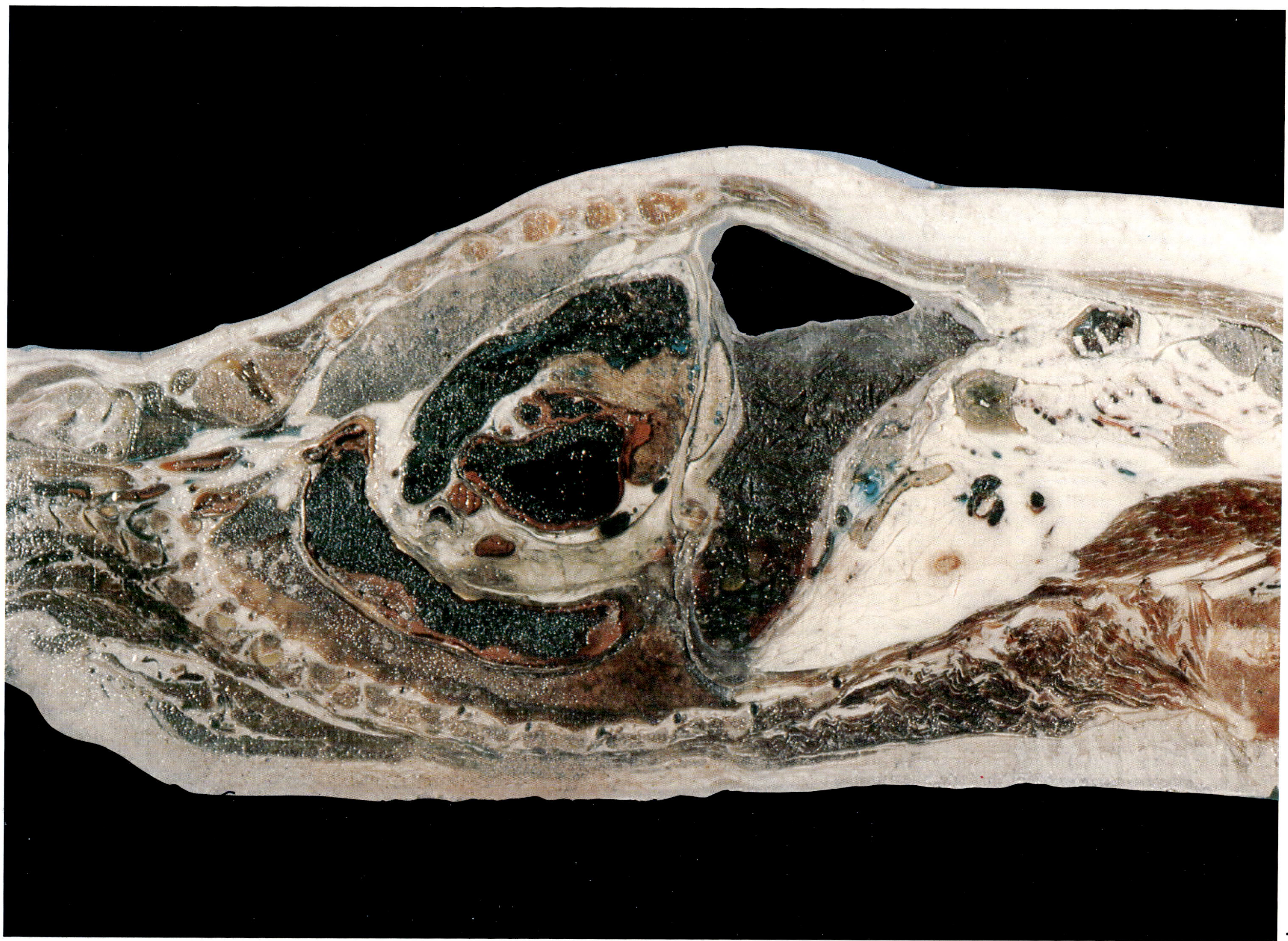

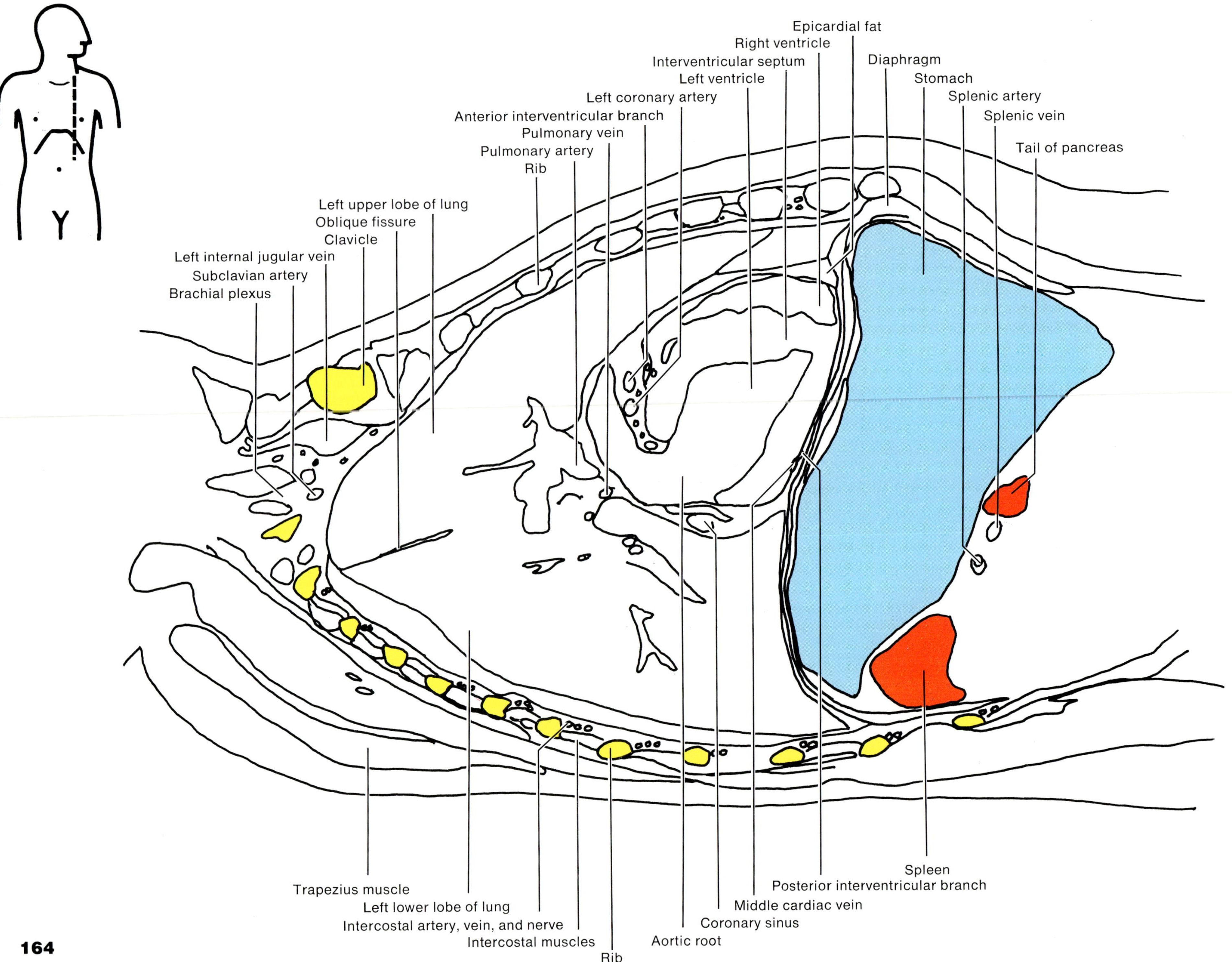
Epicardial fat
Right ventricle
Interventricular septum
Diaphragm
Left ventricle
Stomach
Left coronary artery
Splenic artery
Anterior interventricular branch
Splenic vein
Pulmonary vein
Tail of pancreas
Pulmonary artery
Rib
Left upper lobe of lung
Oblique fissure
Clavicle
Left internal jugular vein
Subclavian artery
Brachial plexus
Trapezius muscle
Spleen
Left lower lobe of lung
Posterior interventricular branch
Intercostal artery, vein, and nerve
Middle cardiac vein
Intercostal muscles
Coronary sinus
Rib
Aortic root

PARASAGITTAL **Chest**

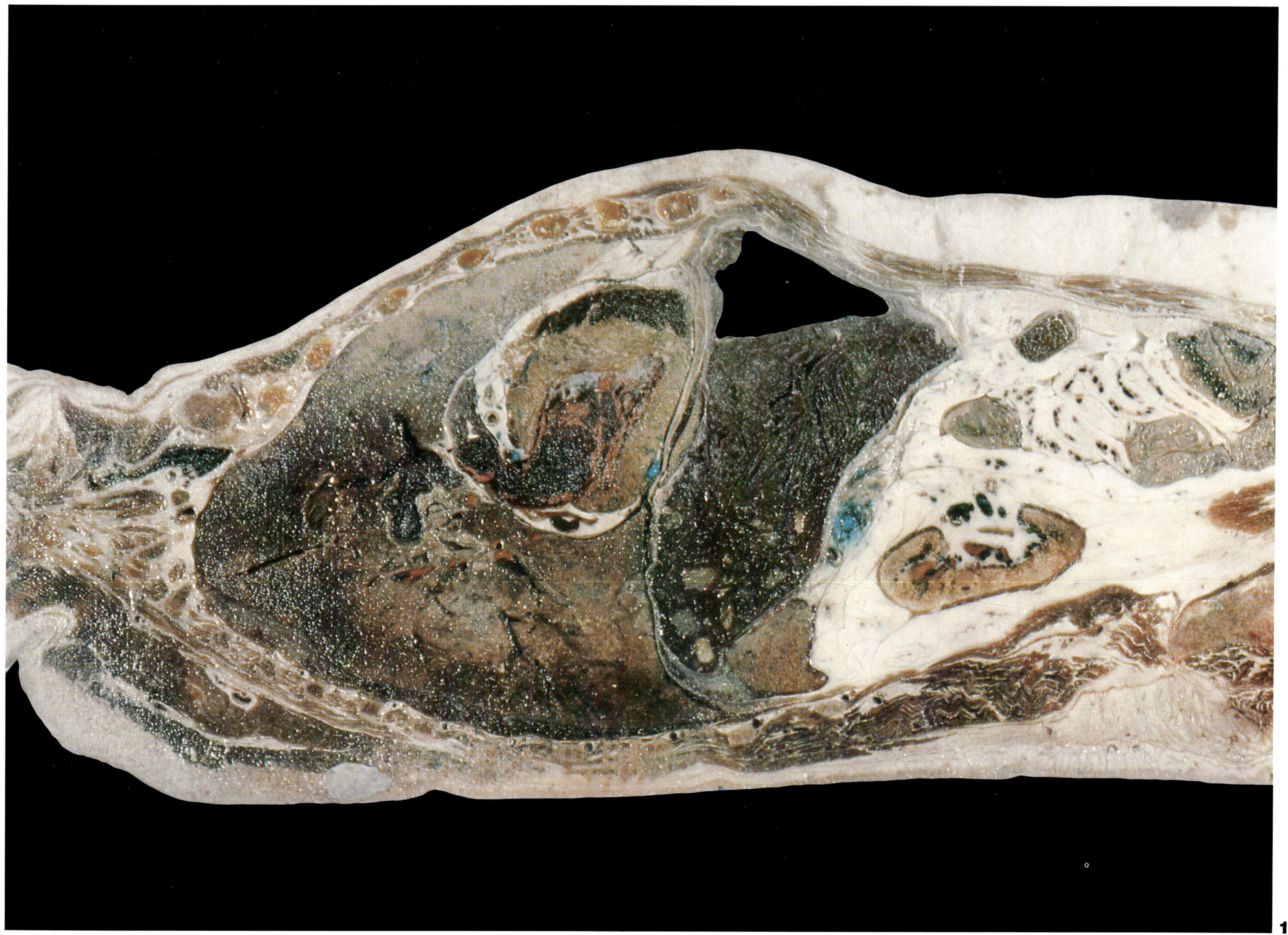

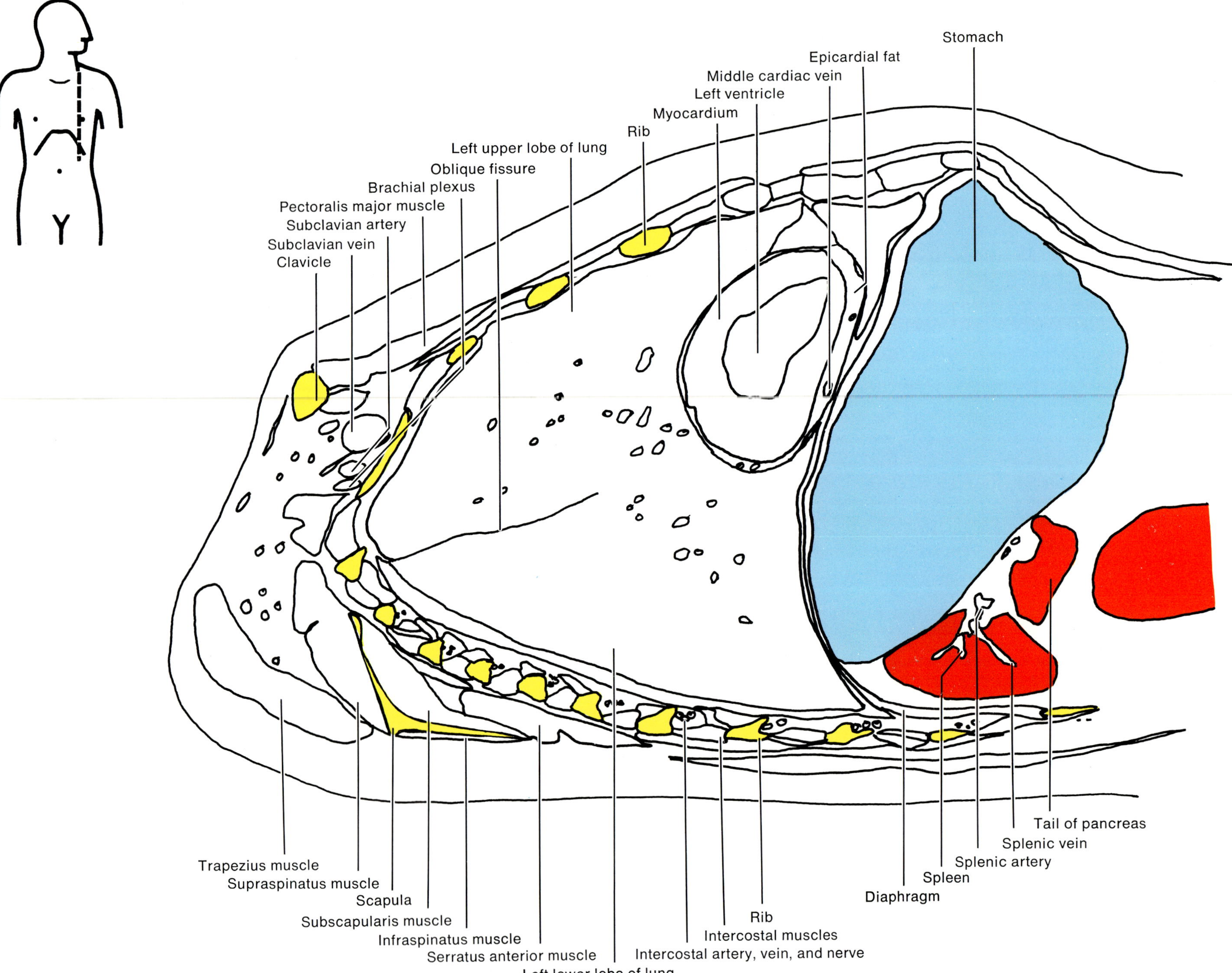
Stomach
Epicardial fat
Middle cardiac vein
Left ventricle
Myocardium
Rib
Left upper lobe of lung
Oblique fissure
Brachial plexus
Pectoralis major muscle
Subclavian artery
Subclavian vein
Clavicle
Tail of pancreas
Splenic vein
Splenic artery
Spleen
Diaphragm
Trapezius muscle
Supraspinatus muscle
Scapula
Subscapularis muscle
Infraspinatus muscle
Serratus anterior muscle
Left lower lobe of lung
Rib
Intercostal muscles
Intercostal artery, vein, and nerve

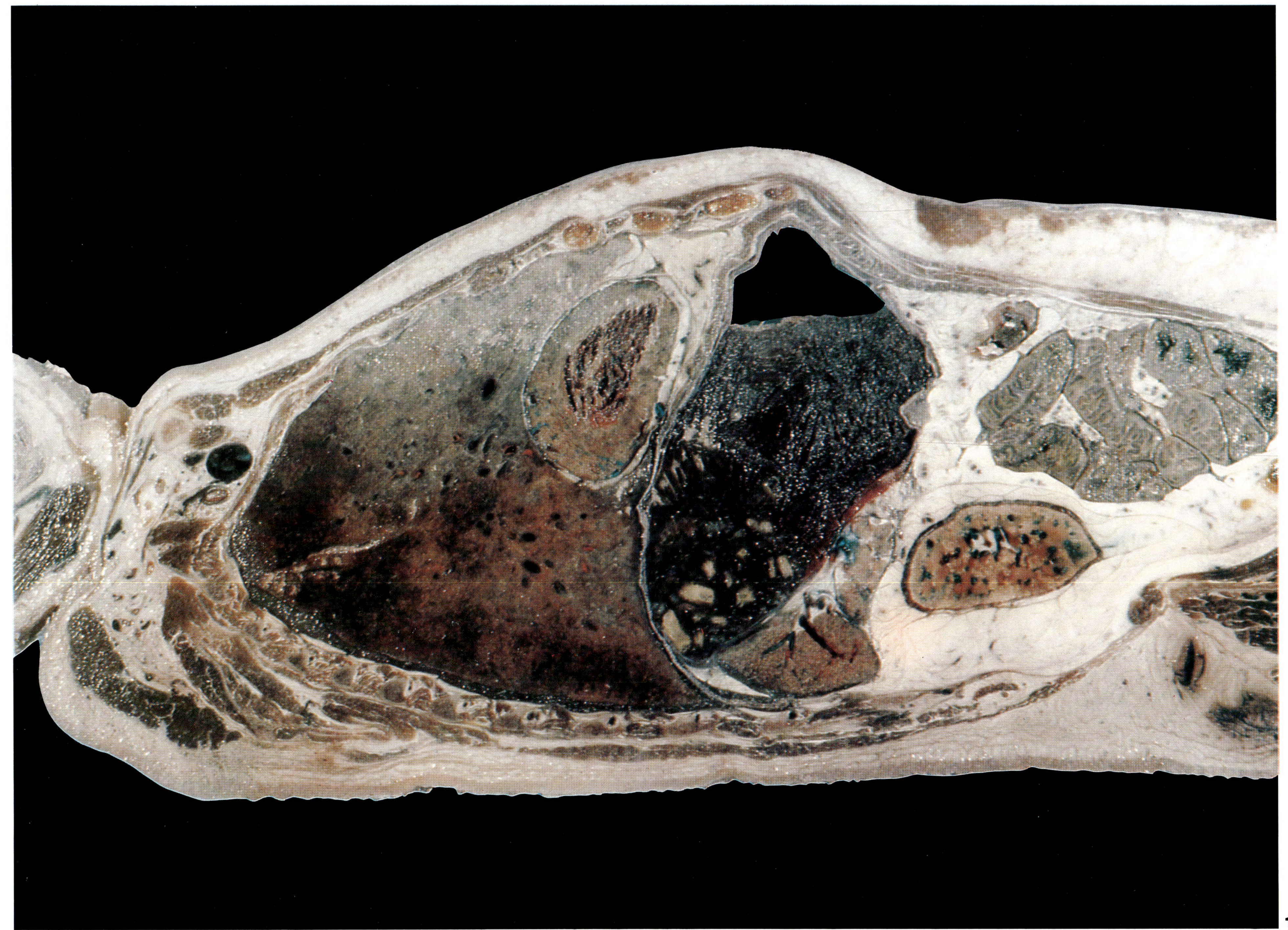

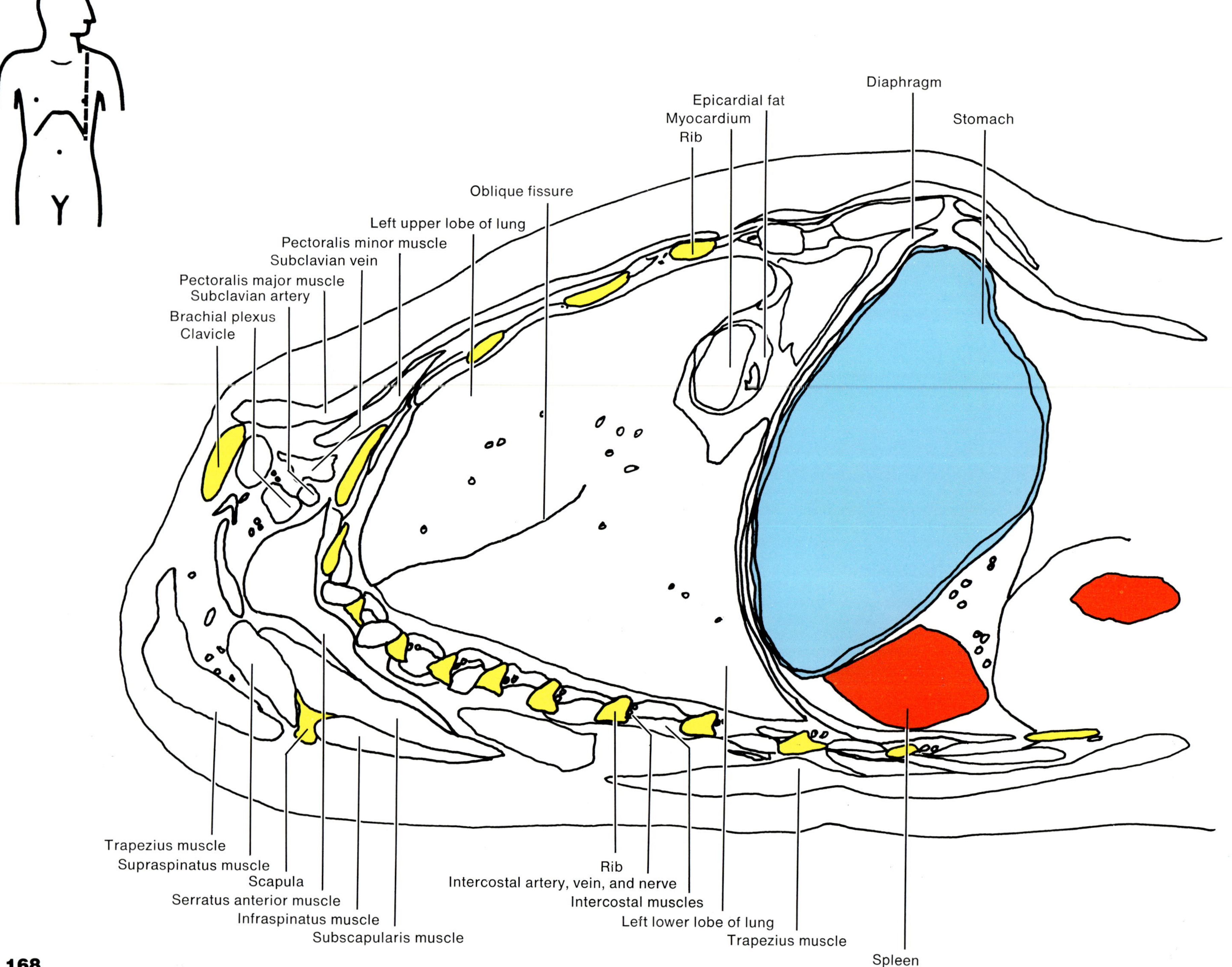

Epicardial fat
Myocardium
Rib
Diaphragm
Stomach
Oblique fissure
Left upper lobe of lung
Pectoralis minor muscle
Subclavian vein
Pectoralis major muscle
Subclavian artery
Brachial plexus
Clavicle
Trapezius muscle
Supraspinatus muscle
Scapula
Serratus anterior muscle
Infraspinatus muscle
Subscapularis muscle
Rib
Intercostal artery, vein, and nerve
Intercostal muscles
Left lower lobe of lung
Trapezius muscle
Spleen

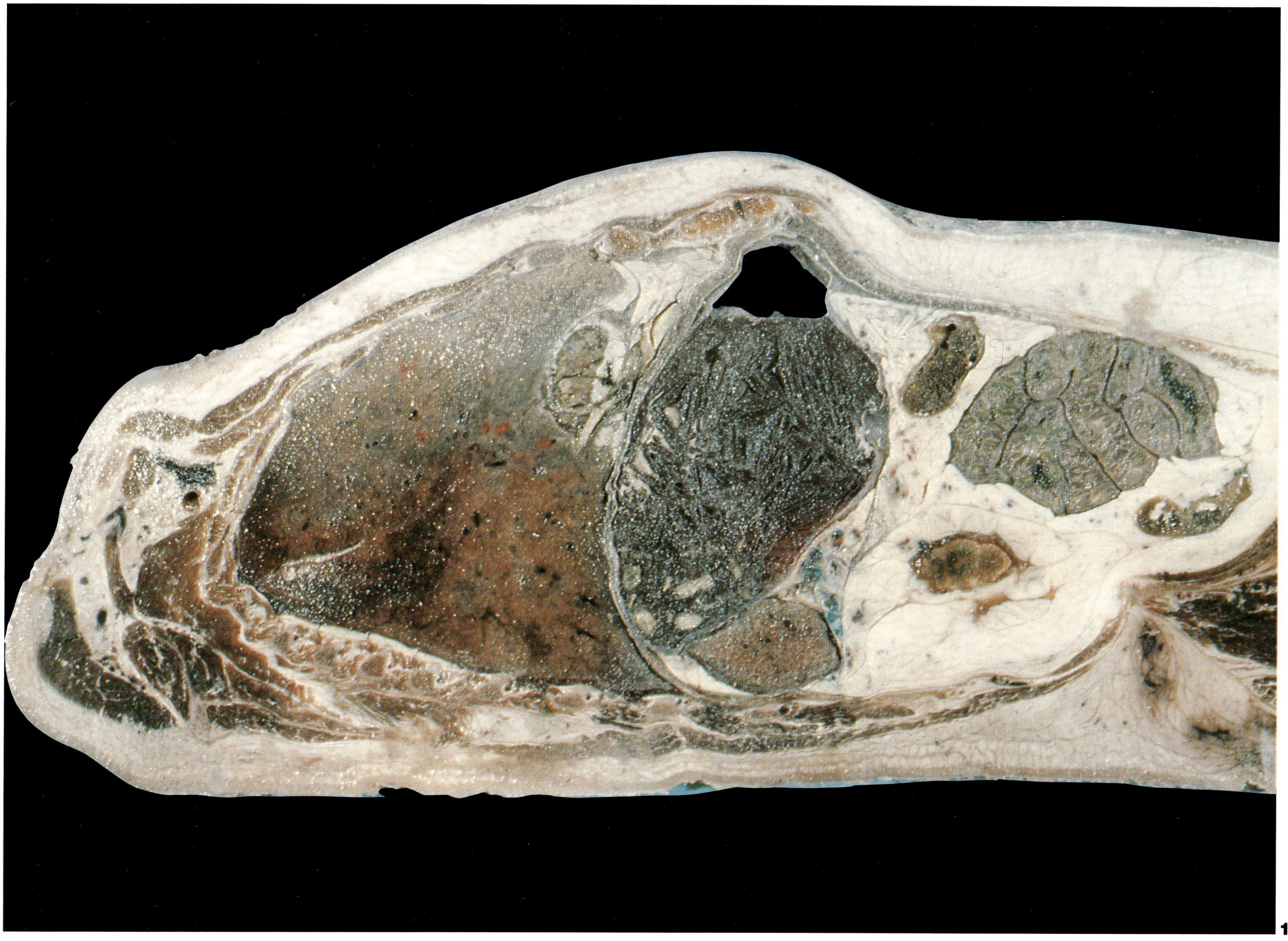

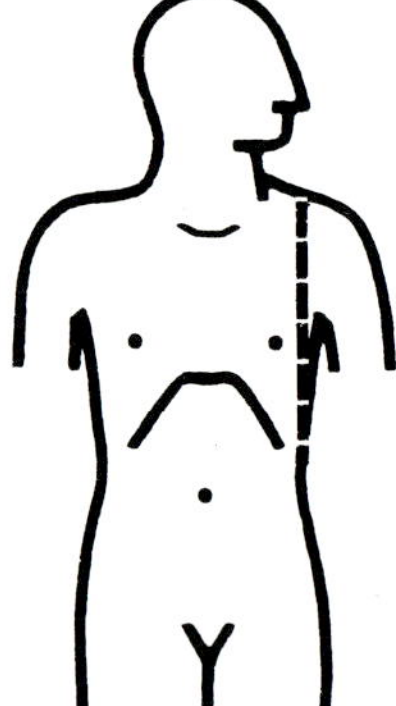

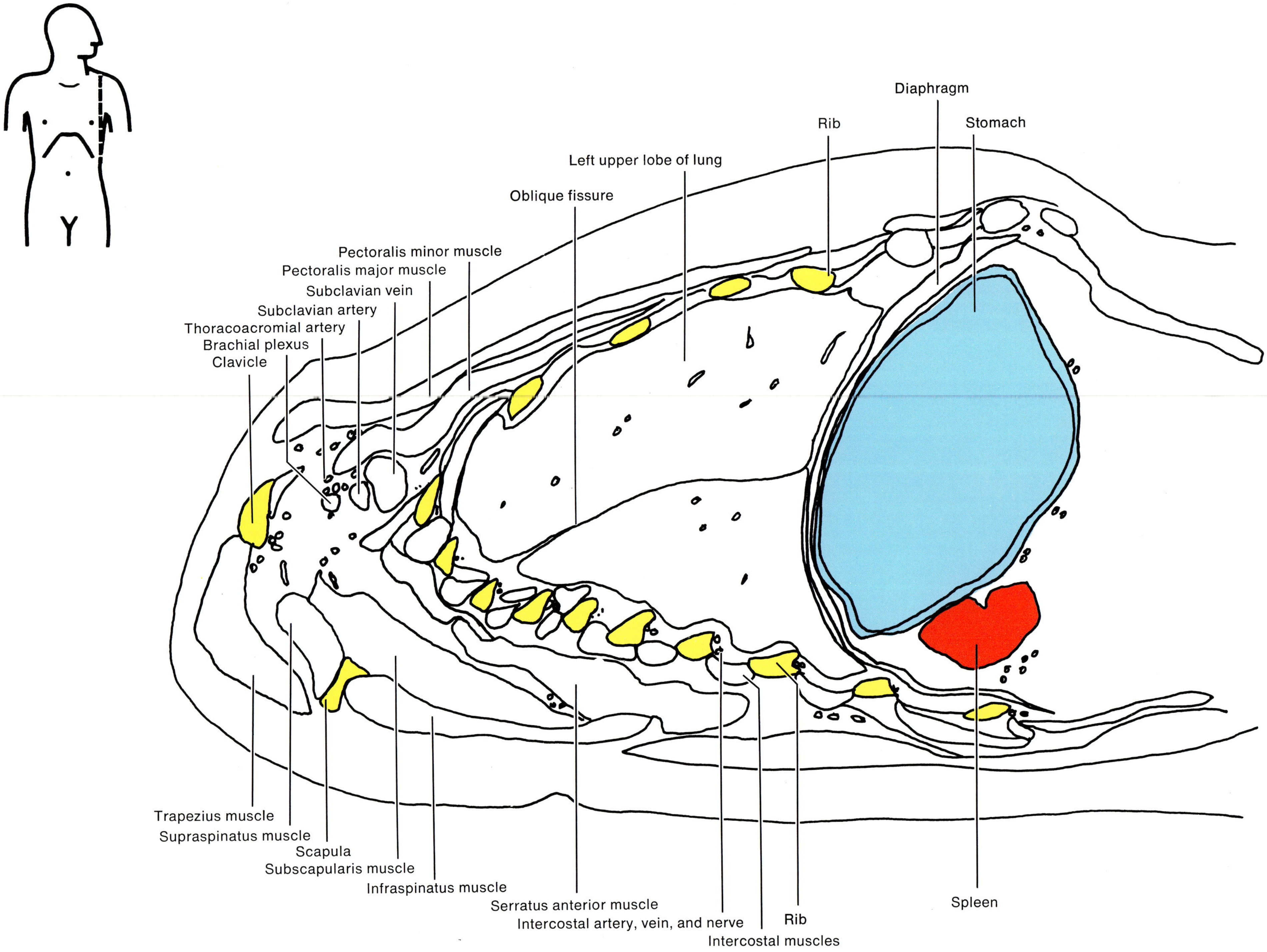

Diaphragm
Rib
Stomach
Left upper lobe of lung
Oblique fissure
Pectoralis minor muscle
Pectoralis major muscle
Subclavian vein
Subclavian artery
Thoracoacromial artery
Brachial plexus
Clavicle
Trapezius muscle
Supraspinatus muscle
Scapula
Subscapularis muscle
Infraspinatus muscle
Serratus anterior muscle
Intercostal artery, vein, and nerve
Intercostal muscles
Rib
Spleen

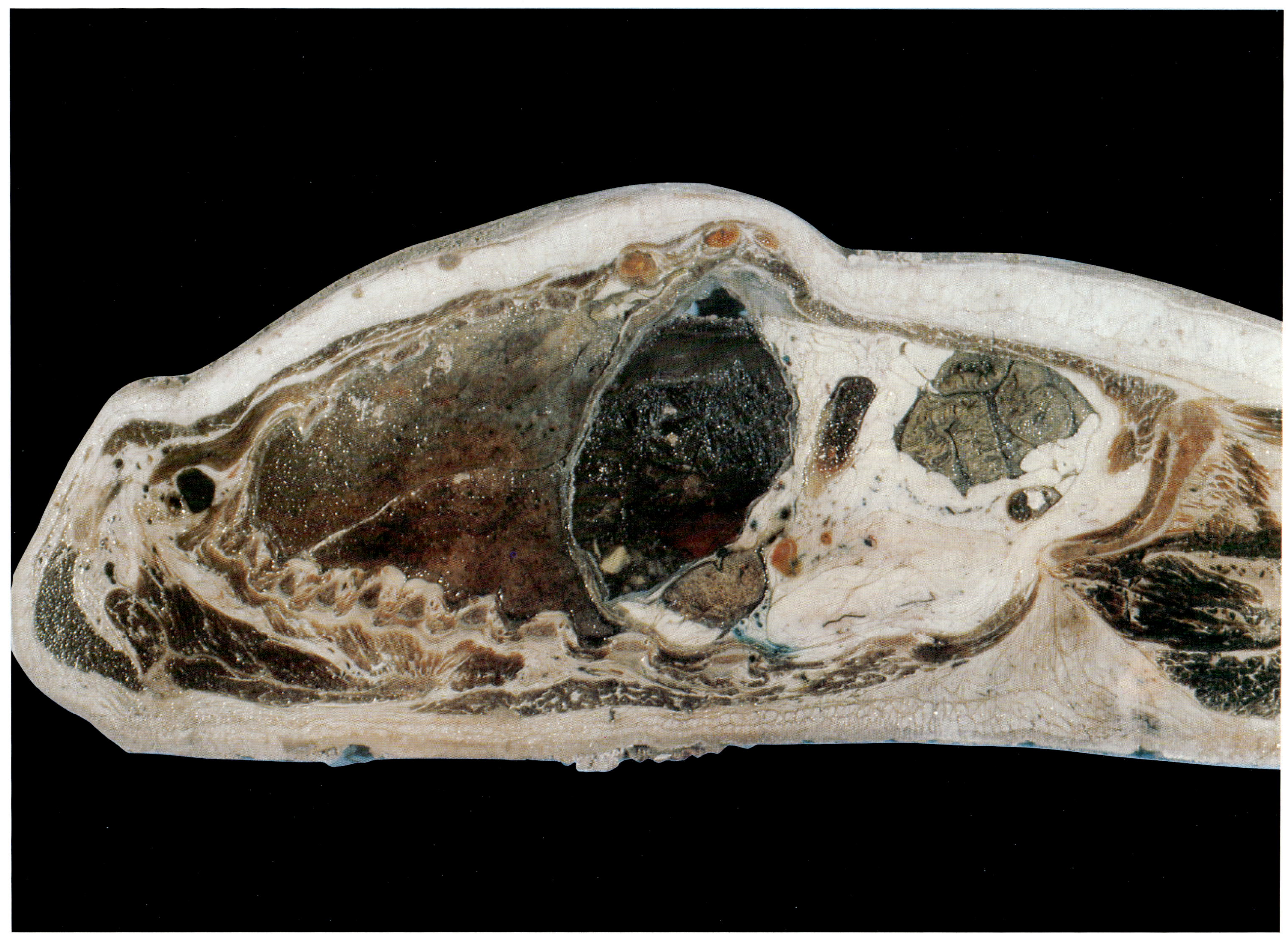

Abdomen and pelvis—male

PLATES 76-105

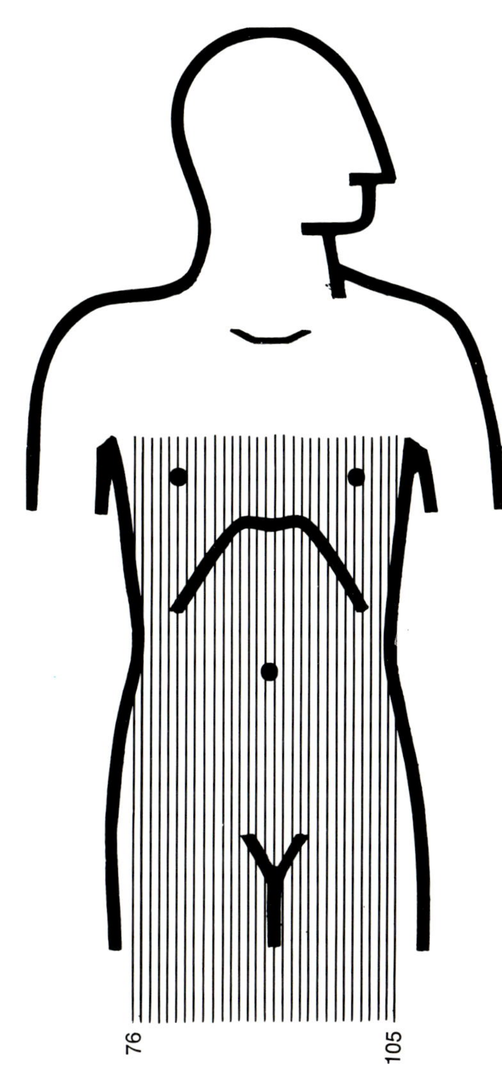

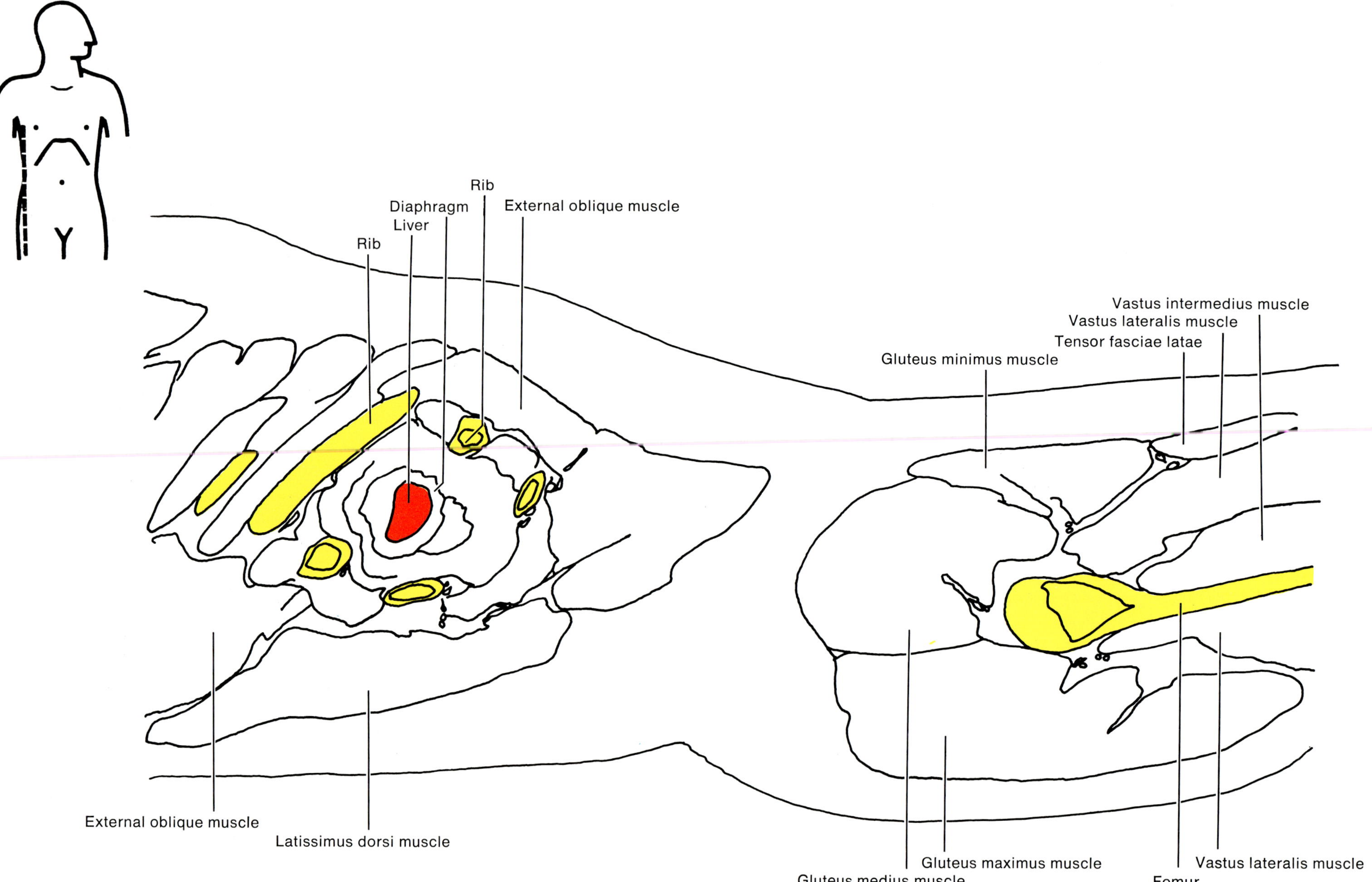
Rib
Diaphragm
Liver
Rib
External oblique muscle
Rib
Gluteus minimus muscle
Vastus intermedius muscle
Vastus lateralis muscle
Tensor fasciae latae
External oblique muscle
Latissimus dorsi muscle
Gluteus medius muscle
Gluteus maximus muscle
Femur
Vastus lateralis muscle

PARASAGITTAL **Abdomen and pelvis—male**

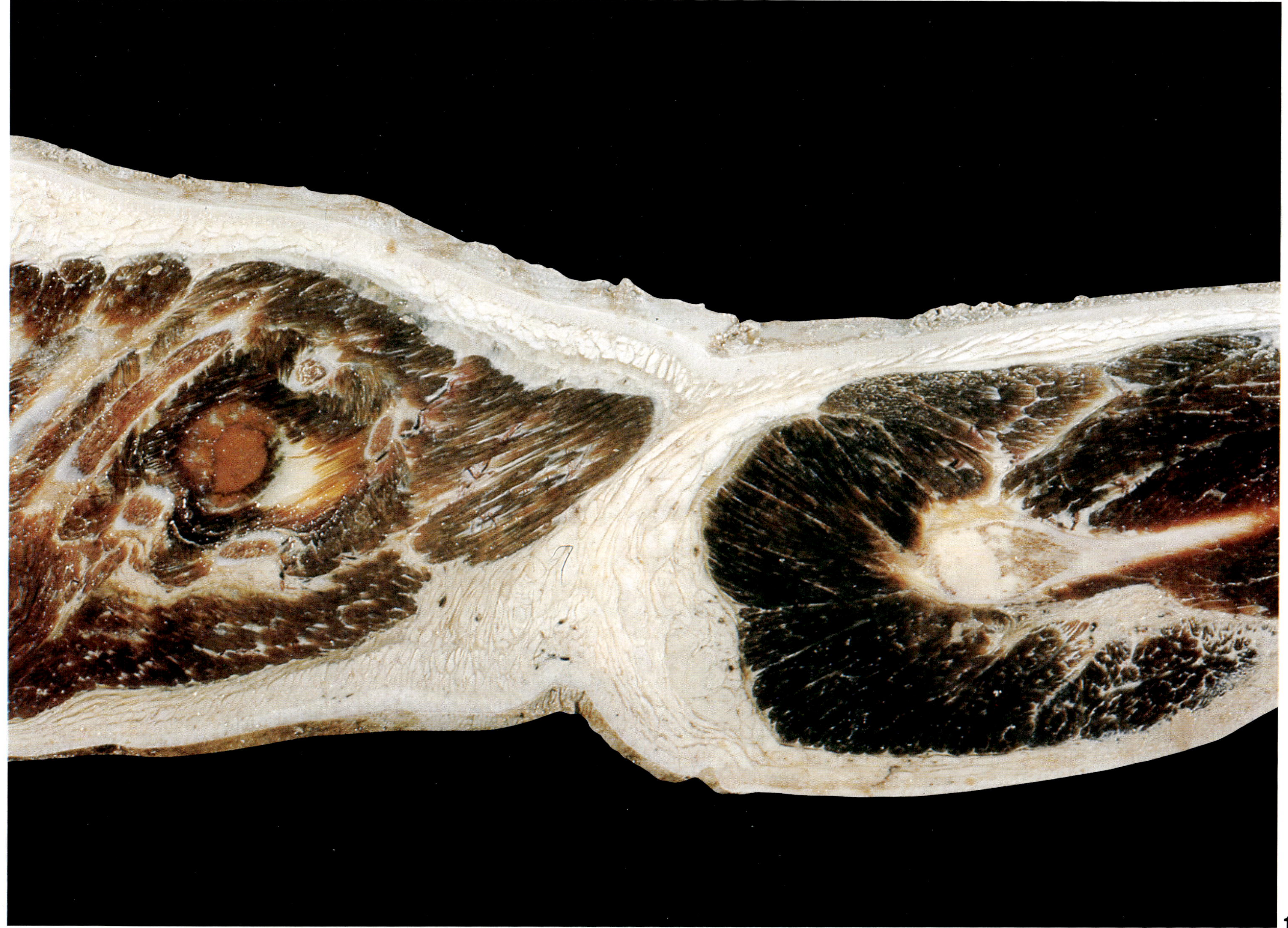

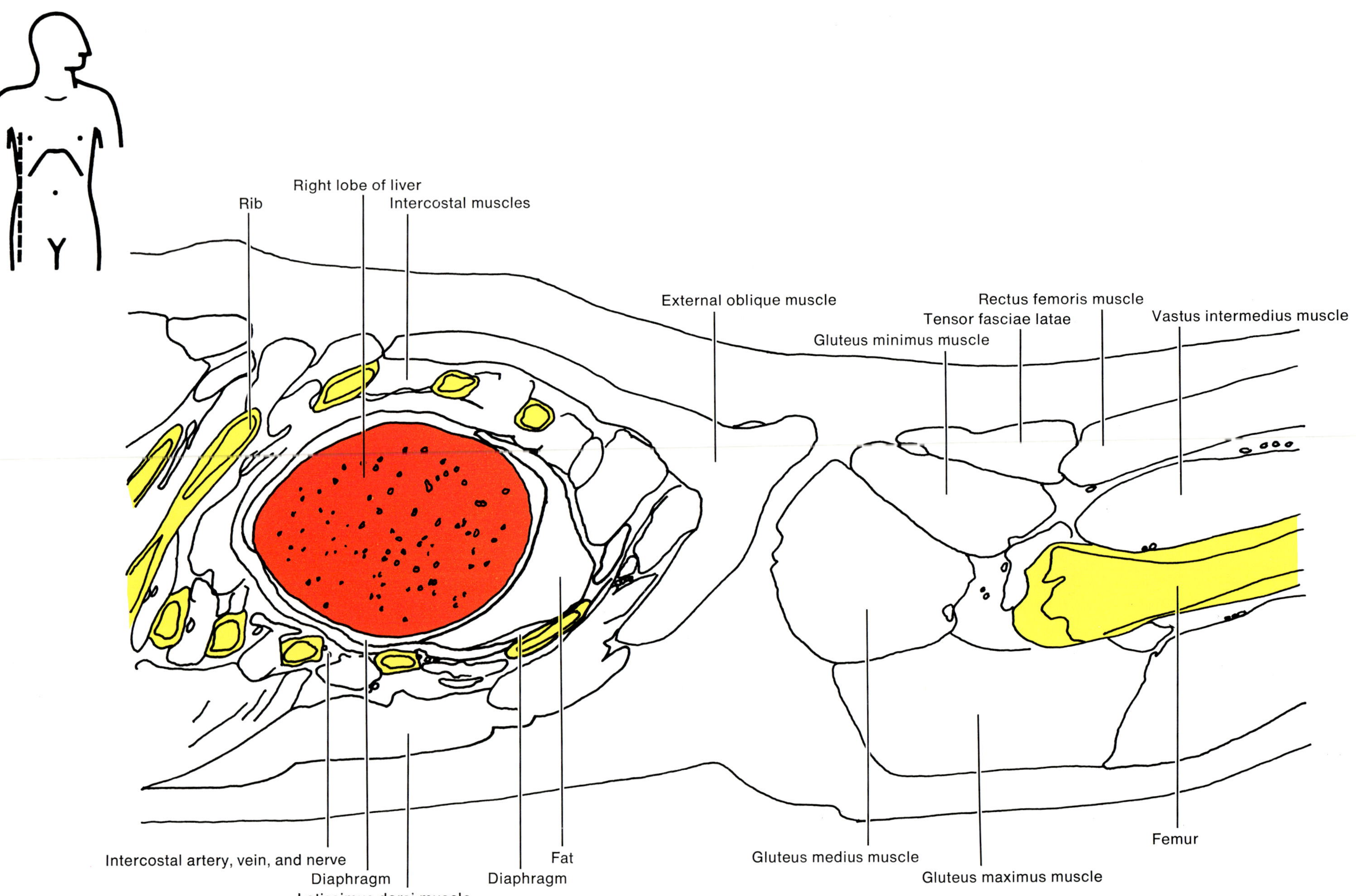

Rib
Right lobe of liver
Intercostal muscles
External oblique muscle
Rectus femoris muscle
Tensor fasciae latae
Vastus intermedius muscle
Gluteus minimus muscle
Intercostal artery, vein, and nerve
Diaphragm
Latissimus dorsi muscle
Fat
Diaphragm
Gluteus medius muscle
Gluteus maximus muscle
Femur

PARASAGITTAL **Abdomen and pelvis—male**

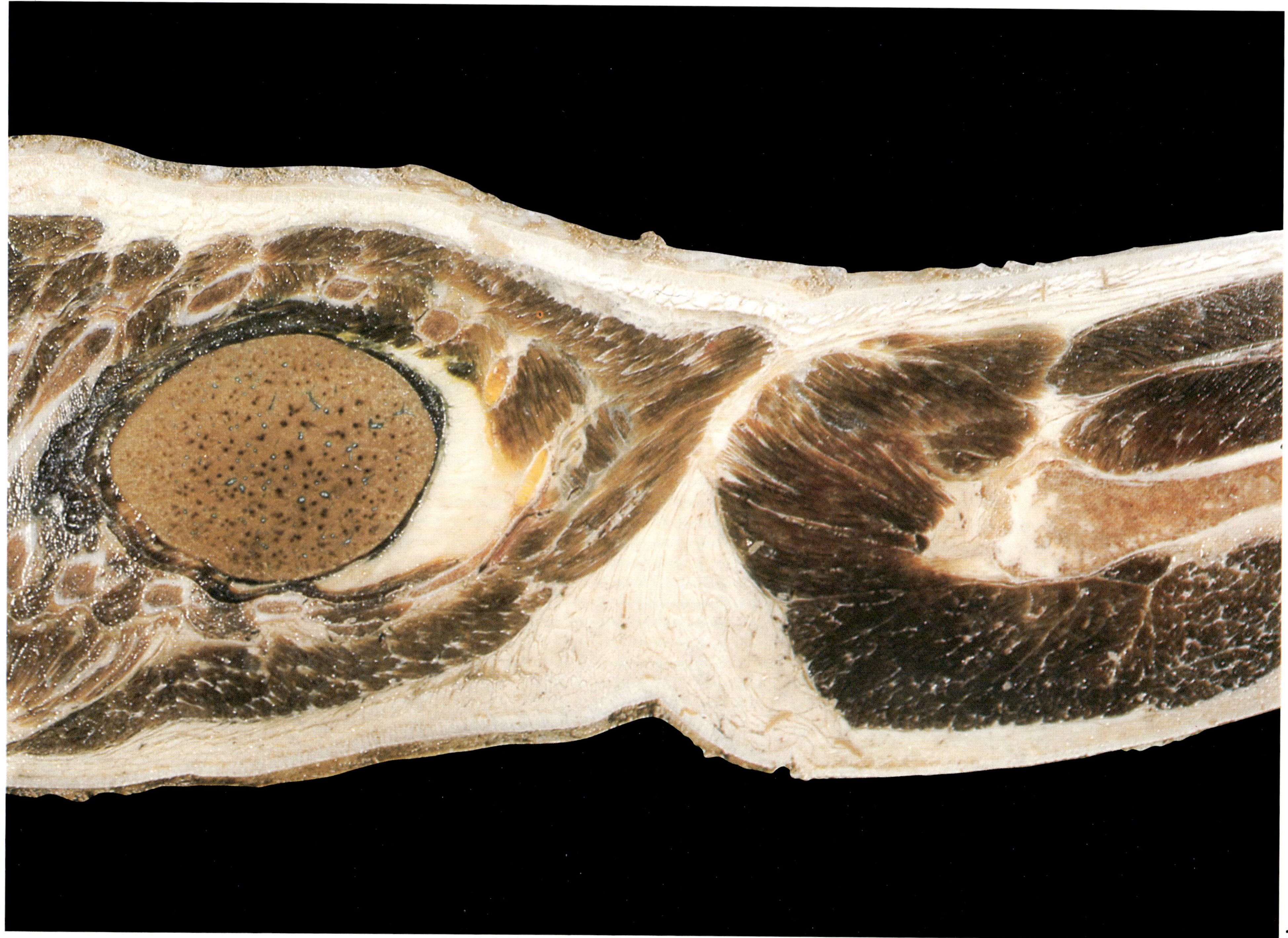

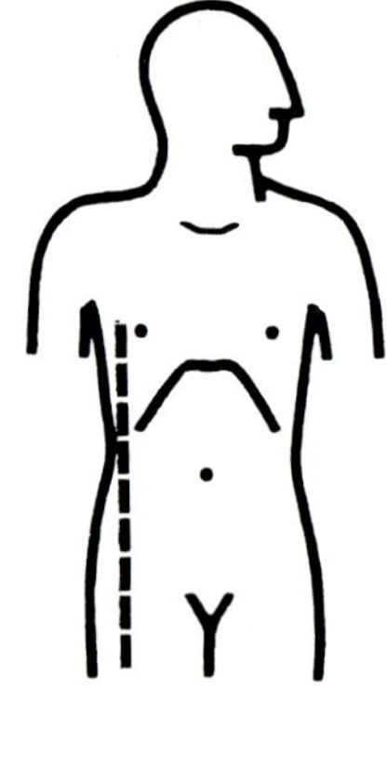

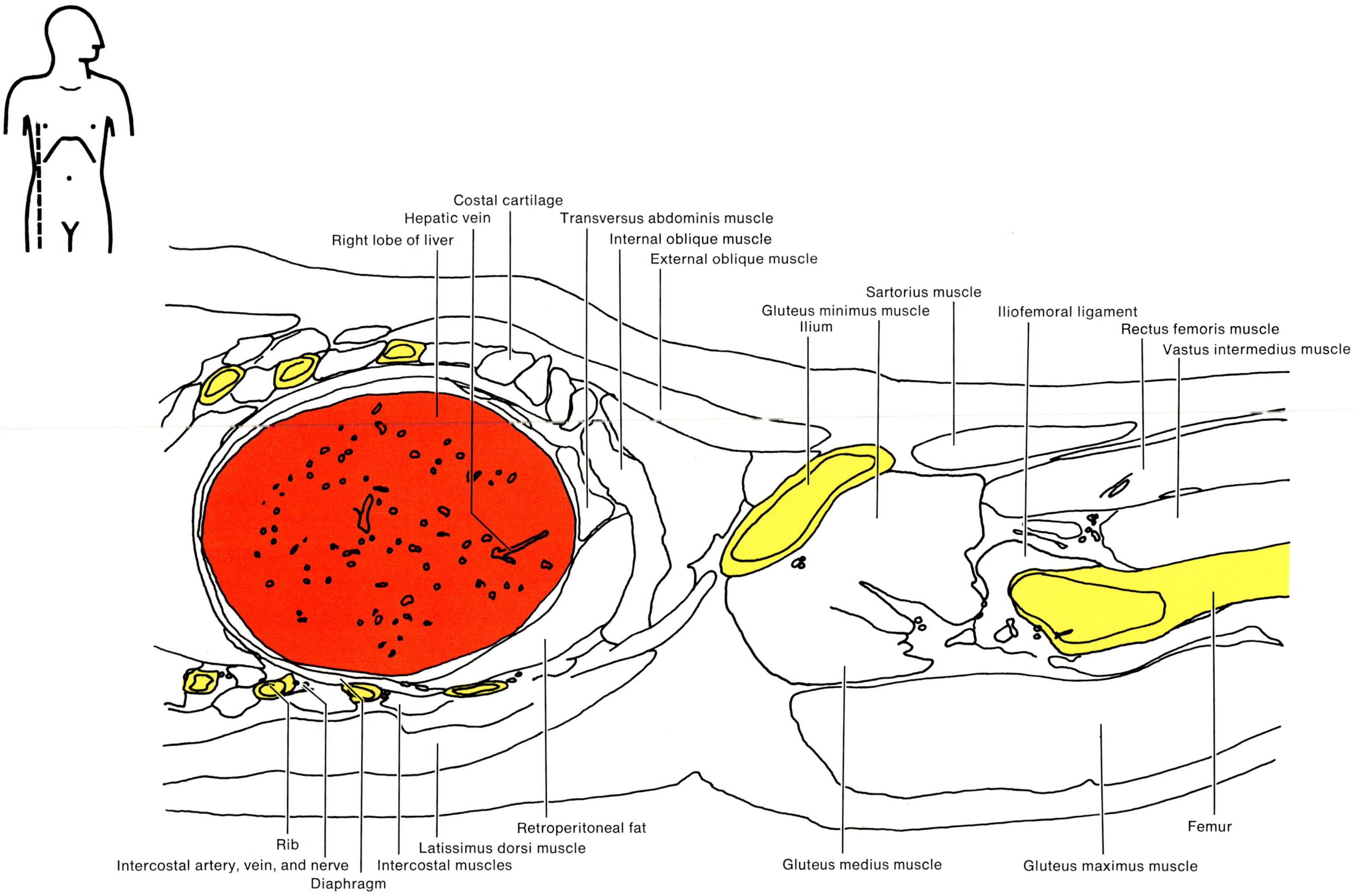

Costal cartilage
Hepatic vein
Right lobe of liver
Transversus abdominis muscle
Internal oblique muscle
External oblique muscle
Sartorius muscle
Gluteus minimus muscle
Ilium
Iliofemoral ligament
Rectus femoris muscle
Vastus intermedius muscle
Rib
Intercostal artery, vein, and nerve
Diaphragm
Intercostal muscles
Latissimus dorsi muscle
Retroperitoneal fat
Gluteus medius muscle
Gluteus maximus muscle
Femur

PARASAGITTAL **Abdomen and pelvis—male**

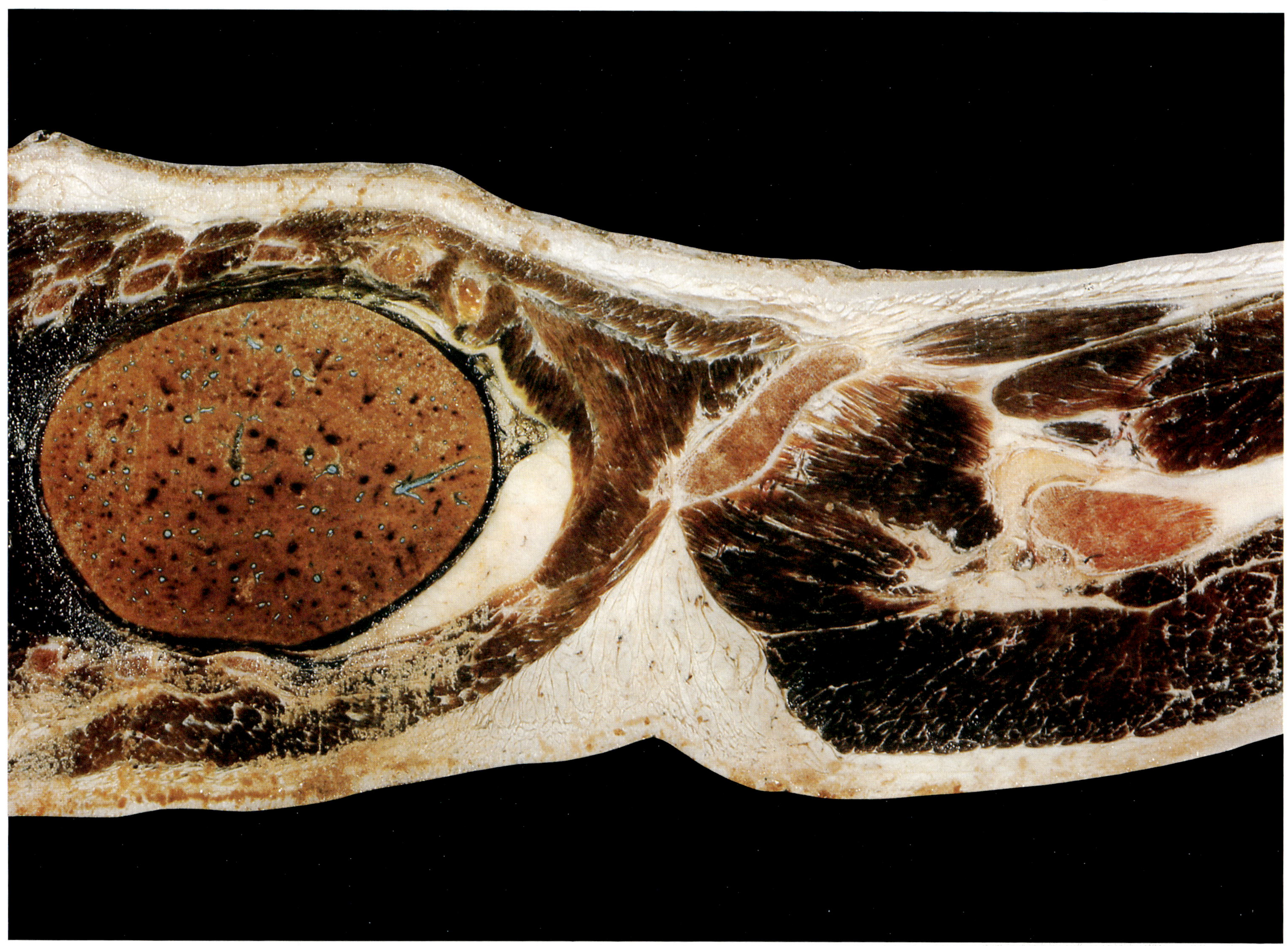

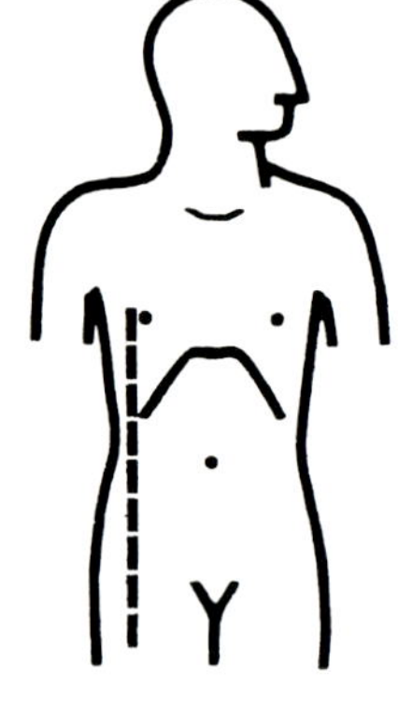

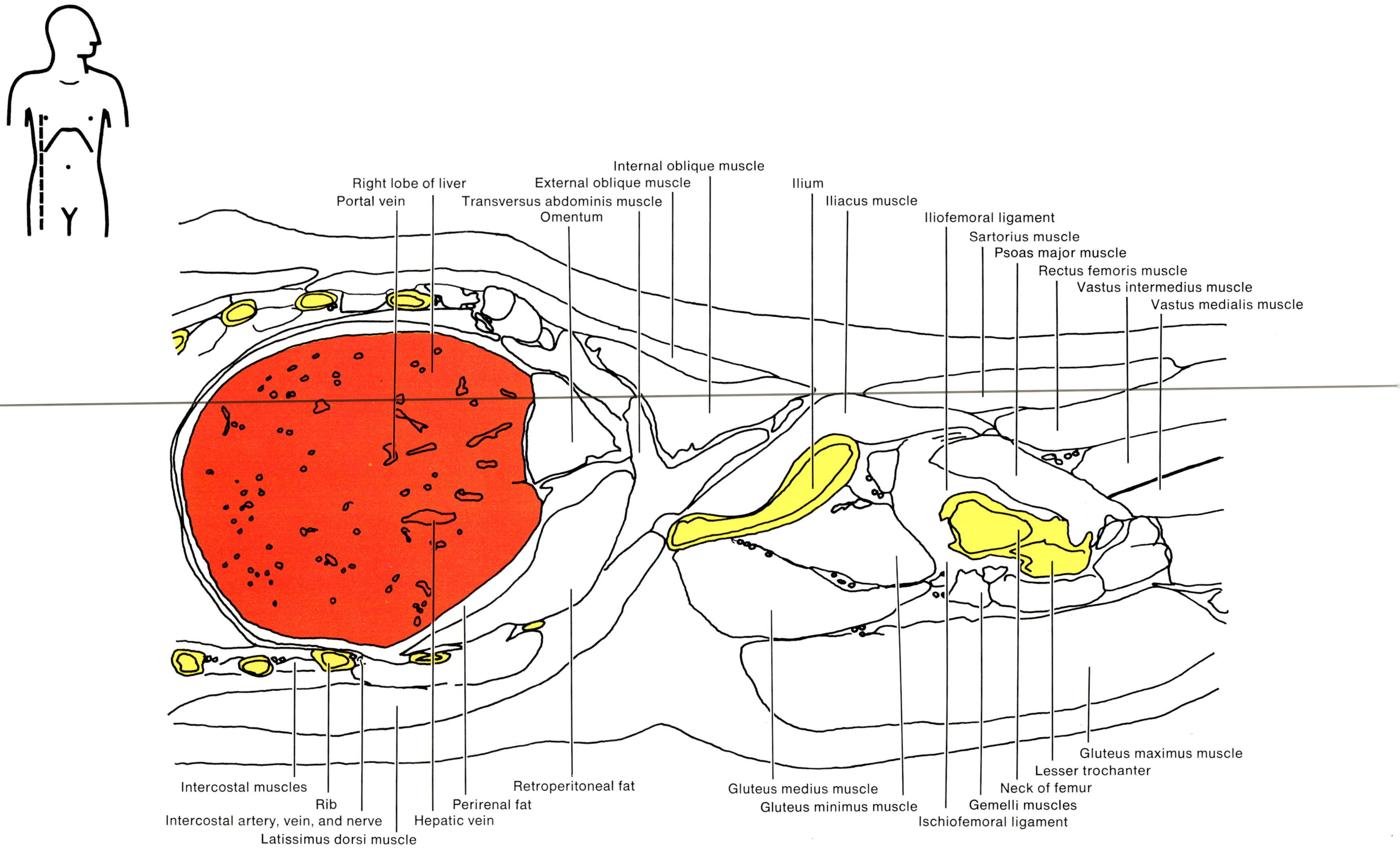

Right lobe of liver
Portal vein
Internal oblique muscle
External oblique muscle
Transversus abdominis muscle
Omentum
Ilium
Iliacus muscle
Iliofemoral ligament
Sartorius muscle
Psoas major muscle
Rectus femoris muscle
Vastus intermedius muscle
Vastus medialis muscle
Intercostal muscles
Rib
Intercostal artery, vein, and nerve
Latissimus dorsi muscle
Perirenal fat
Hepatic vein
Retroperitoneal fat
Gluteus medius muscle
Gluteus minimus muscle
Gluteus maximus muscle
Lesser trochanter
Neck of femur
Gemelli muscles
Ischiofemoral ligament

PARASAGITTAL **Abdomen and pelvis—male**

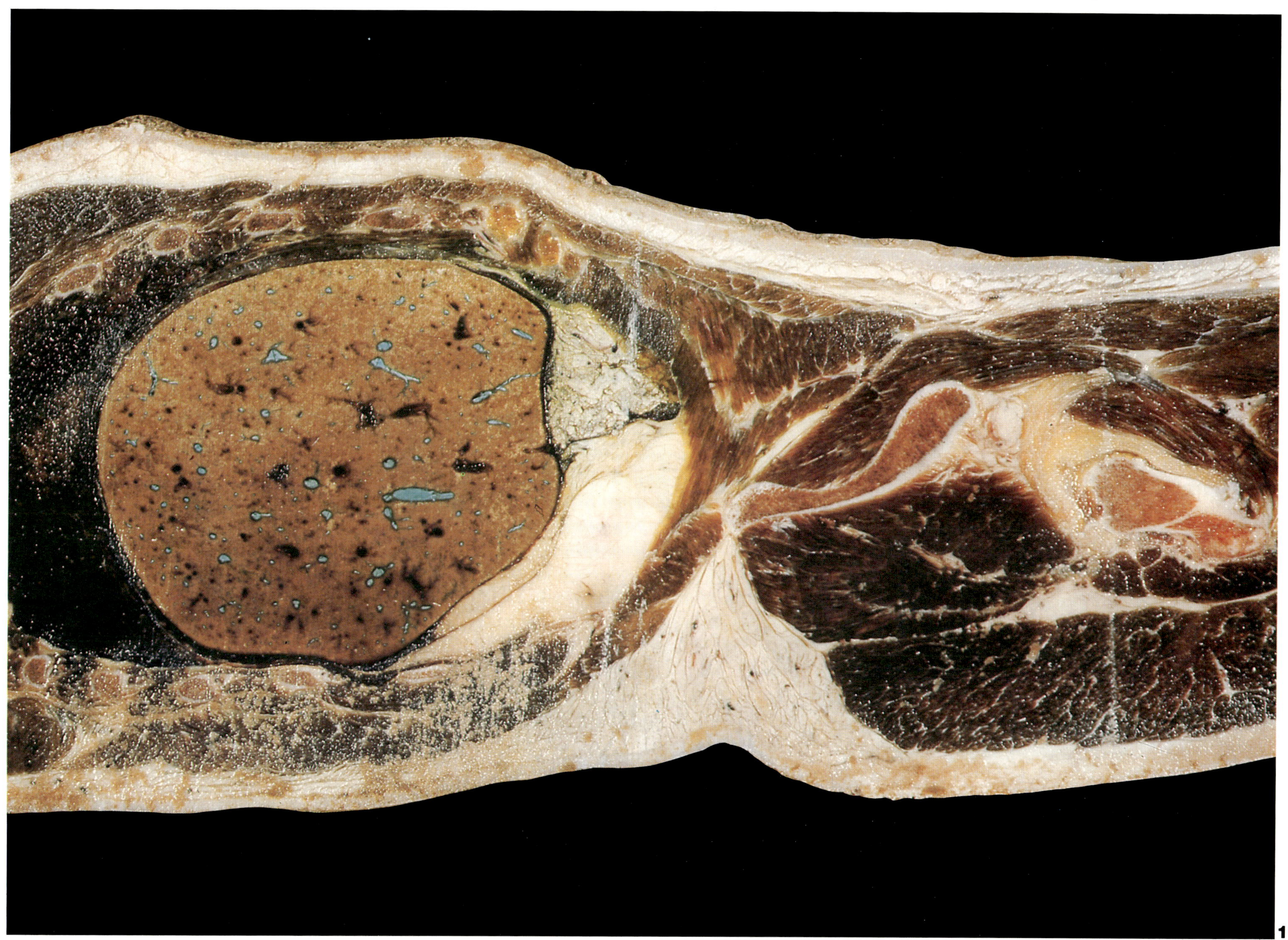

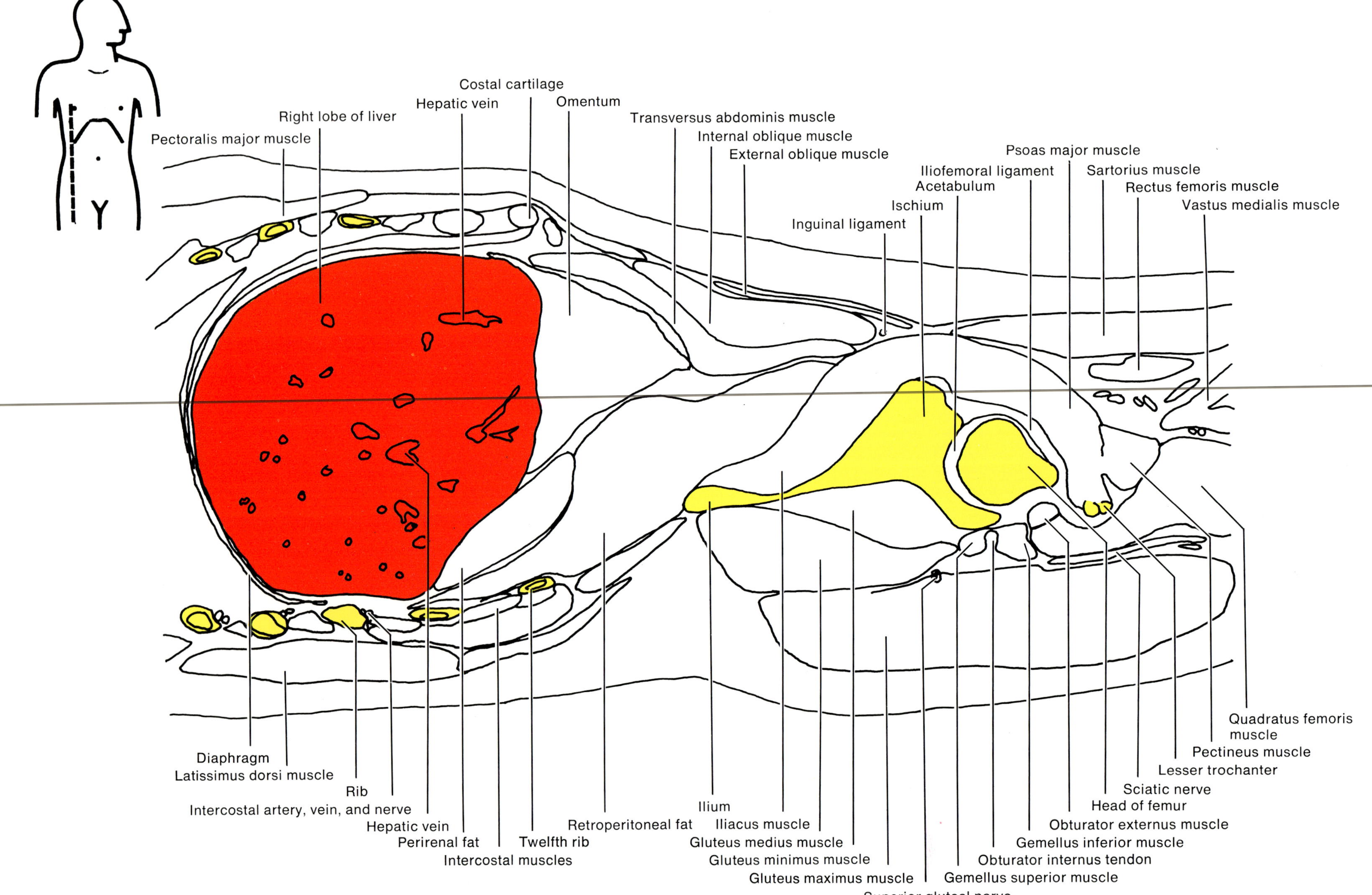

Costal cartilage
Hepatic vein
Right lobe of liver
Omentum
Pectoralis major muscle
Transversus abdominis muscle
Internal oblique muscle
External oblique muscle
Psoas major muscle
Iliofemoral ligament
Sartorius muscle
Acetabulum
Rectus femoris muscle
Vastus medialis muscle
Ischium
Inguinal ligament
Diaphragm
Latissimus dorsi muscle
Rib
Intercostal artery, vein, and nerve
Hepatic vein
Perirenal fat
Twelfth rib
Intercostal muscles
Retroperitoneal fat
Ilium
Iliacus muscle
Gluteus medius muscle
Gluteus minimus muscle
Gluteus maximus muscle
Superior gluteal nerve
Quadratus femoris muscle
Pectineus muscle
Lesser trochanter
Sciatic nerve
Head of femur
Obturator externus muscle
Gemellus inferior muscle
Obturator internus tendon
Gemellus superior muscle

PARASAGITTAL **Abdomen and pelvis—male**

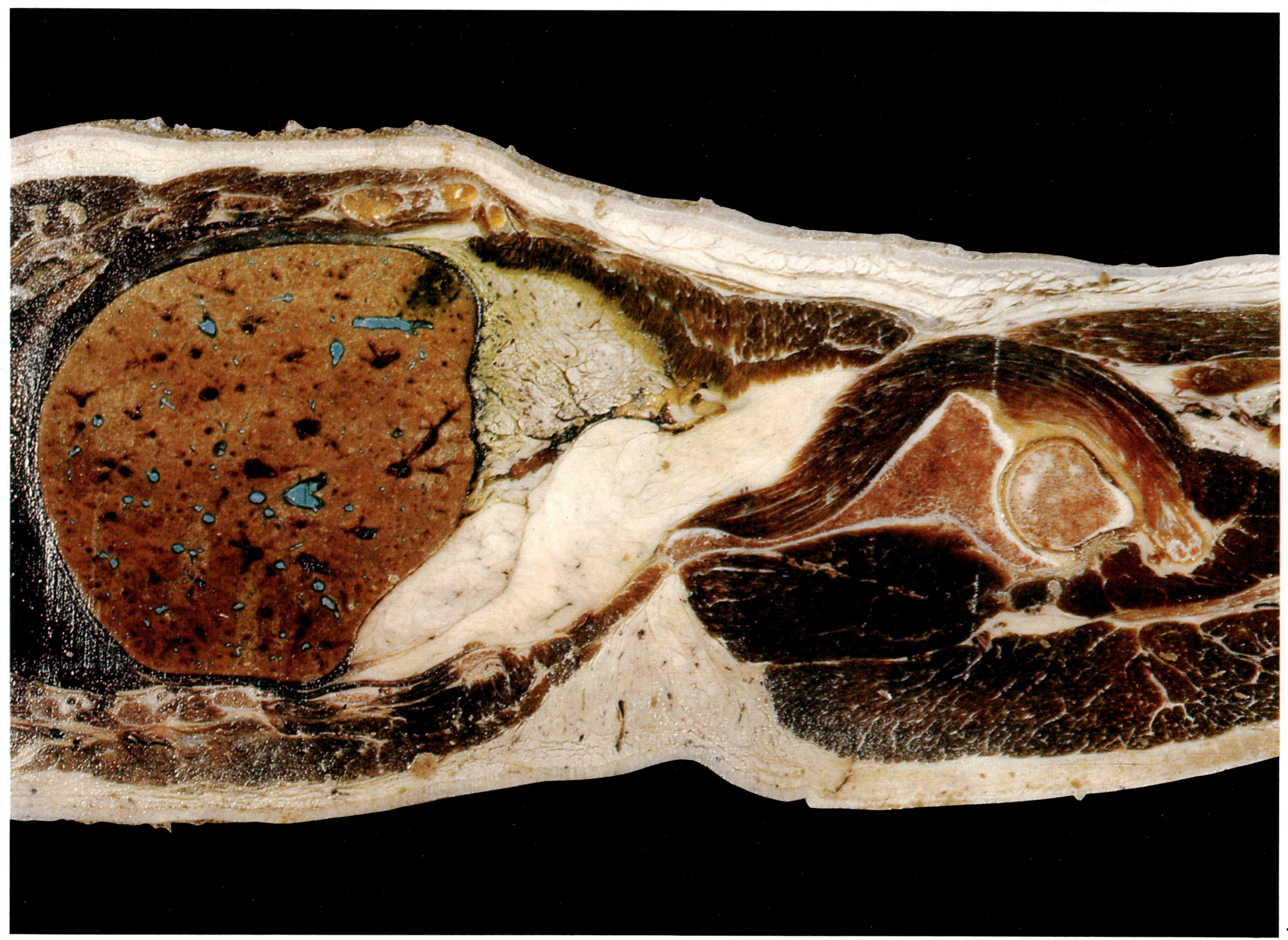

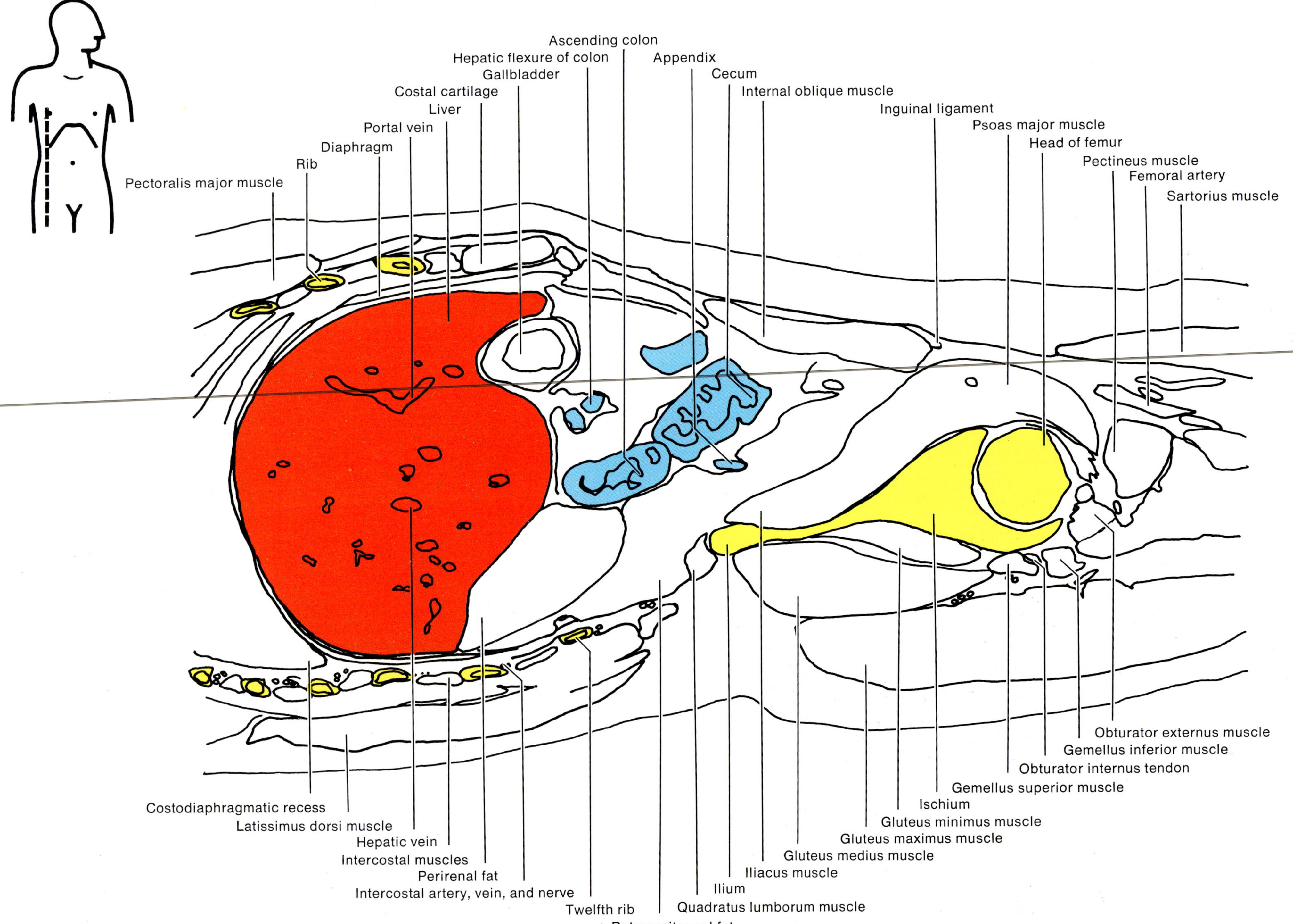
Pectoralis major muscle
Rib
Diaphragm
Portal vein
Liver
Costal cartilage
Gallbladder
Hepatic flexure of colon
Ascending colon
Appendix
Cecum
Internal oblique muscle
Inguinal ligament
Psoas major muscle
Head of femur
Pectineus muscle
Femoral artery
Sartorius muscle
Obturator externus muscle
Gemellus inferior muscle
Obturator internus tendon
Gemellus superior muscle
Ischium
Gluteus minimus muscle
Gluteus maximus muscle
Gluteus medius muscle
Iliacus muscle
Ilium
Quadratus lumborum muscle
Retroperitoneal fat
Twelfth rib
Perirenal fat
Intercostal artery, vein, and nerve
Intercostal muscles
Hepatic vein
Latissimus dorsi muscle
Costodiaphragmatic recess

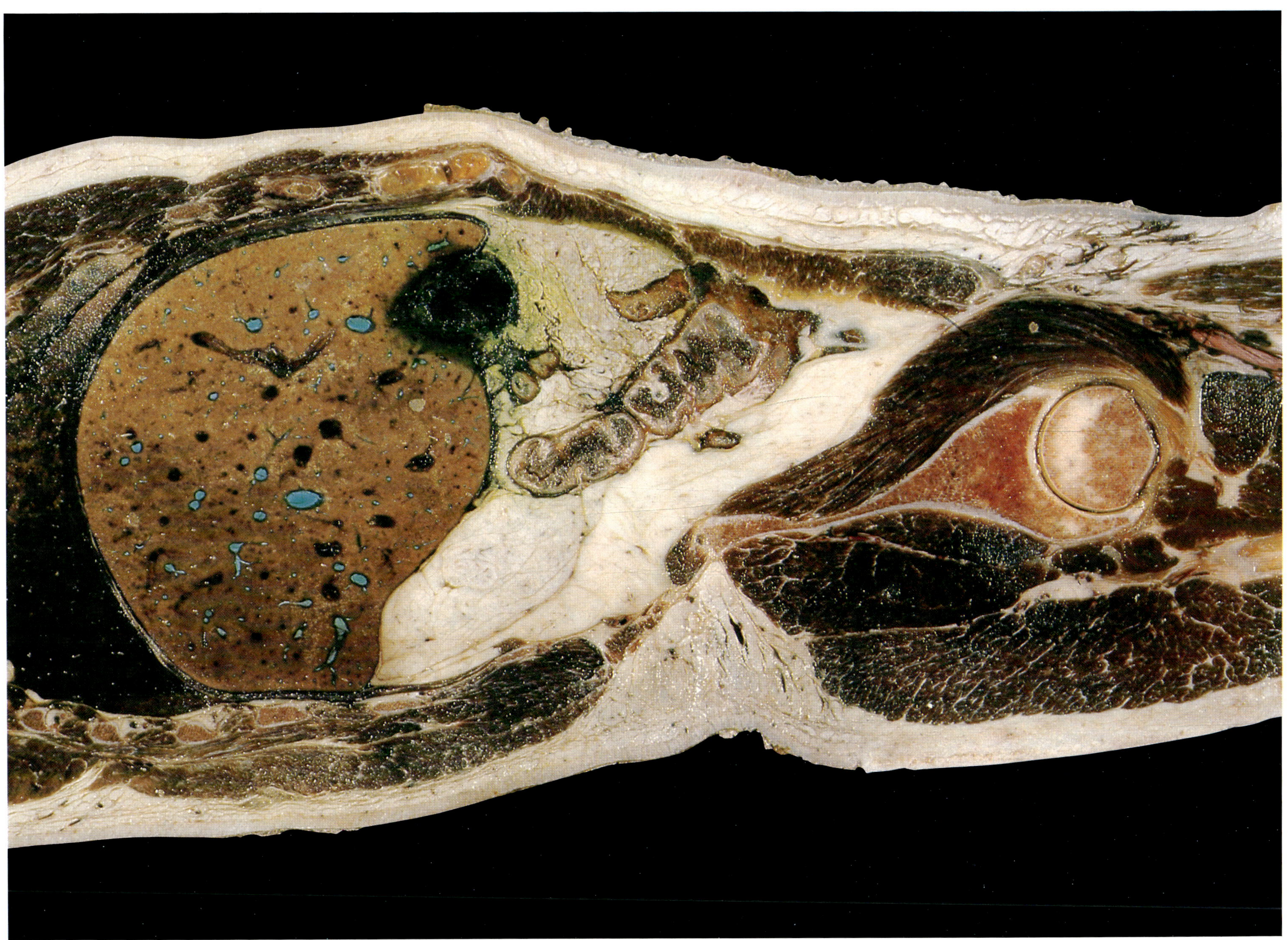

PARASAGITTAL **Abdomen and pelvis—male**

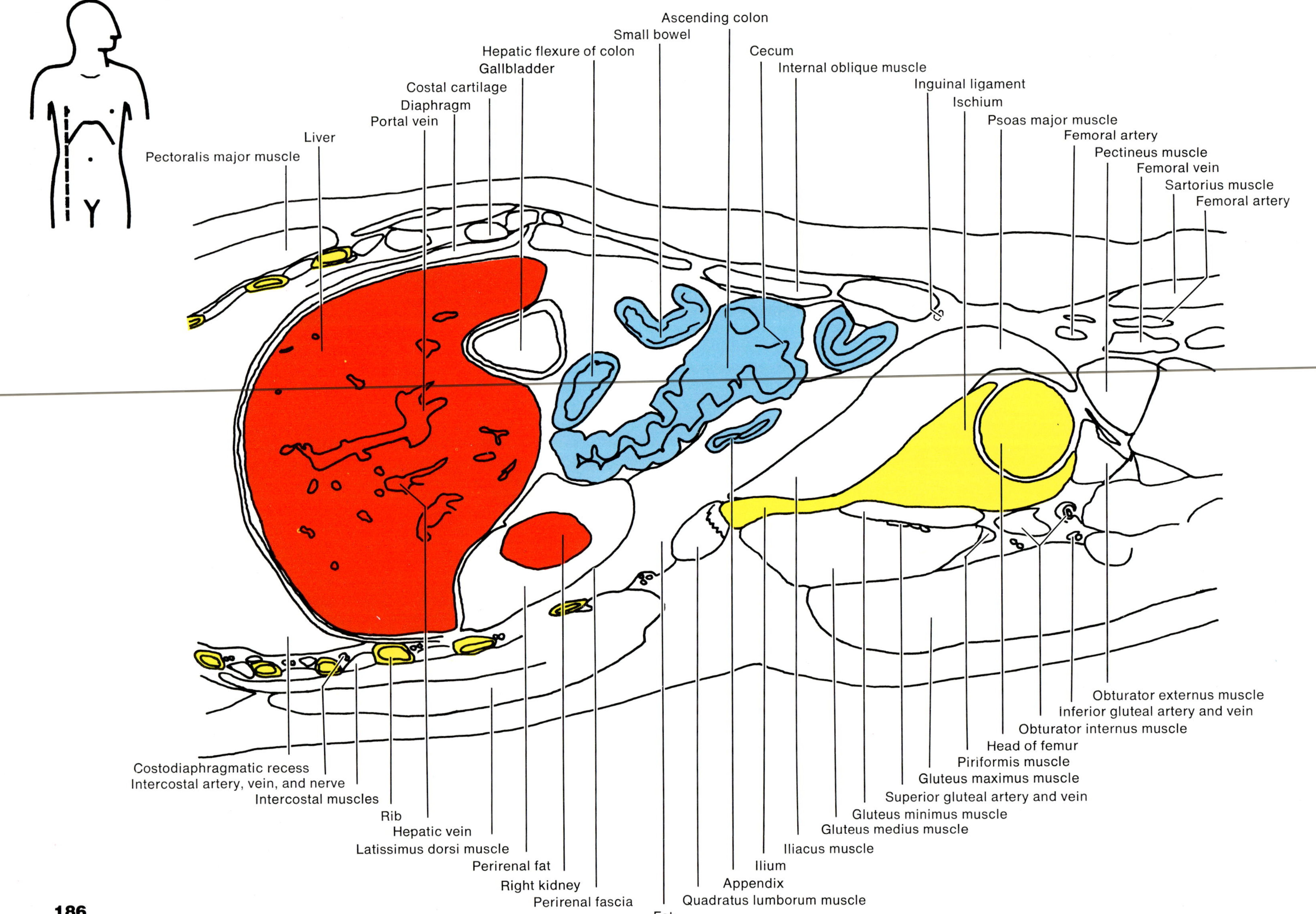
Pectoralis major muscle
Liver
Portal vein
Diaphragm
Costal cartilage
Gallbladder
Hepatic flexure of colon
Small bowel
Ascending colon
Cecum
Internal oblique muscle
Inguinal ligament
Ischium
Psoas major muscle
Femoral artery
Pectineus muscle
Femoral vein
Sartorius muscle
Femoral artery
Costodiaphragmatic recess
Intercostal artery, vein, and nerve
Intercostal muscles
Rib
Hepatic vein
Latissimus dorsi muscle
Perirenal fat
Right kidney
Perirenal fascia
Fat
Quadratus lumborum muscle
Appendix
Ilium
Iliacus muscle
Gluteus medius muscle
Gluteus minimus muscle
Superior gluteal artery and vein
Gluteus maximus muscle
Piriformis muscle
Head of femur
Obturator internus muscle
Inferior gluteal artery and vein
Obturator externus muscle

PARASAGITTAL **Abdomen and pelvis—male**

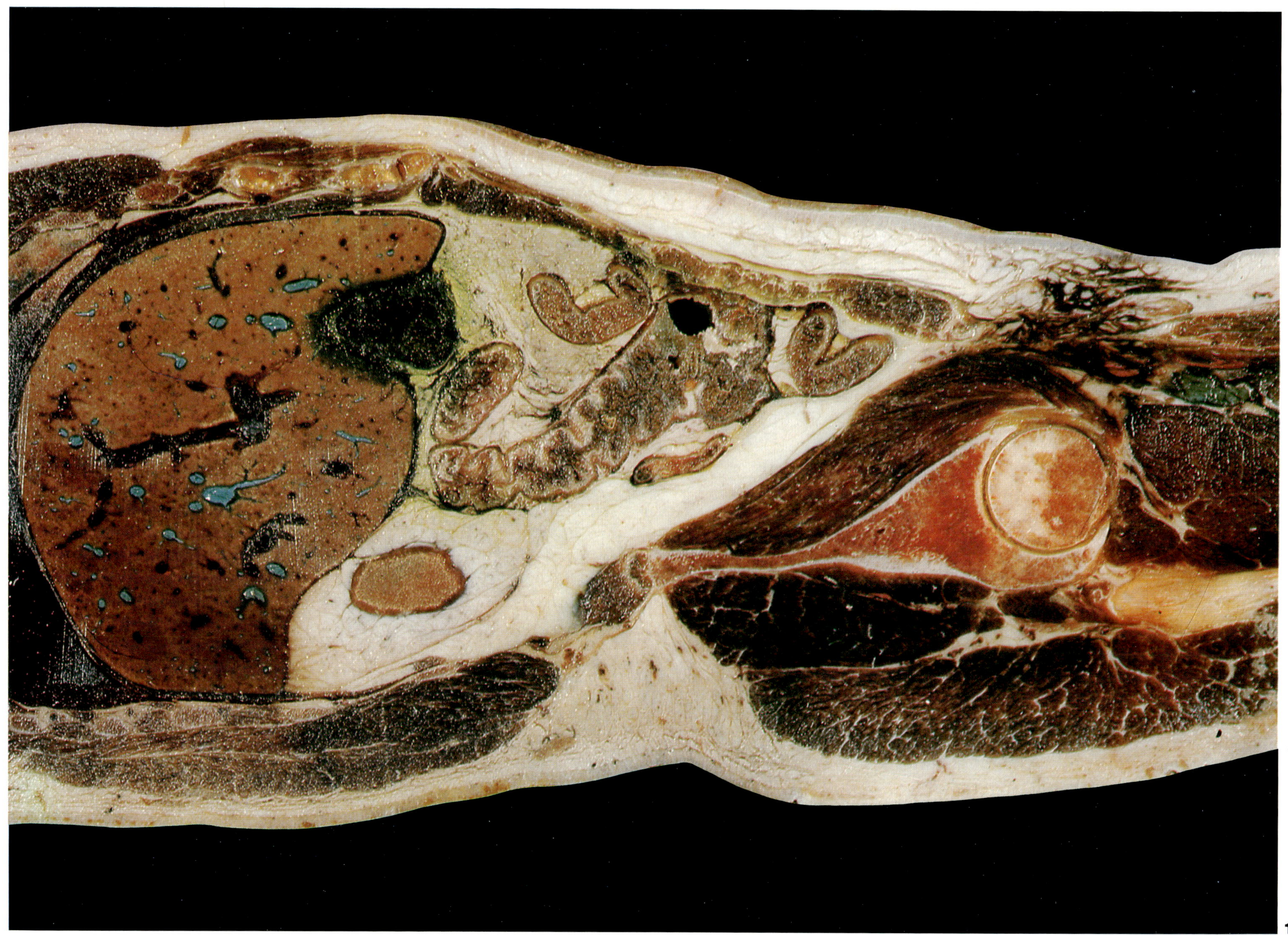

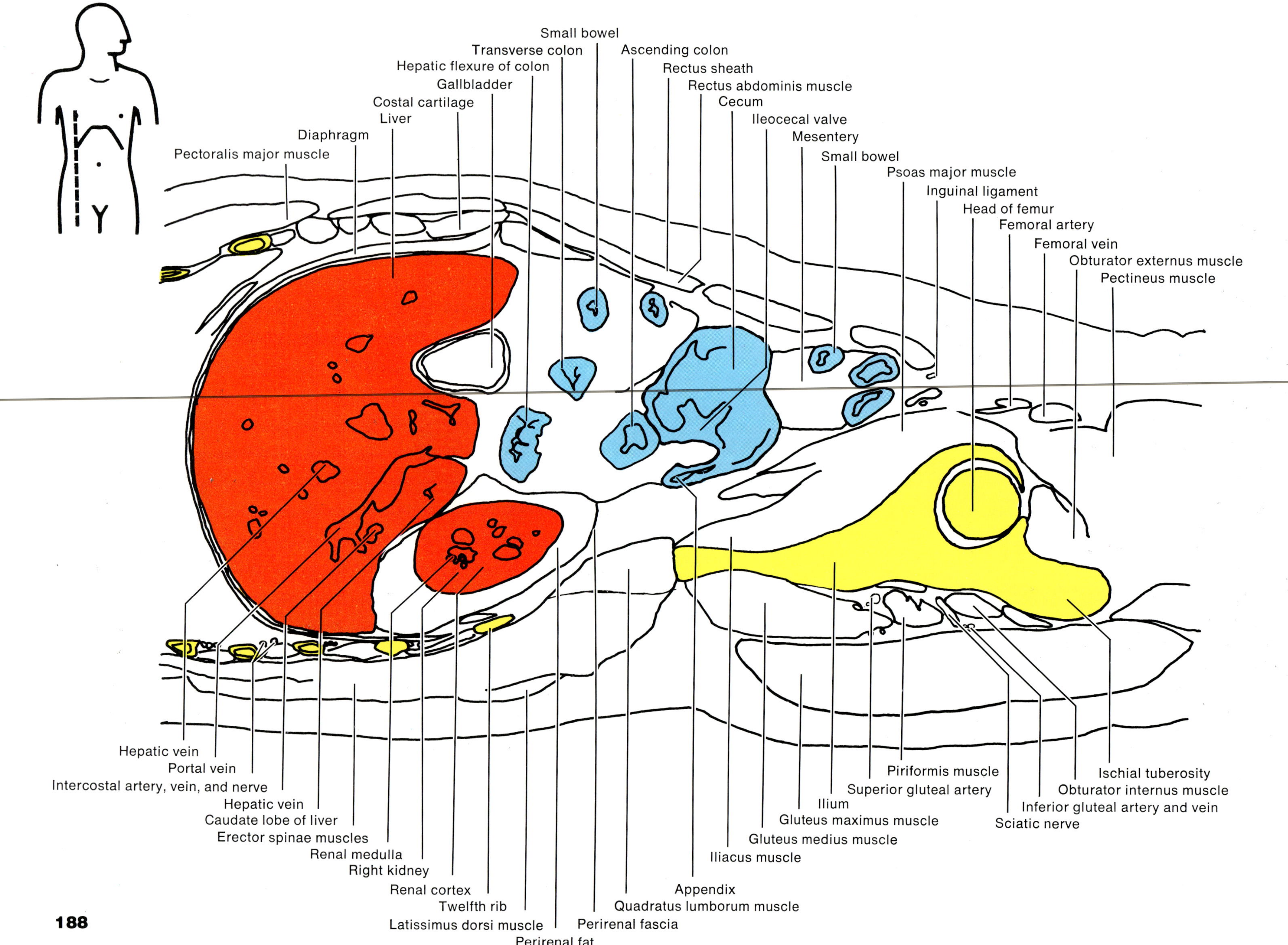

Pectoralis major muscle
Diaphragm
Costal cartilage
Liver
Gallbladder
Hepatic flexure of colon
Transverse colon
Small bowel
Ascending colon
Rectus sheath
Rectus abdominis muscle
Cecum
Ileocecal valve
Mesentery
Small bowel
Psoas major muscle
Inguinal ligament
Head of femur
Femoral artery
Femoral vein
Obturator externus muscle
Pectineus muscle
Hepatic vein
Portal vein
Intercostal artery, vein, and nerve
Hepatic vein
Caudate lobe of liver
Erector spinae muscles
Renal medulla
Right kidney
Renal cortex
Twelfth rib
Latissimus dorsi muscle
Perirenal fat
Perirenal fascia
Quadratus lumborum muscle
Appendix
Iliacus muscle
Gluteus medius muscle
Gluteus maximus muscle
Ilium
Superior gluteal artery
Piriformis muscle
Sciatic nerve
Inferior gluteal artery and vein
Obturator internus muscle
Ischial tuberosity

PARASAGITTAL **Abdomen and pelvis—male**

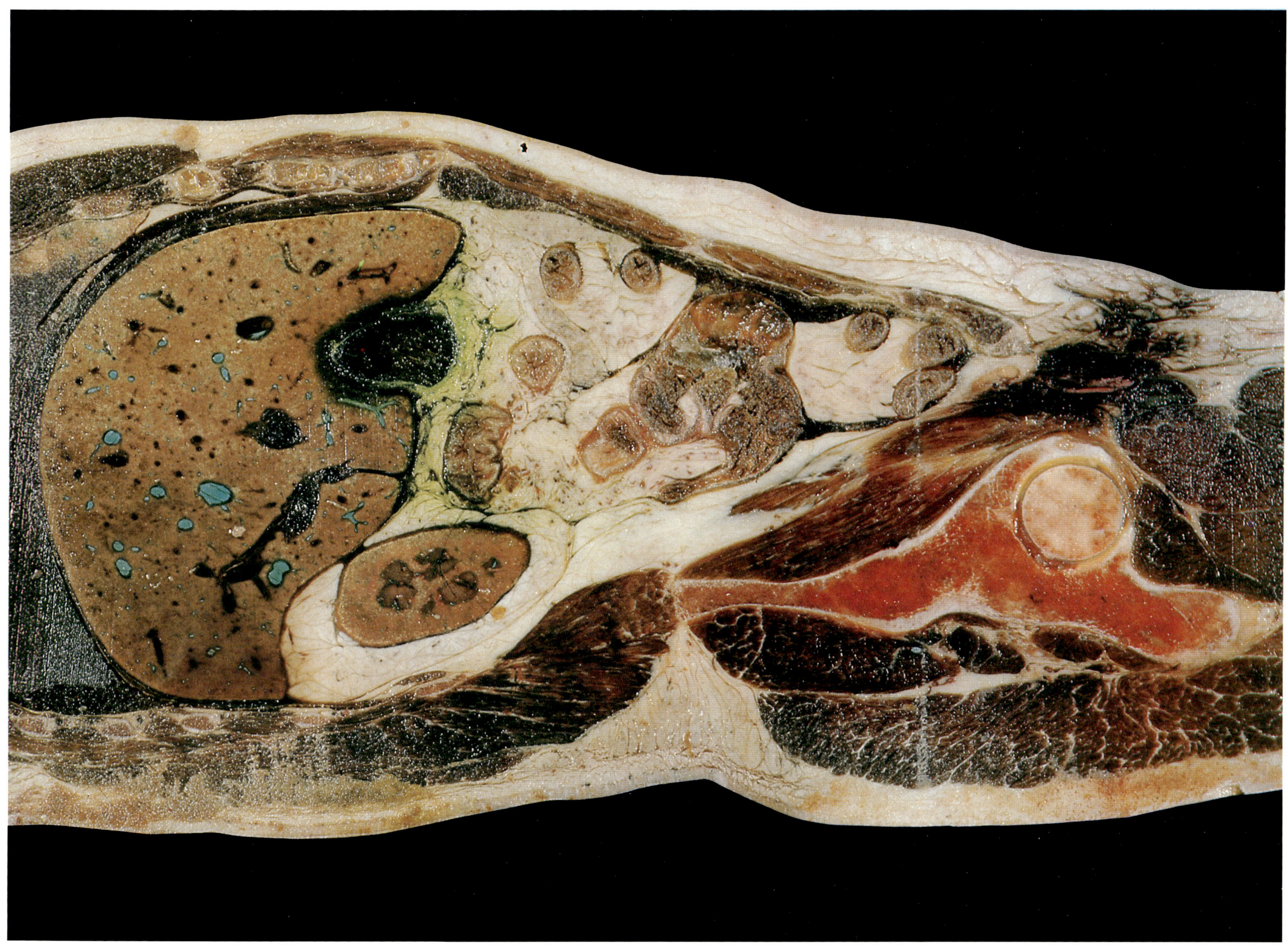

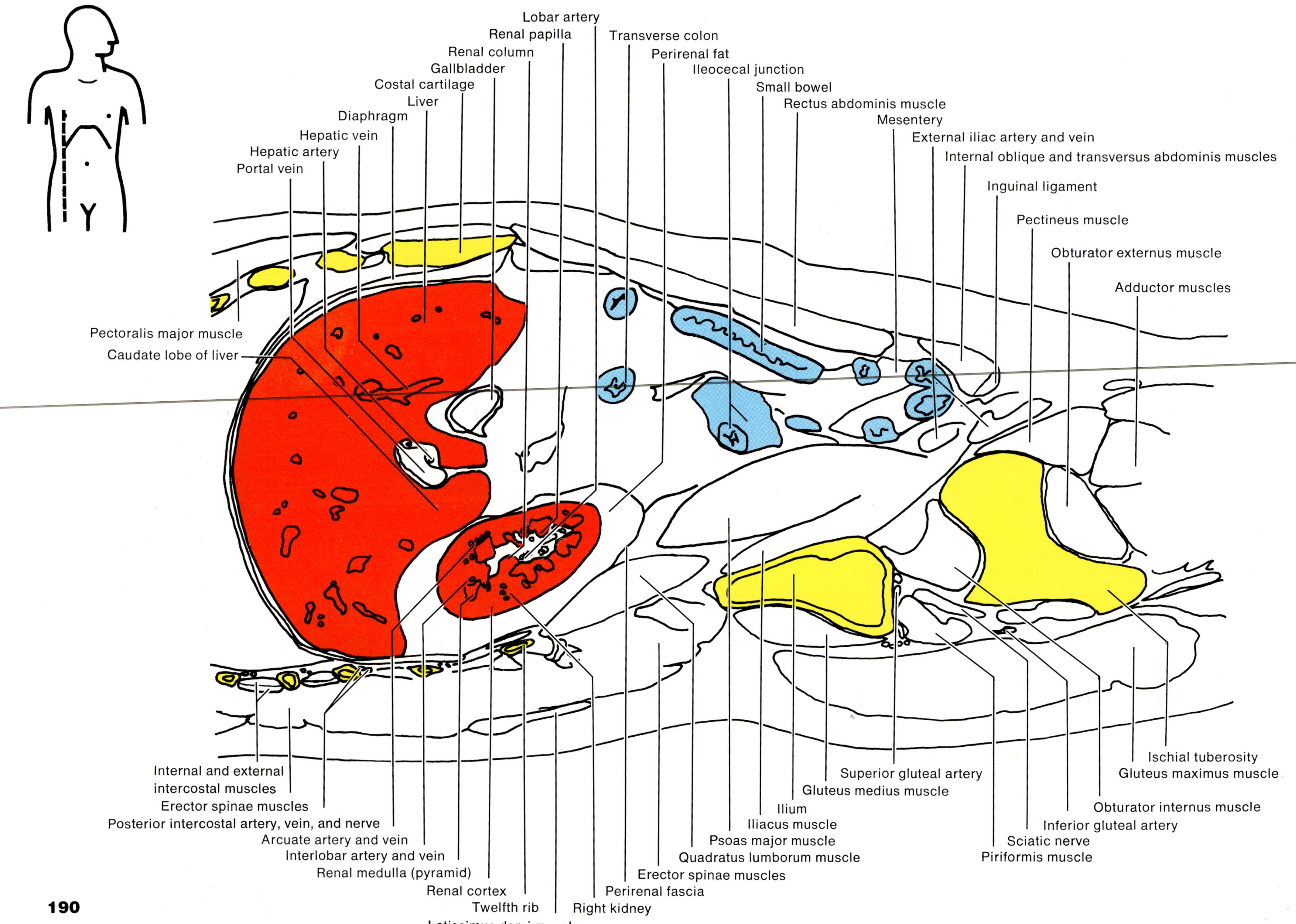

Lobar artery
Renal papilla
Renal column
Gallbladder
Costal cartilage
Liver
Diaphragm
Hepatic vein
Hepatic artery
Portal vein
Transverse colon
Perirenal fat
Ileocecal junction
Small bowel
Rectus abdominis muscle
Mesentery
External iliac artery and vein
Internal oblique and transversus abdominis muscles
Inguinal ligament
Pectineus muscle
Obturator externus muscle
Adductor muscles
Pectoralis major muscle
Caudate lobe of liver
Internal and external intercostal muscles
Erector spinae muscles
Posterior intercostal artery, vein, and nerve
Arcuate artery and vein
Interlobar artery and vein
Renal medulla (pyramid)
Renal cortex
Twelfth rib
Right kidney
Latissimus dorsi muscle
Perirenal fascia
Erector spinae muscles
Quadratus lumborum muscle
Psoas major muscle
Iliacus muscle
Ilium
Gluteus medius muscle
Superior gluteal artery
Sciatic nerve
Piriformis muscle
Inferior gluteal artery
Obturator internus muscle
Gluteus maximus muscle
Ischial tuberosity

PARASAGITTAL **Abdomen and pelvis—male**

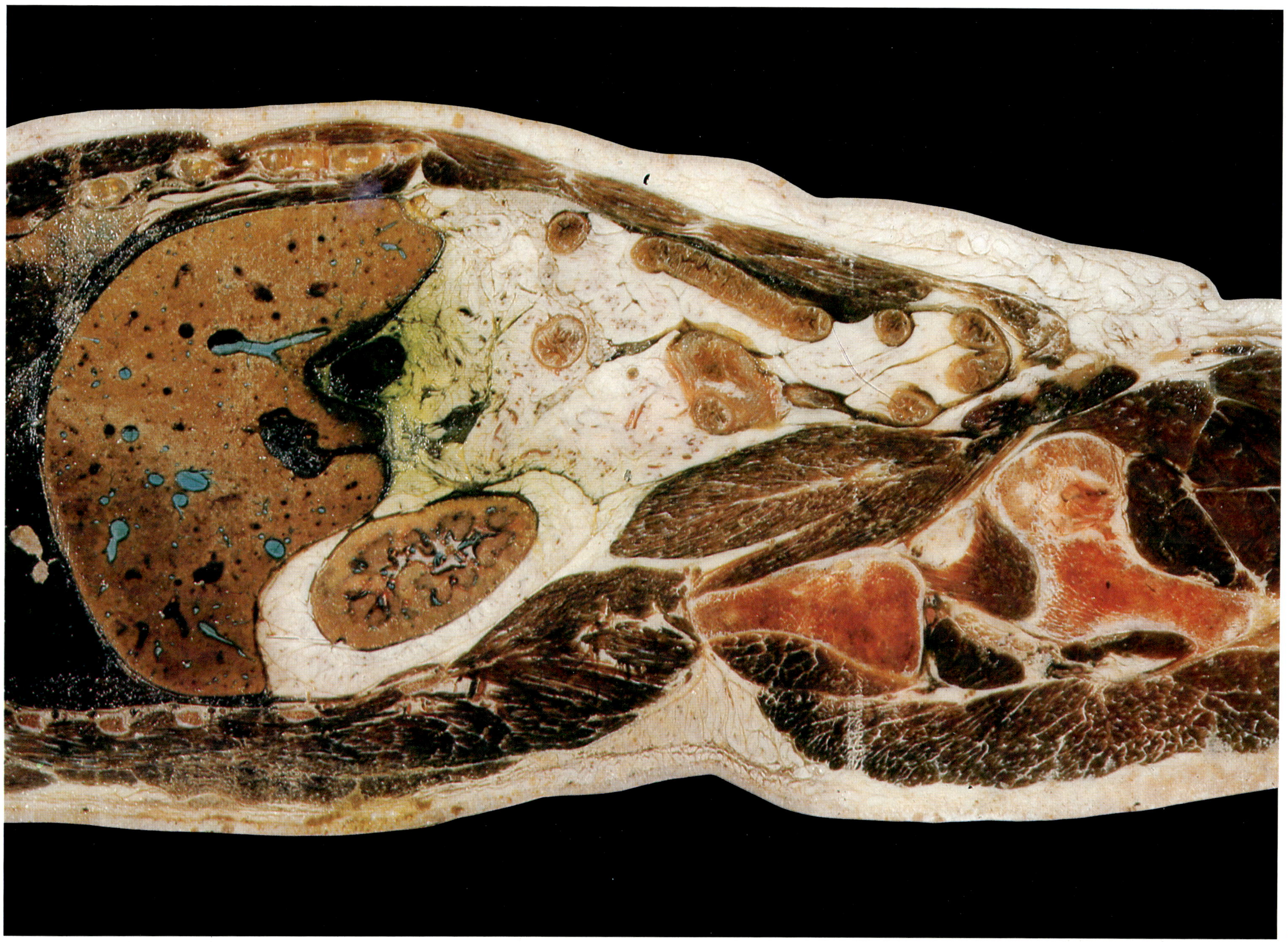

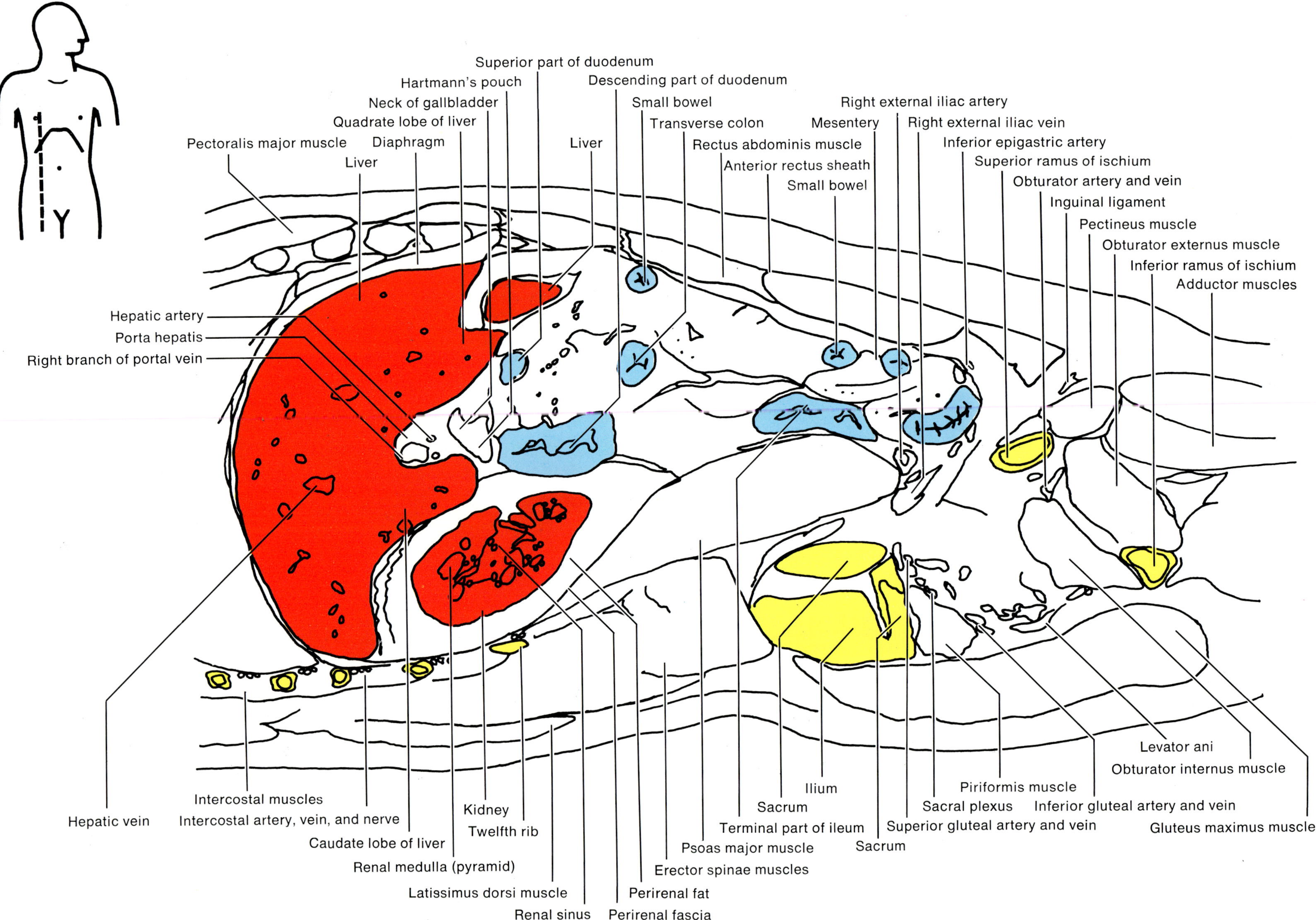

Superior part of duodenum
Hartmann's pouch
Neck of gallbladder
Quadrate lobe of liver
Pectoralis major muscle
Diaphragm
Liver
Descending part of duodenum
Small bowel
Transverse colon
Liver
Rectus abdominis muscle
Anterior rectus sheath
Small bowel
Right external iliac artery
Mesentery
Right external iliac vein
Inferior epigastric artery
Superior ramus of ischium
Obturator artery and vein
Inguinal ligament
Pectineus muscle
Obturator externus muscle
Inferior ramus of ischium
Adductor muscles
Hepatic artery
Porta hepatis
Right branch of portal vein
Levator ani
Obturator internus muscle
Hepatic vein
Intercostal muscles
Intercostal artery, vein, and nerve
Caudate lobe of liver
Renal medulla (pyramid)
Latissimus dorsi muscle
Renal sinus
Kidney
Twelfth rib
Perirenal fat
Perirenal fascia
Ilium
Terminal part of ileum
Psoas major muscle
Erector spinae muscles
Sacrum
Piriformis muscle
Sacral plexus
Superior gluteal artery and vein
Sacrum
Inferior gluteal artery and vein
Gluteus maximus muscle

PARASAGITTAL **Abdomen and pelvis—male**

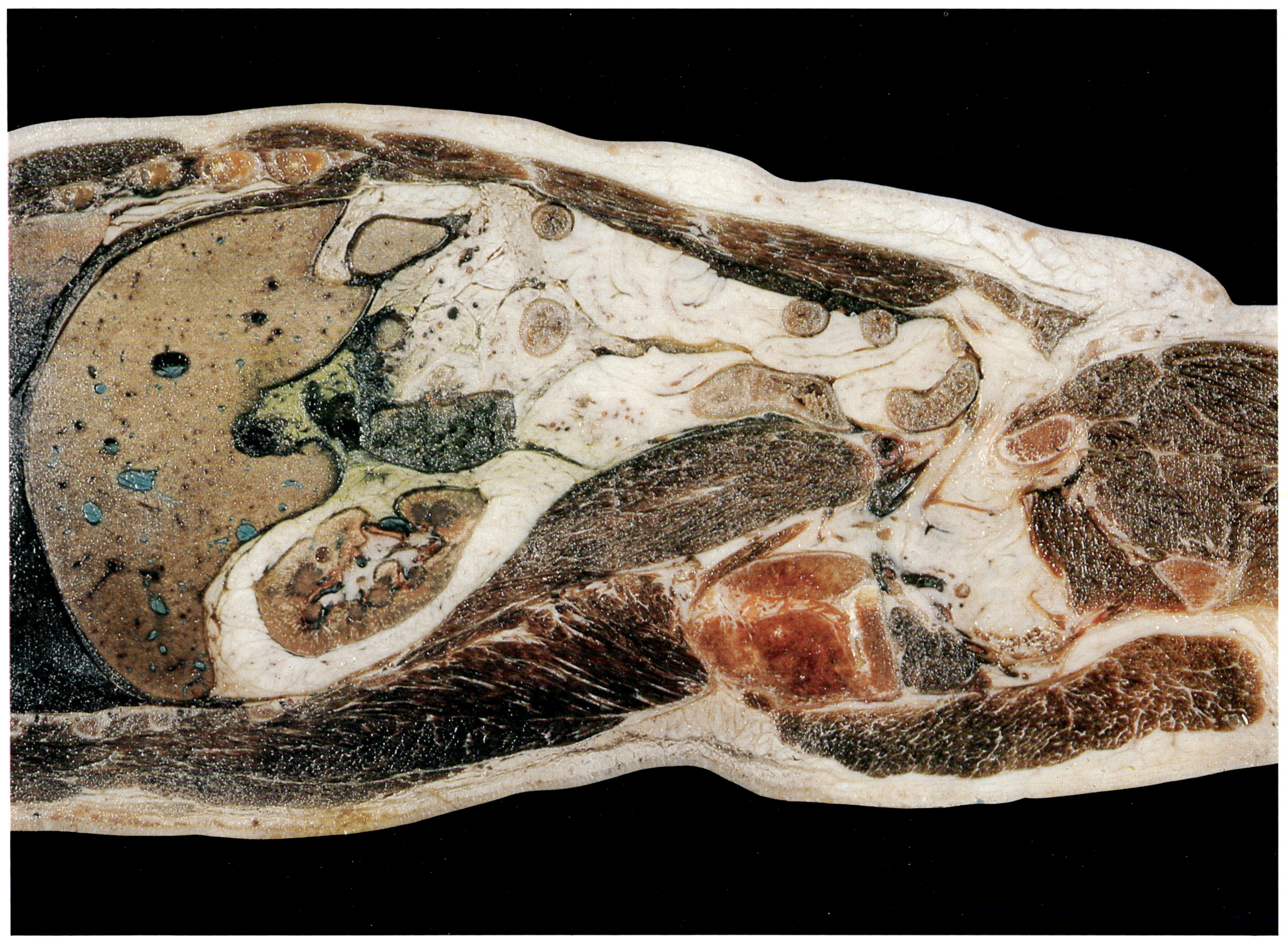

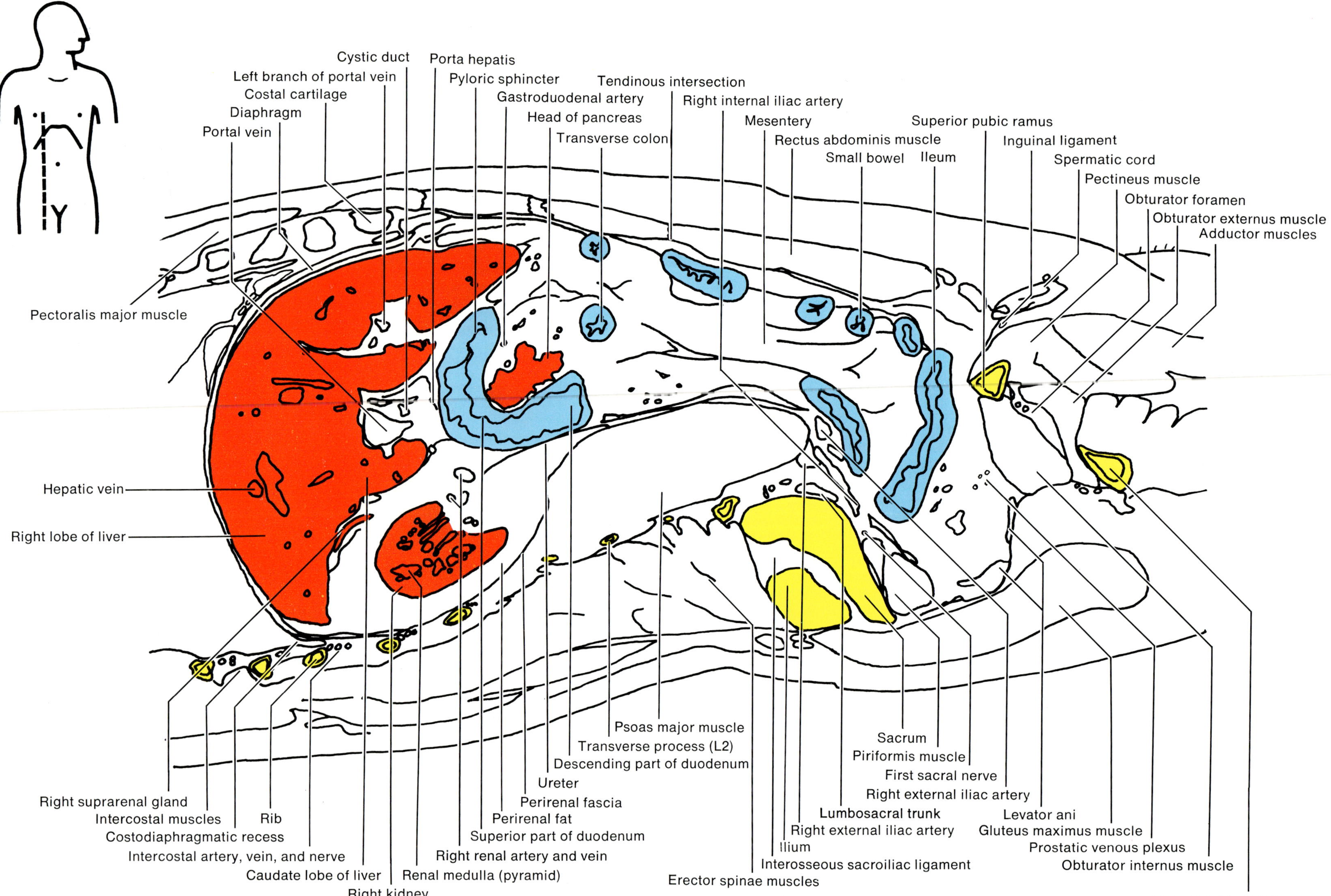
Cystic duct
Porta hepatis
Left branch of portal vein
Pyloric sphincter
Tendinous intersection
Costal cartilage
Gastroduodenal artery
Right internal iliac artery
Diaphragm
Head of pancreas
Mesentery
Superior pubic ramus
Portal vein
Transverse colon
Rectus abdominis muscle
Inguinal ligament
Small bowel
Ileum
Spermatic cord
Pectineus muscle
Obturator foramen
Obturator externus muscle
Adductor muscles
Pectoralis major muscle
Hepatic vein
Right lobe of liver
Psoas major muscle
Transverse process (L2)
Descending part of duodenum
Sacrum
Piriformis muscle
First sacral nerve
Ureter
Right external iliac artery
Right suprarenal gland
Perirenal fascia
Intercostal muscles
Rib
Lumbosacral trunk
Levator ani
Costodiaphragmatic recess
Perirenal fat
Right external iliac artery
Gluteus maximus muscle
Intercostal artery, vein, and nerve
Superior part of duodenum
Ilium
Prostatic venous plexus
Caudate lobe of liver
Right renal artery and vein
Interosseous sacroiliac ligament
Obturator internus muscle
Renal medulla (pyramid)
Right kidney
Erector spinae muscles
Inferior pubic ramus

PARASAGITTAL **Abdomen and pelvis—male**

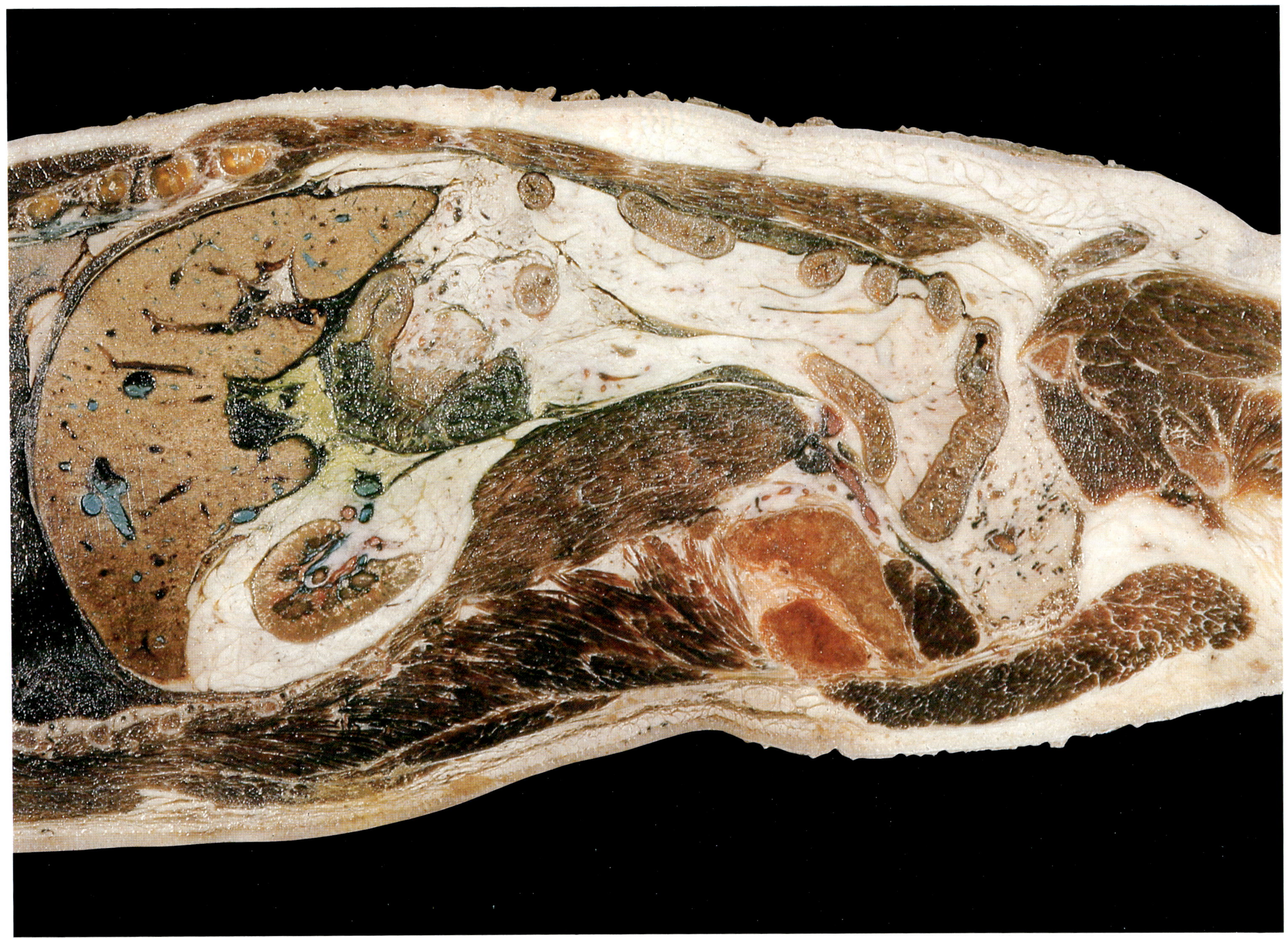

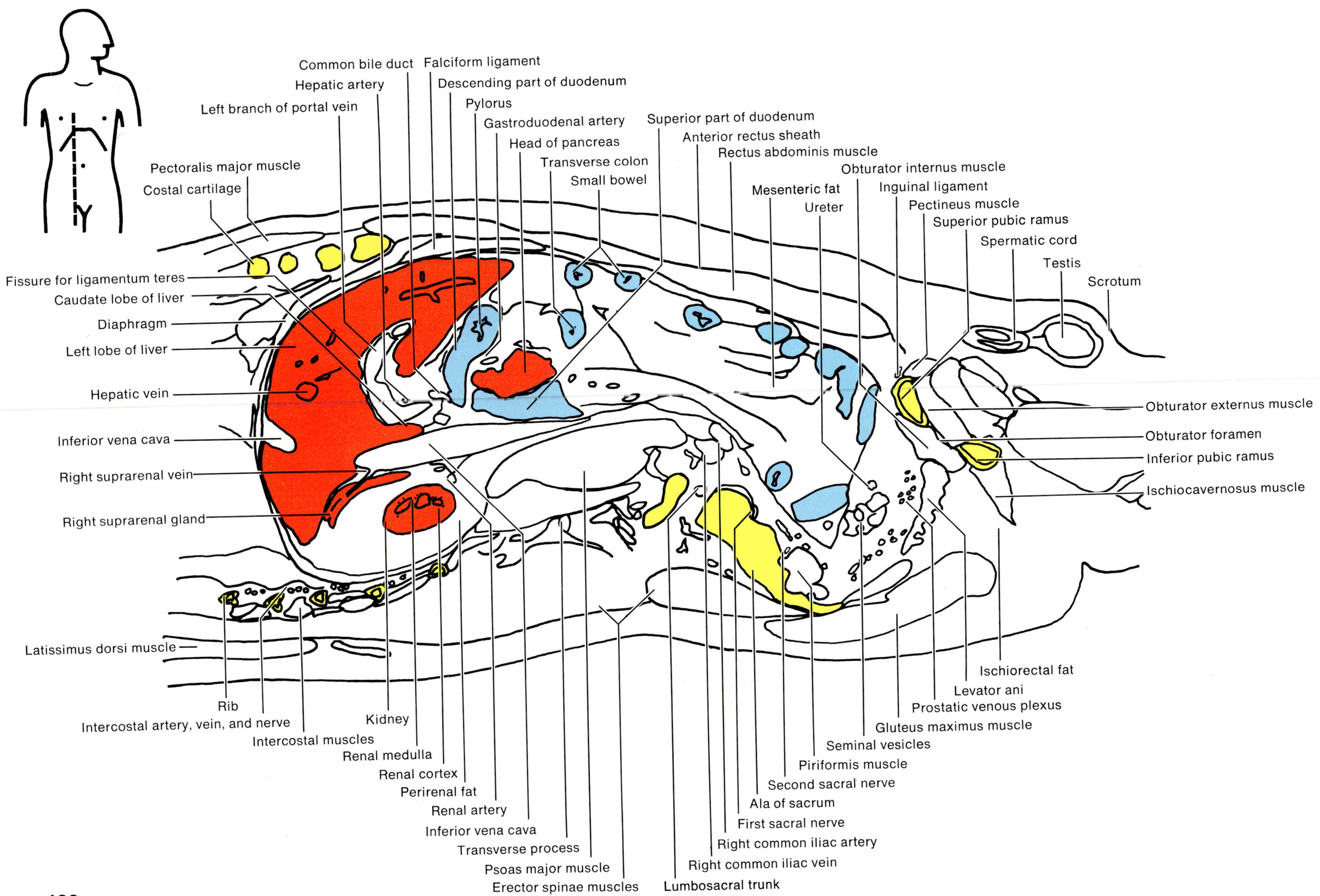

Common bile duct
Hepatic artery
Left branch of portal vein
Falciform ligament
Descending part of duodenum
Pylorus
Gastroduodenal artery
Head of pancreas
Transverse colon
Small bowel
Superior part of duodenum
Anterior rectus sheath
Rectus abdominis muscle
Obturator internus muscle
Inguinal ligament
Pectineus muscle
Superior pubic ramus
Spermatic cord
Testis
Scrotum
Mesenteric fat
Ureter
Pectoralis major muscle
Costal cartilage
Fissure for ligamentum teres
Caudate lobe of liver
Diaphragm
Left lobe of liver
Hepatic vein
Inferior vena cava
Right suprarenal vein
Right suprarenal gland
Obturator externus muscle
Obturator foramen
Inferior pubic ramus
Ischiocavernosus muscle
Latissimus dorsi muscle
Rib
Intercostal artery, vein, and nerve
Intercostal muscles
Kidney
Renal medulla
Renal cortex
Perirenal fat
Renal artery
Inferior vena cava
Transverse process
Psoas major muscle
Erector spinae muscles
Lumbosacral trunk
Right common iliac vein
Right common iliac artery
First sacral nerve
Ala of sacrum
Second sacral nerve
Piriformis muscle
Seminal vesicles
Gluteus maximus muscle
Prostatic venous plexus
Levator ani
Ischiorectal fat

PARASAGITTAL **Abdomen and pelvis—male**

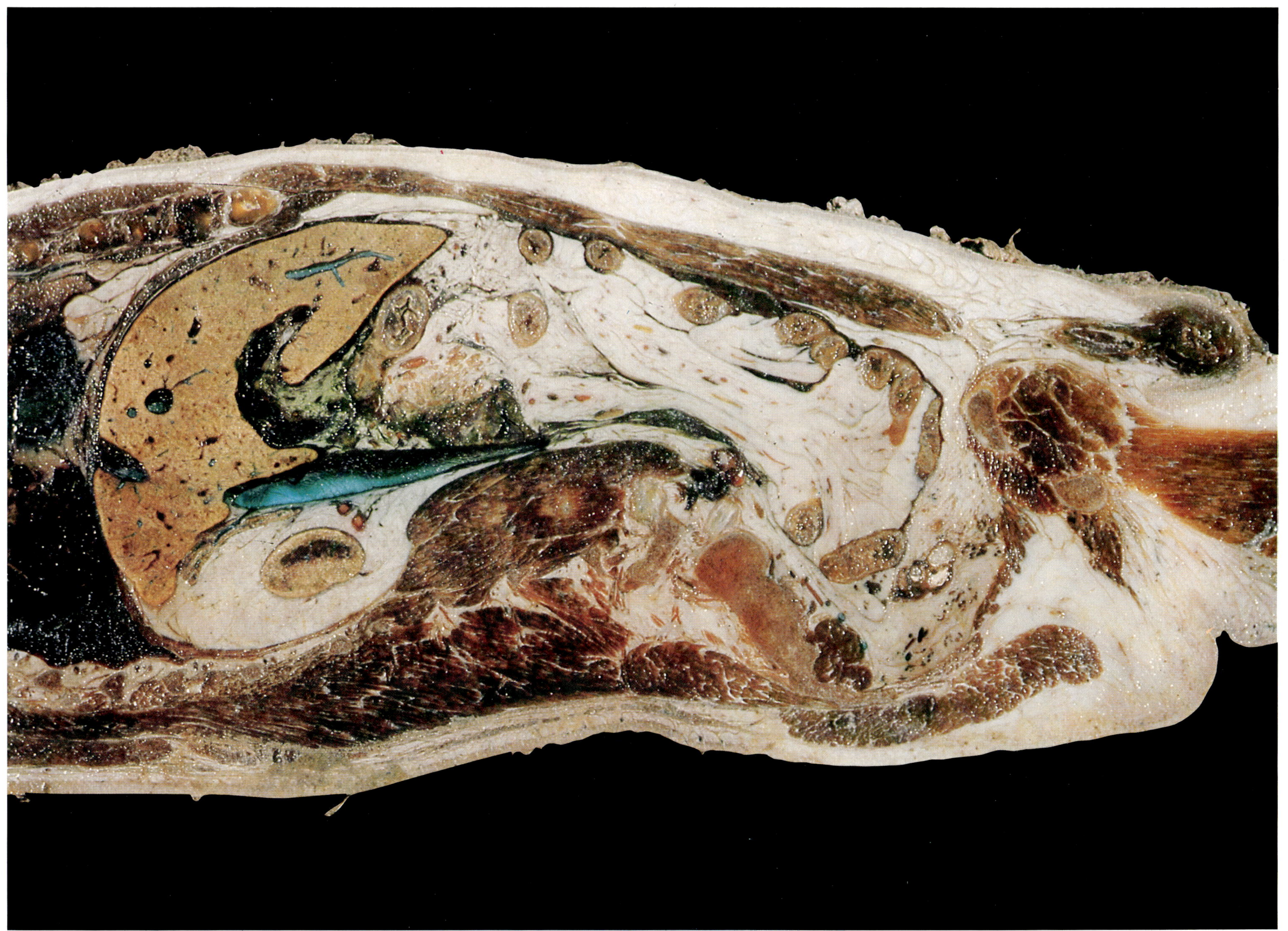

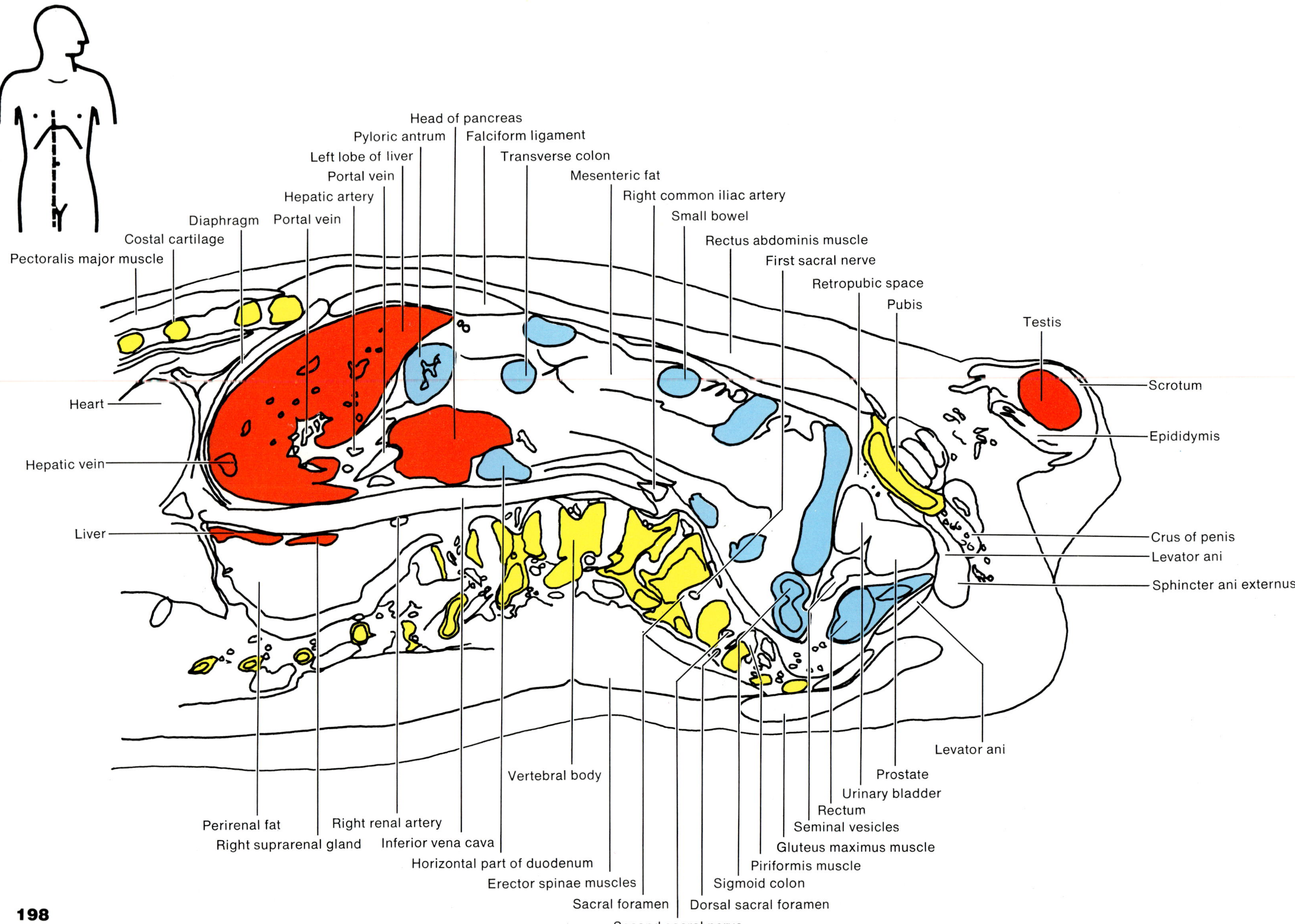
Pectoralis major muscle
Costal cartilage
Diaphragm
Portal vein
Hepatic artery
Portal vein
Left lobe of liver
Pyloric antrum
Head of pancreas
Falciform ligament
Transverse colon
Mesenteric fat
Right common iliac artery
Small bowel
Rectus abdominis muscle
First sacral nerve
Retropubic space
Pubis
Testis
Heart
Scrotum
Hepatic vein
Epididymis
Liver
Crus of penis
Levator ani
Sphincter ani externus
Perirenal fat
Right renal artery
Right suprarenal gland
Inferior vena cava
Horizontal part of duodenum
Erector spinae muscles
Vertebral body
Sacral foramen
Second sacral nerve
Dorsal sacral foramen
Sigmoid colon
Piriformis muscle
Gluteus maximus muscle
Seminal vesicles
Rectum
Urinary bladder
Prostate
Levator ani

PARASAGITTAL **Abdomen and pelvis—male**

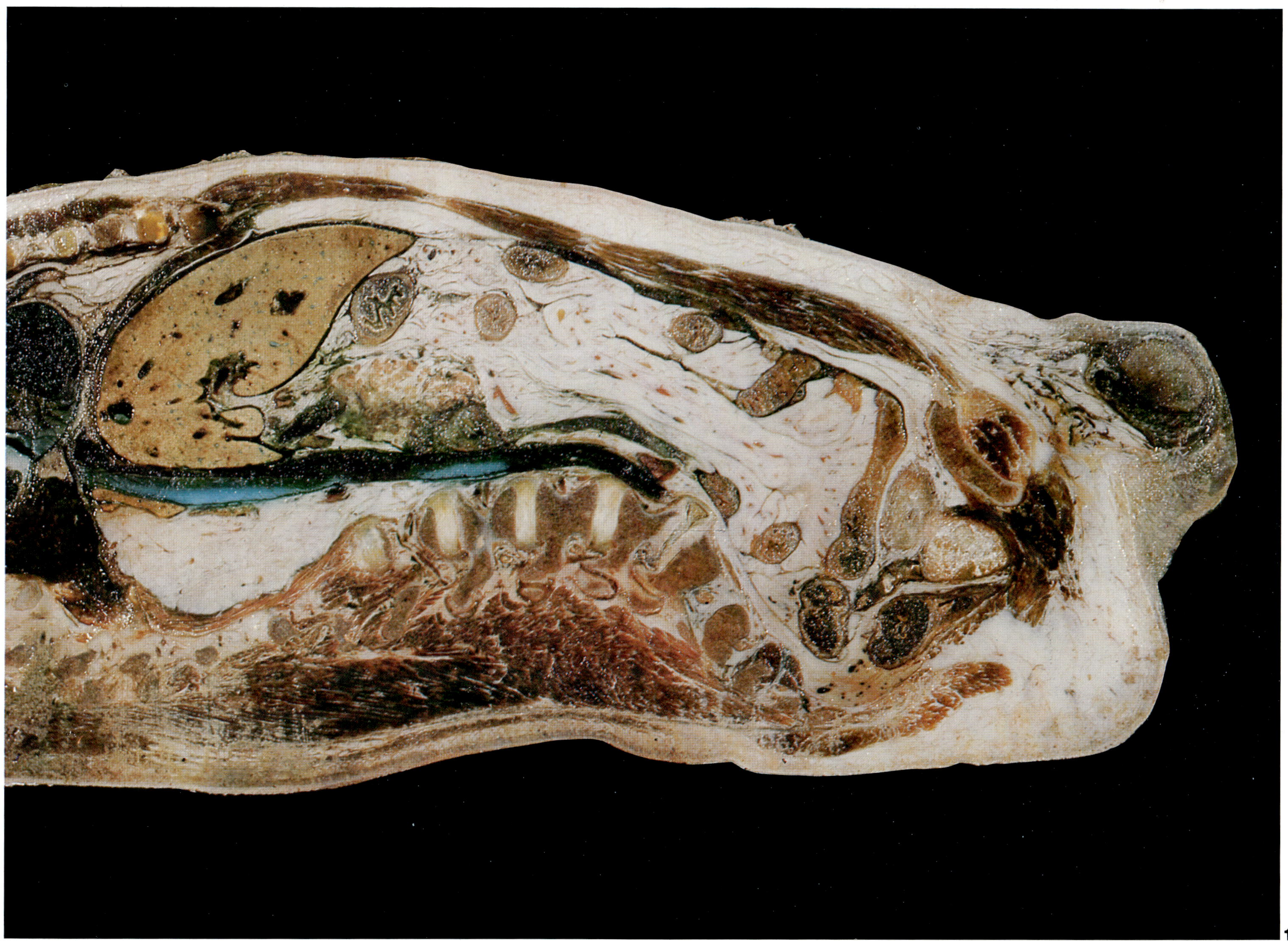

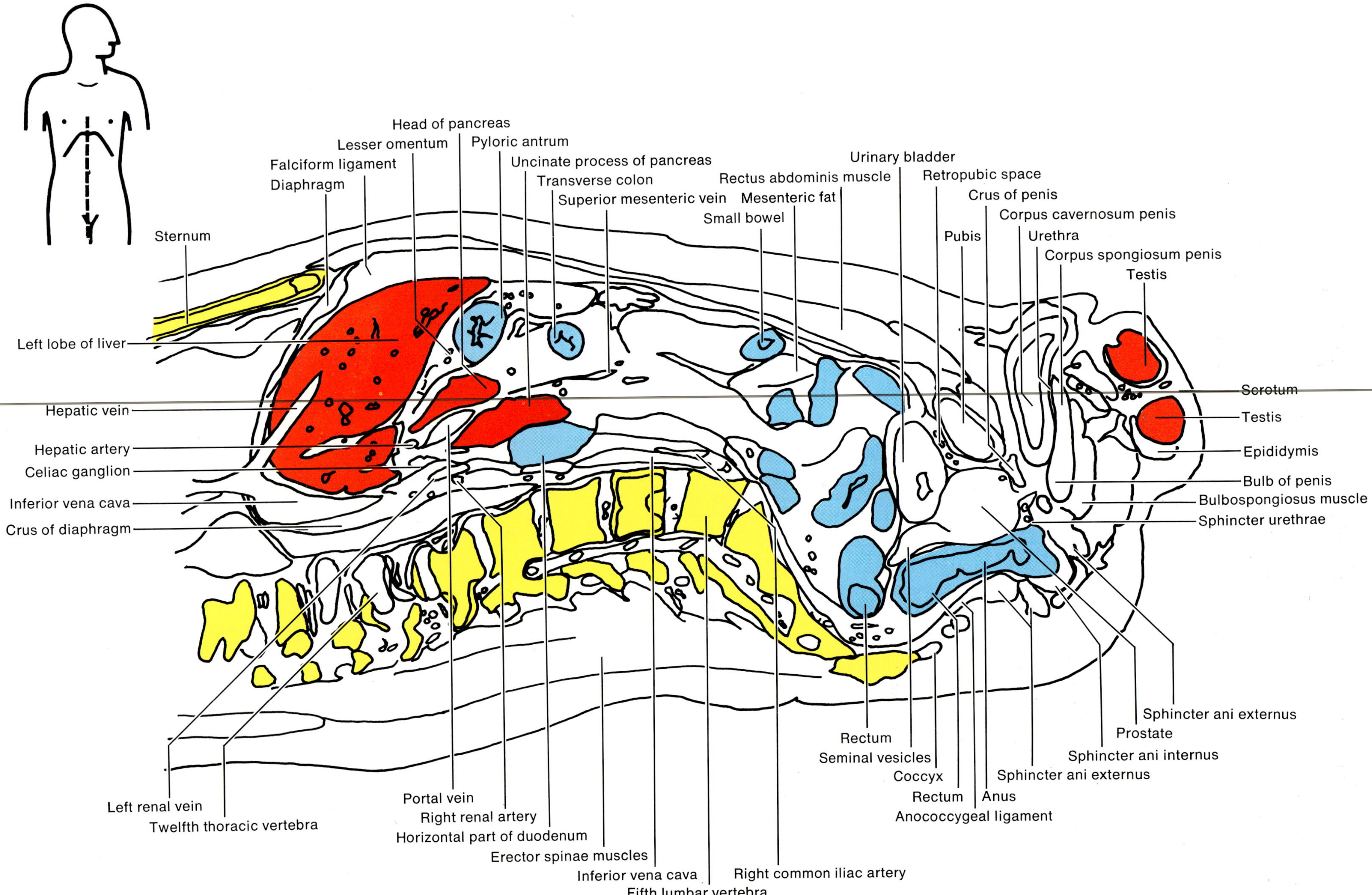

Sternum
Left lobe of liver
Hepatic vein
Hepatic artery
Celiac ganglion
Inferior vena cava
Crus of diaphragm
Left renal vein
Twelfth thoracic vertebra
Falciform ligament
Diaphragm
Lesser omentum
Head of pancreas
Pyloric antrum
Uncinate process of pancreas
Transverse colon
Superior mesenteric vein
Small bowel
Rectus abdominis muscle
Mesenteric fat
Urinary bladder
Retropubic space
Crus of penis
Pubis
Corpus cavernosum penis
Urethra
Corpus spongiosum penis
Testis
Scrotum
Testis
Epididymis
Bulb of penis
Bulbospongiosus muscle
Sphincter urethrae
Sphincter ani externus
Prostate
Sphincter ani internus
Sphincter ani externus
Rectum
Seminal vesicles
Coccyx
Rectum
Anus
Anococcygeal ligament
Portal vein
Right renal artery
Horizontal part of duodenum
Erector spinae muscles
Inferior vena cava
Fifth lumbar vertebra
Right common iliac artery

PARASAGITTAL **Abdomen and pelvis—male**

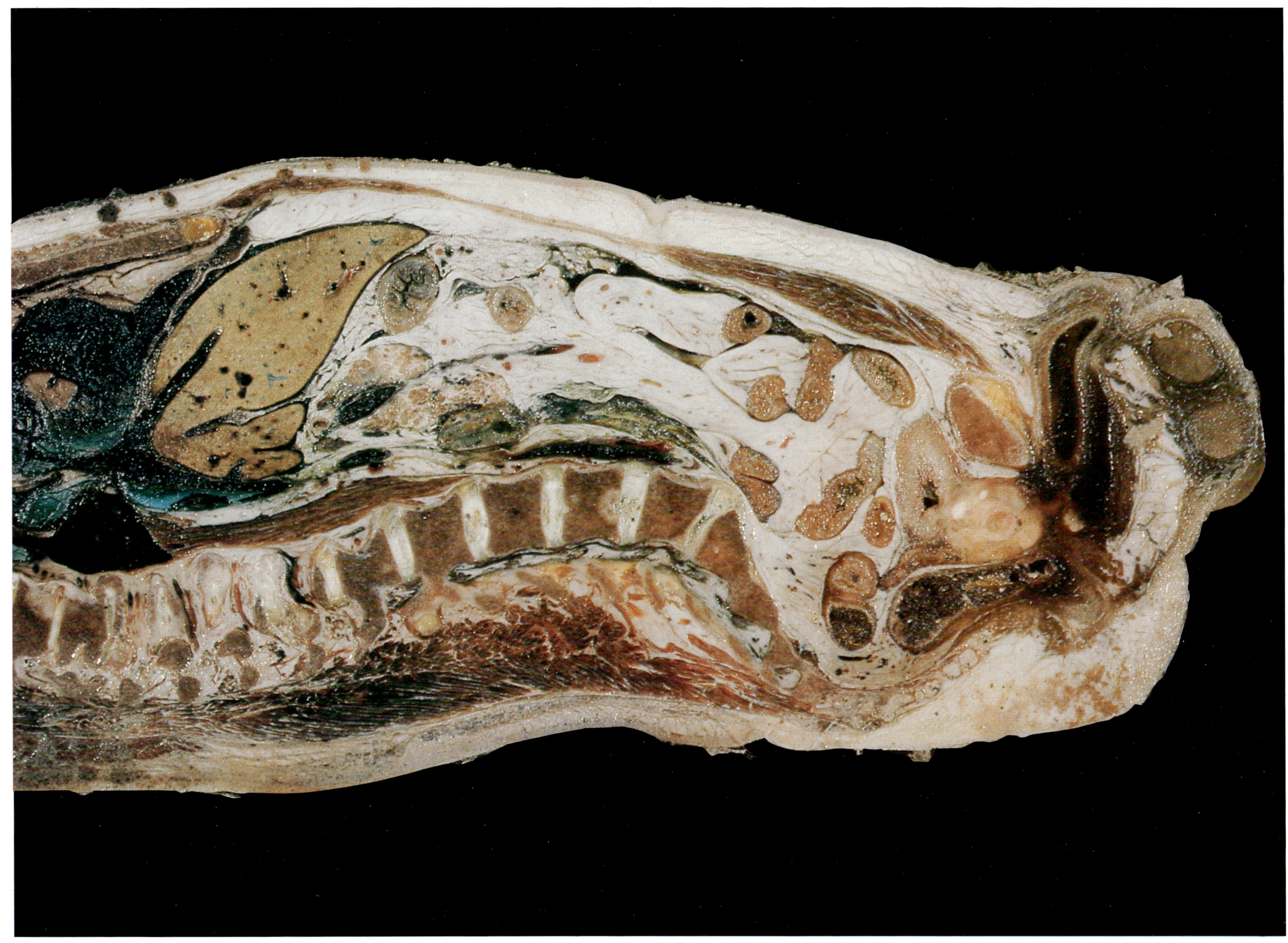

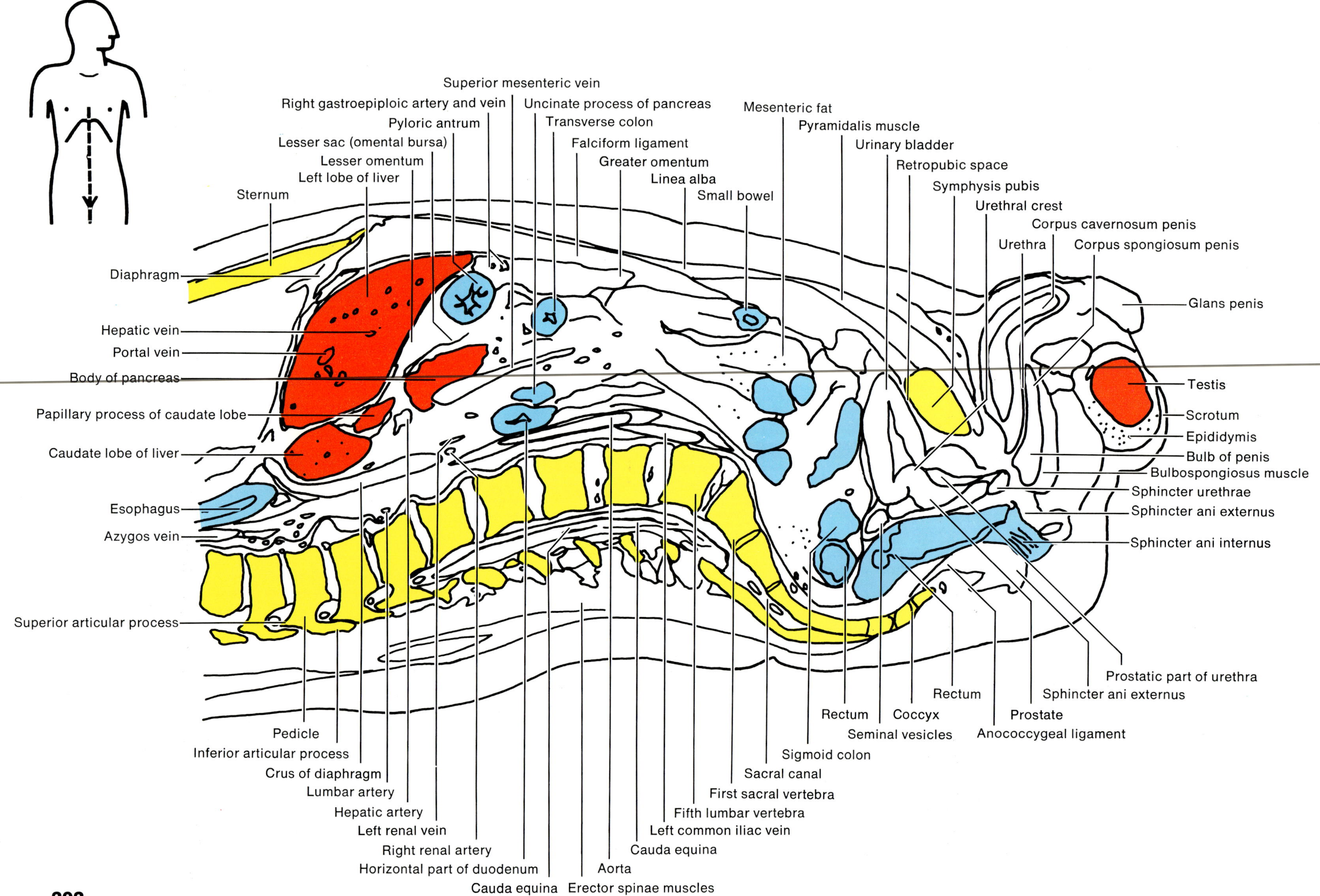

Superior mesenteric vein
Right gastroepiploic artery and vein
Uncinate process of pancreas
Mesenteric fat
Pyloric antrum
Transverse colon
Pyramidalis muscle
Urinary bladder
Lesser sac (omental bursa)
Falciform ligament
Retropubic space
Lesser omentum
Greater omentum
Symphysis pubis
Left lobe of liver
Linea alba
Urethral crest
Sternum
Small bowel
Corpus cavernosum penis
Urethra
Corpus spongiosum penis
Diaphragm
Glans penis
Hepatic vein
Portal vein
Body of pancreas
Testis
Papillary process of caudate lobe
Scrotum
Epididymis
Caudate lobe of liver
Bulb of penis
Bulbospongiosus muscle
Sphincter urethrae
Esophagus
Sphincter ani externus
Azygos vein
Sphincter ani internus
Superior articular process
Prostatic part of urethra
Sphincter ani externus
Rectum
Rectum
Coccyx
Prostate
Seminal vesicles
Anococcygeal ligament
Pedicle
Sigmoid colon
Inferior articular process
Sacral canal
Crus of diaphragm
First sacral vertebra
Lumbar artery
Fifth lumbar vertebra
Hepatic artery
Left common iliac vein
Left renal vein
Cauda equina
Right renal artery
Horizontal part of duodenum
Aorta
Cauda equina
Erector spinae muscles

PARASAGITTAL **Abdomen and pelvis—male**

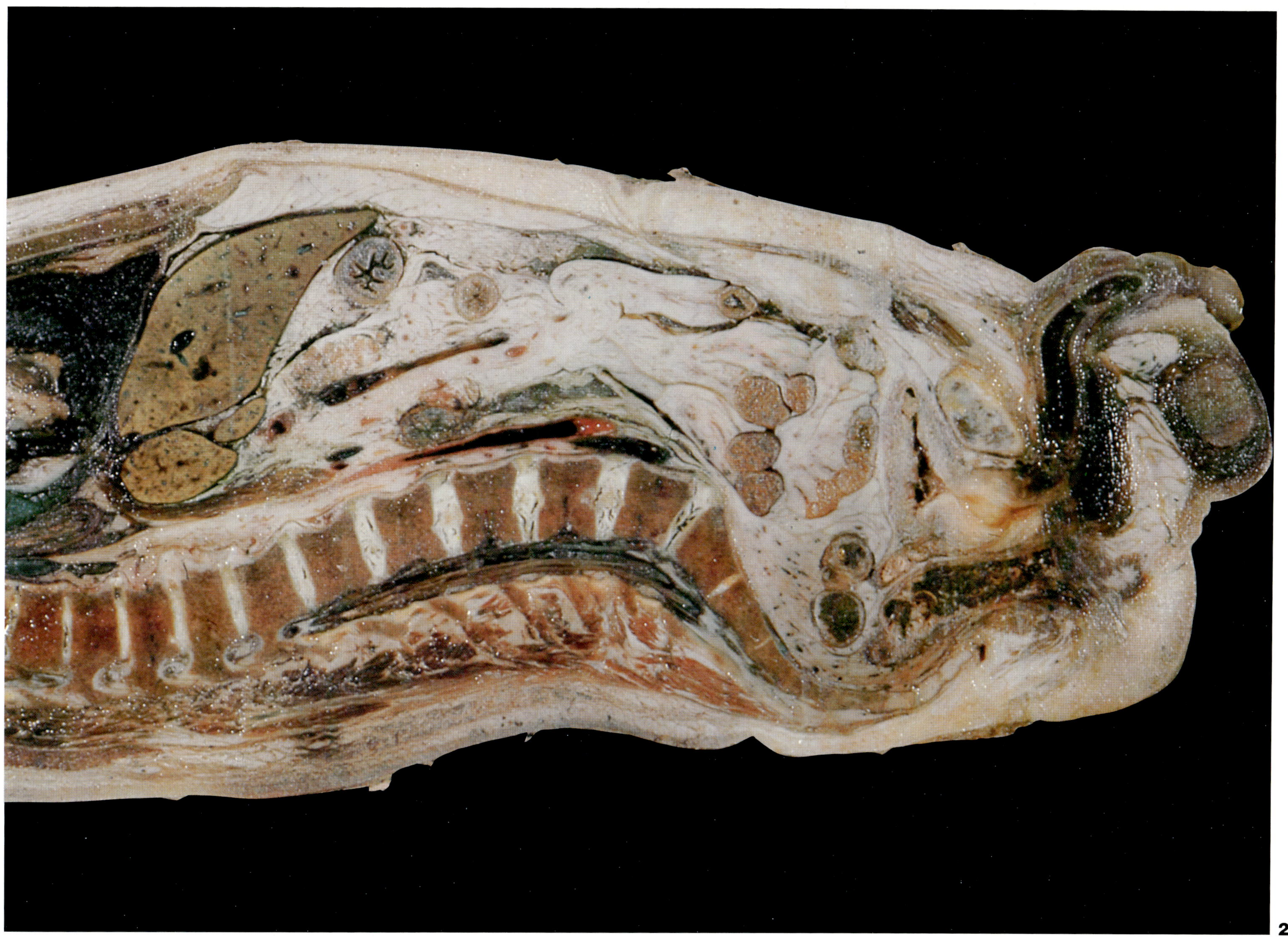

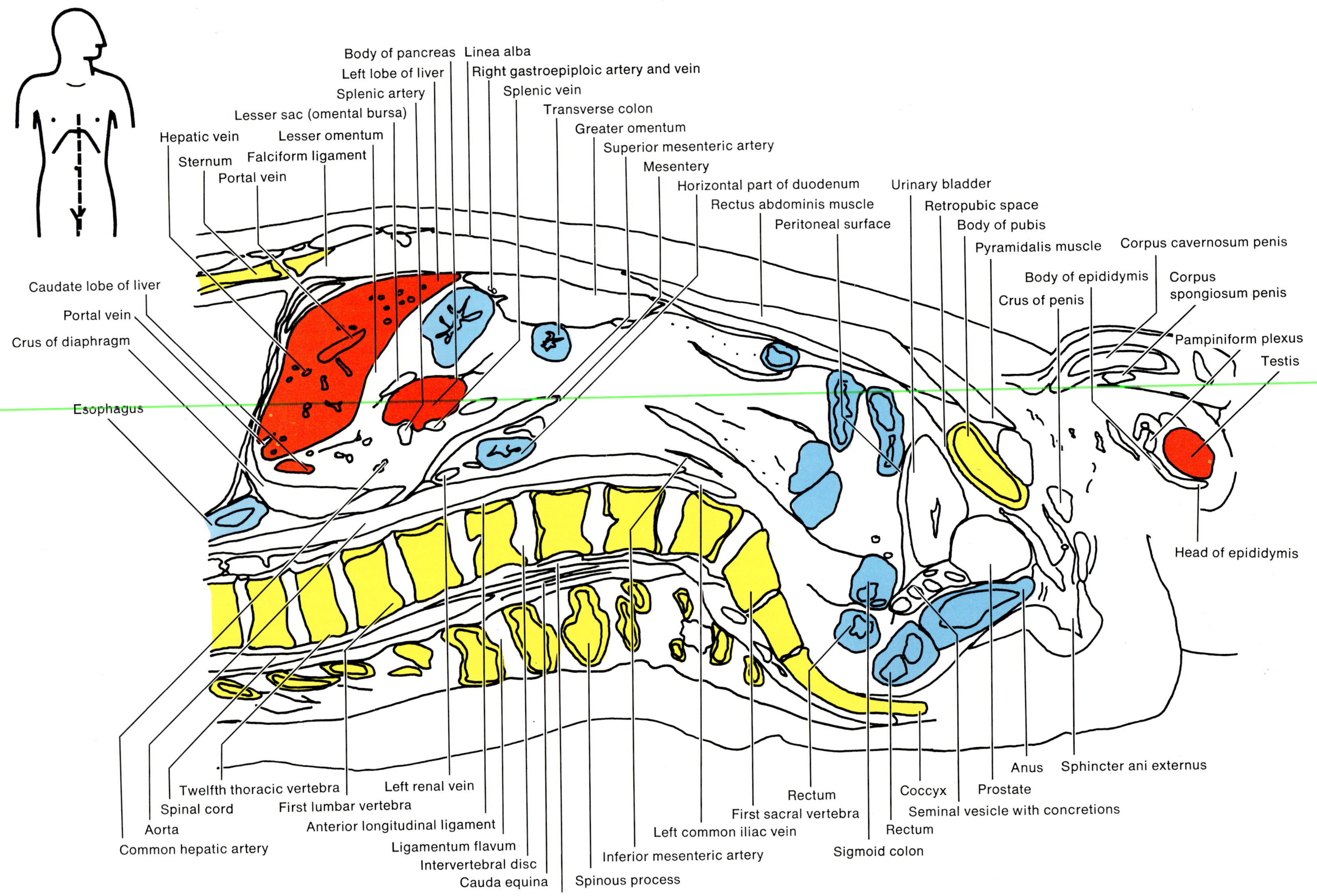

Body of pancreas
Linea alba
Left lobe of liver
Right gastroepiploic artery and vein
Splenic artery
Splenic vein
Lesser sac (omental bursa)
Transverse colon
Hepatic vein
Lesser omentum
Greater omentum
Sternum
Falciform ligament
Superior mesenteric artery
Portal vein
Mesentery
Horizontal part of duodenum
Urinary bladder
Rectus abdominis muscle
Retropubic space
Peritoneal surface
Body of pubis
Pyramidalis muscle
Corpus cavernosum penis
Caudate lobe of liver
Body of epididymis
Corpus spongiosum penis
Portal vein
Crus of penis
Crus of diaphragm
Pampiniform plexus
Testis
Esophagus
Head of epididymis
Twelfth thoracic vertebra
Left renal vein
Spinal cord
First lumbar vertebra
Anterior longitudinal ligament
Rectum
Aorta
First sacral vertebra
Coccyx
Prostate
Anus
Sphincter ani externus
Common hepatic artery
Ligamentum flavum
Left common iliac vein
Rectum
Seminal vesicle with concretions
Intervertebral disc
Inferior mesenteric artery
Sigmoid colon
Cauda equina
Spinous process
Posterior longitudinal ligament

PARASAGITTAL **Abdomen and pelvis—male**

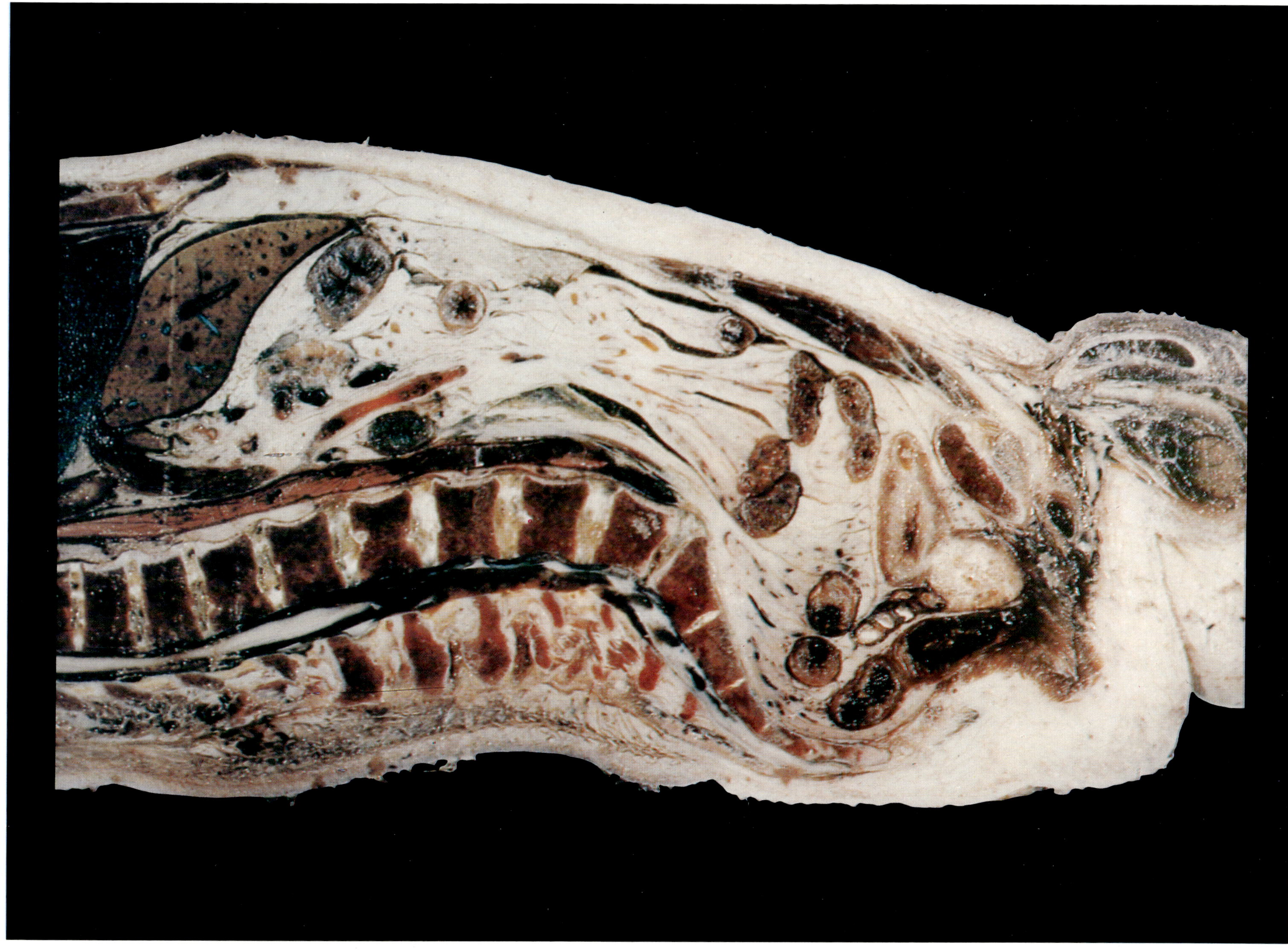

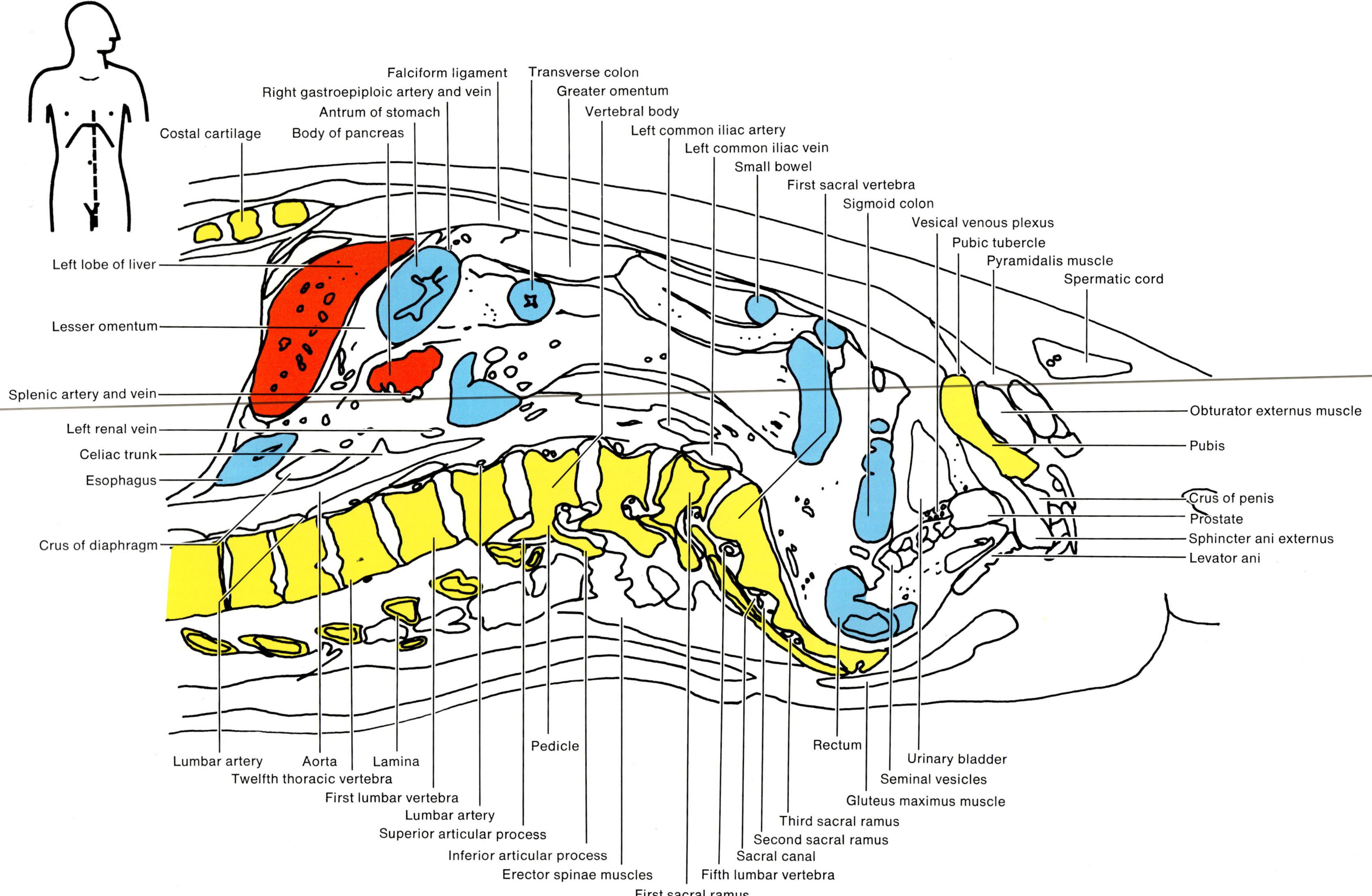
Costal cartilage
Right gastroepiploic artery and vein
Falciform ligament
Antrum of stomach
Body of pancreas
Transverse colon
Greater omentum
Vertebral body
Left common iliac artery
Left common iliac vein
Small bowel
First sacral vertebra
Sigmoid colon
Vesical venous plexus
Pubic tubercle
Pyramidalis muscle
Spermatic cord
Left lobe of liver
Lesser omentum
Splenic artery and vein
Obturator externus muscle
Left renal vein
Pubis
Celiac trunk
Esophagus
Crus of penis
Prostate
Sphincter ani externus
Levator ani
Crus of diaphragm
Lumbar artery
Aorta
Lamina
Twelfth thoracic vertebra
First lumbar vertebra
Lumbar artery
Superior articular process
Inferior articular process
Erector spinae muscles
First sacral ramus
Pedicle
Fifth lumbar vertebra
Sacral canal
Second sacral ramus
Third sacral ramus
Gluteus maximus muscle
Seminal vesicles
Urinary bladder
Rectum

PARASAGITTAL **Abdomen and pelvis—male**

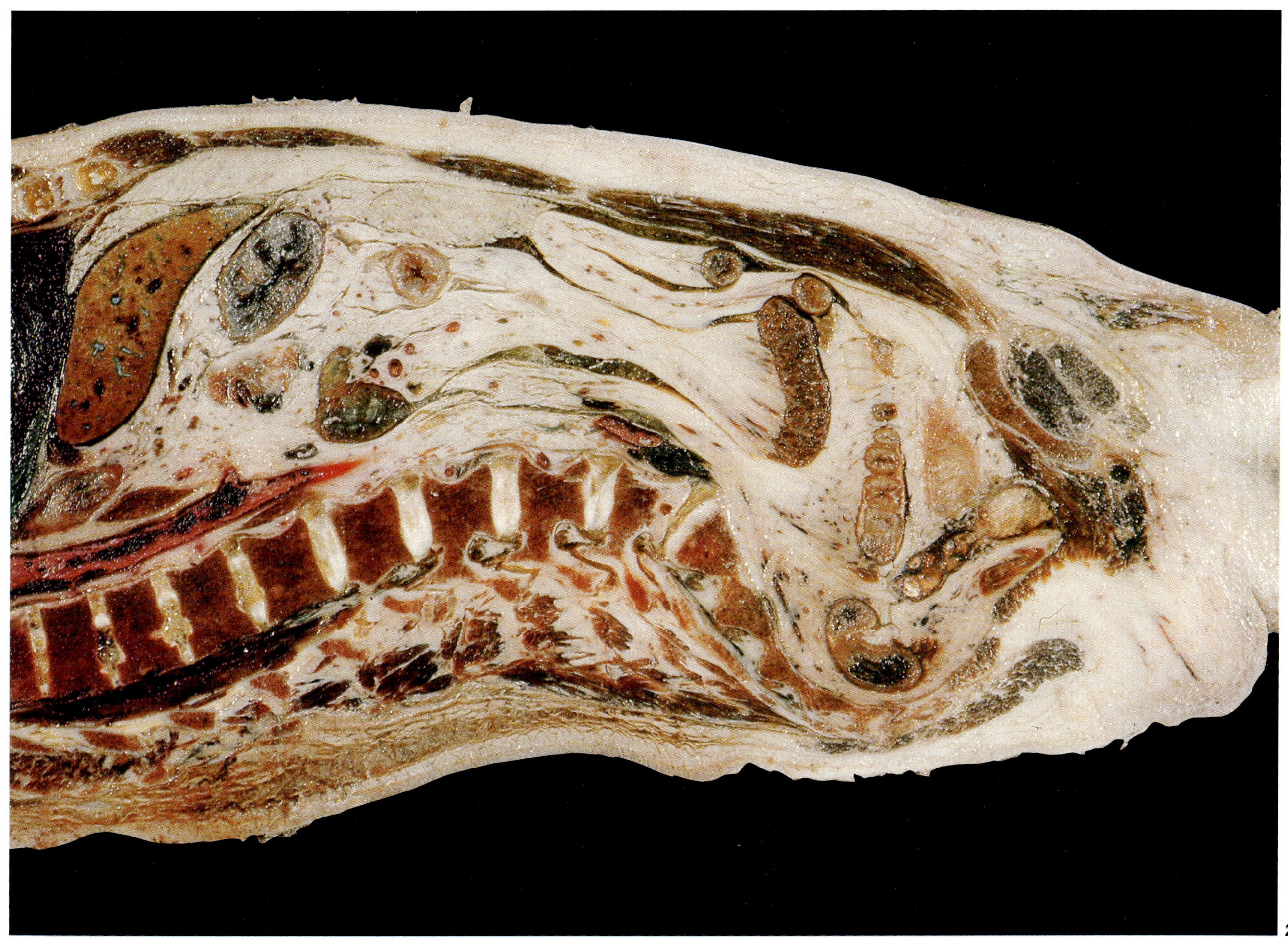

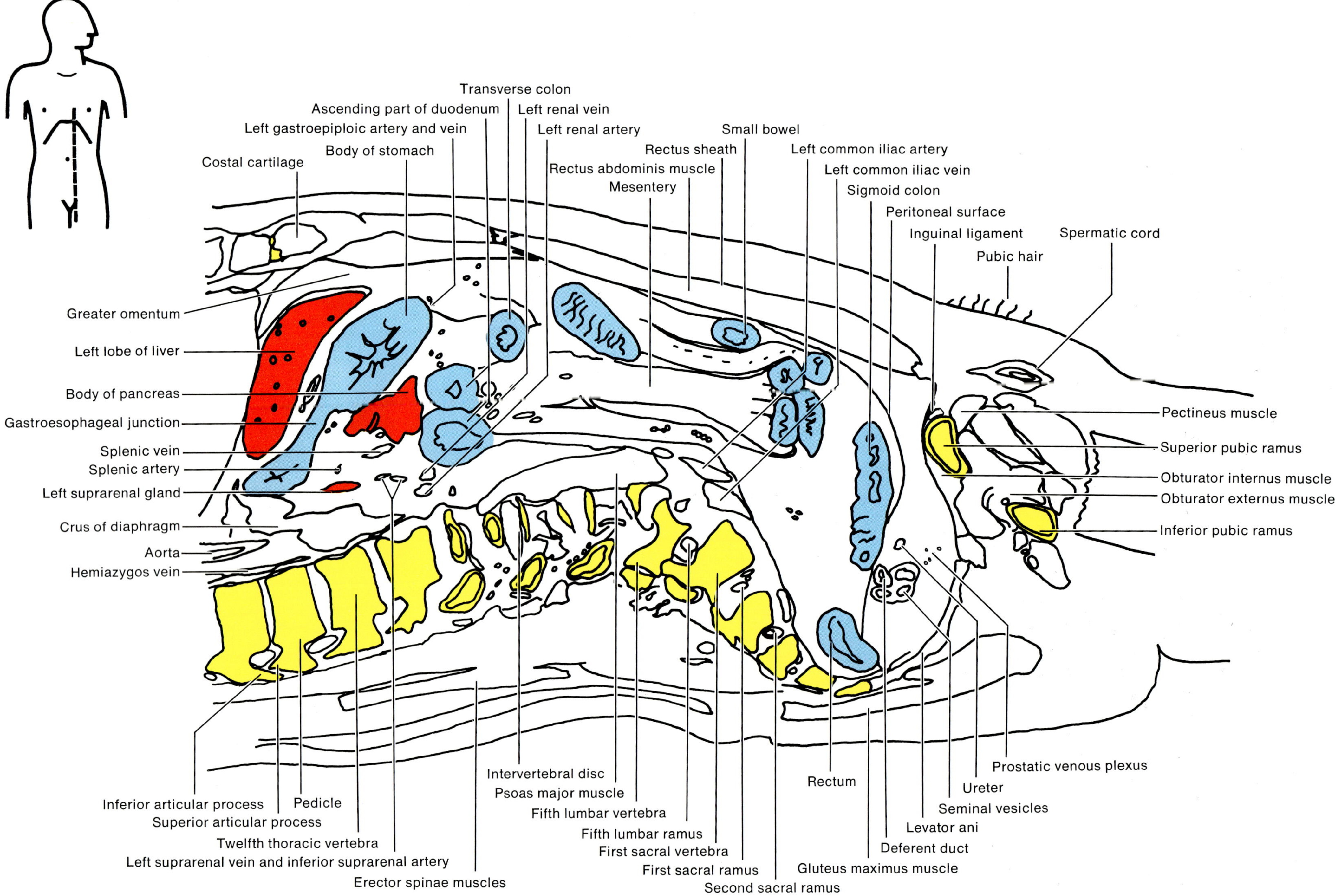

Costal cartilage
Ascending part of duodenum
Left gastroepiploic artery and vein
Body of stomach
Transverse colon
Left renal vein
Left renal artery
Rectus sheath
Rectus abdominis muscle
Mesentery
Small bowel
Left common iliac artery
Left common iliac vein
Sigmoid colon
Peritoneal surface
Inguinal ligament
Pubic hair
Spermatic cord
Greater omentum
Left lobe of liver
Body of pancreas
Gastroesophageal junction
Splenic vein
Splenic artery
Left suprarenal gland
Crus of diaphragm
Aorta
Hemiazygos vein
Pectineus muscle
Superior pubic ramus
Obturator internus muscle
Obturator externus muscle
Inferior pubic ramus
Inferior articular process
Pedicle
Superior articular process
Twelfth thoracic vertebra
Left suprarenal vein and inferior suprarenal artery
Erector spinae muscles
Intervertebral disc
Psoas major muscle
Fifth lumbar vertebra
Fifth lumbar ramus
First sacral vertebra
First sacral ramus
Second sacral ramus
Rectum
Gluteus maximus muscle
Levator ani
Deferent duct
Seminal vesicles
Ureter
Prostatic venous plexus

PARASAGITTAL **Abdomen and pelvis—male**

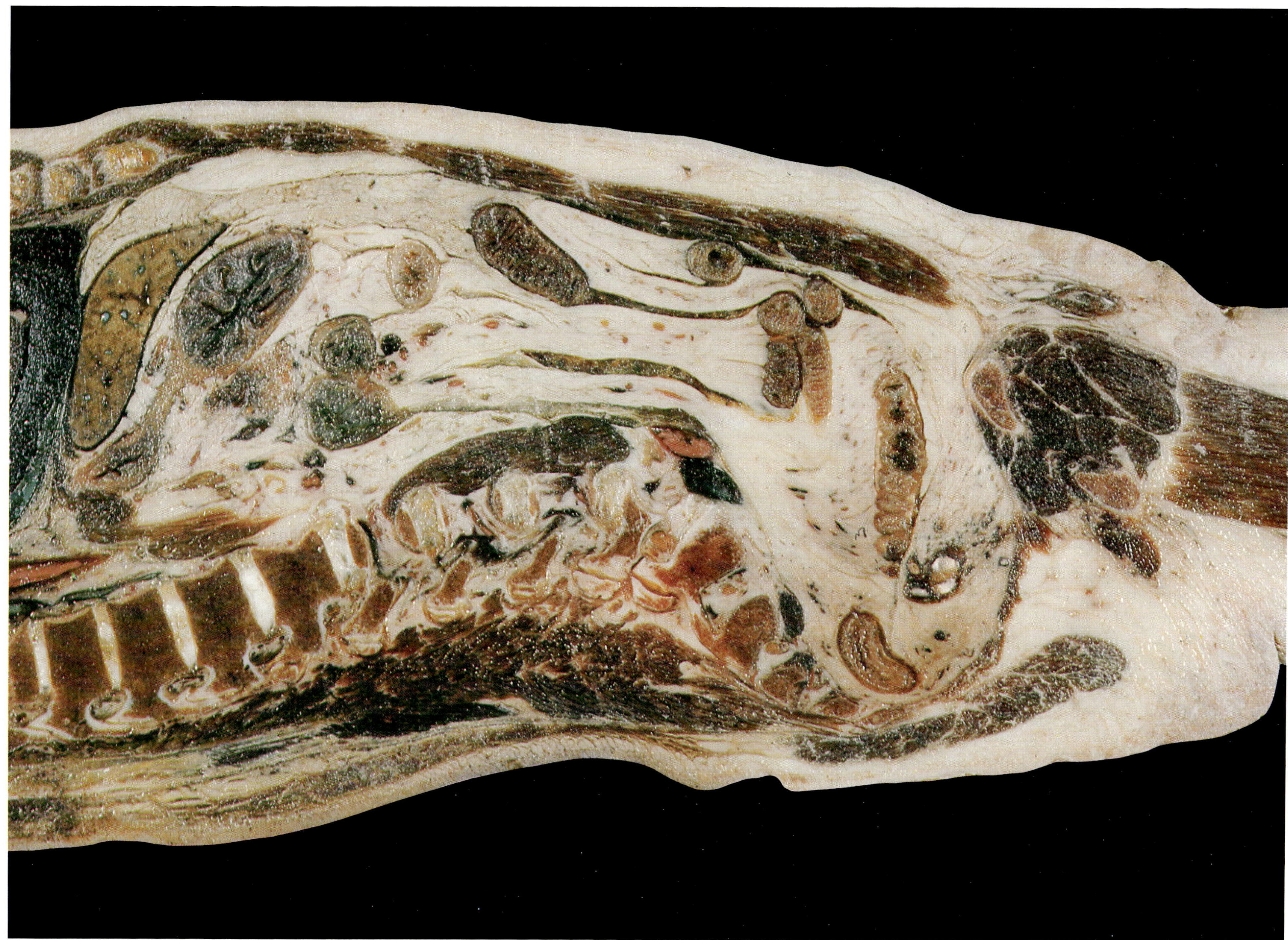

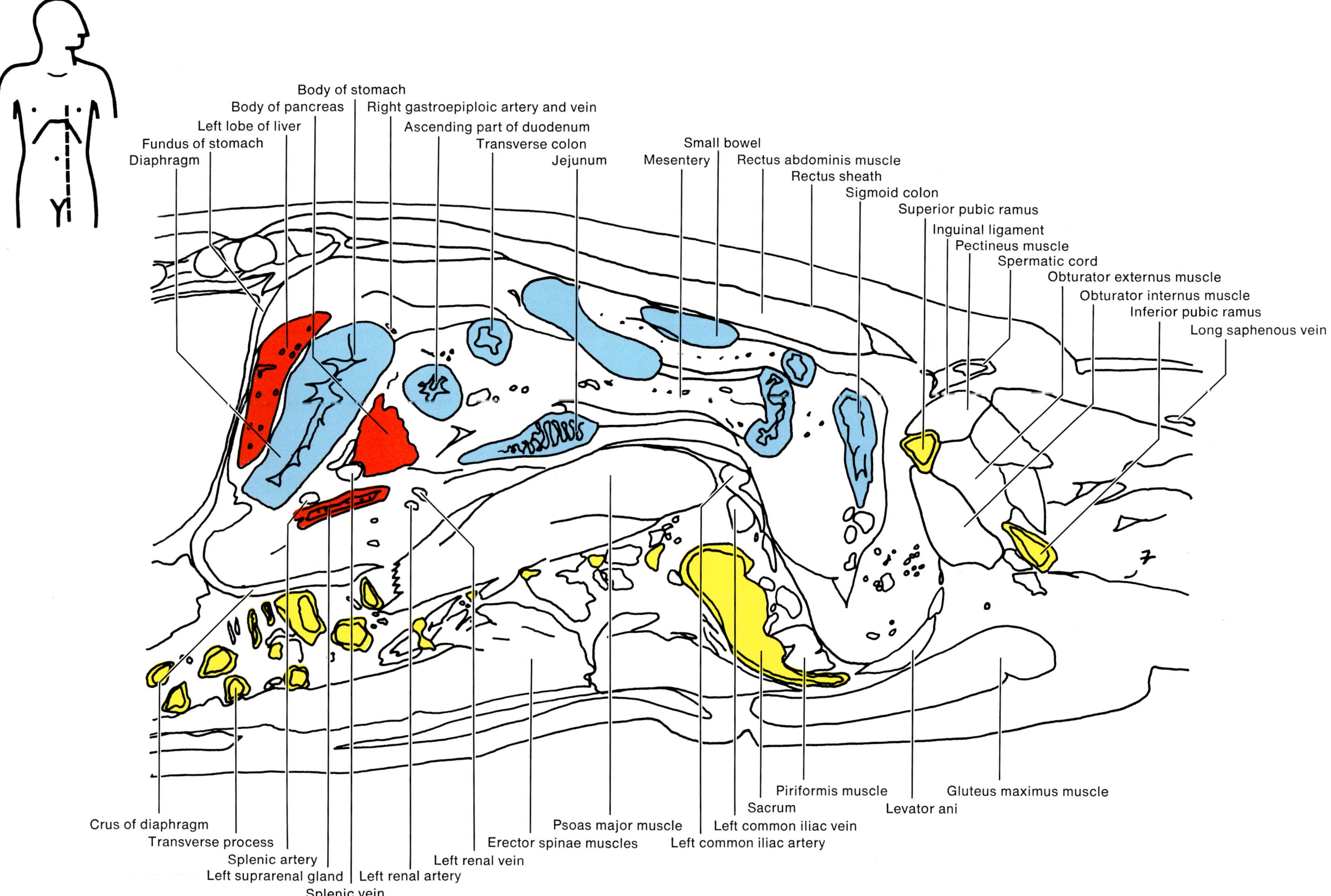

Body of stomach
Body of pancreas
Right gastroepiploic artery and vein
Left lobe of liver
Ascending part of duodenum
Fundus of stomach
Transverse colon
Diaphragm
Jejunum
Small bowel
Mesentery
Rectus abdominis muscle
Rectus sheath
Sigmoid colon
Superior pubic ramus
Inguinal ligament
Pectineus muscle
Spermatic cord
Obturator externus muscle
Obturator internus muscle
Inferior pubic ramus
Long saphenous vein
Crus of diaphragm
Transverse process
Splenic artery
Left suprarenal gland
Left renal artery
Splenic vein
Left renal vein
Psoas major muscle
Erector spinae muscles
Piriformis muscle
Gluteus maximus muscle
Sacrum
Levator ani
Left common iliac vein
Left common iliac artery

PARASAGITTAL **Abdomen and pelvis—male**

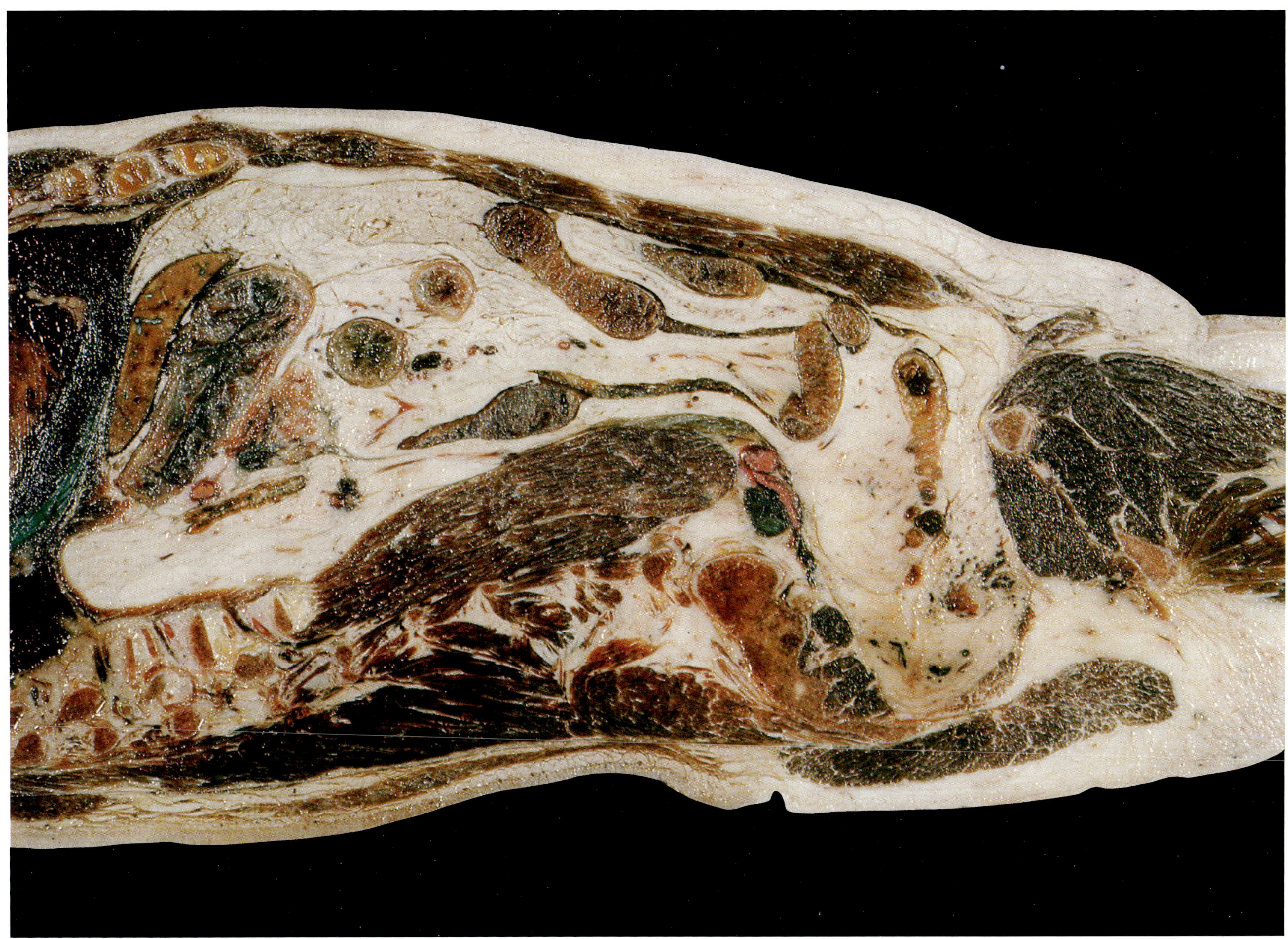

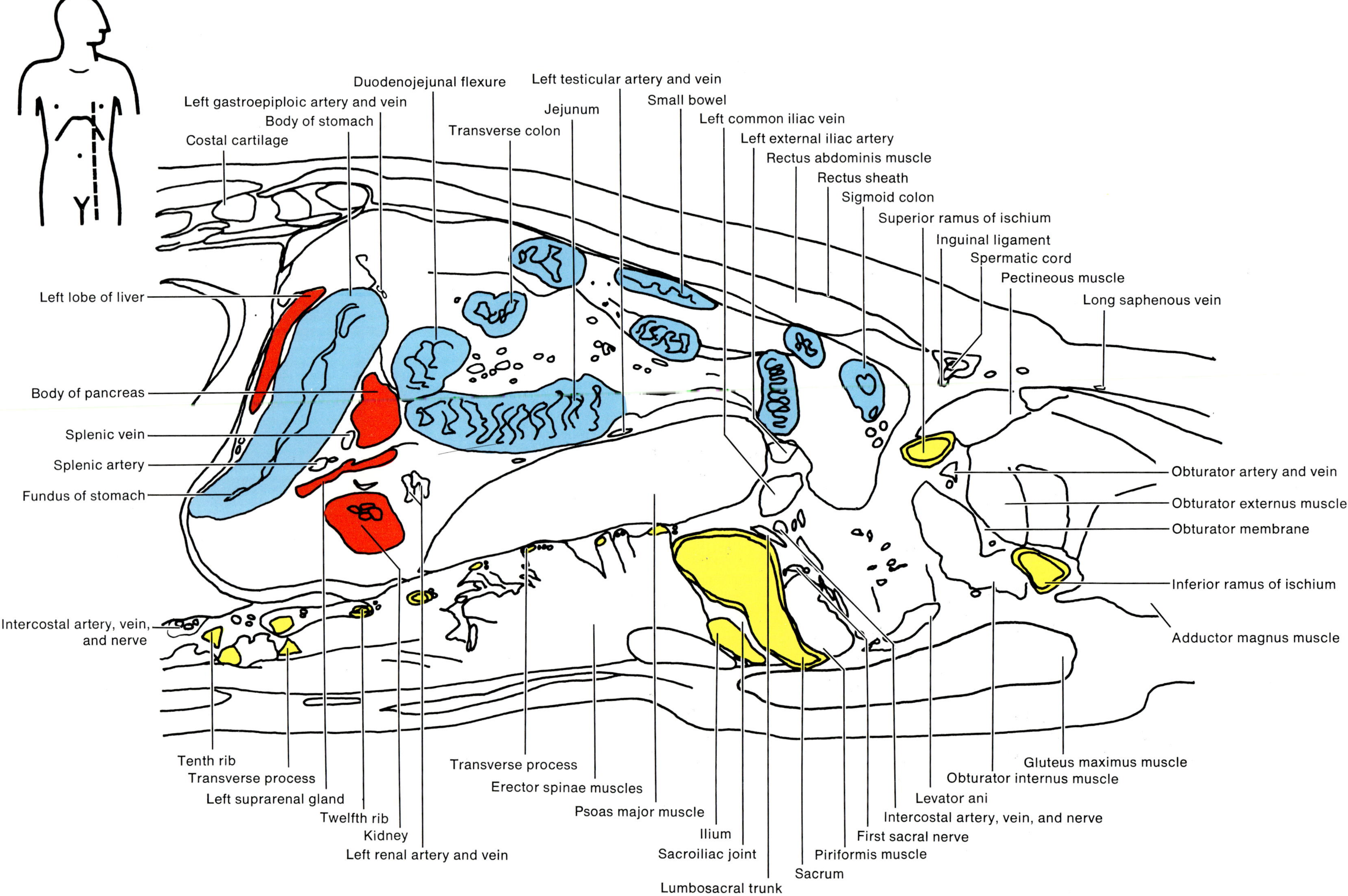

Duodenojejunal flexure
Left gastroepiploic artery and vein
Body of stomach
Costal cartilage
Left testicular artery and vein
Jejunum
Small bowel
Transverse colon
Left common iliac vein
Left external iliac artery
Rectus abdominis muscle
Rectus sheath
Sigmoid colon
Superior ramus of ischium
Inguinal ligament
Spermatic cord
Pectineous muscle
Long saphenous vein
Left lobe of liver
Body of pancreas
Splenic vein
Splenic artery
Fundus of stomach
Obturator artery and vein
Obturator externus muscle
Obturator membrane
Inferior ramus of ischium
Intercostal artery, vein, and nerve
Adductor magnus muscle
Tenth rib
Transverse process
Left suprarenal gland
Twelfth rib
Kidney
Left renal artery and vein
Transverse process
Erector spinae muscles
Psoas major muscle
Ilium
Sacroiliac joint
Lumbosacral trunk
Sacrum
Piriformis muscle
First sacral nerve
Intercostal artery, vein, and nerve
Levator ani
Obturator internus muscle
Gluteus maximus muscle

PARASAGITTAL **Abdomen and pelvis—male**

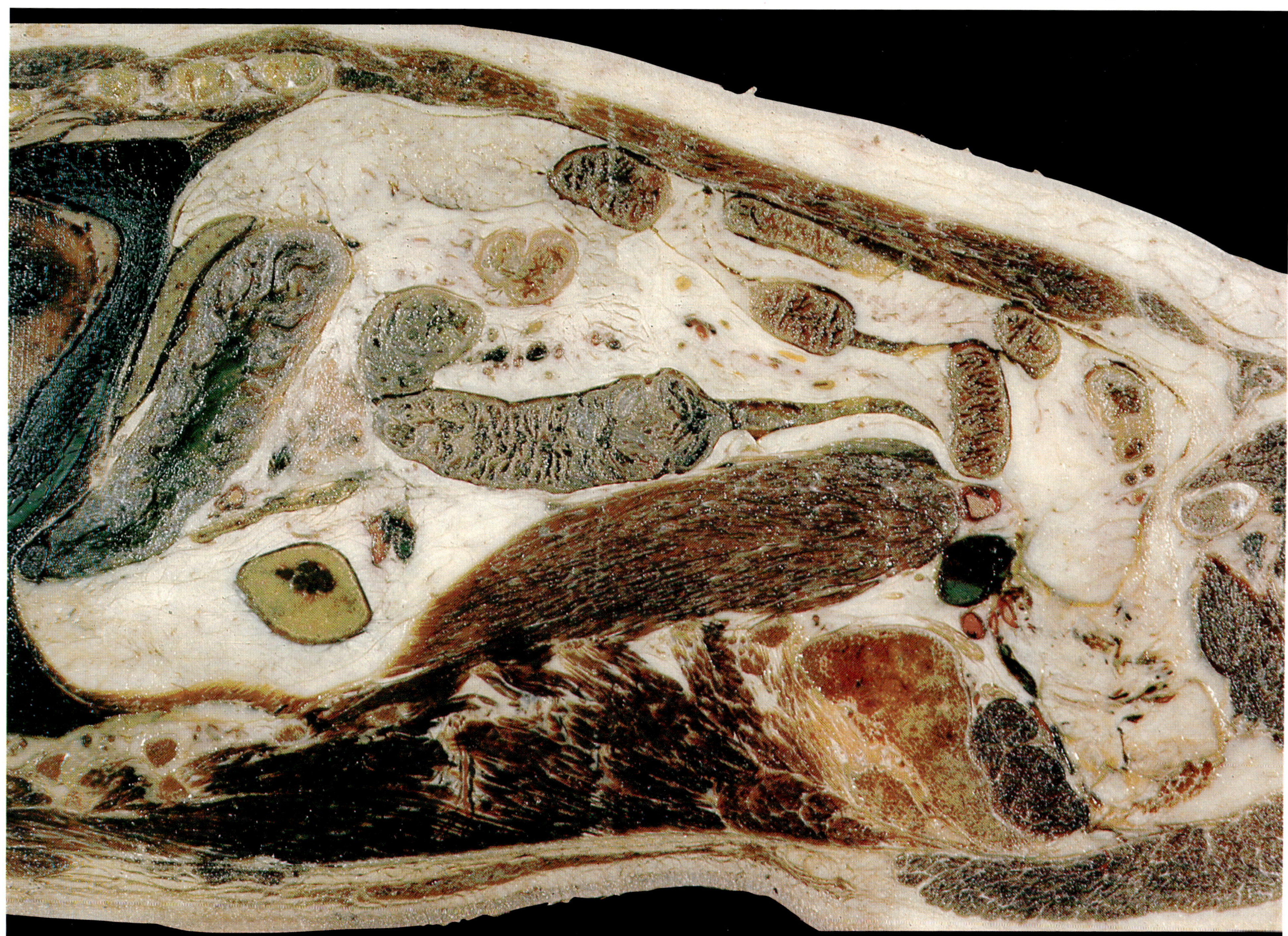

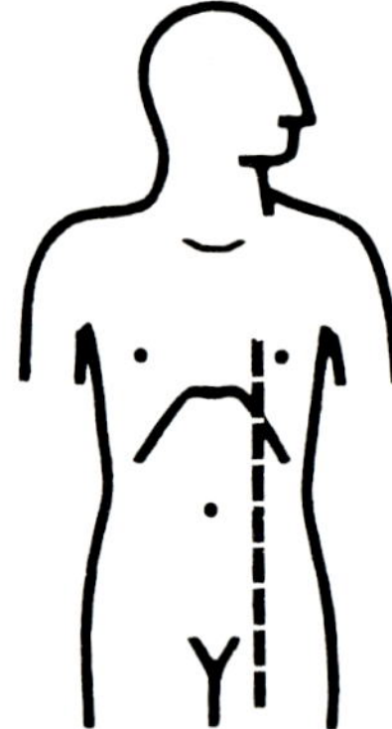

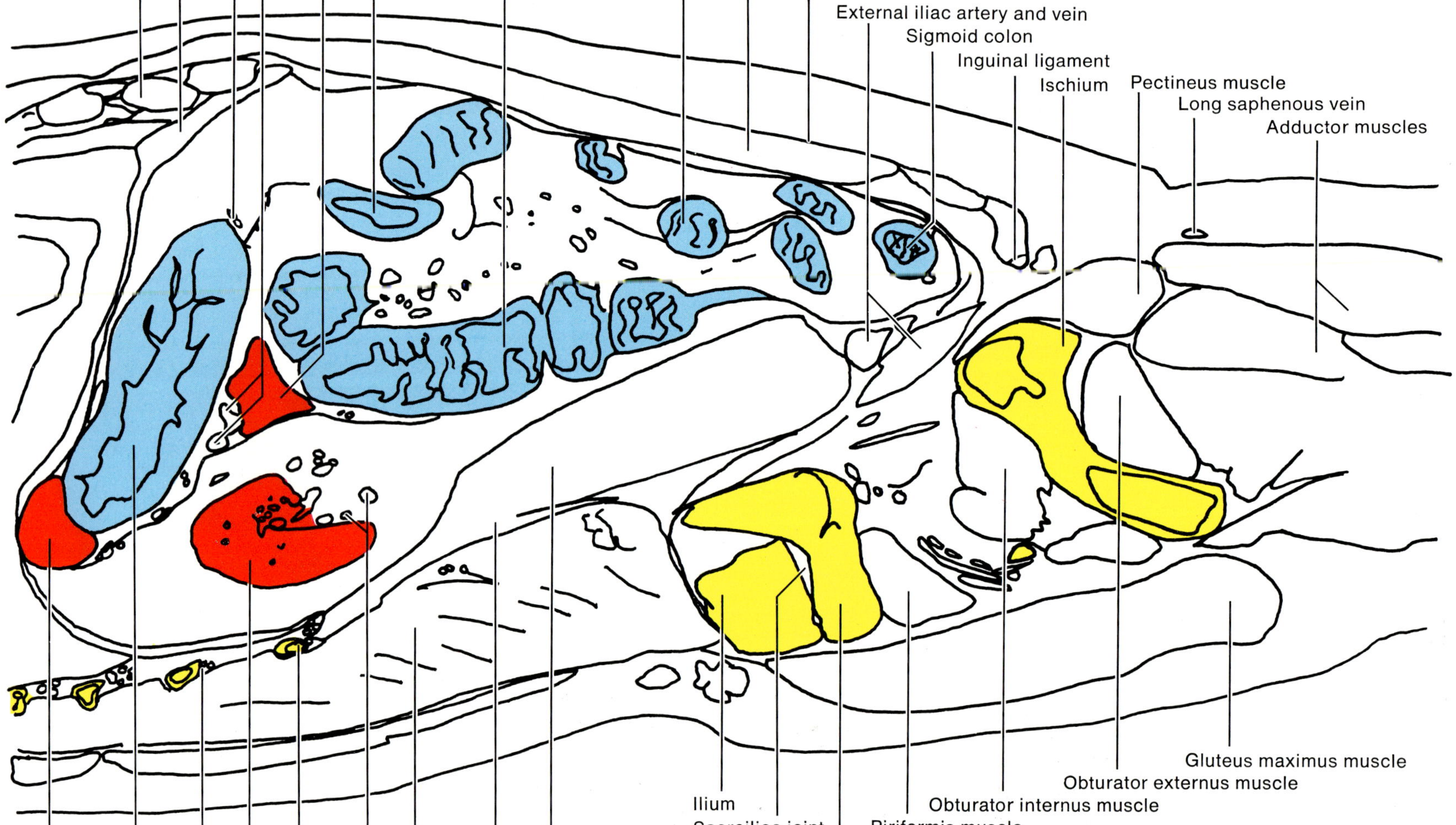

Left gastroepiploic artery and vein
Diaphragm
Splenic artery and vein
Costal cartilage
Body of pancreas
Transverse colon
Jejunum

Small bowel
Rectus abdominis muscle
Rectus sheath
External iliac artery and vein
Sigmoid colon
Inguinal ligament
Ischium
Pectineus muscle
Long saphenous vein
Adductor muscles

Gluteus maximus muscle
Obturator externus muscle
Obturator internus muscle
Ilium
Piriformis muscle
Sacroiliac joint
Sacrum

Spleen
Fundus of stomach
Intercostal artery, vein, and nerve
Left kidney
Renal artery and vein
Twelfth rib
Erector spinae muscles
Quadratus lumborum muscle
Psoas major muscle

PARASAGITTAL **Abdomen and pelvis—male**

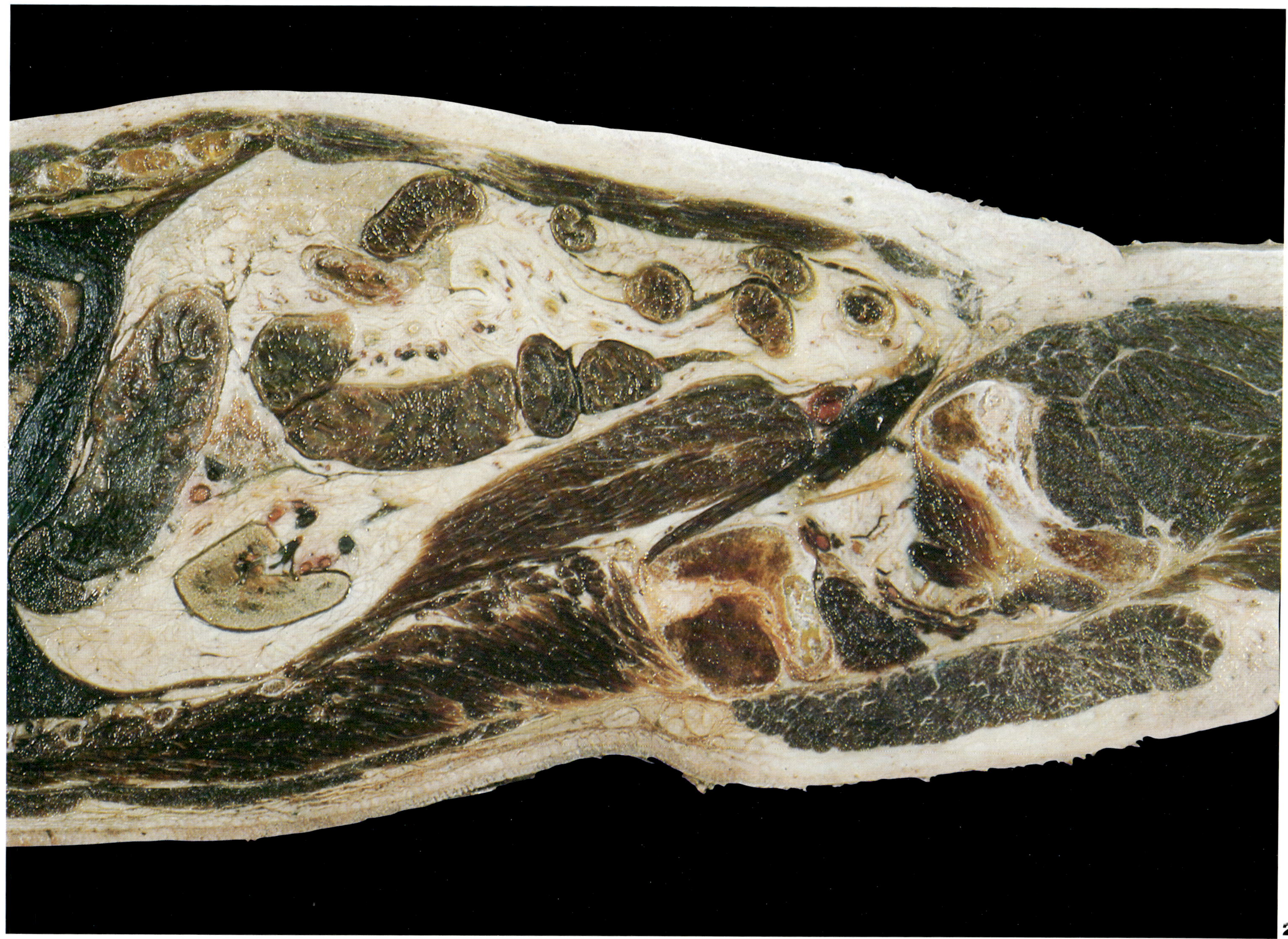

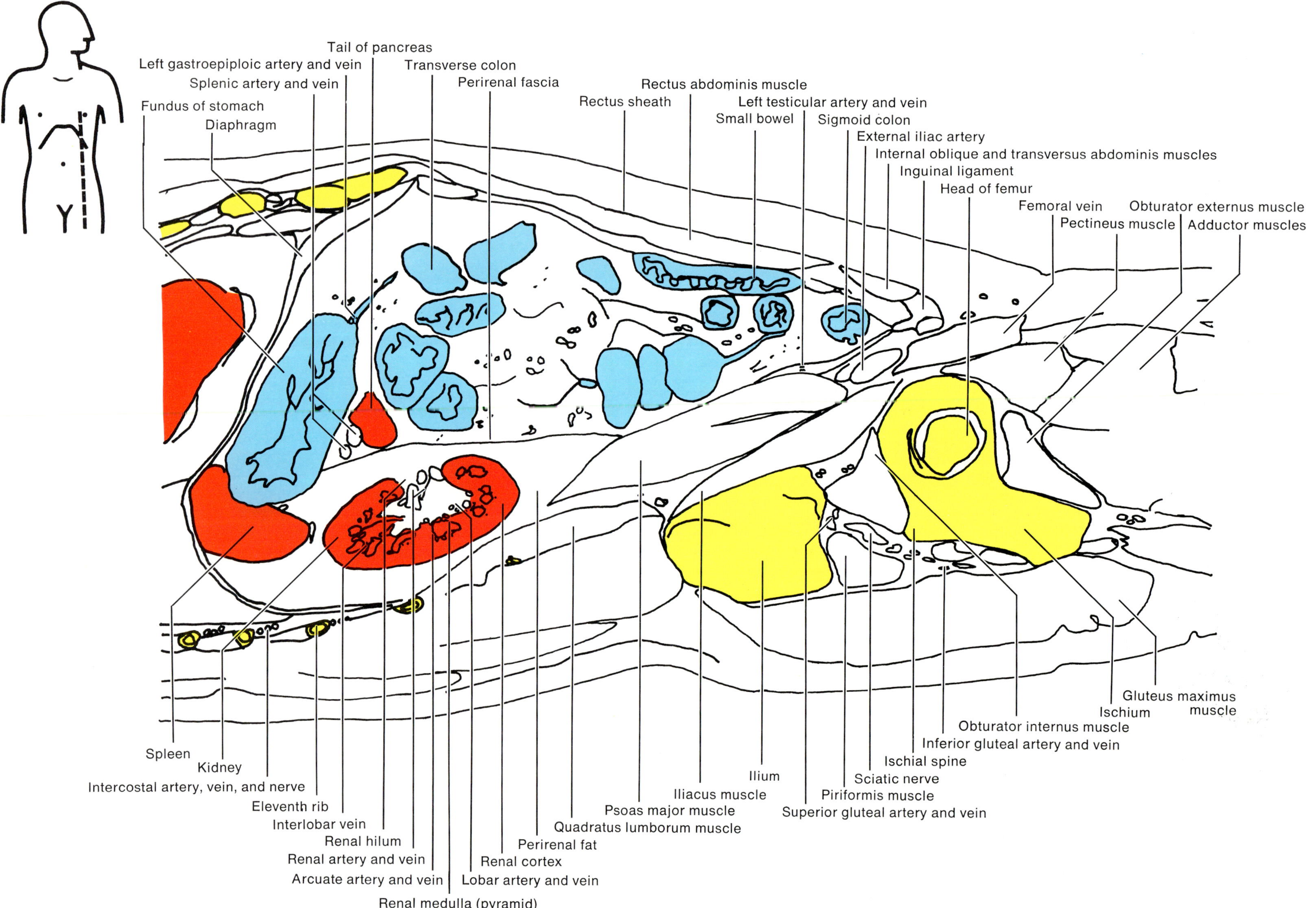
Tail of pancreas
Left gastroepiploic artery and vein
Splenic artery and vein
Fundus of stomach
Diaphragm
Transverse colon
Perirenal fascia
Rectus abdominis muscle
Rectus sheath
Left testicular artery and vein
Small bowel
Sigmoid colon
External iliac artery
Internal oblique and transversus abdominis muscles
Inguinal ligament
Head of femur
Femoral vein
Pectineus muscle
Obturator externus muscle
Adductor muscles
Gluteus maximus muscle
Ischium
Obturator internus muscle
Inferior gluteal artery and vein
Ischial spine
Sciatic nerve
Piriformis muscle
Superior gluteal artery and vein
Ilium
Iliacus muscle
Psoas major muscle
Quadratus lumborum muscle
Perirenal fat
Renal cortex
Lobar artery and vein
Renal medulla (pyramid)
Arcuate artery and vein
Renal artery and vein
Renal hilum
Interlobar vein
Eleventh rib
Intercostal artery, vein, and nerve
Kidney
Spleen

PARASAGITTAL **Abdomen and pelvis—male**

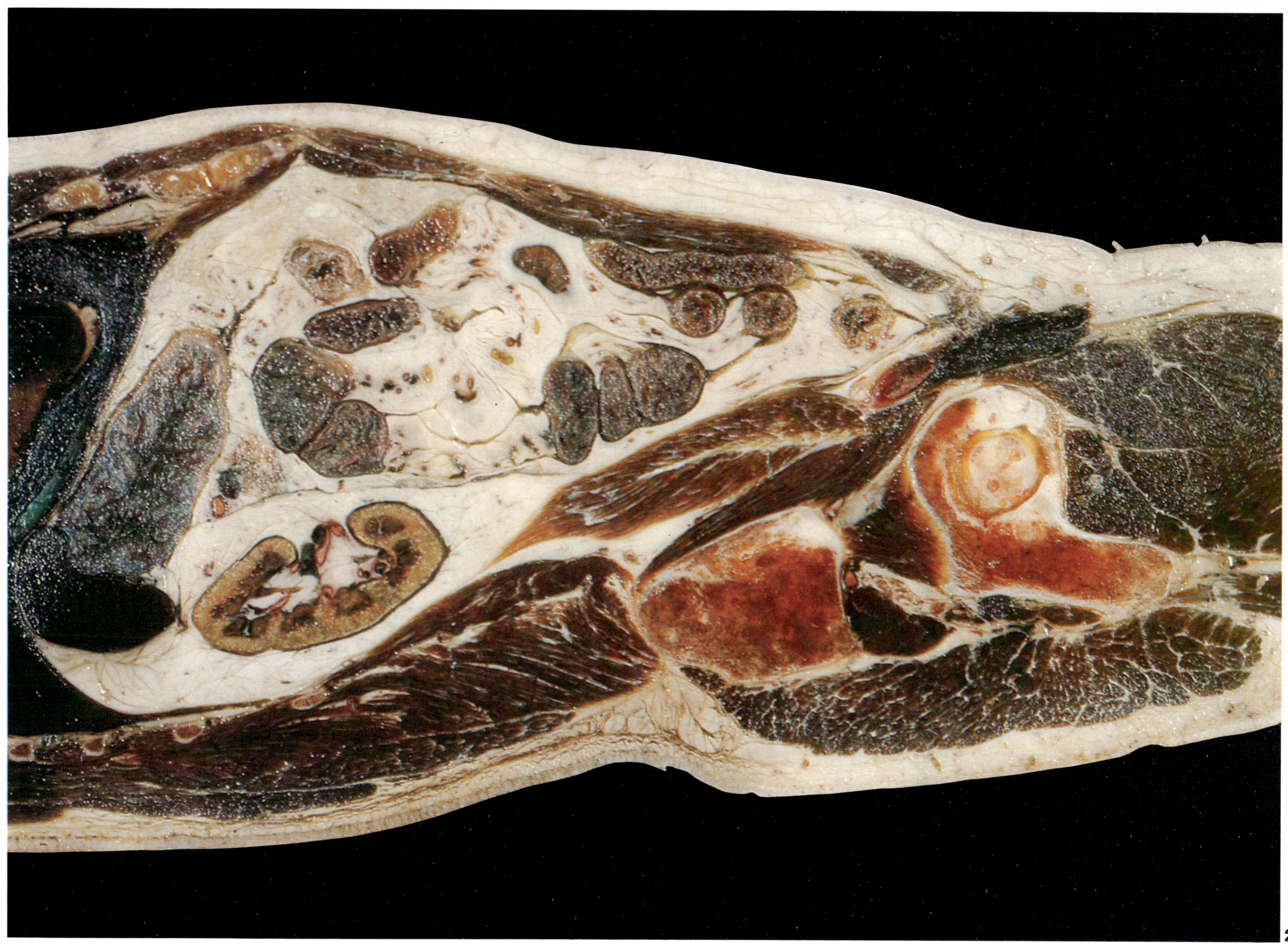

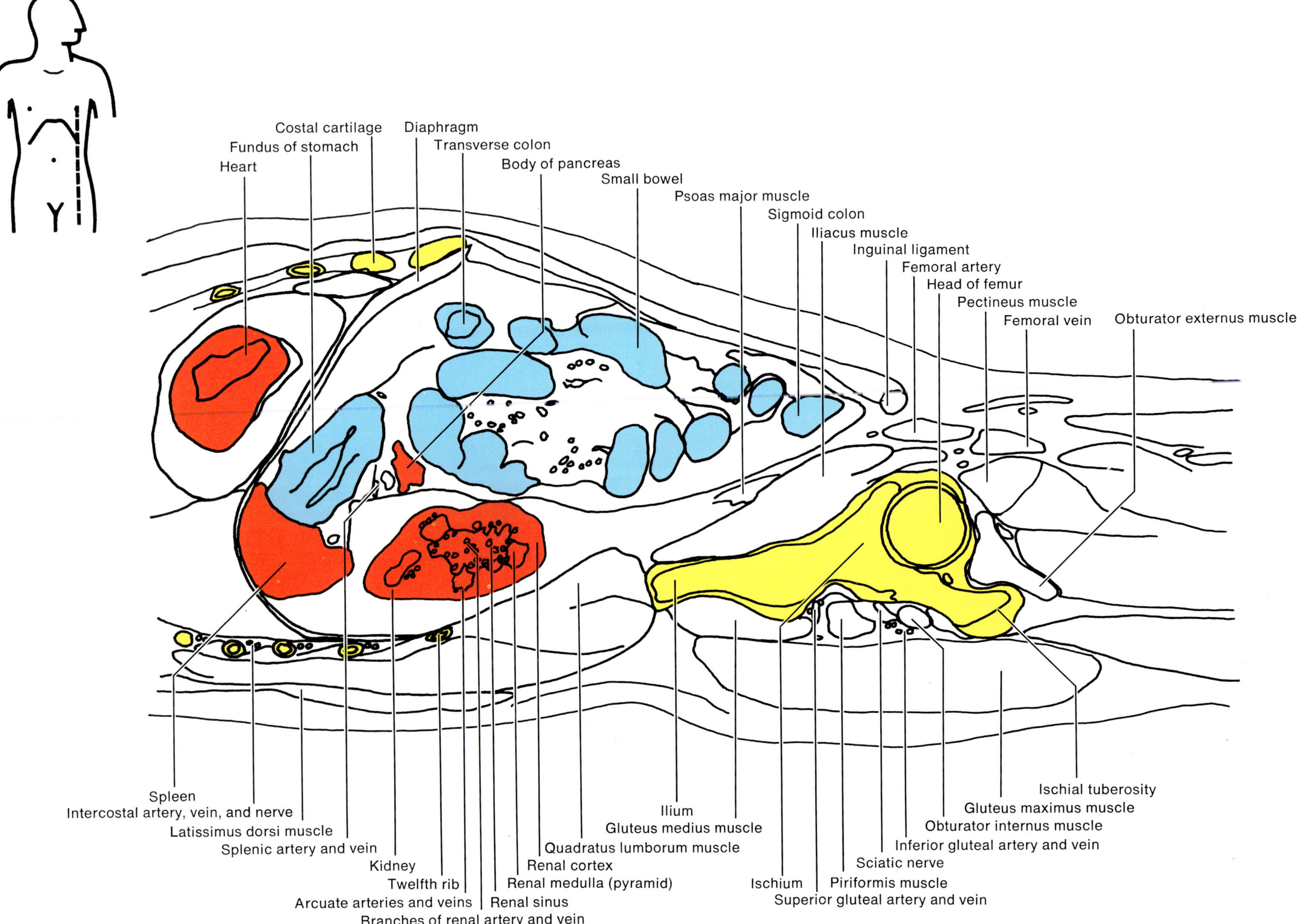
Costal cartilage
Fundus of stomach
Heart
Diaphragm
Transverse colon
Body of pancreas
Small bowel
Psoas major muscle
Sigmoid colon
Iliacus muscle
Inguinal ligament
Femoral artery
Head of femur
Pectineus muscle
Femoral vein
Obturator externus muscle
Spleen
Intercostal artery, vein, and nerve
Latissimus dorsi muscle
Splenic artery and vein
Kidney
Twelfth rib
Arcuate arteries and veins
Branches of renal artery and vein
Renal sinus
Renal medulla (pyramid)
Renal cortex
Quadratus lumborum muscle
Gluteus medius muscle
Ilium
Ischium
Superior gluteal artery and vein
Piriformis muscle
Sciatic nerve
Inferior gluteal artery and vein
Obturator internus muscle
Gluteus maximus muscle
Ischial tuberosity

PARASAGITTAL **Abdomen and pelvis—male**

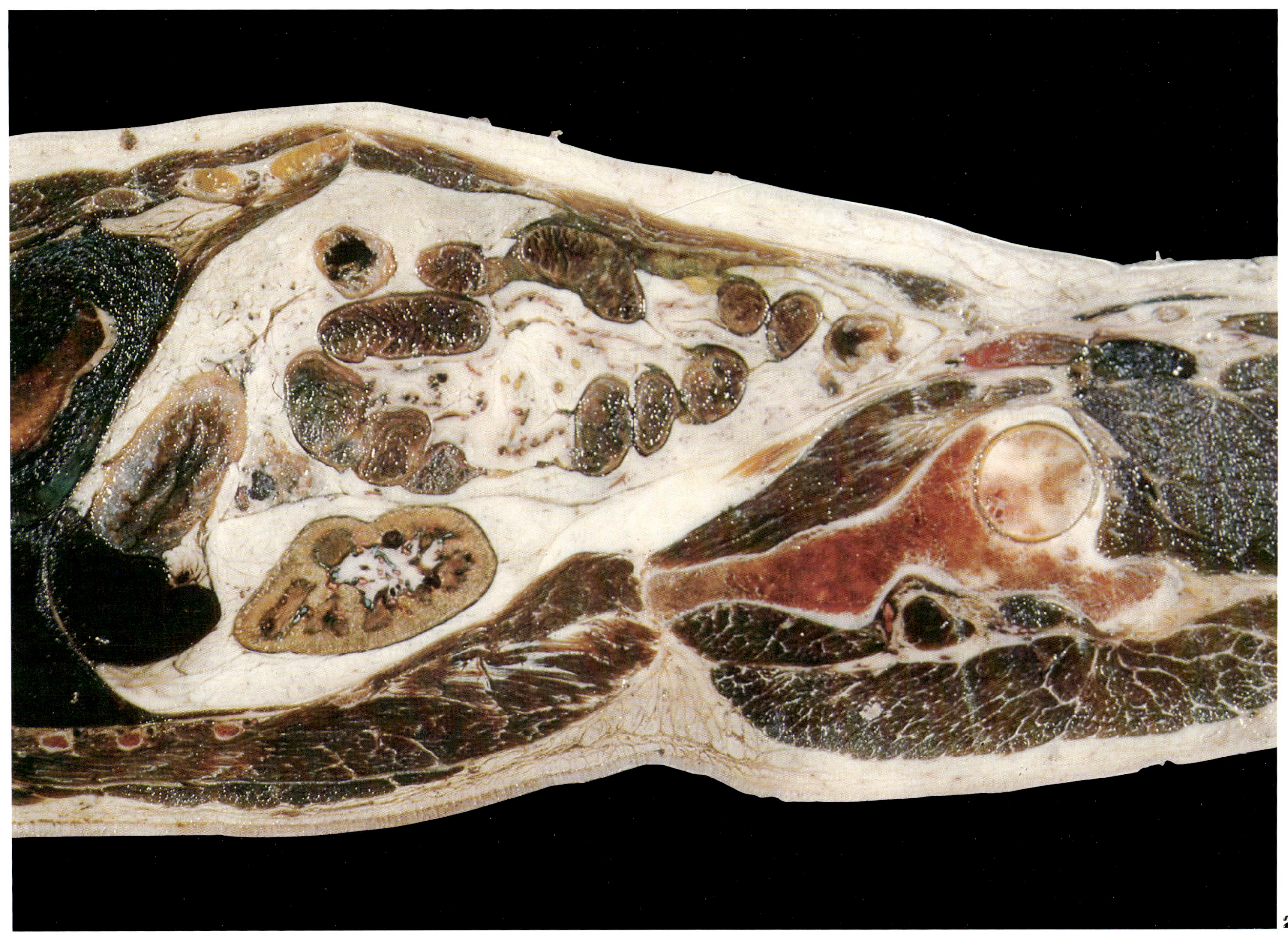

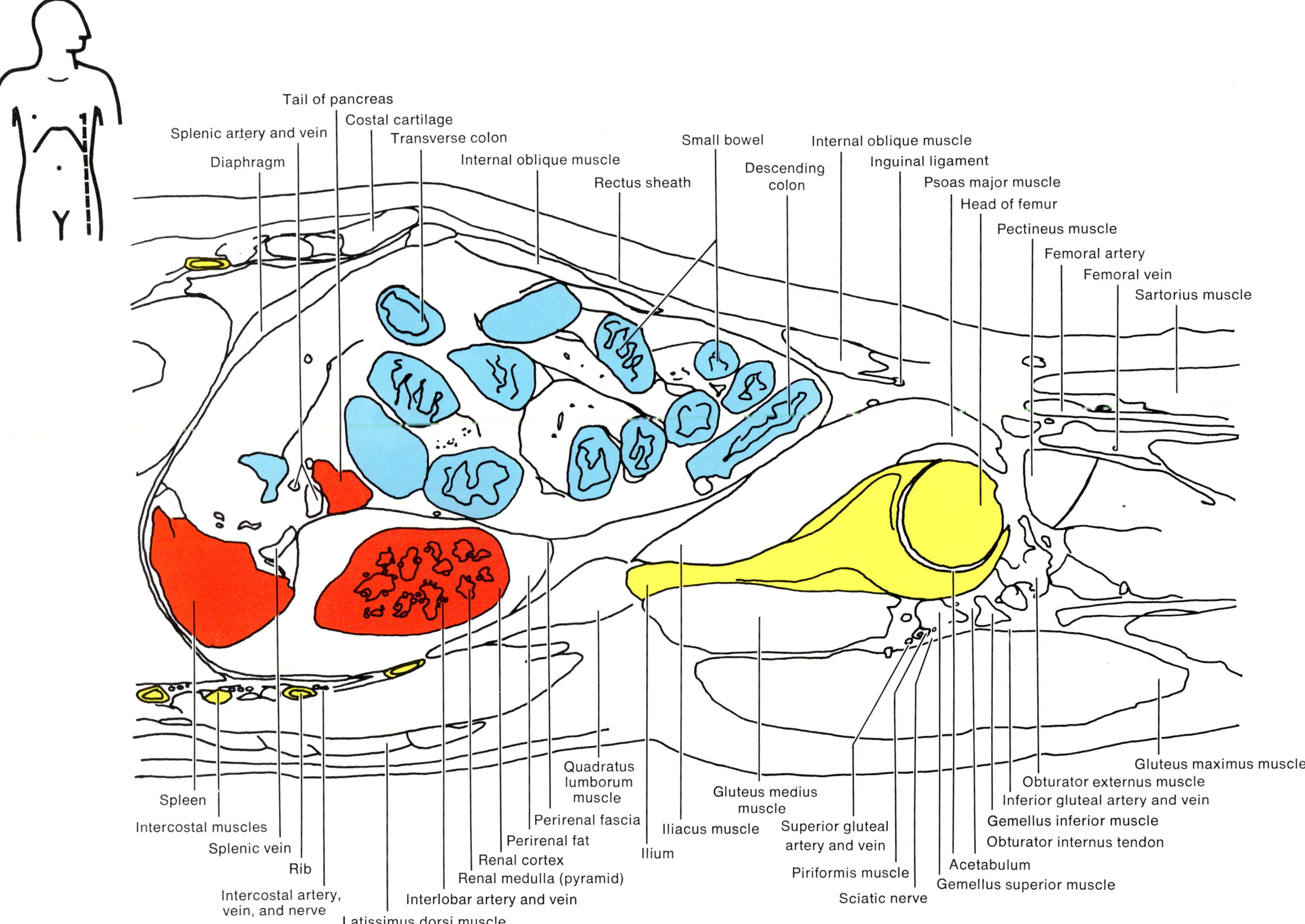

Tail of pancreas
Splenic artery and vein
Costal cartilage
Transverse colon
Diaphragm
Internal oblique muscle
Small bowel
Internal oblique muscle
Rectus sheath
Descending colon
Inguinal ligament
Psoas major muscle
Head of femur
Pectineus muscle
Femoral artery
Femoral vein
Sartorius muscle
Spleen
Intercostal muscles
Splenic vein
Rib
Intercostal artery, vein, and nerve
Latissimus dorsi muscle
Interlobar artery and vein
Renal medulla (pyramid)
Renal cortex
Perirenal fat
Perirenal fascia
Quadratus lumborum muscle
Iliacus muscle
Ilium
Gluteus medius muscle
Superior gluteal artery and vein
Piriformis muscle
Sciatic nerve
Gemellus superior muscle
Acetabulum
Obturator internus tendon
Gemellus inferior muscle
Inferior gluteal artery and vein
Obturator externus muscle
Gluteus maximus muscle

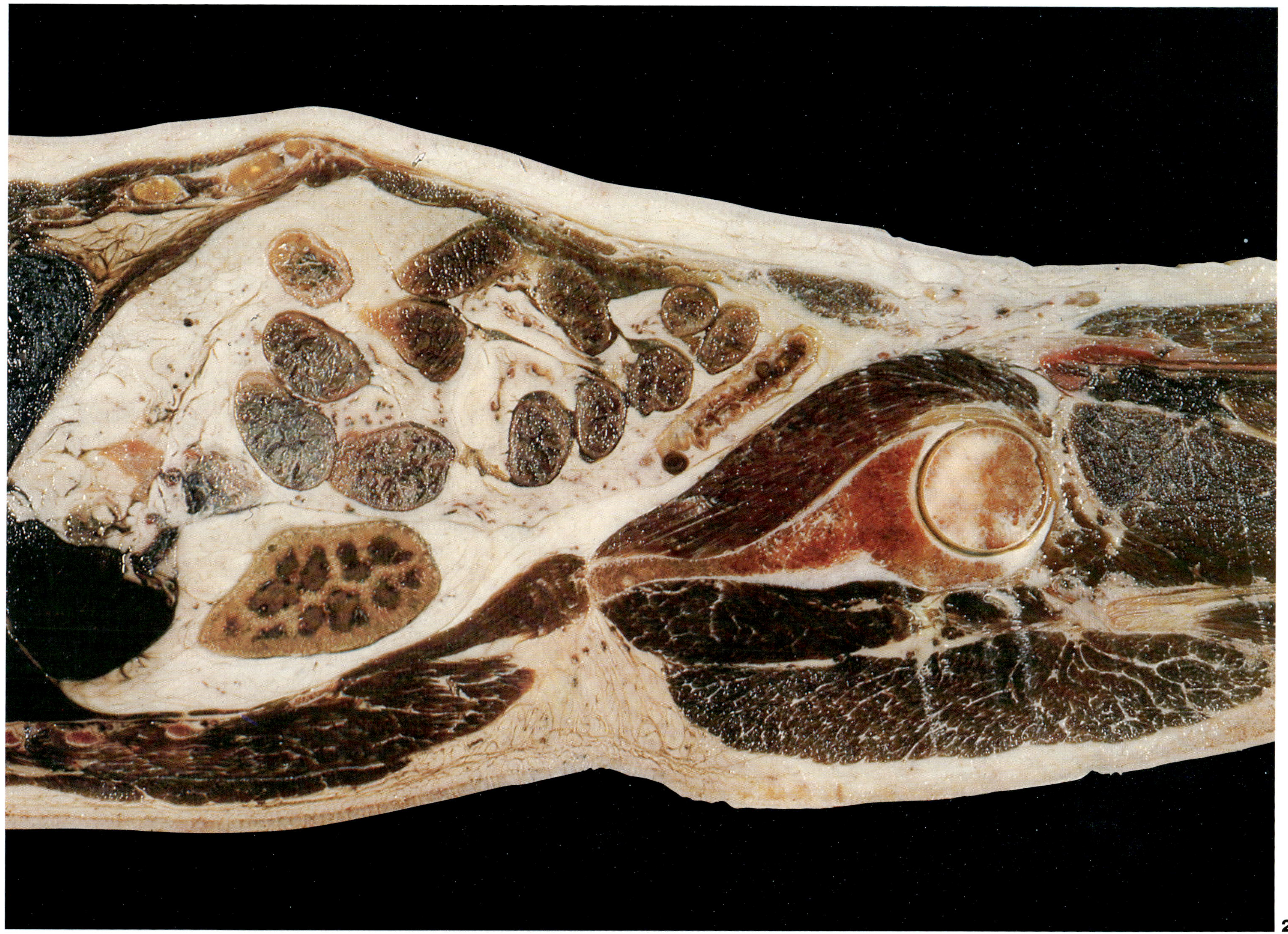

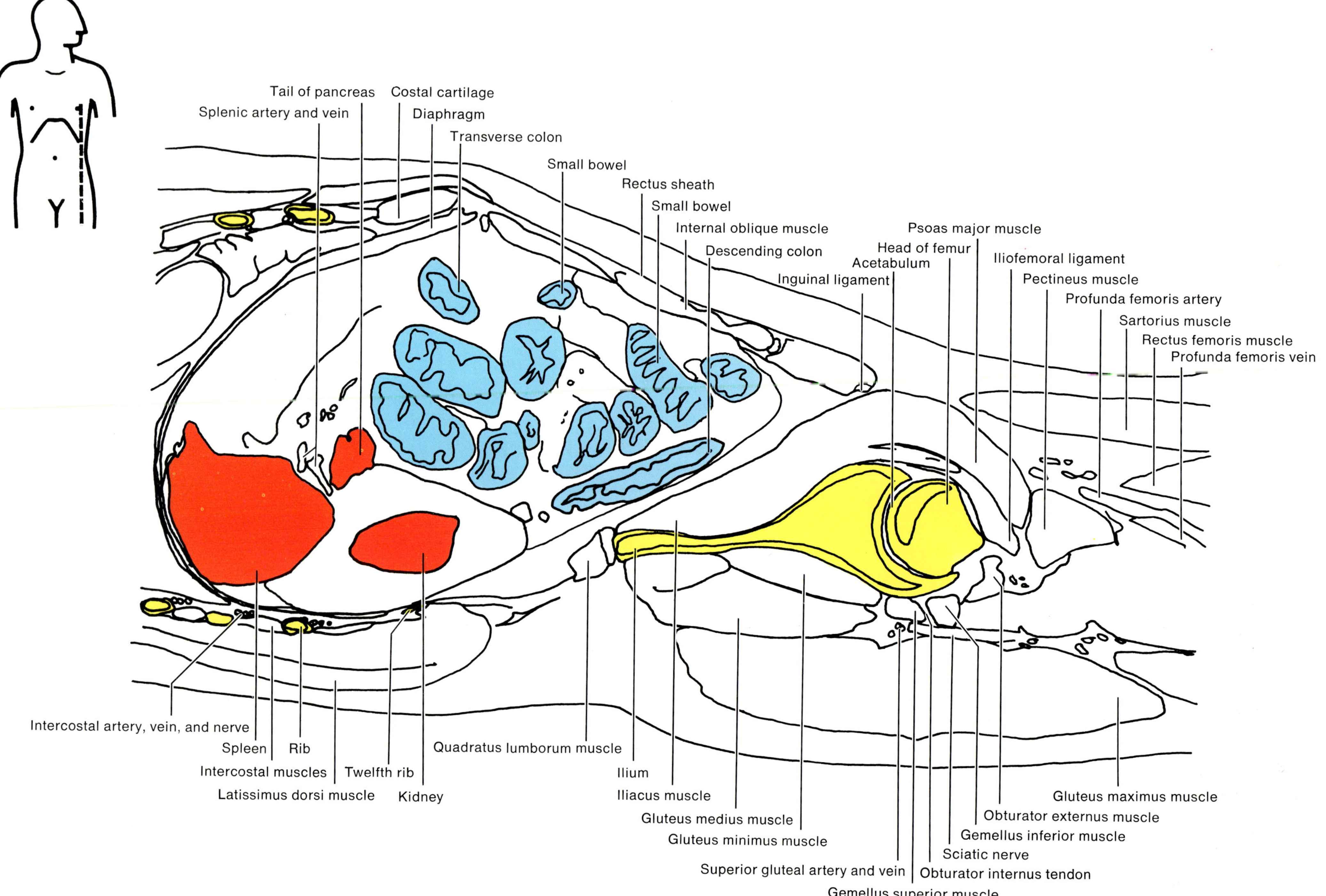

Tail of pancreas
Splenic artery and vein
Costal cartilage
Diaphragm
Transverse colon
Small bowel
Rectus sheath
Small bowel
Internal oblique muscle
Descending colon
Inguinal ligament
Acetabulum
Head of femur
Psoas major muscle
Iliofemoral ligament
Pectineus muscle
Profunda femoris artery
Sartorius muscle
Rectus femoris muscle
Profunda femoris vein
Intercostal artery, vein, and nerve
Spleen
Rib
Intercostal muscles
Twelfth rib
Latissimus dorsi muscle
Kidney
Quadratus lumborum muscle
Ilium
Iliacus muscle
Gluteus medius muscle
Gluteus minimus muscle
Superior gluteal artery and vein
Gemellus superior muscle
Obturator internus tendon
Sciatic nerve
Gemellus inferior muscle
Obturator externus muscle
Gluteus maximus muscle

PARASAGITTAL **Abdomen and pelvis—male**

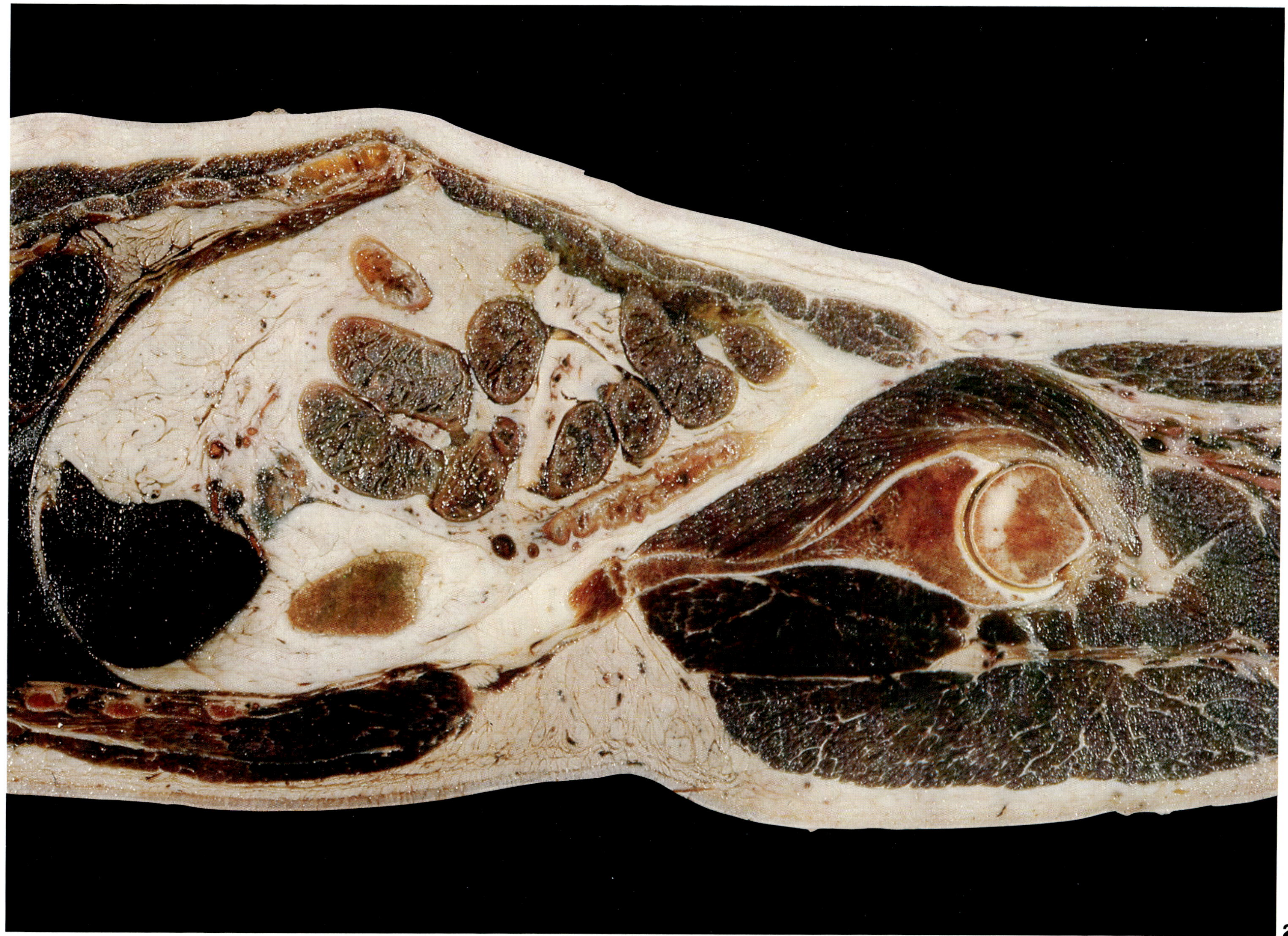

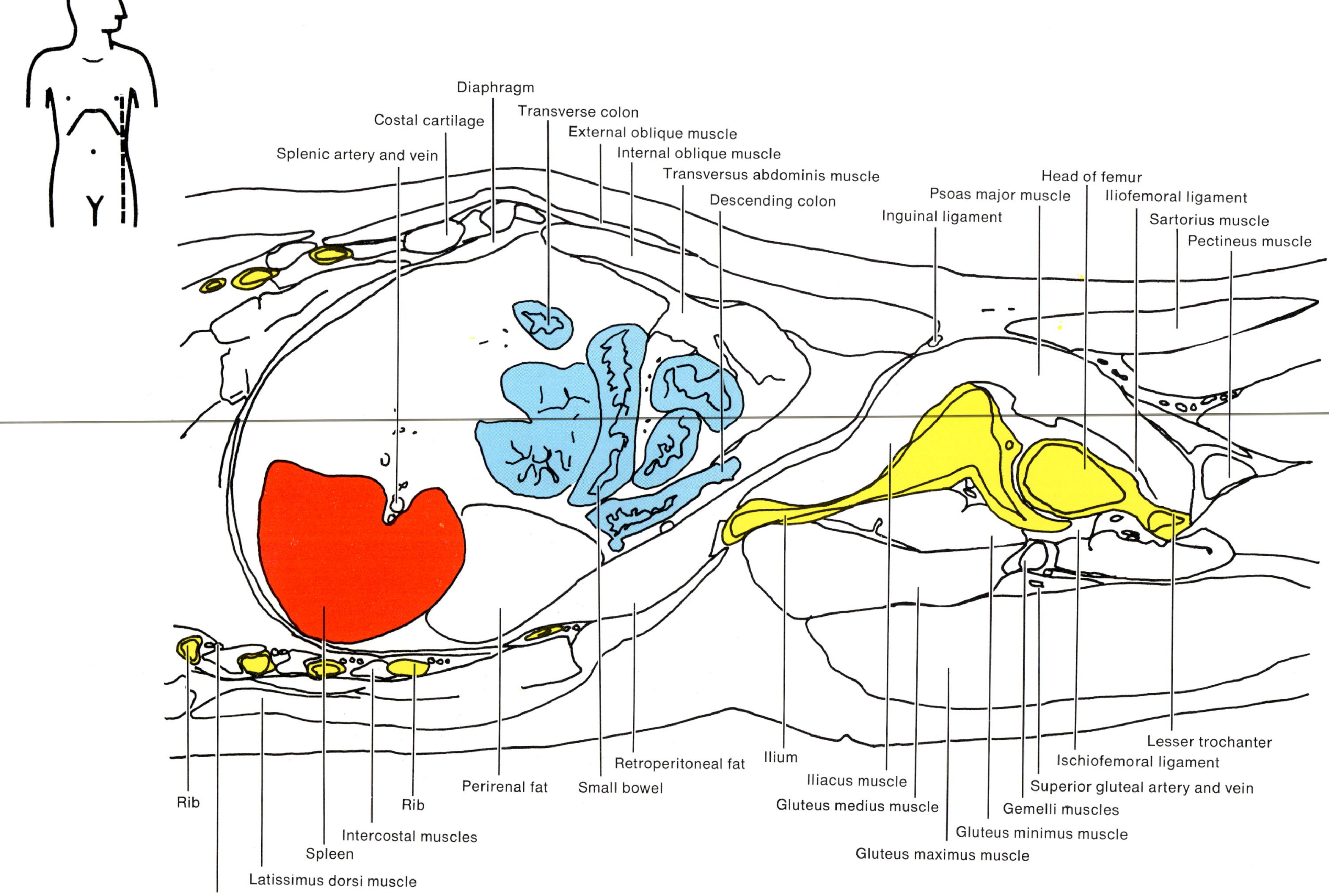

Diaphragm
Transverse colon
Costal cartilage
External oblique muscle
Splenic artery and vein
Internal oblique muscle
Transversus abdominis muscle
Head of femur
Descending colon
Psoas major muscle
Iliofemoral ligament
Inguinal ligament
Sartorius muscle
Pectineus muscle
Lesser trochanter
Retroperitoneal fat
Ilium
Ischiofemoral ligament
Perirenal fat
Small bowel
Iliacus muscle
Superior gluteal artery and vein
Rib
Gluteus medius muscle
Gemelli muscles
Rib
Intercostal muscles
Gluteus minimus muscle
Spleen
Gluteus maximus muscle
Latissimus dorsi muscle
Intercostal artery, vein, and nerve

PARASAGITTAL **Abdomen and pelvis—male**

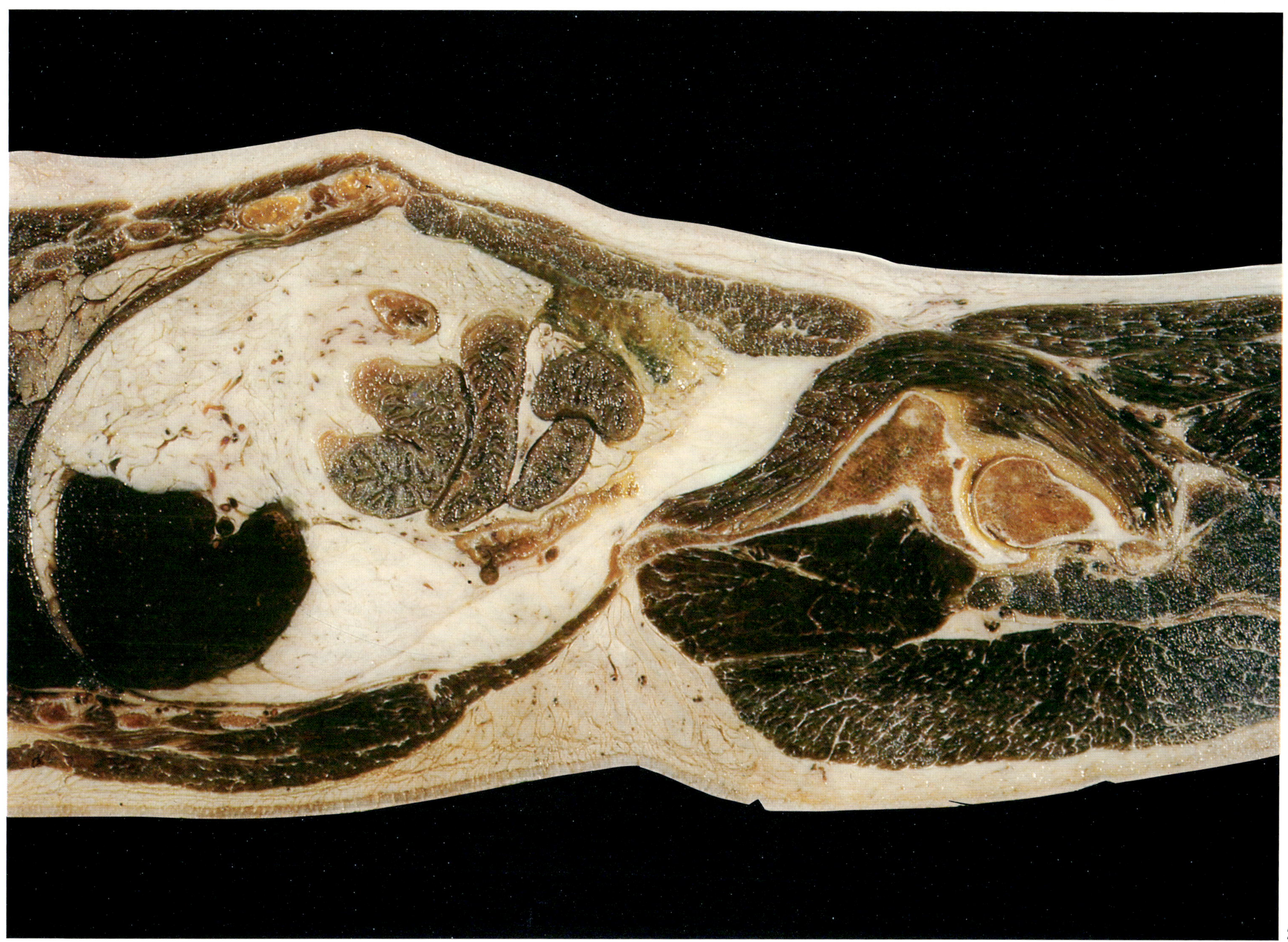

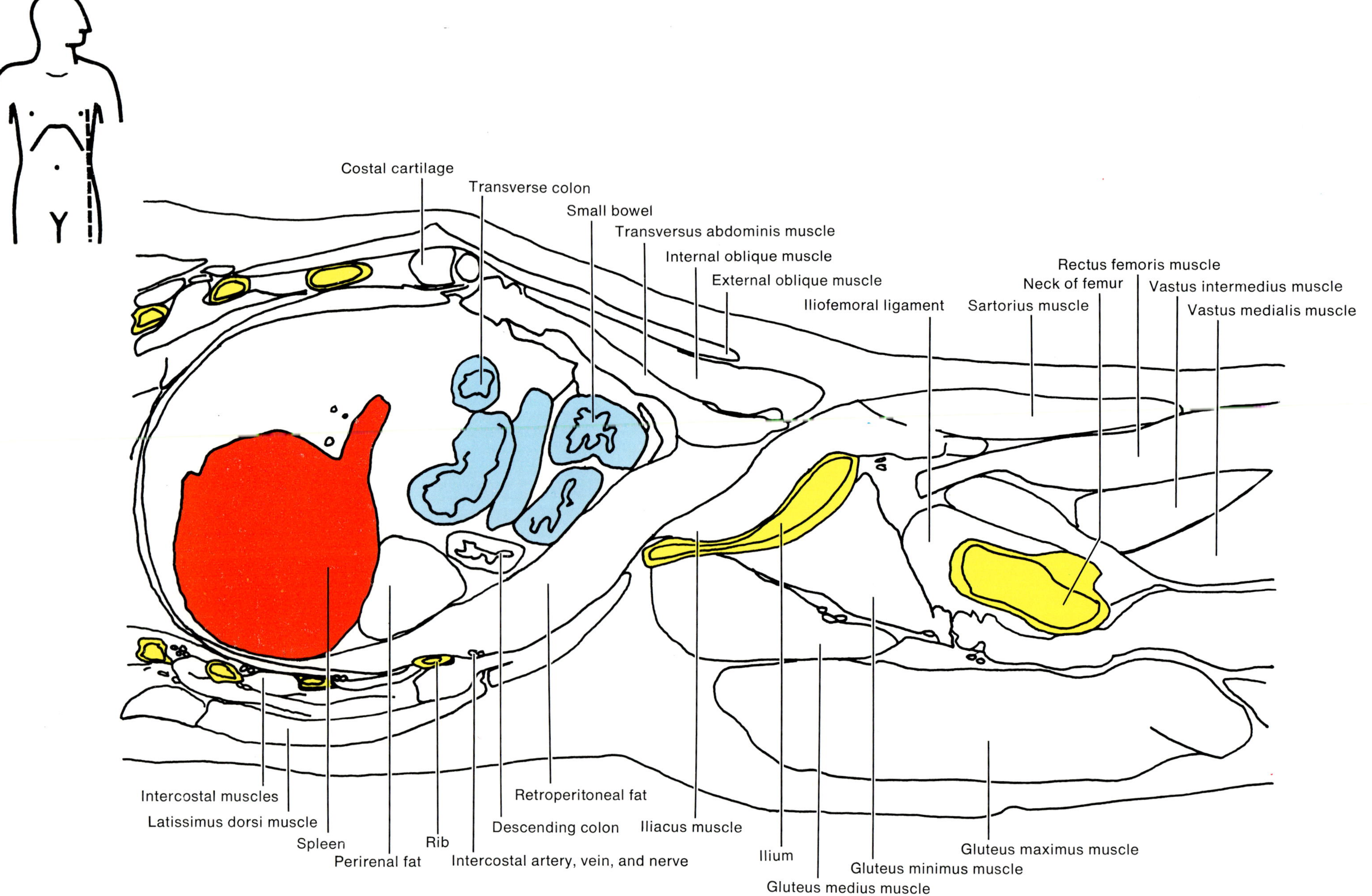

Costal cartilage
Transverse colon
Small bowel
Transversus abdominis muscle
Internal oblique muscle
External oblique muscle
Iliofemoral ligament
Rectus femoris muscle
Neck of femur
Vastus intermedius muscle
Vastus medialis muscle
Sartorius muscle
Intercostal muscles
Latissimus dorsi muscle
Spleen
Rib
Retroperitoneal fat
Descending colon
Iliacus muscle
Ilium
Gluteus maximus muscle
Gluteus minimus muscle
Gluteus medius muscle
Perirenal fat
Intercostal artery, vein, and nerve

PARASAGITTAL **Abdomen and pelvis—male**

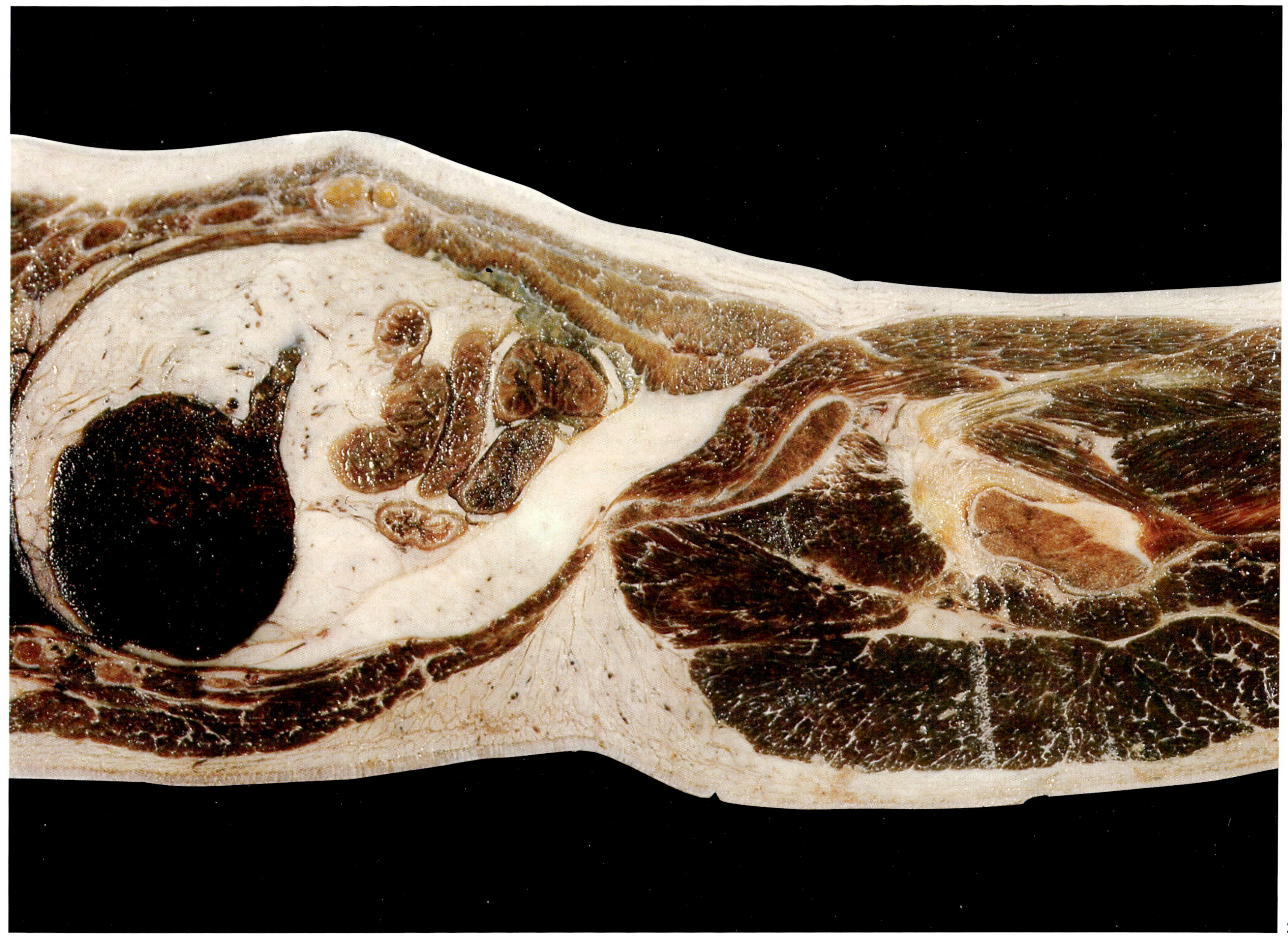

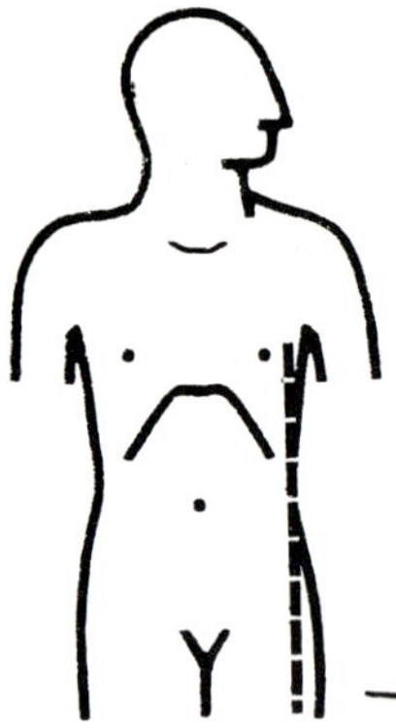

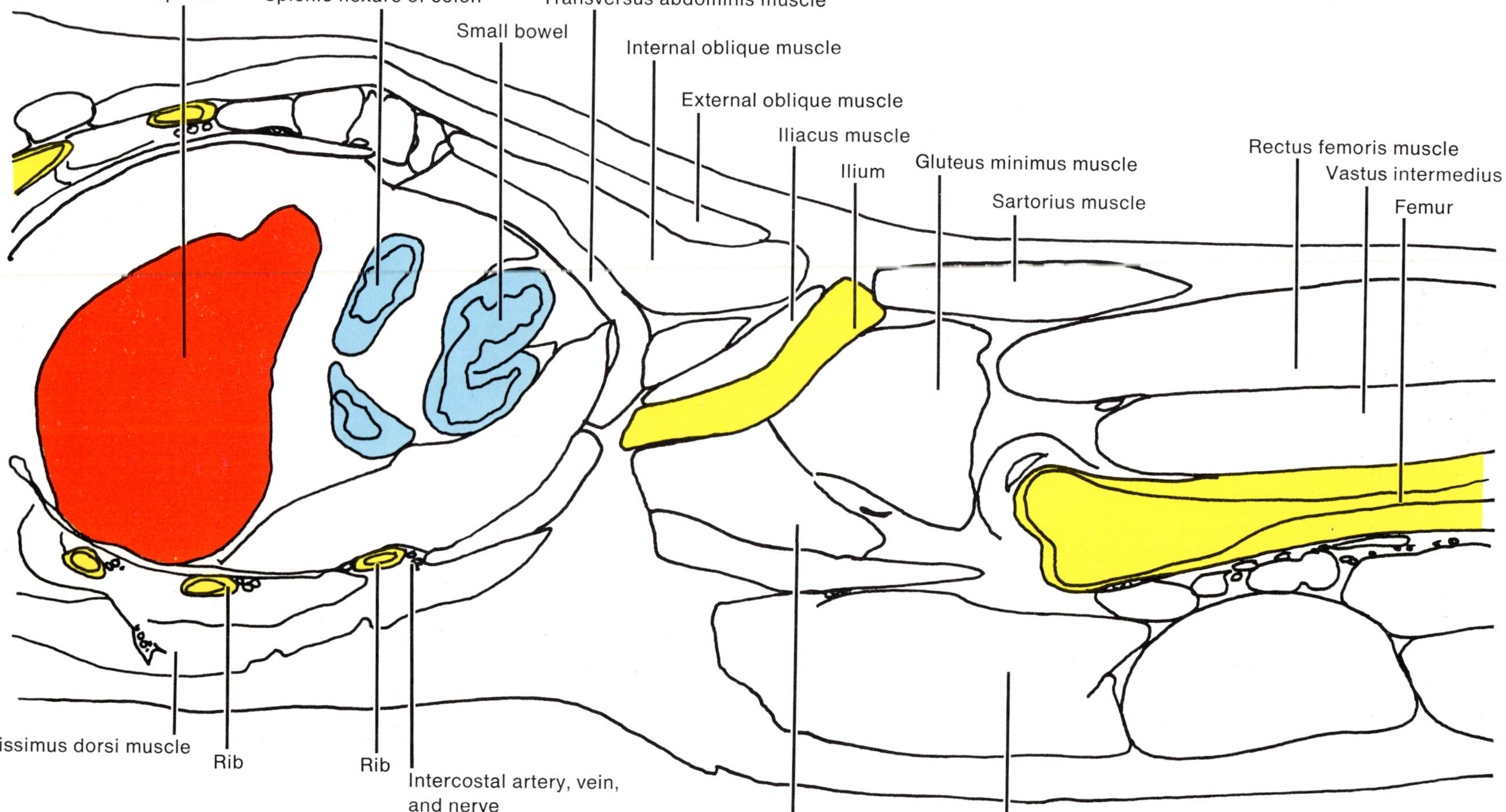

Spleen
Splenic flexure of colon
Small bowel
Transversus abdominis muscle
Internal oblique muscle
External oblique muscle
Iliacus muscle
Ilium
Gluteus minimus muscle
Sartorius muscle
Rectus femoris muscle
Vastus intermedius muscle
Femur
Latissimus dorsi muscle
Rib
Rib
Intercostal artery, vein, and nerve
Gluteus medius muscle
Gluteus maximus muscle

PARASAGITTAL **Abdomen and pelvis—male**

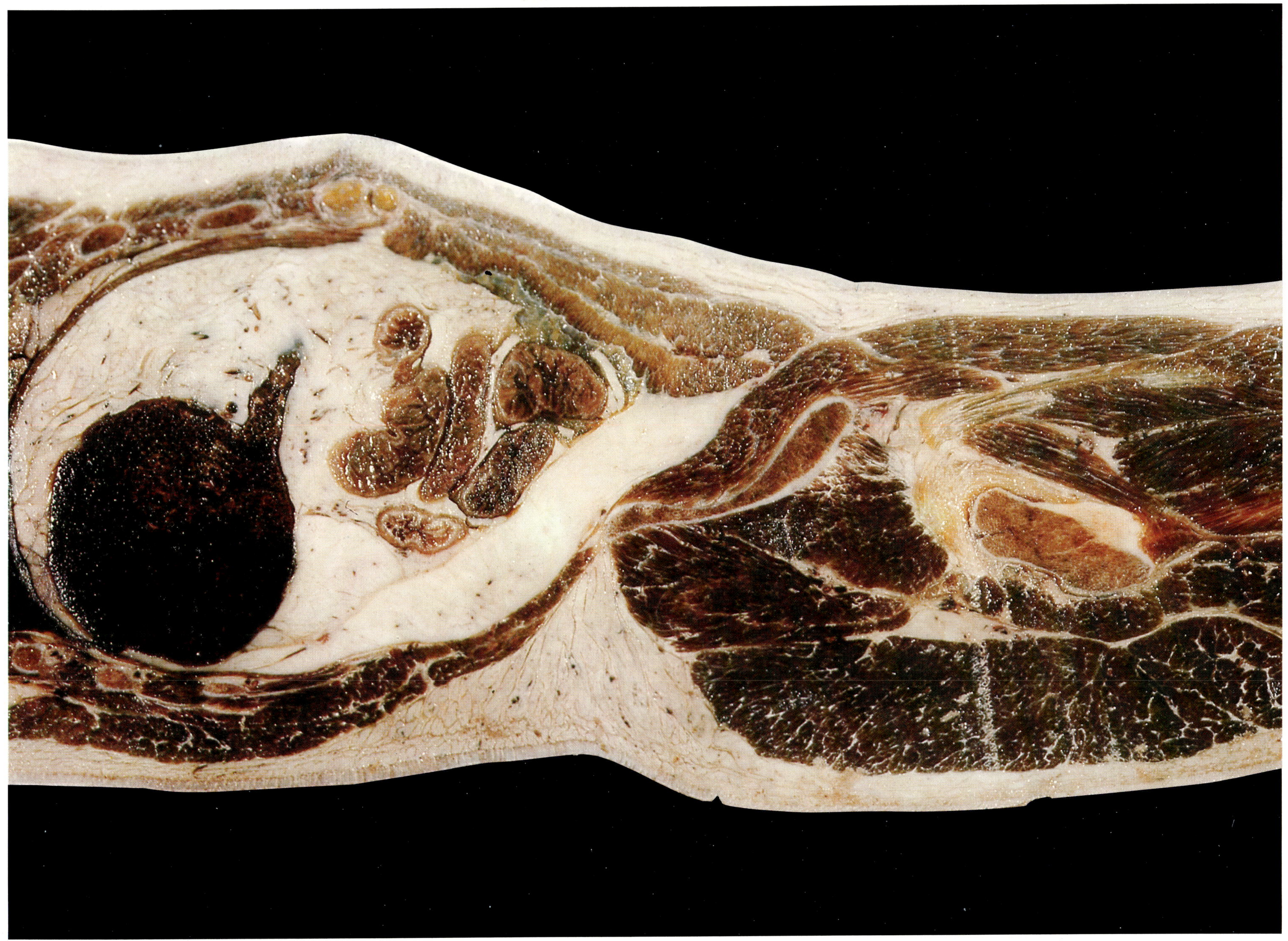

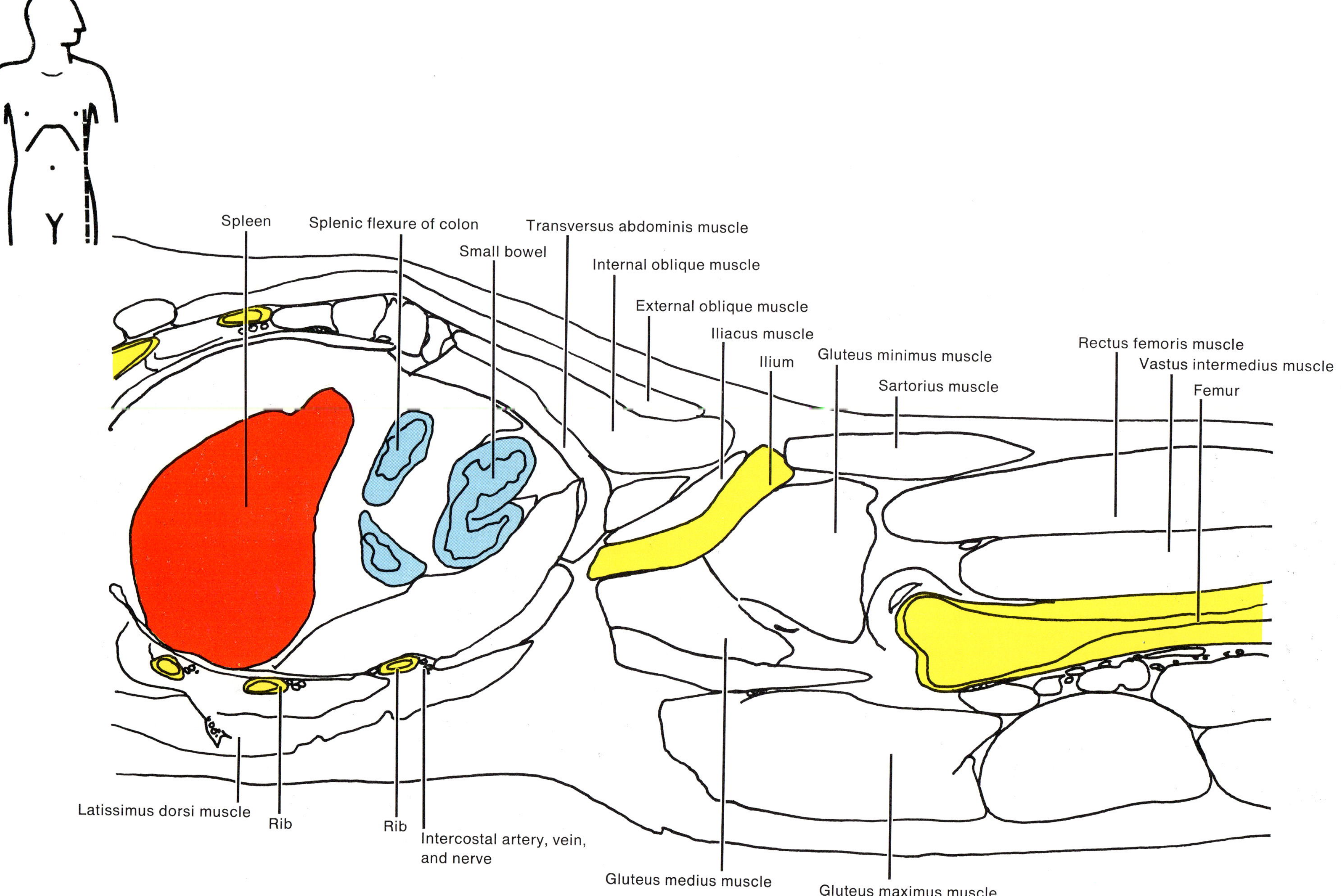

Spleen
Splenic flexure of colon
Small bowel
Transversus abdominis muscle
Internal oblique muscle
External oblique muscle
Iliacus muscle
Ilium
Gluteus minimus muscle
Sartorius muscle
Rectus femoris muscle
Vastus intermedius muscle
Femur
Latissimus dorsi muscle
Rib
Rib
Intercostal artery, vein, and nerve
Gluteus medius muscle
Gluteus maximus muscle

PARASAGITTAL **Abdomen and pelvis—male**

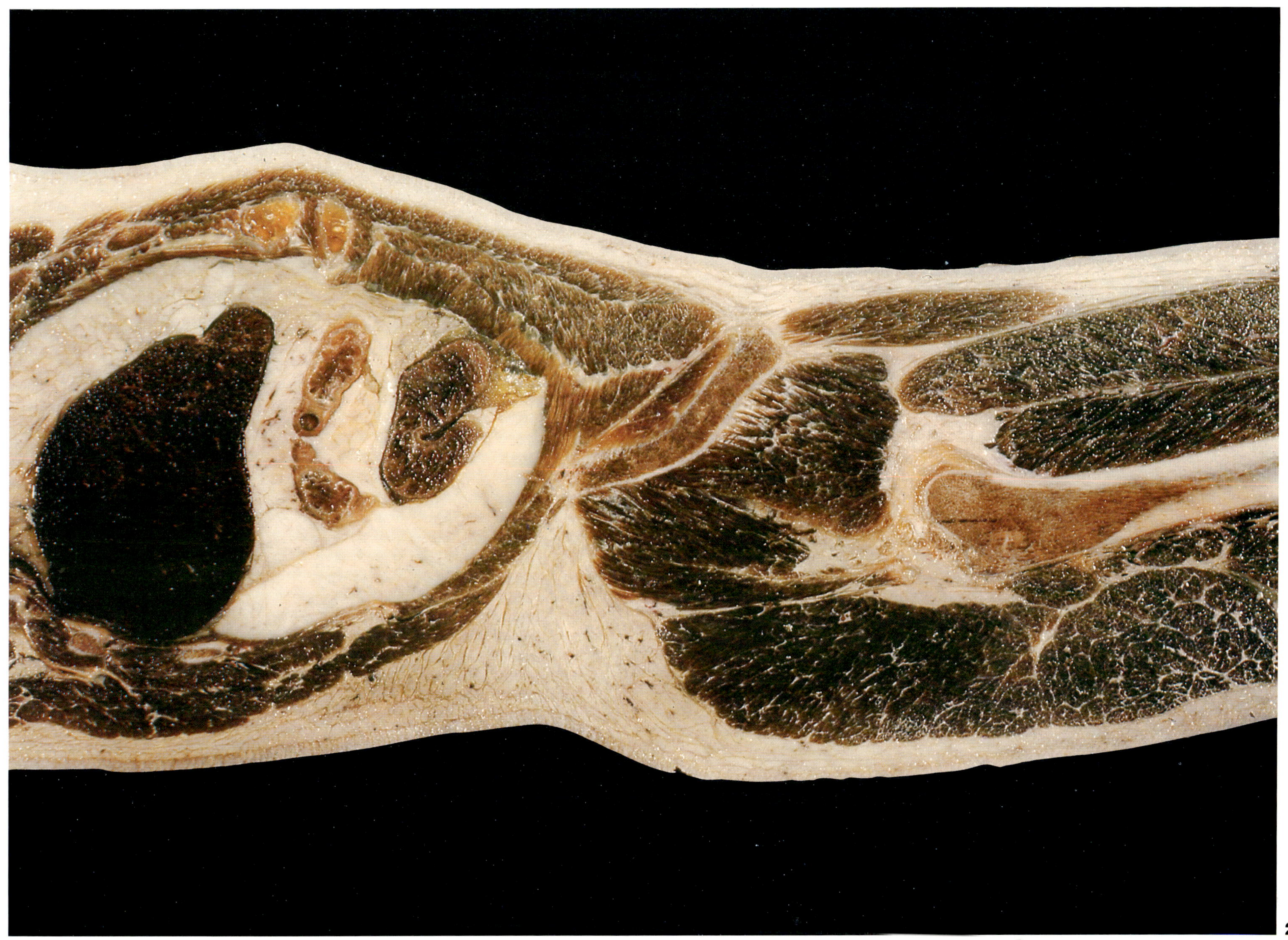

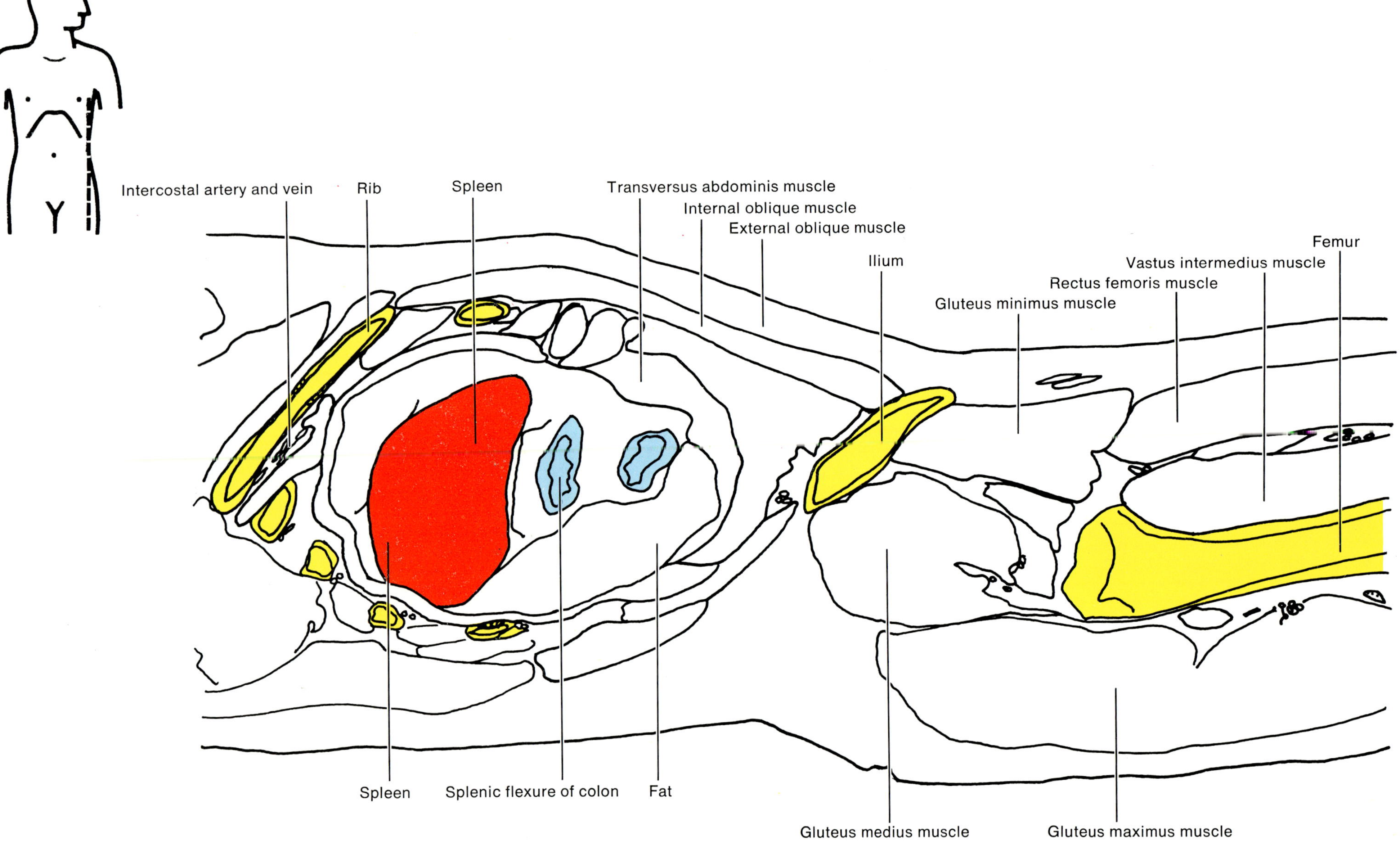

Intercostal artery and vein
Rib
Spleen
Transversus abdominis muscle
Internal oblique muscle
External oblique muscle
Ilium
Femur
Vastus intermedius muscle
Rectus femoris muscle
Gluteus minimus muscle
Spleen
Splenic flexure of colon
Fat
Gluteus medius muscle
Gluteus maximus muscle

PARASAGITTAL **Abdomen and pelvis—male**

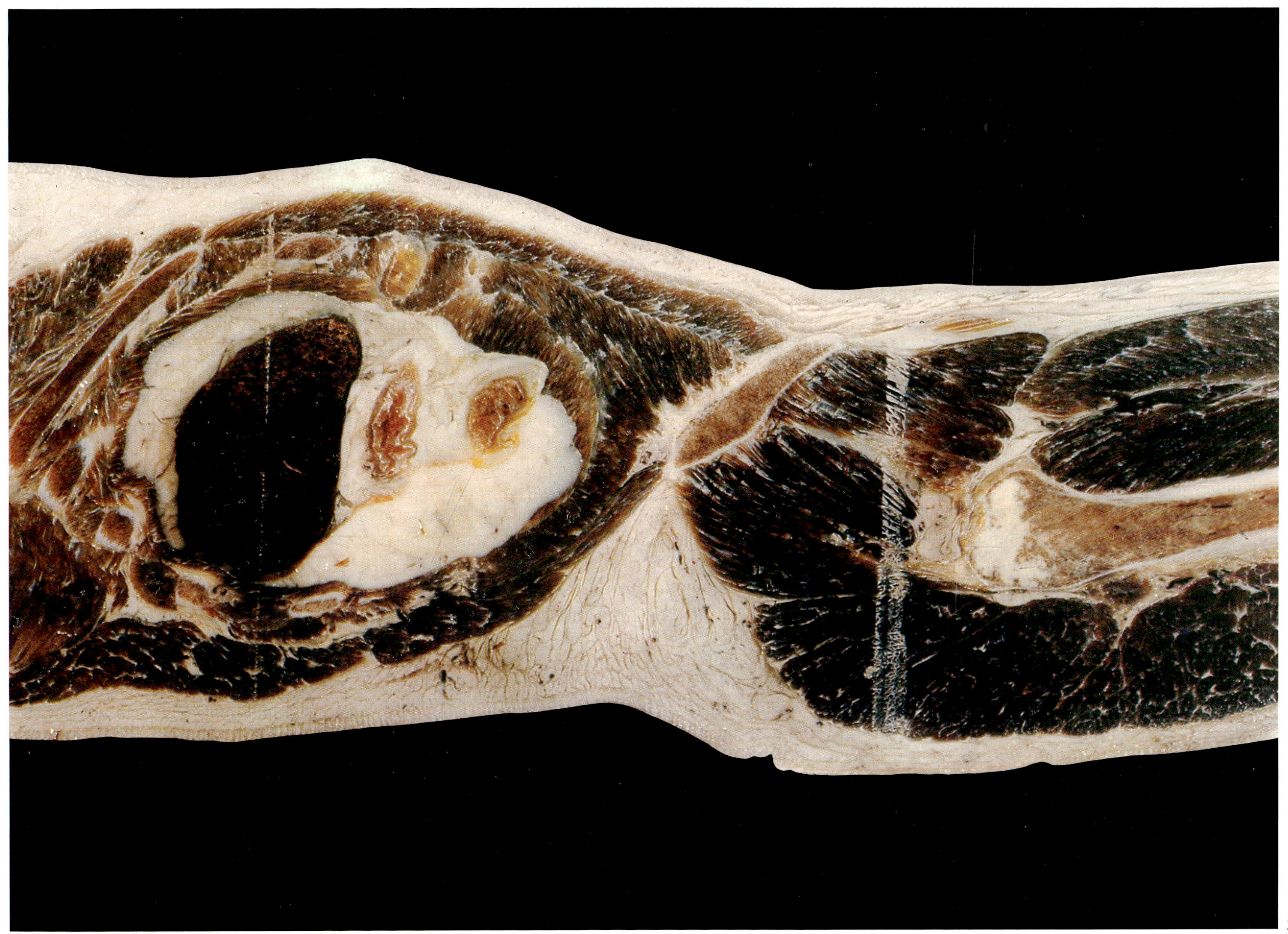

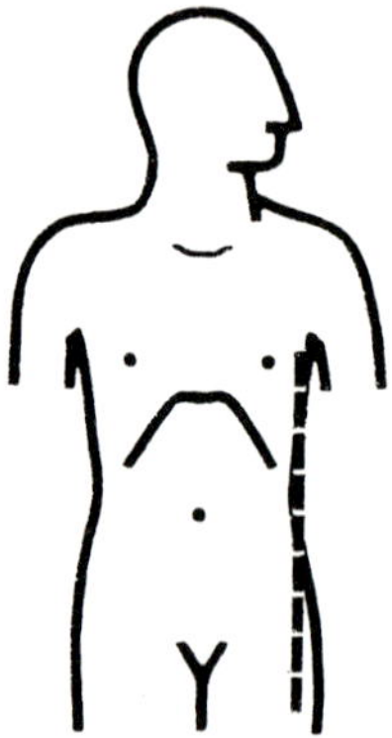

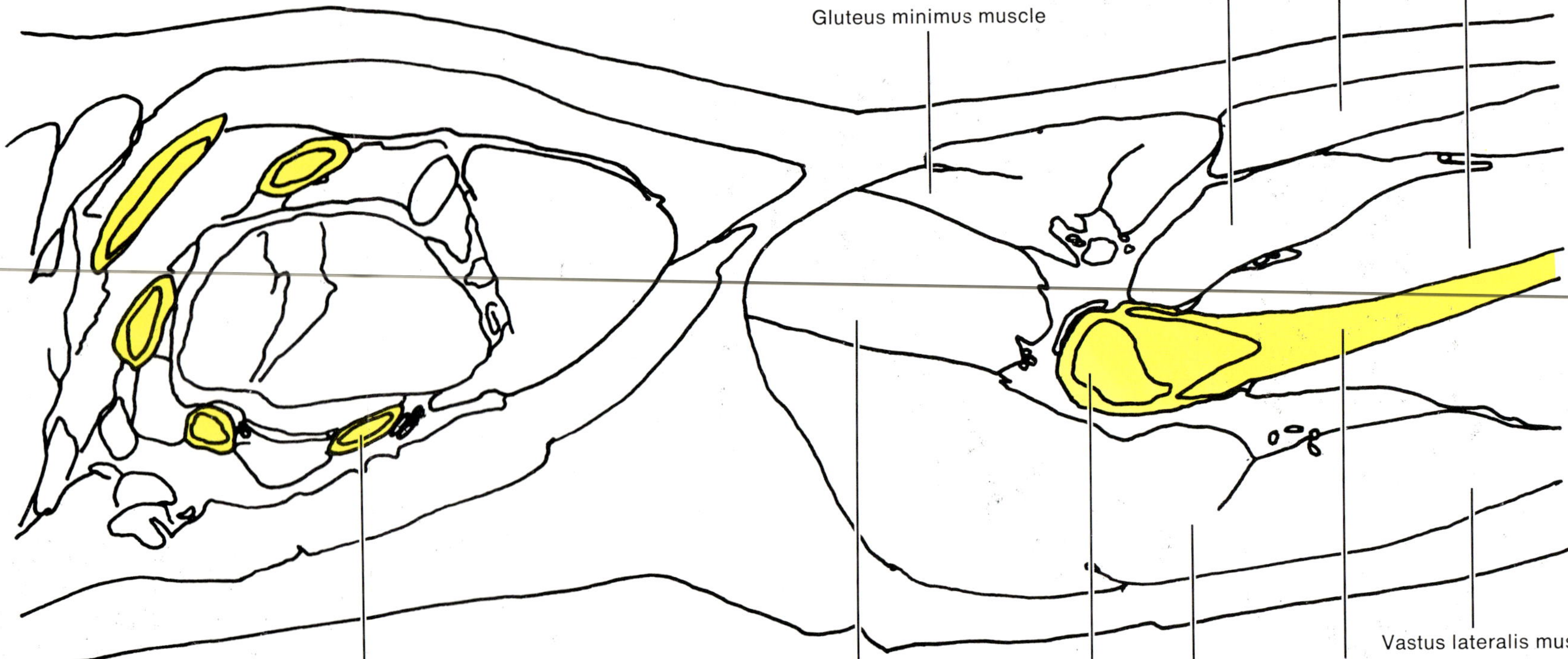

Rectus femoris muscle

Vastus lateralis muscle

Vastus intermedius muscle

Gluteus minimus muscle

Rib

Gluteus medius muscle

Greater trochanter

Gluteus maximus muscle

Vastus lateralis muscle

Femur

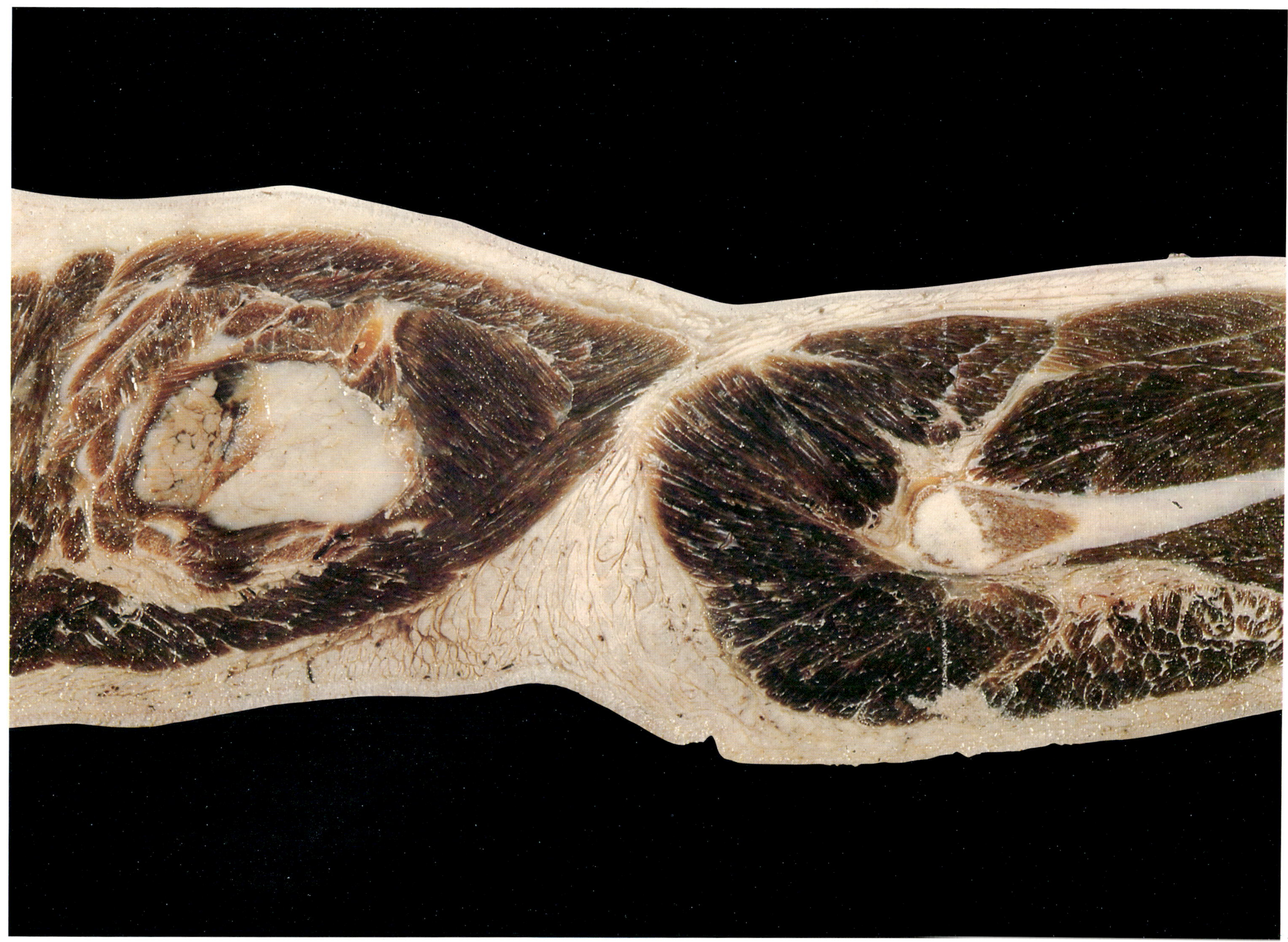

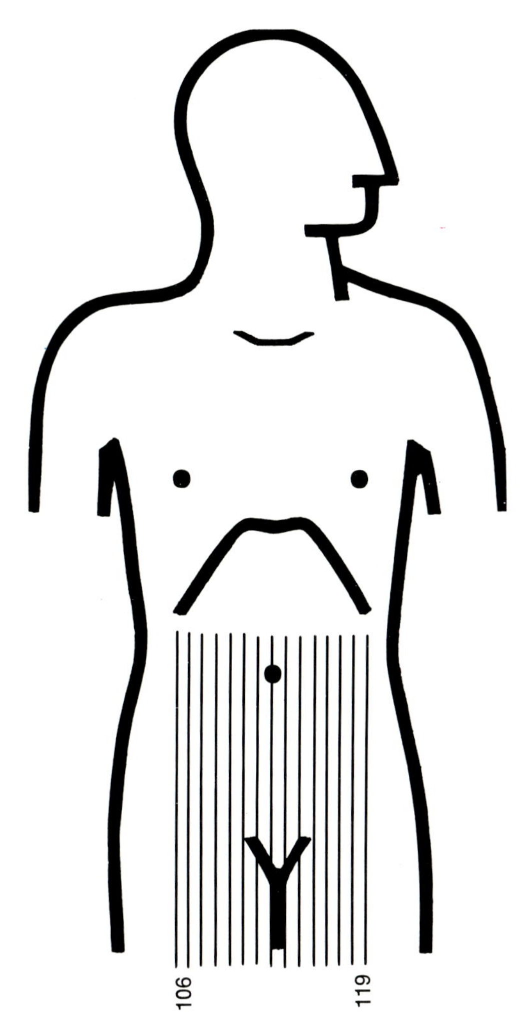

106
119

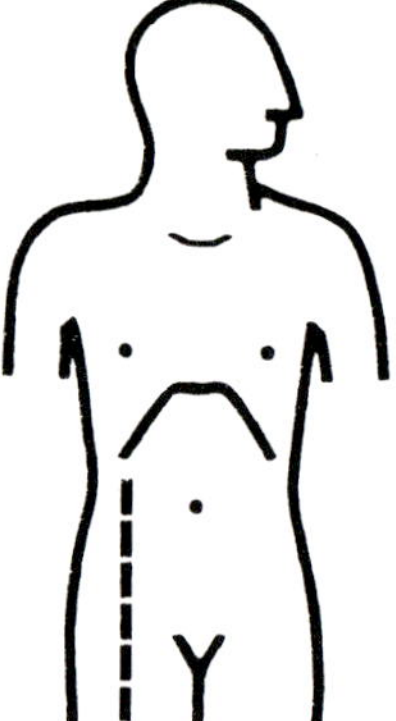

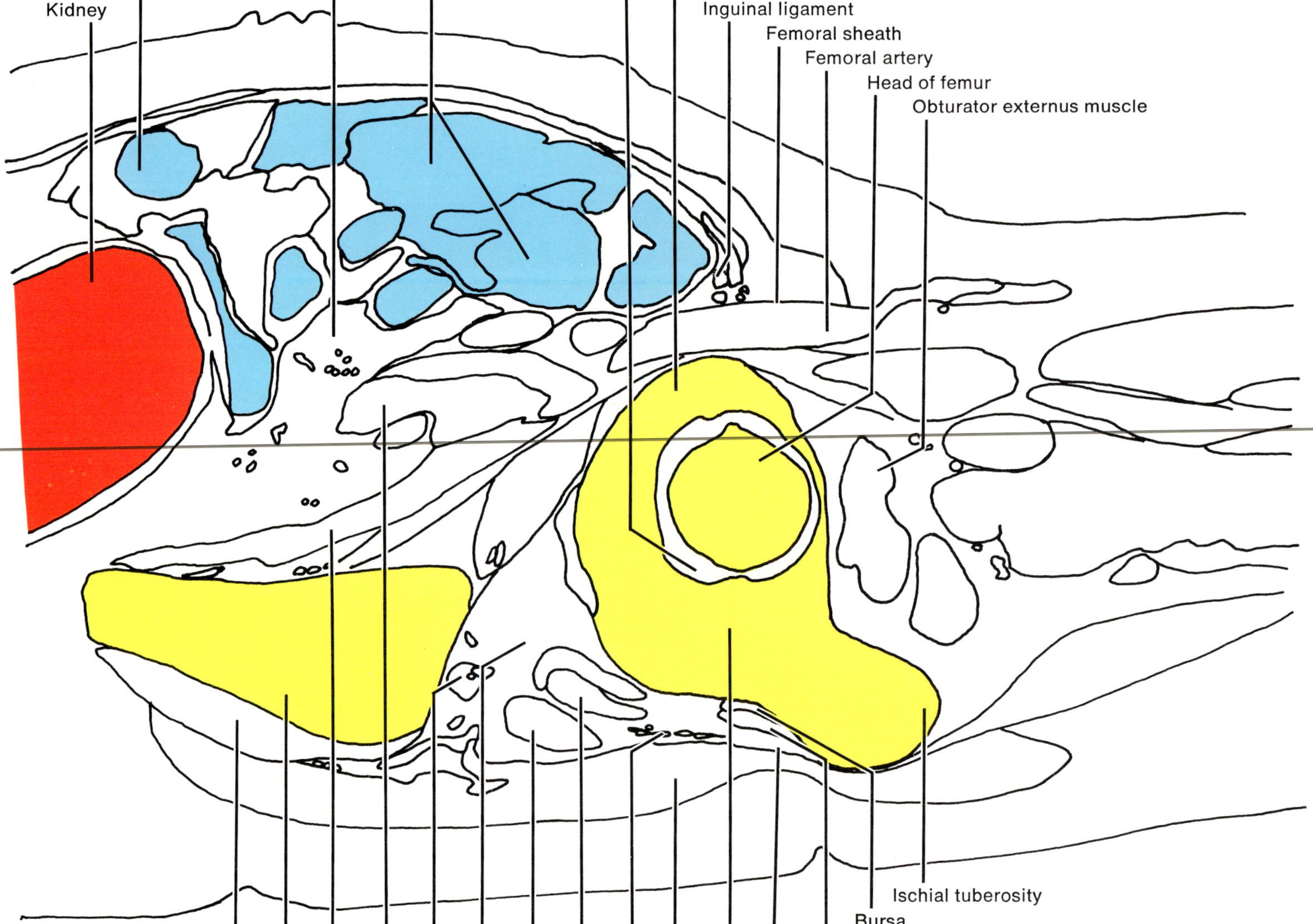

Transverse colon
Kidney
Mesentery
Small bowel
Acetabulum
Pubis
Inguinal ligament
Femoral sheath
Femoral artery
Head of femur
Obturator externus muscle

Gluteus medius muscle
Ilium
Iliacus muscle
Psoas muscle
Superior gluteal artery and vein
Greater sciatic foramen
Piriformis muscle
Sciatic nerve
Inferior gluteal artery and vein
Gluteus maximus muscle
Ischium
Lesser sciatic foramen
Obturator internus muscle
Bursa
Ischial tuberosity

PARASAGITTAL **Pelvis—female**

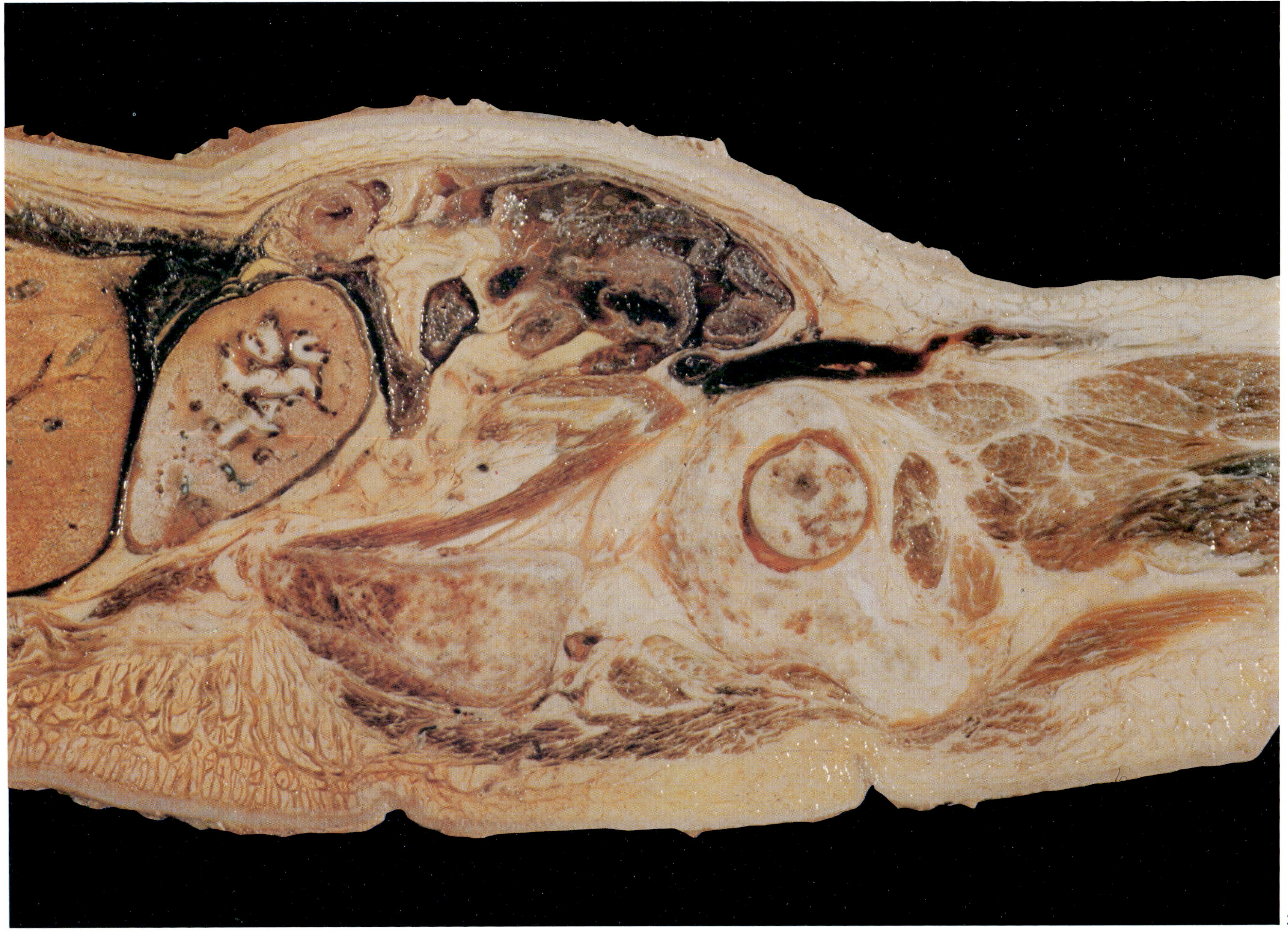

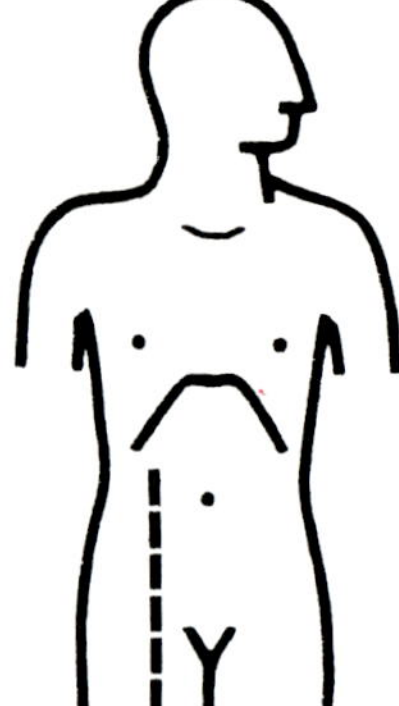

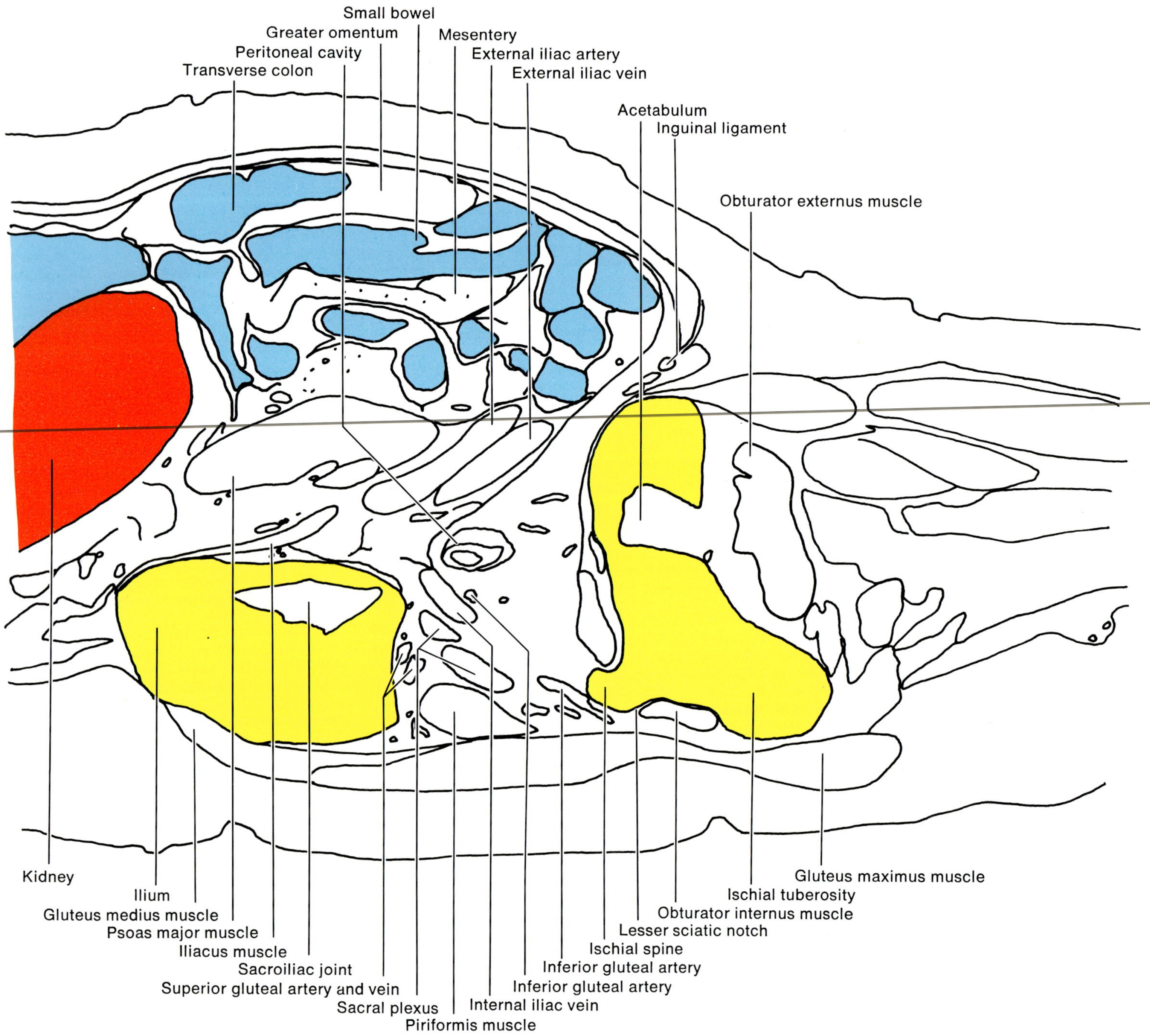

Small bowel
Greater omentum
Mesentery
Peritoneal cavity
External iliac artery
Transverse colon
External iliac vein
Acetabulum
Inguinal ligament
Obturator externus muscle
Kidney
Ilium
Gluteus maximus muscle
Gluteus medius muscle
Ischial tuberosity
Psoas major muscle
Obturator internus muscle
Iliacus muscle
Lesser sciatic notch
Sacroiliac joint
Ischial spine
Superior gluteal artery and vein
Inferior gluteal artery
Sacral plexus
Inferior gluteal artery
Piriformis muscle
Internal iliac vein

PARASAGITTAL **Pelvis—female**

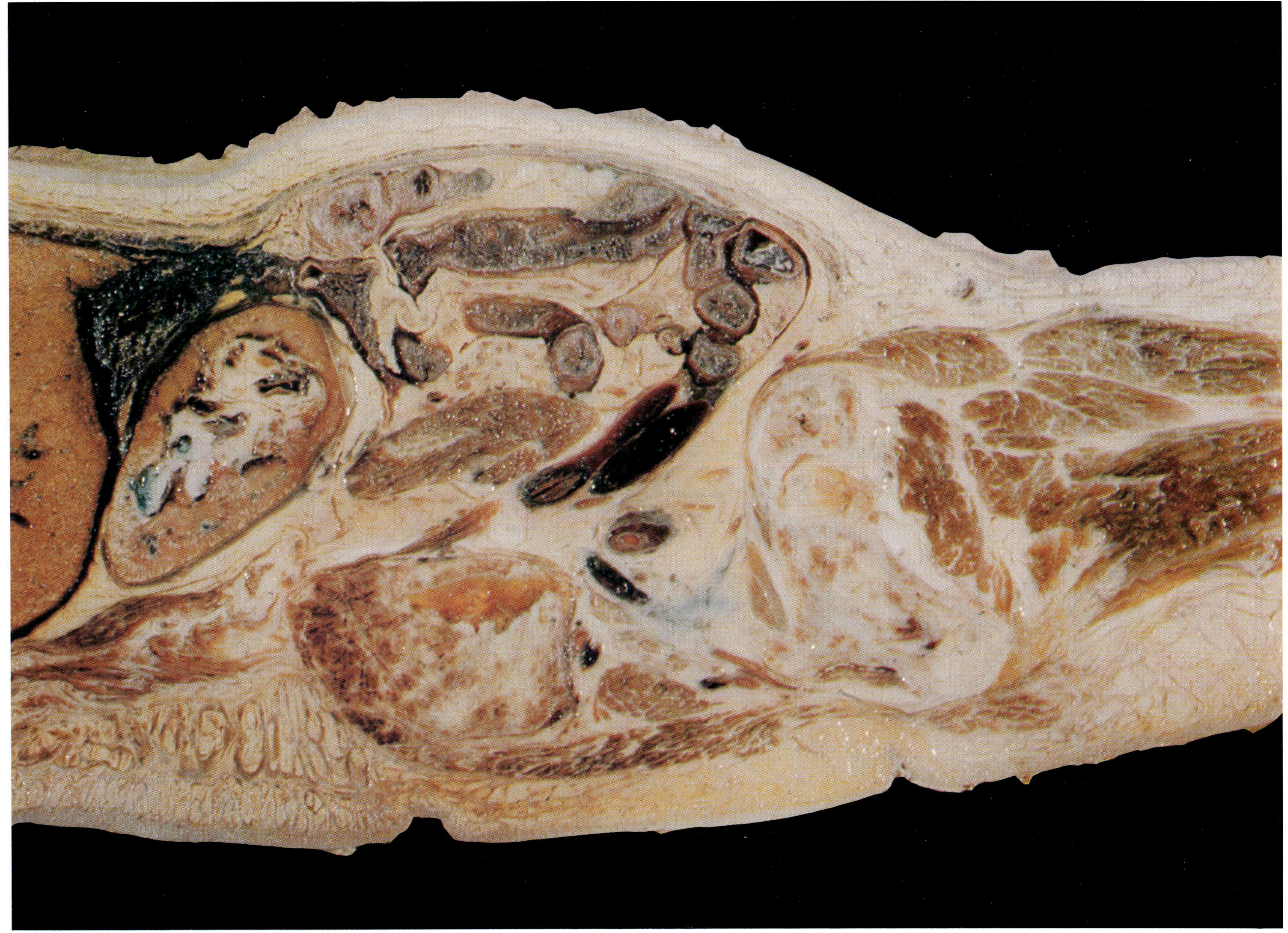

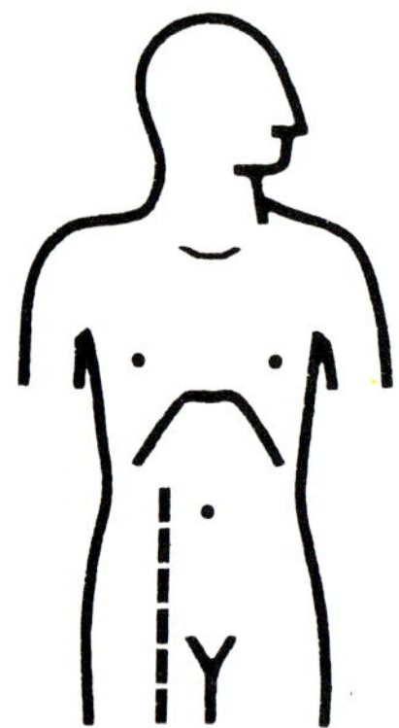

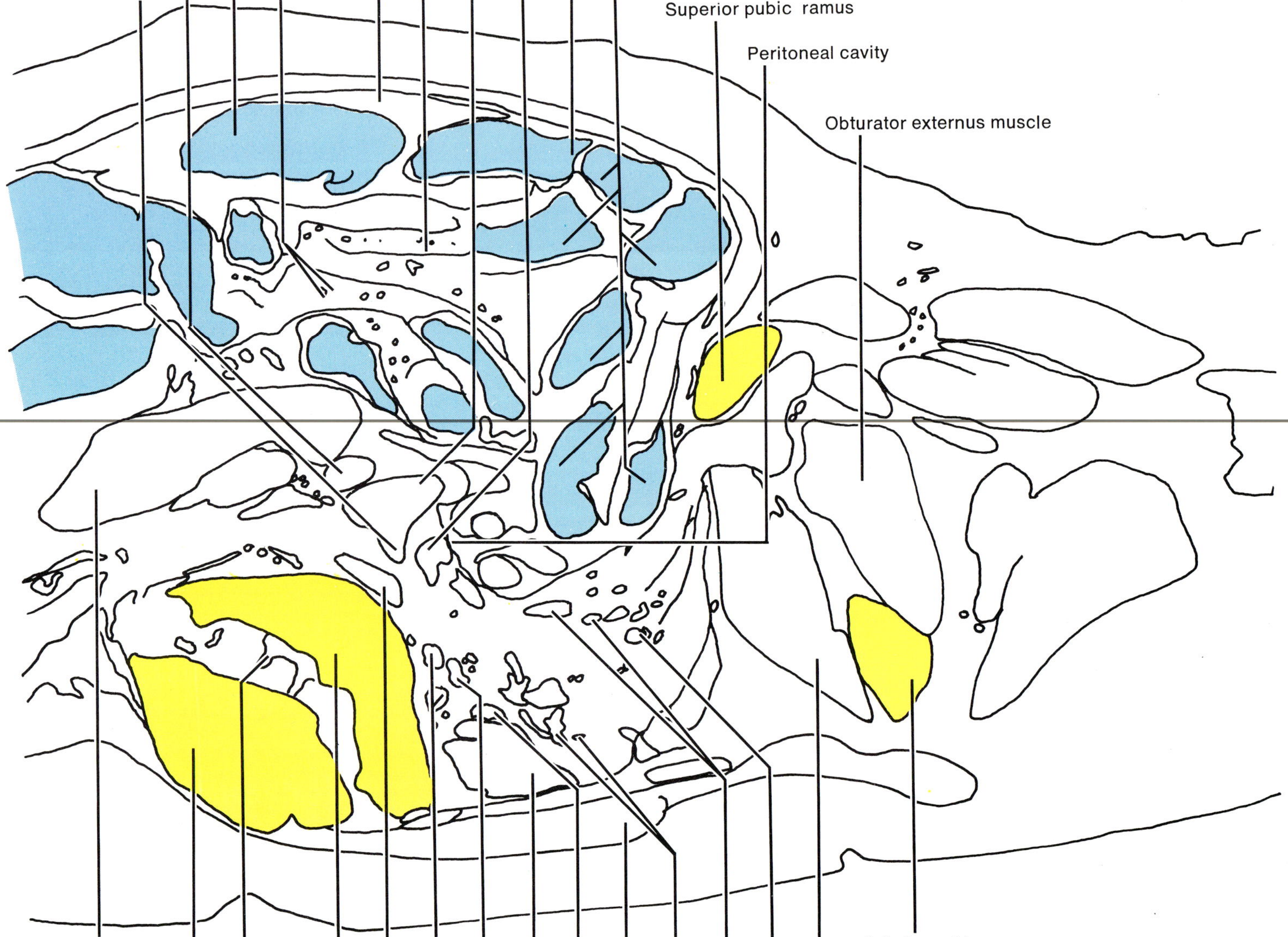

Mesentery
Greater omentum
Transverse colon
External iliac vein
Internal iliac artery
Small bowel
Right common iliac artery
Ileal arteries
Small bowel
Internal iliac vein
Superior pubic ramus
Peritoneal cavity
Obturator externus muscle
Psoas major muscle
Ilium
Interosseous sacroiliac ligament
Lateral part of sacrum
Lumbosacral trunk
Superior gluteal artery and vein
First sacral ramus
Piriformis muscle
Second sacral ramus
Gluteus maximus muscle
Inferior gluteal artery and vein
Internal pudendal artery and vein
Uterine vein
Obturator internus muscle
Inferior pubic ramus

PARASAGITTAL **Pelvis—female**

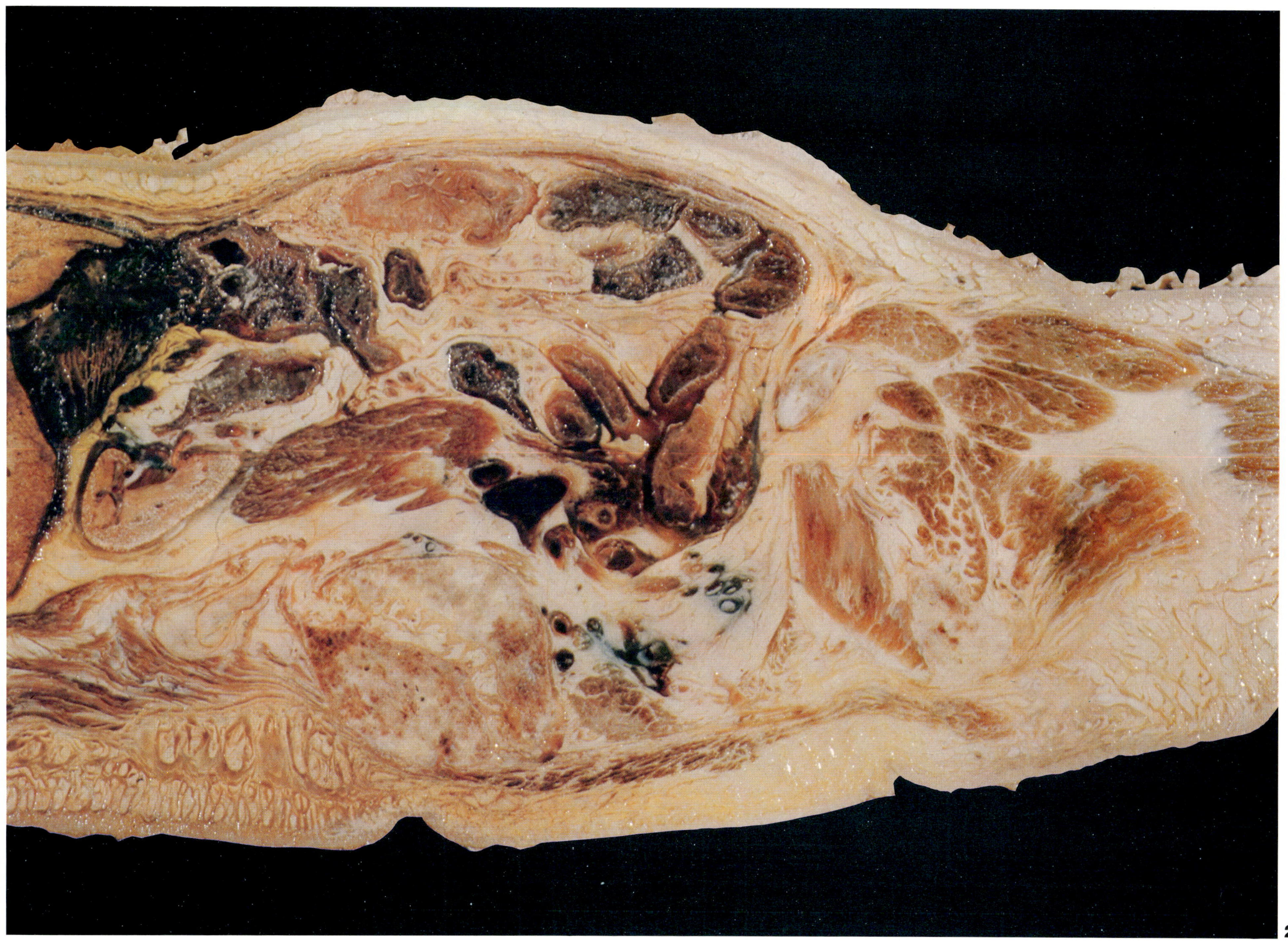

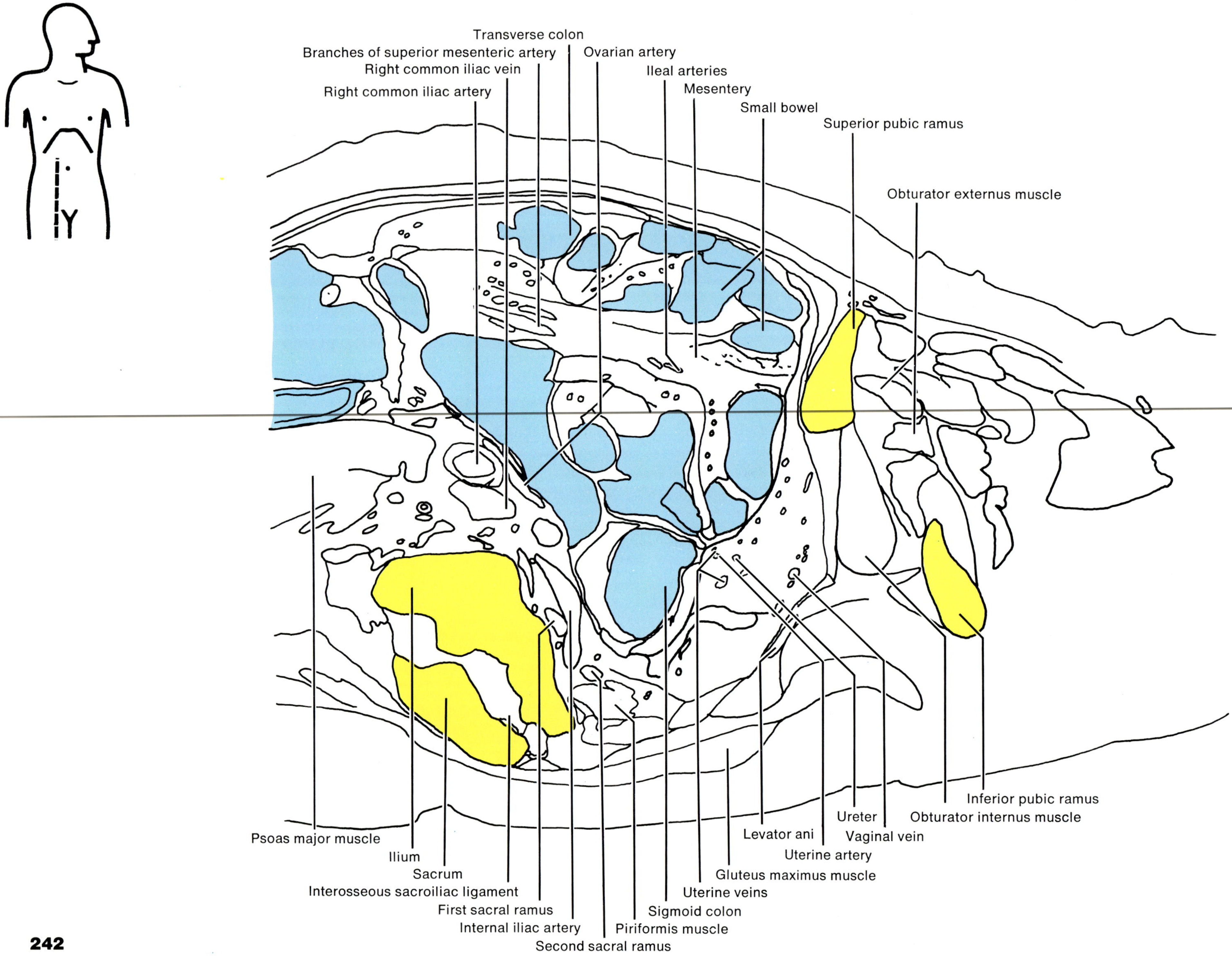

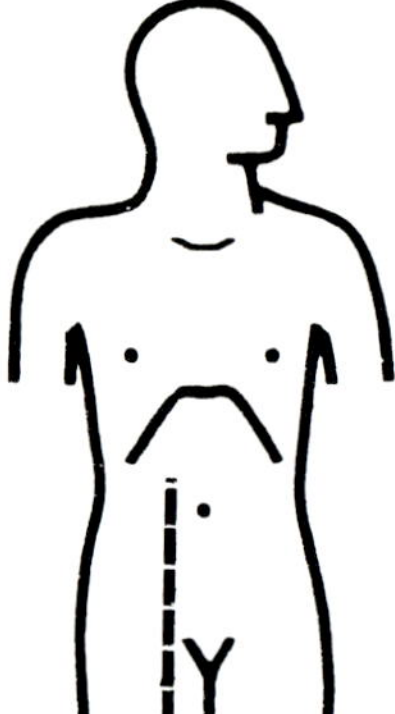

Transverse colon
Branches of superior mesenteric artery
Right common iliac vein
Right common iliac artery
Ovarian artery
Ileal arteries
Mesentery
Small bowel
Superior pubic ramus
Obturator externus muscle
Psoas major muscle
Ilium
Sacrum
Interosseous sacroiliac ligament
First sacral ramus
Internal iliac artery
Second sacral ramus
Piriformis muscle
Sigmoid colon
Uterine veins
Gluteus maximus muscle
Uterine artery
Levator ani
Vaginal vein
Ureter
Obturator internus muscle
Inferior pubic ramus

PARASAGITTAL **Pelvis—female**

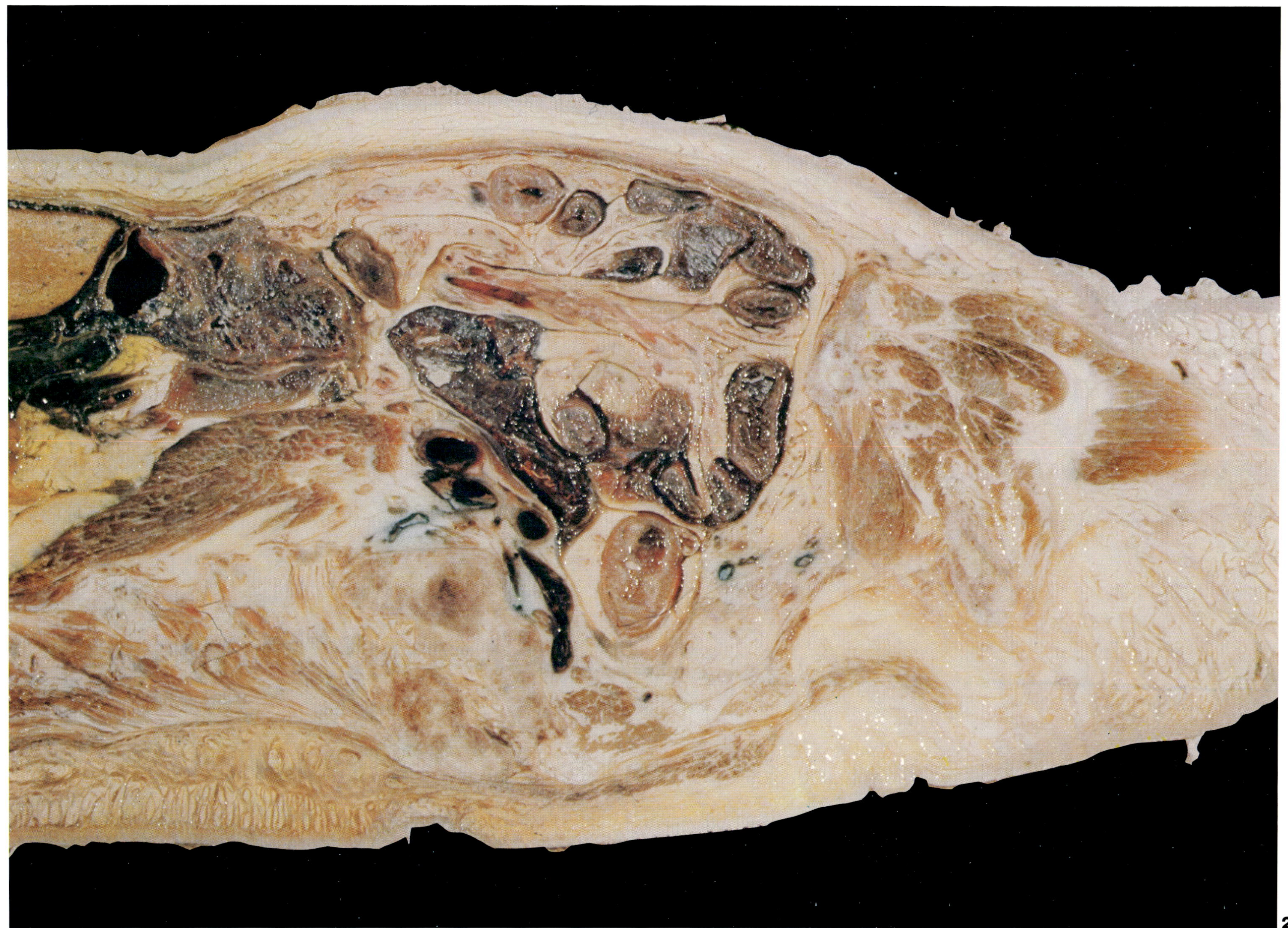

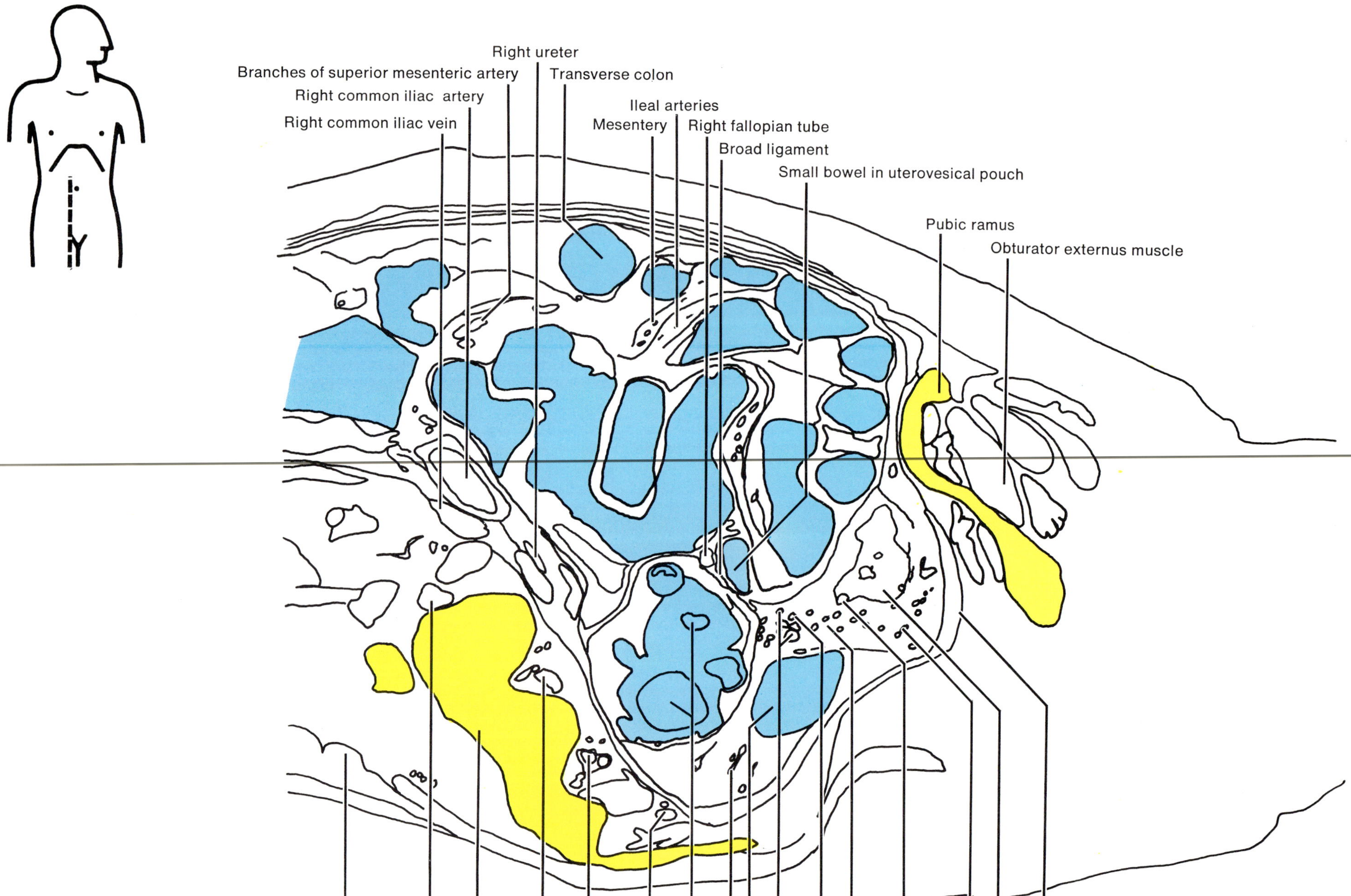

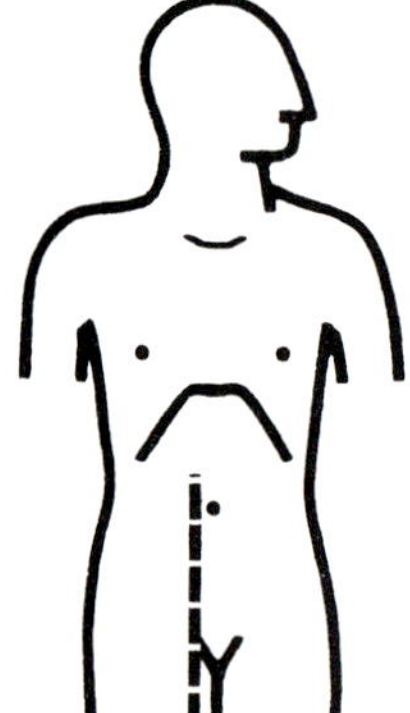

Branches of superior mesenteric artery
Right common iliac artery
Right common iliac vein
Right ureter
Transverse colon
Ileal arteries
Mesentery
Right fallopian tube
Broad ligament
Small bowel in uterovesical pouch
Pubic ramus
Obturator externus muscle

Erector spinae muscles
Fifth lumbar ramus
Second sacral vertebra
First sacral ramus
Second sacral ramus
Third sacral ramus
Sigmoid colon
Rectum
Superior rectal artery
Uterine veins
Uterine artery
Vaginal venous plexus
Ureter
Vesical venous plexus
Urinary bladder
Levator ani

PARASAGITTAL **Pelvis—female**

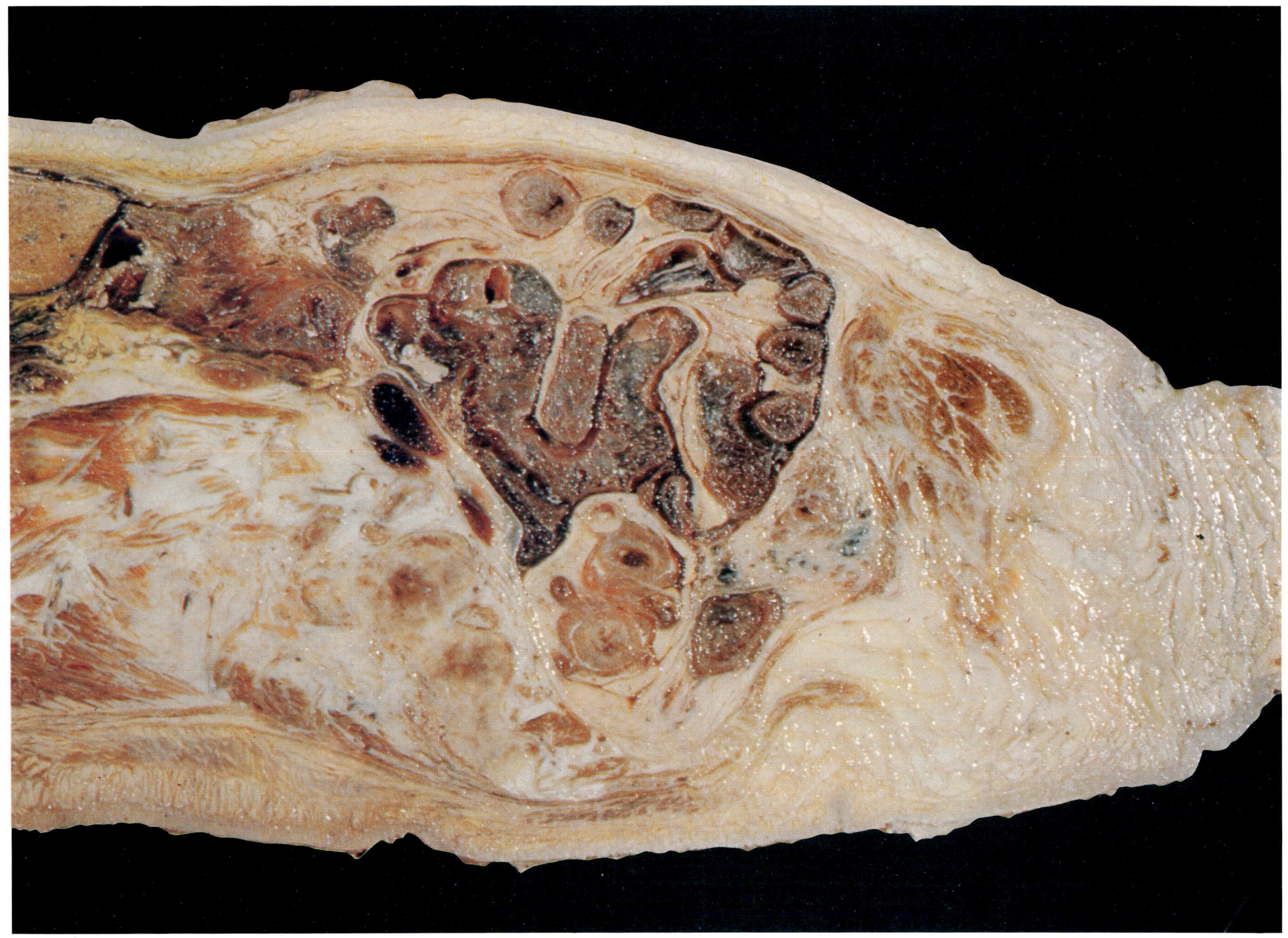

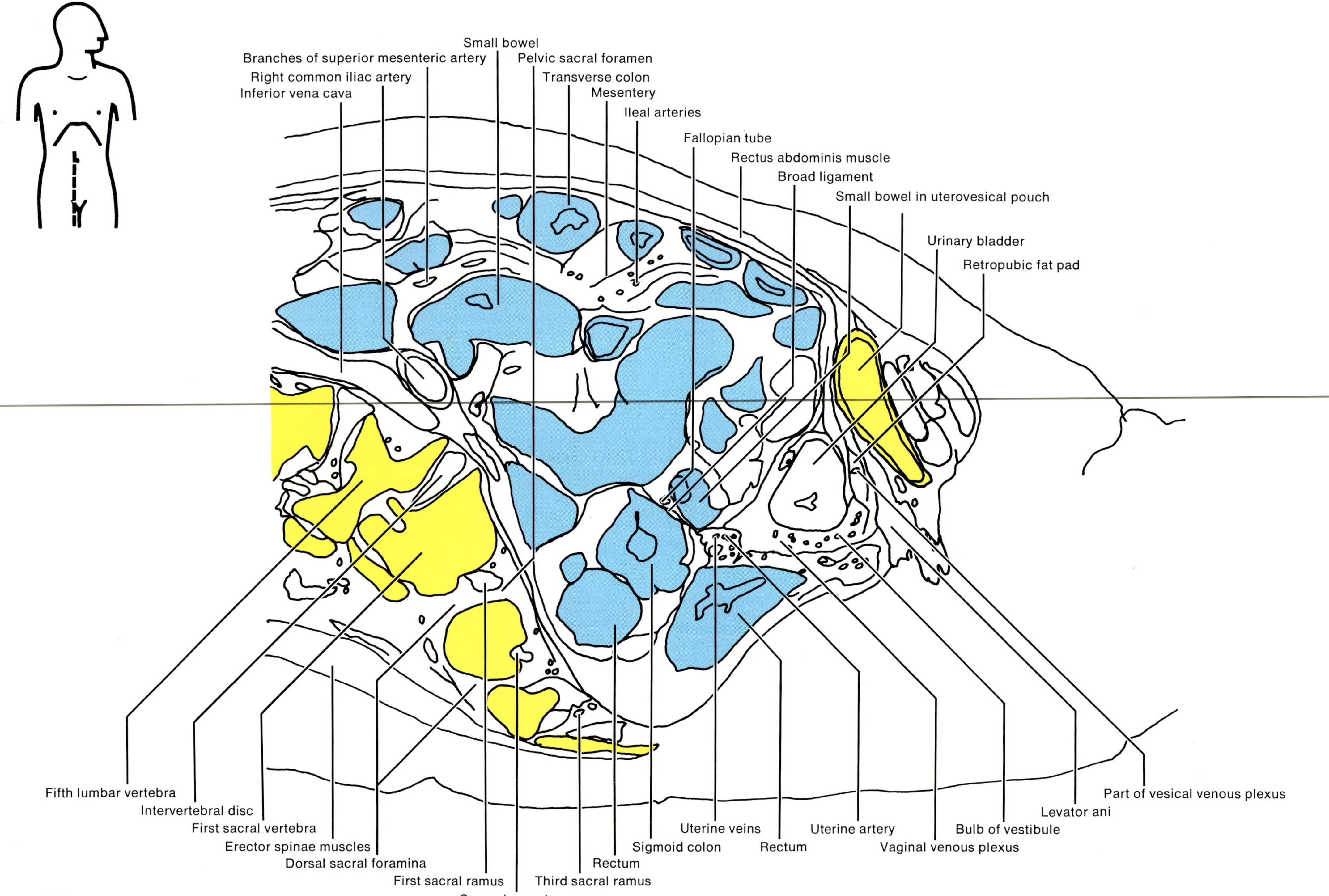

Branches of superior mesenteric artery
Right common iliac artery
Inferior vena cava
Small bowel
Pelvic sacral foramen
Transverse colon
Mesentery
Ileal arteries
Fallopian tube
Rectus abdominis muscle
Broad ligament
Small bowel in uterovesical pouch
Urinary bladder
Retropubic fat pad
Fifth lumbar vertebra
Intervertebral disc
First sacral vertebra
Erector spinae muscles
Dorsal sacral foramina
First sacral ramus
Second sacral ramus
Third sacral ramus
Rectum
Sigmoid colon
Uterine veins
Rectum
Uterine artery
Vaginal venous plexus
Bulb of vestibule
Levator ani
Part of vesical venous plexus

PARASAGITTAL **Pelvis—female**

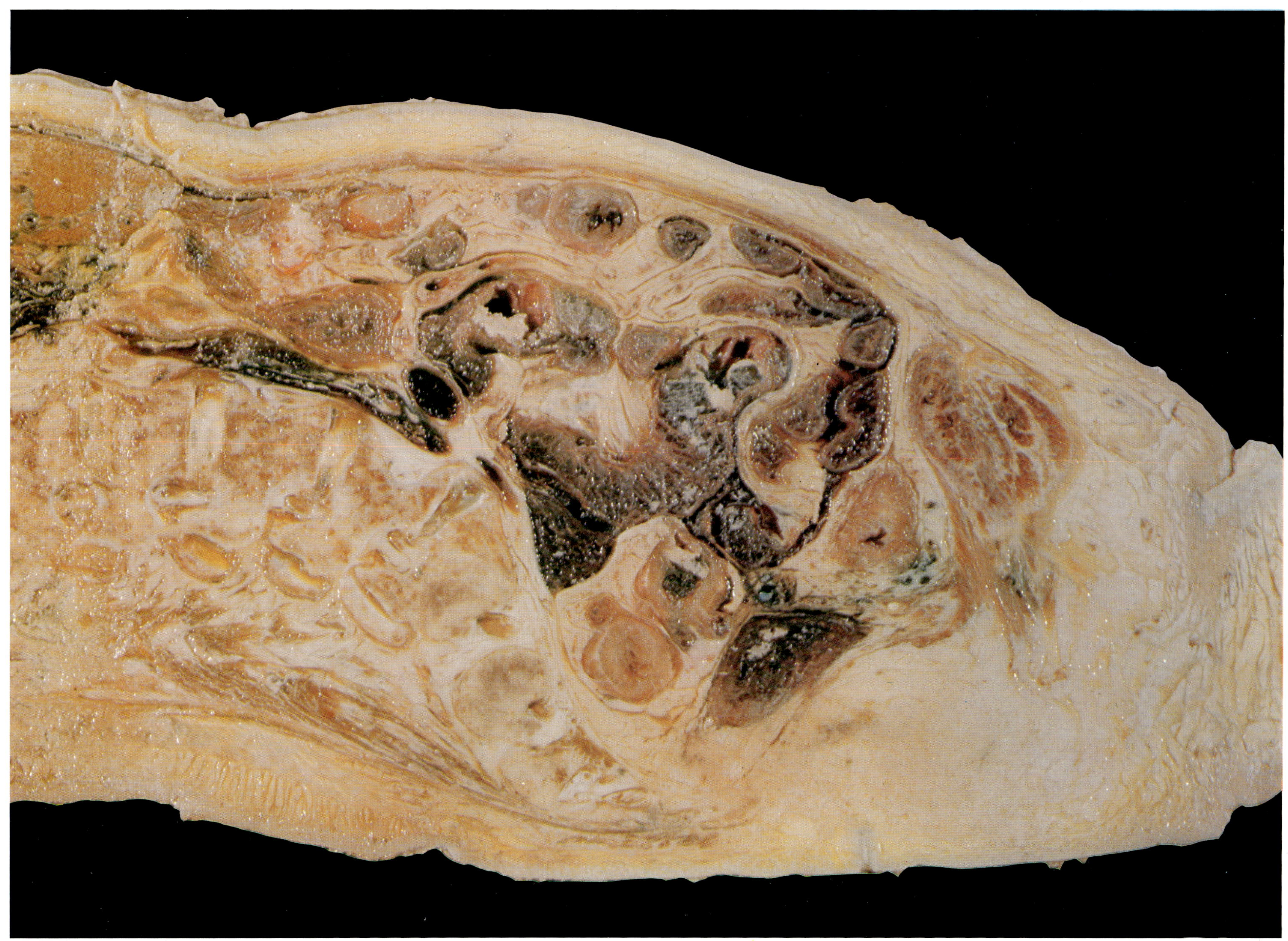

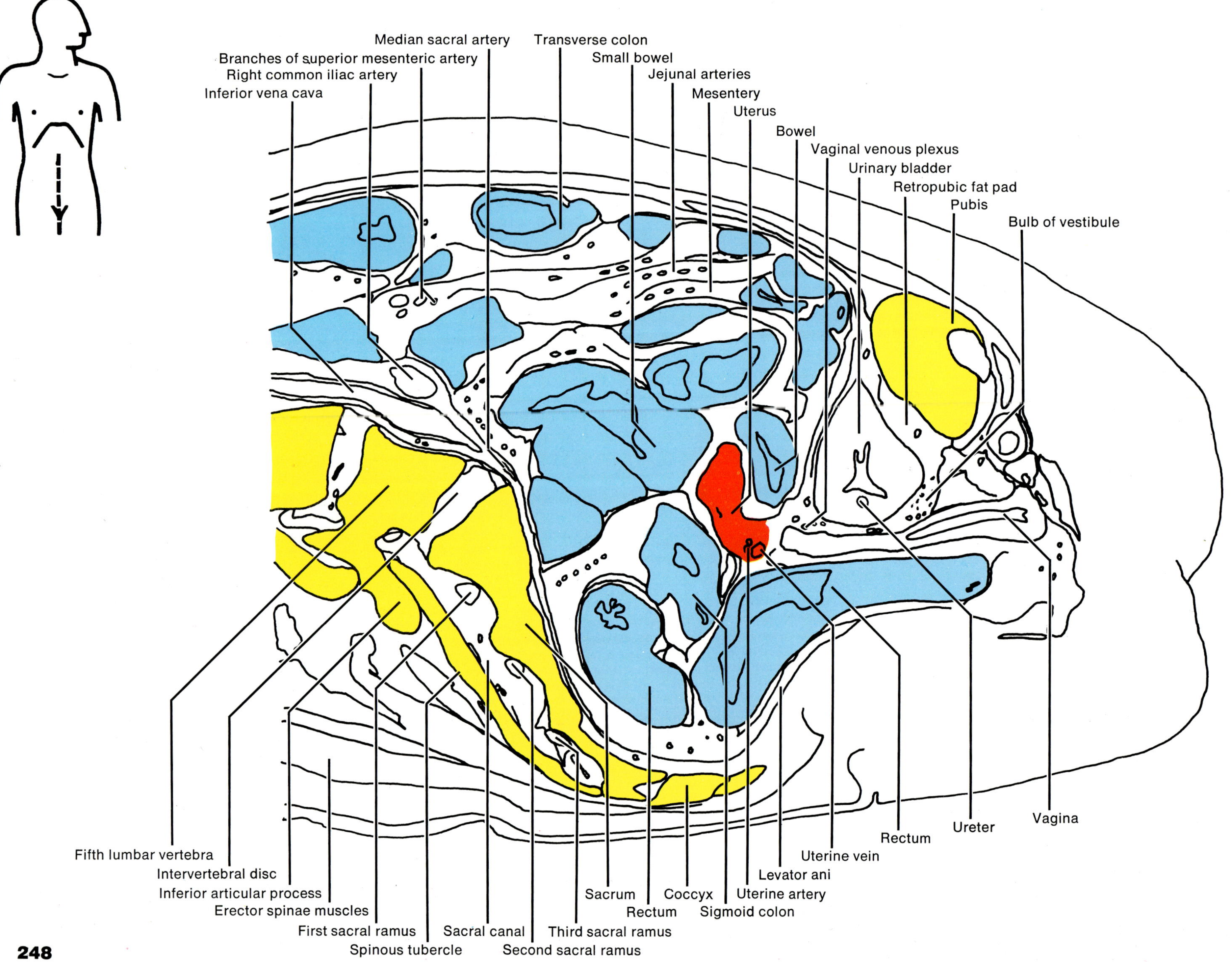
Branches of superior mesenteric artery
Right common iliac artery
Inferior vena cava
Median sacral artery
Transverse colon
Small bowel
Jejunal arteries
Mesentery
Uterus
Bowel
Vaginal venous plexus
Urinary bladder
Retropubic fat pad
Pubis
Bulb of vestibule
Fifth lumbar vertebra
Intervertebral disc
Inferior articular process
Erector spinae muscles
First sacral ramus
Spinous tubercle
Sacral canal
Second sacral ramus
Third sacral ramus
Sacrum
Rectum
Coccyx
Sigmoid colon
Levator ani
Uterine artery
Uterine vein
Rectum
Ureter
Vagina

PARASAGITTAL **Pelvis—female**

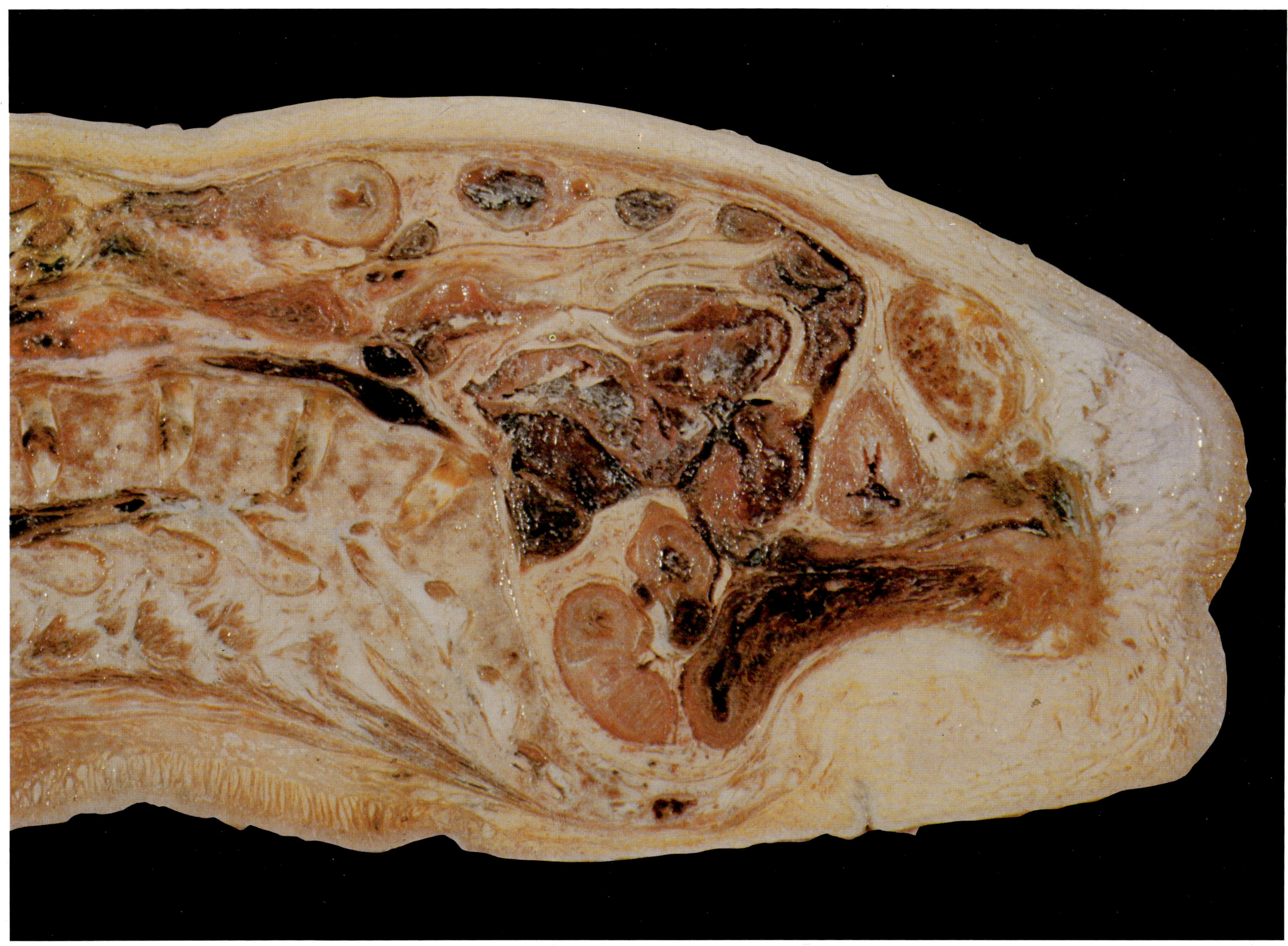

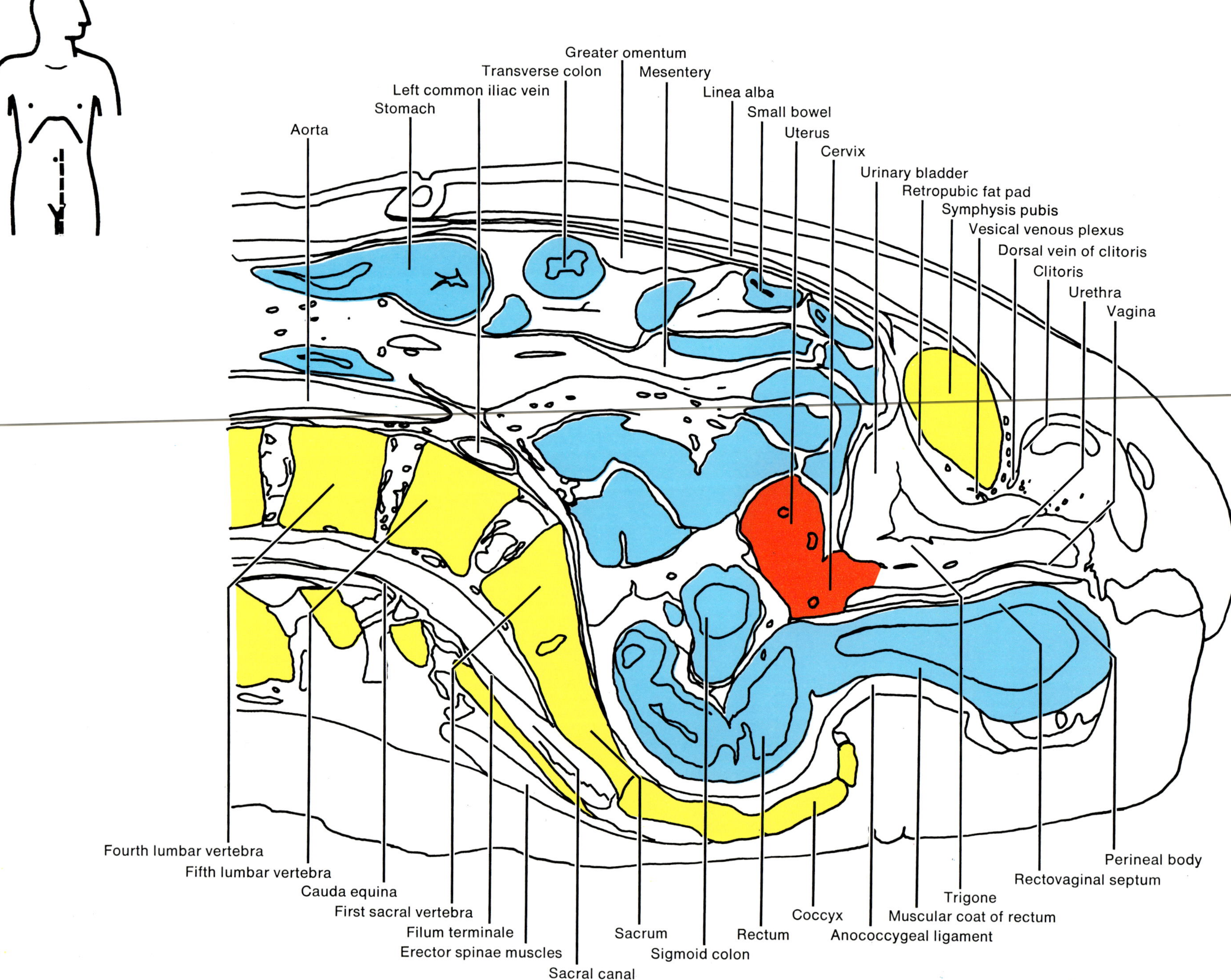

Aorta
Stomach
Left common iliac vein
Transverse colon
Greater omentum
Mesentery
Linea alba
Small bowel
Uterus
Cervix
Urinary bladder
Retropubic fat pad
Symphysis pubis
Vesical venous plexus
Dorsal vein of clitoris
Clitoris
Urethra
Vagina
Fourth lumbar vertebra
Fifth lumbar vertebra
Cauda equina
First sacral vertebra
Filum terminale
Erector spinae muscles
Sacral canal
Sacrum
Sigmoid colon
Rectum
Coccyx
Anococcygeal ligament
Muscular coat of rectum
Trigone
Rectovaginal septum
Perineal body

PARASAGITTAL **Pelvis—female**

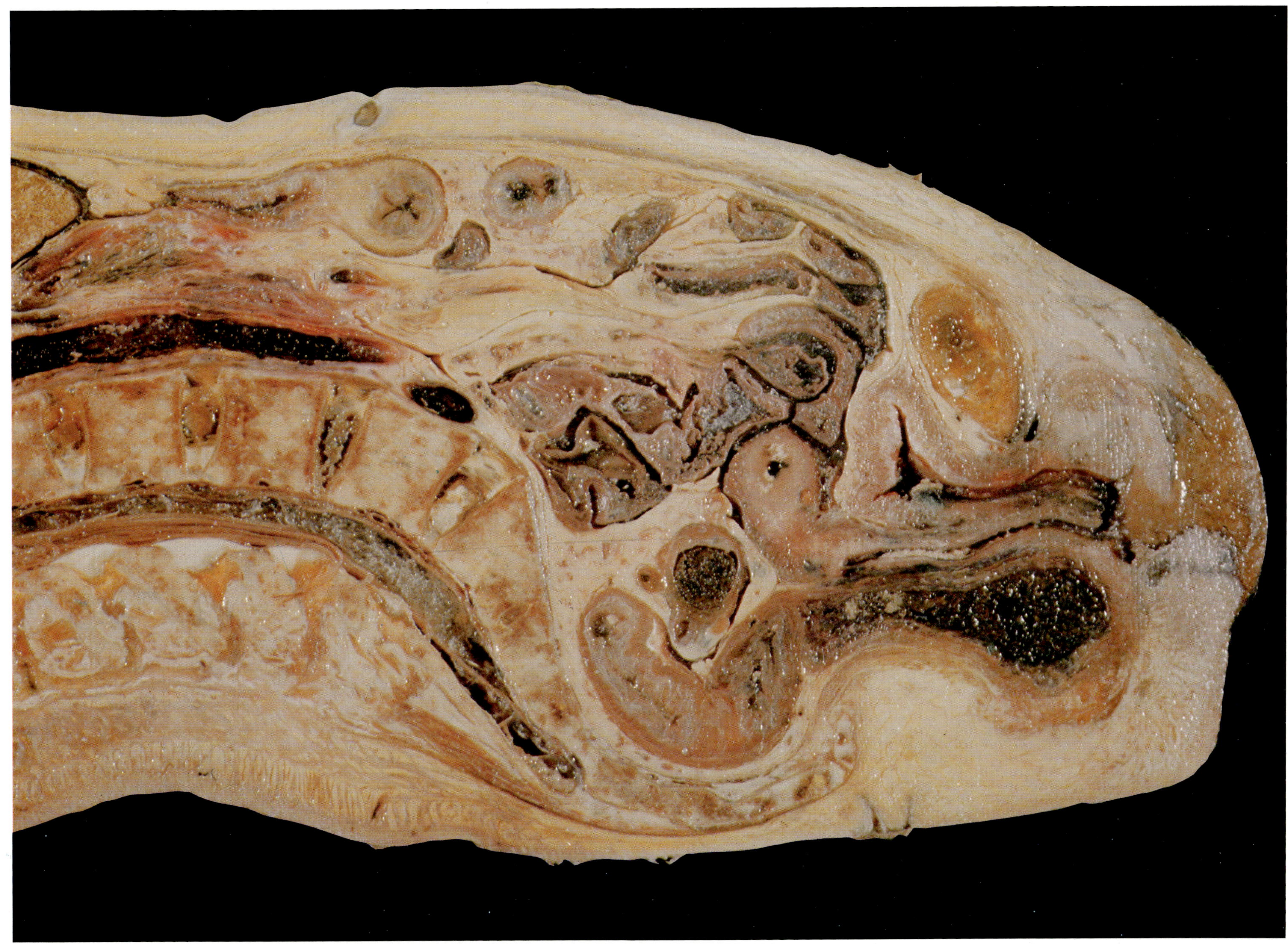

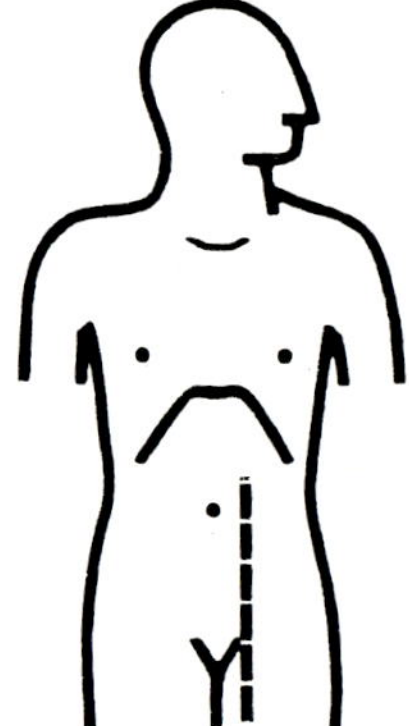

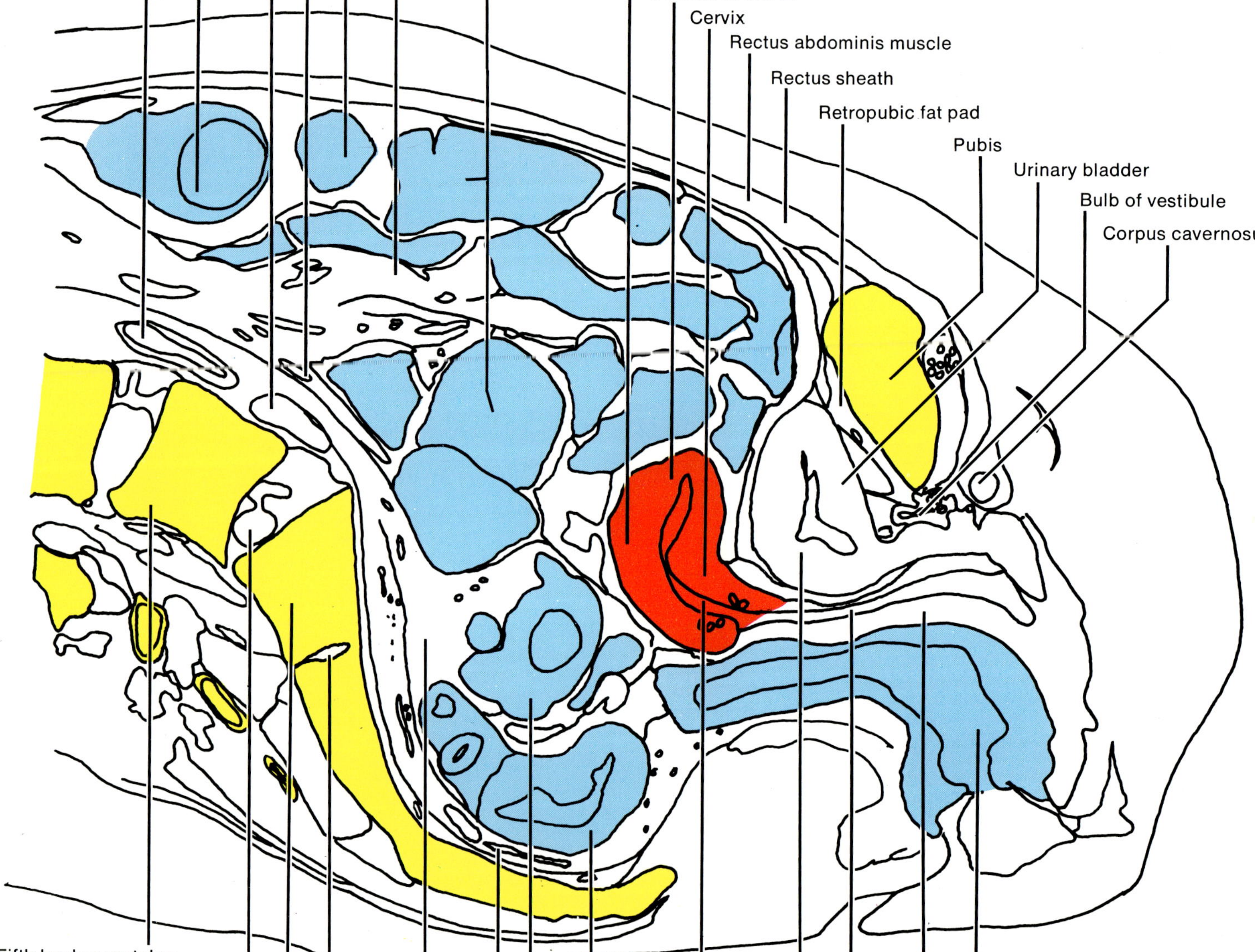

Inferior mesenteric artery
Left common iliac vein
Stomach
Left common iliac artery
Transverse colon
Mesentery
Small bowel
Body of uterus
Fundus of uterus
Cervix
Rectus abdominis muscle
Rectus sheath
Retropubic fat pad
Pubis
Urinary bladder
Bulb of vestibule
Corpus cavernosum clitoris
Fifth lumbar vertebra
Intervertebral disc (L5-S1)
First sacral vertebra
Intervertebral disc (S1-2)
Sigmoid mesocolon
Superior rectal artery
Sigmoid colon
Rectum
Central cavity of uterus
Trigone
Vagina
Rectovaginal septum
Anus

PARASAGITTAL **Pelvis—female**

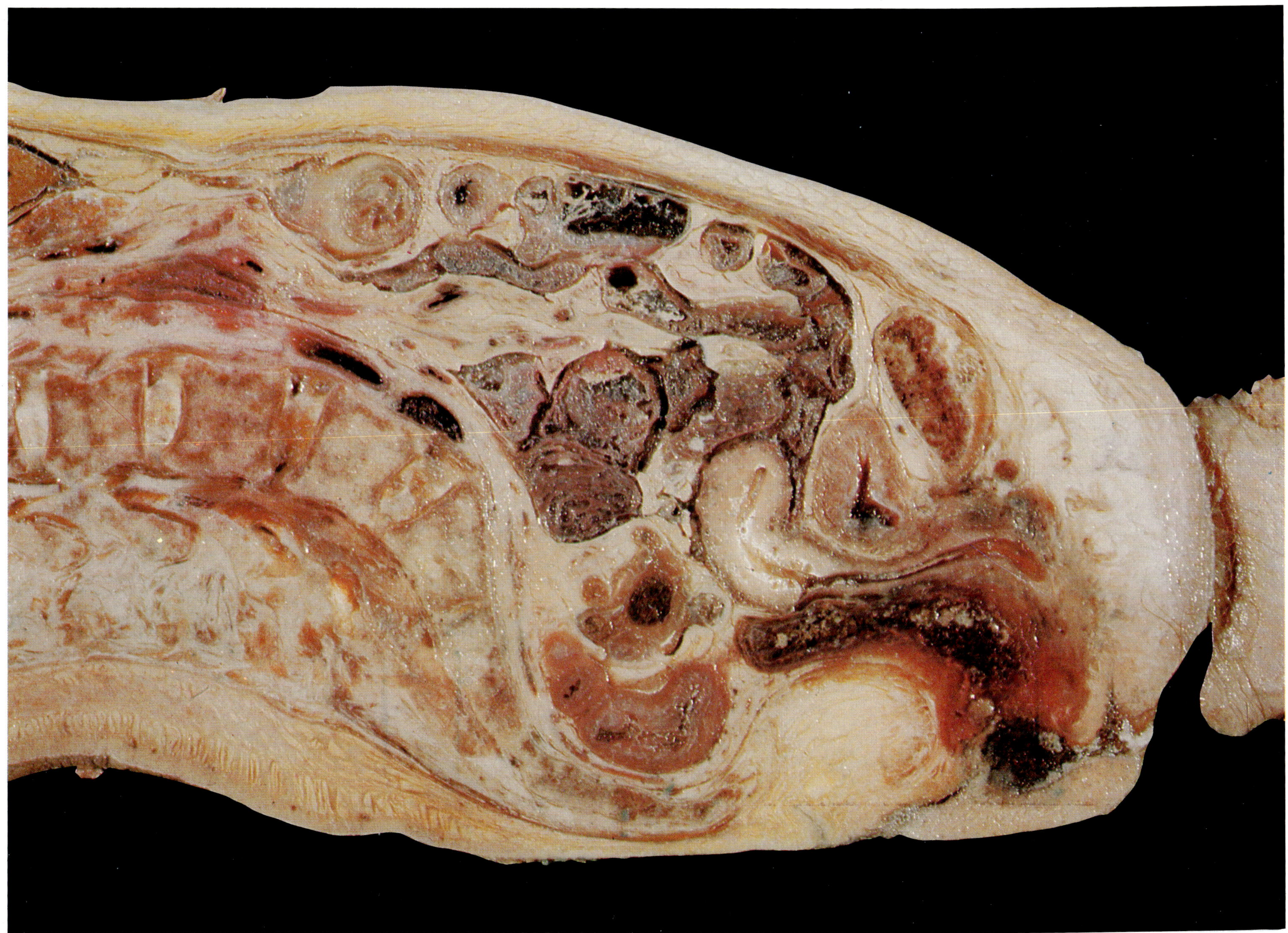

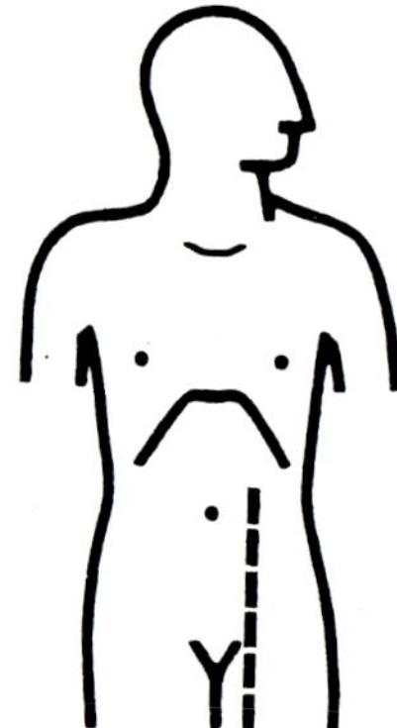

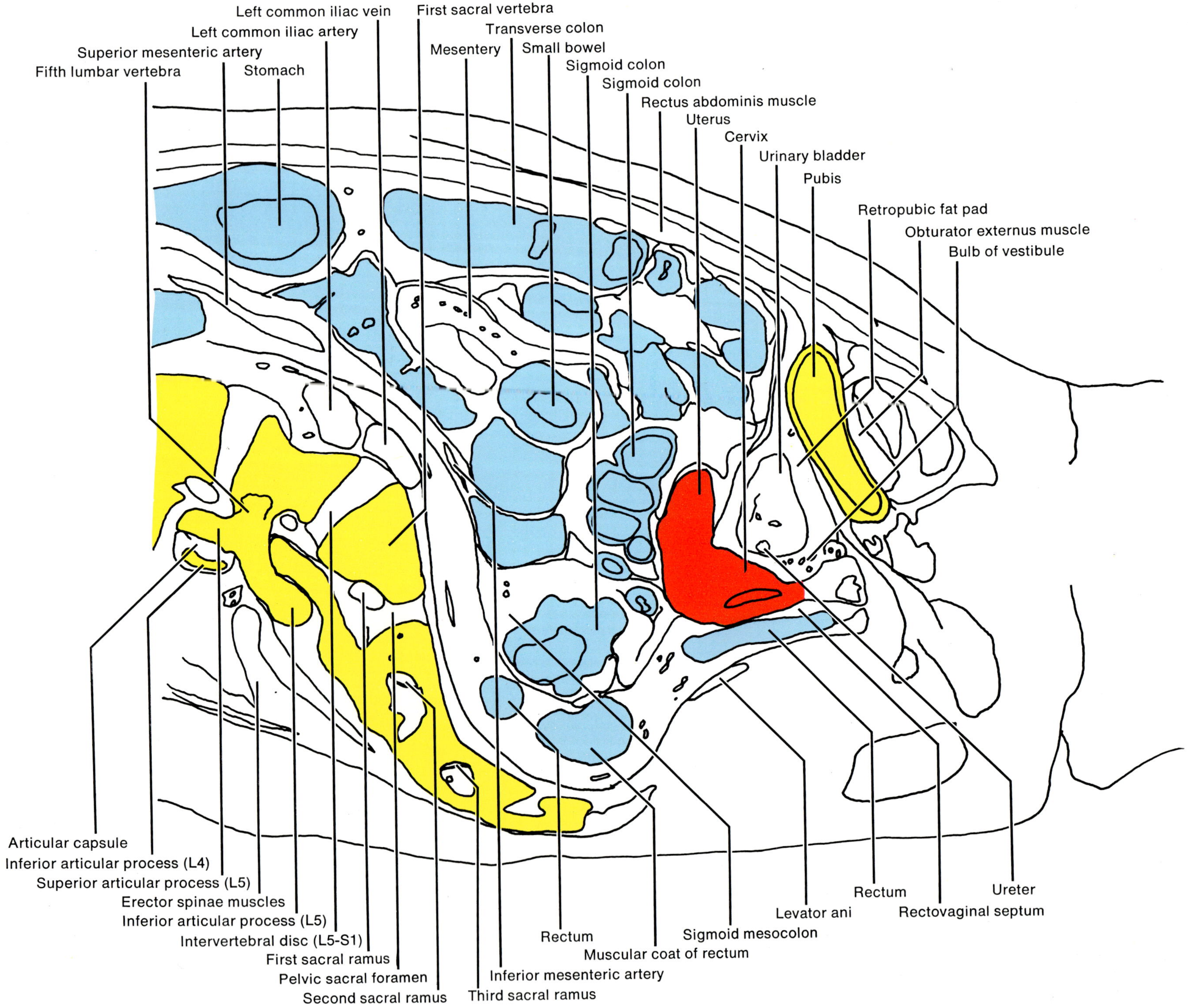

Left common iliac vein
Left common iliac artery
Superior mesenteric artery
Fifth lumbar vertebra
Stomach
First sacral vertebra
Transverse colon
Mesentery
Small bowel
Sigmoid colon
Sigmoid colon
Rectus abdominis muscle
Uterus
Cervix
Urinary bladder
Pubis
Retropubic fat pad
Obturator externus muscle
Bulb of vestibule
Articular capsule
Inferior articular process (L4)
Superior articular process (L5)
Erector spinae muscles
Inferior articular process (L5)
Intervertebral disc (L5-S1)
First sacral ramus
Pelvic sacral foramen
Second sacral ramus
Third sacral ramus
Rectum
Inferior mesenteric artery
Muscular coat of rectum
Sigmoid mesocolon
Levator ani
Rectum
Rectovaginal septum
Ureter

PARASAGITTAL **Pelvis—female**

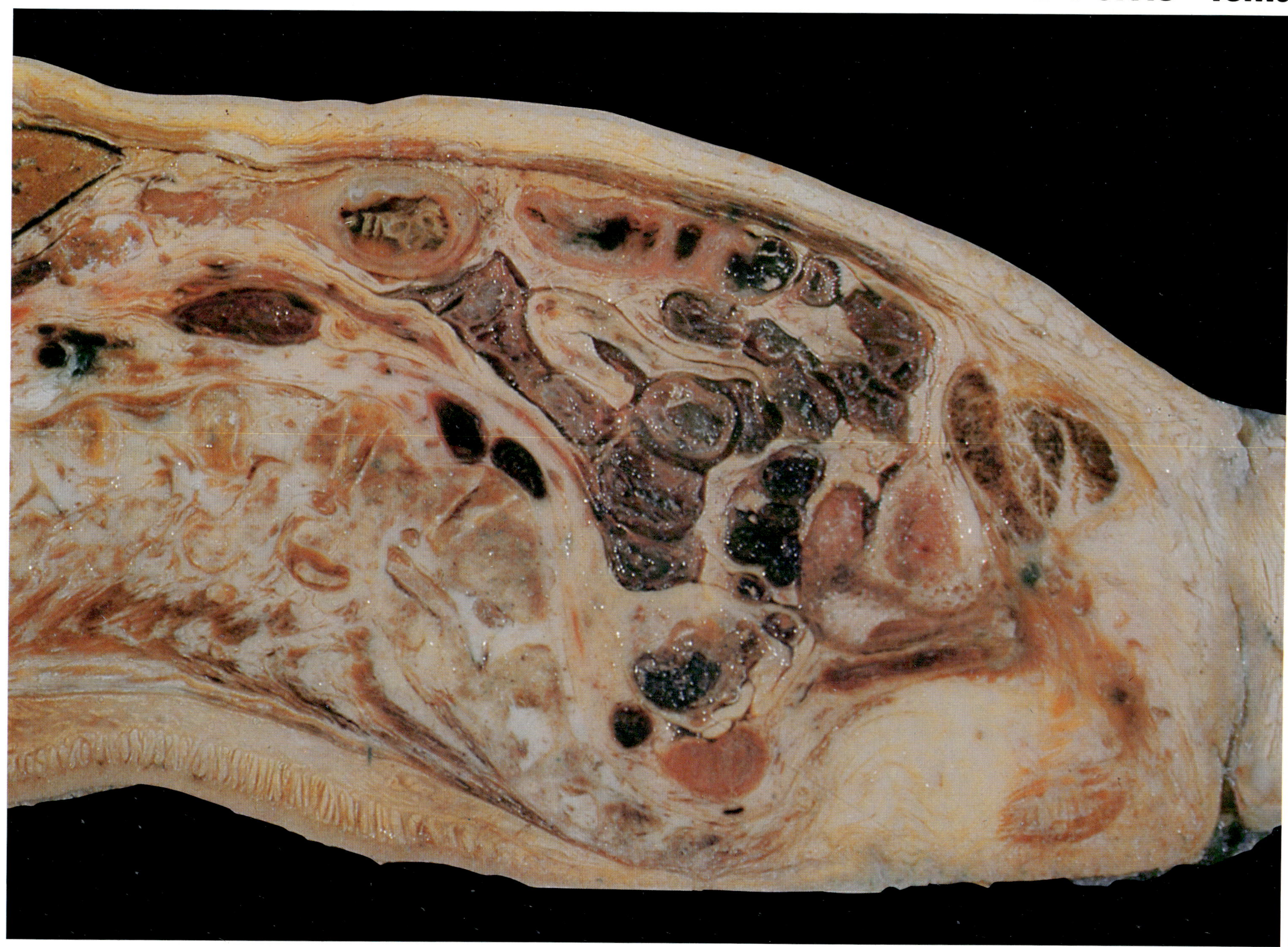

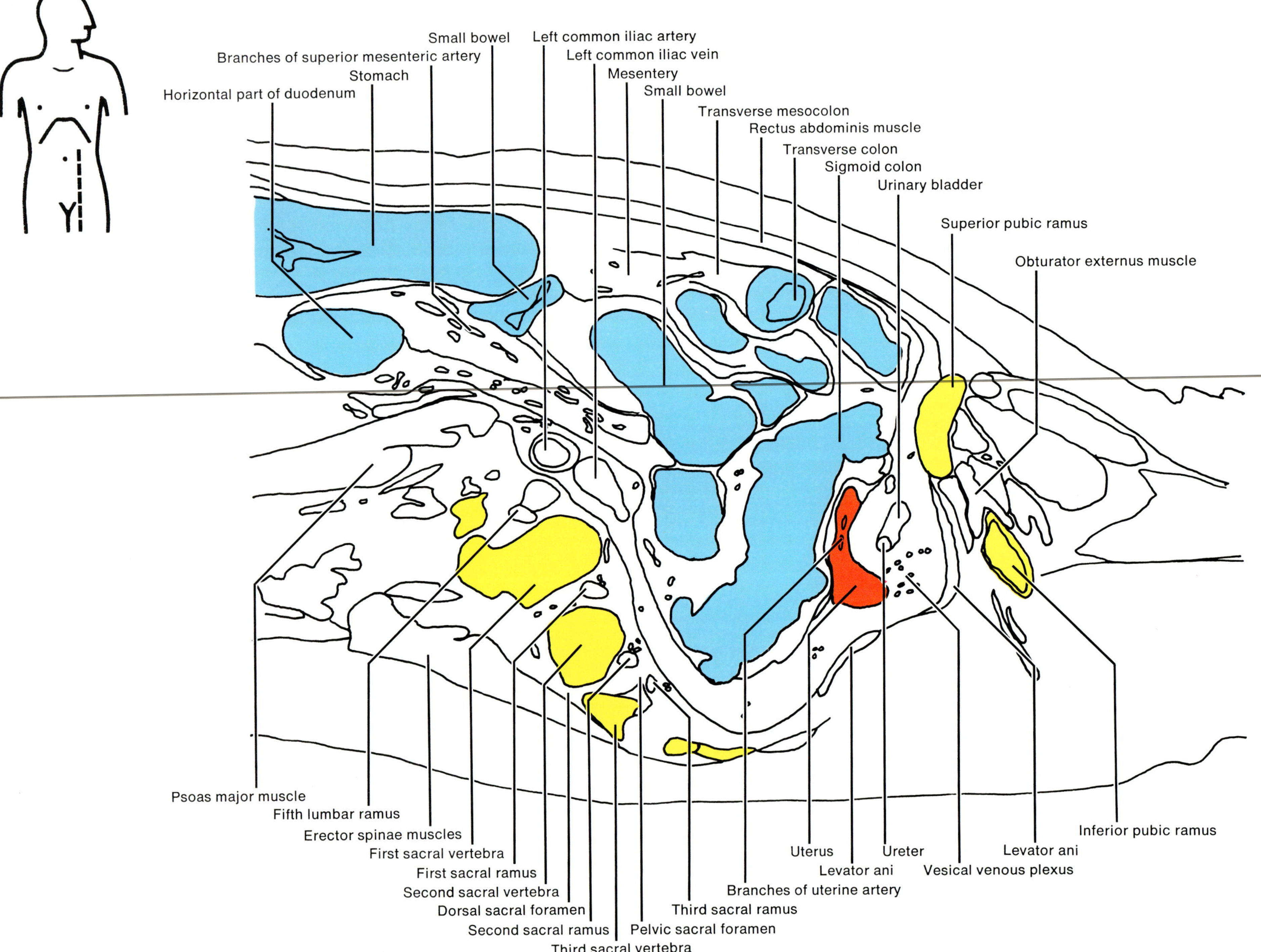

Horizontal part of duodenum
Branches of superior mesenteric artery
Stomach
Small bowel
Left common iliac artery
Left common iliac vein
Mesentery
Small bowel
Transverse mesocolon
Rectus abdominis muscle
Transverse colon
Sigmoid colon
Urinary bladder
Superior pubic ramus
Obturator externus muscle
Psoas major muscle
Fifth lumbar ramus
Erector spinae muscles
First sacral vertebra
First sacral ramus
Second sacral vertebra
Dorsal sacral foramen
Second sacral ramus
Third sacral vertebra
Pelvic sacral foramen
Third sacral ramus
Branches of uterine artery
Uterus
Levator ani
Ureter
Vesical venous plexus
Levator ani
Inferior pubic ramus

PARASAGITTAL **Pelvis—female**

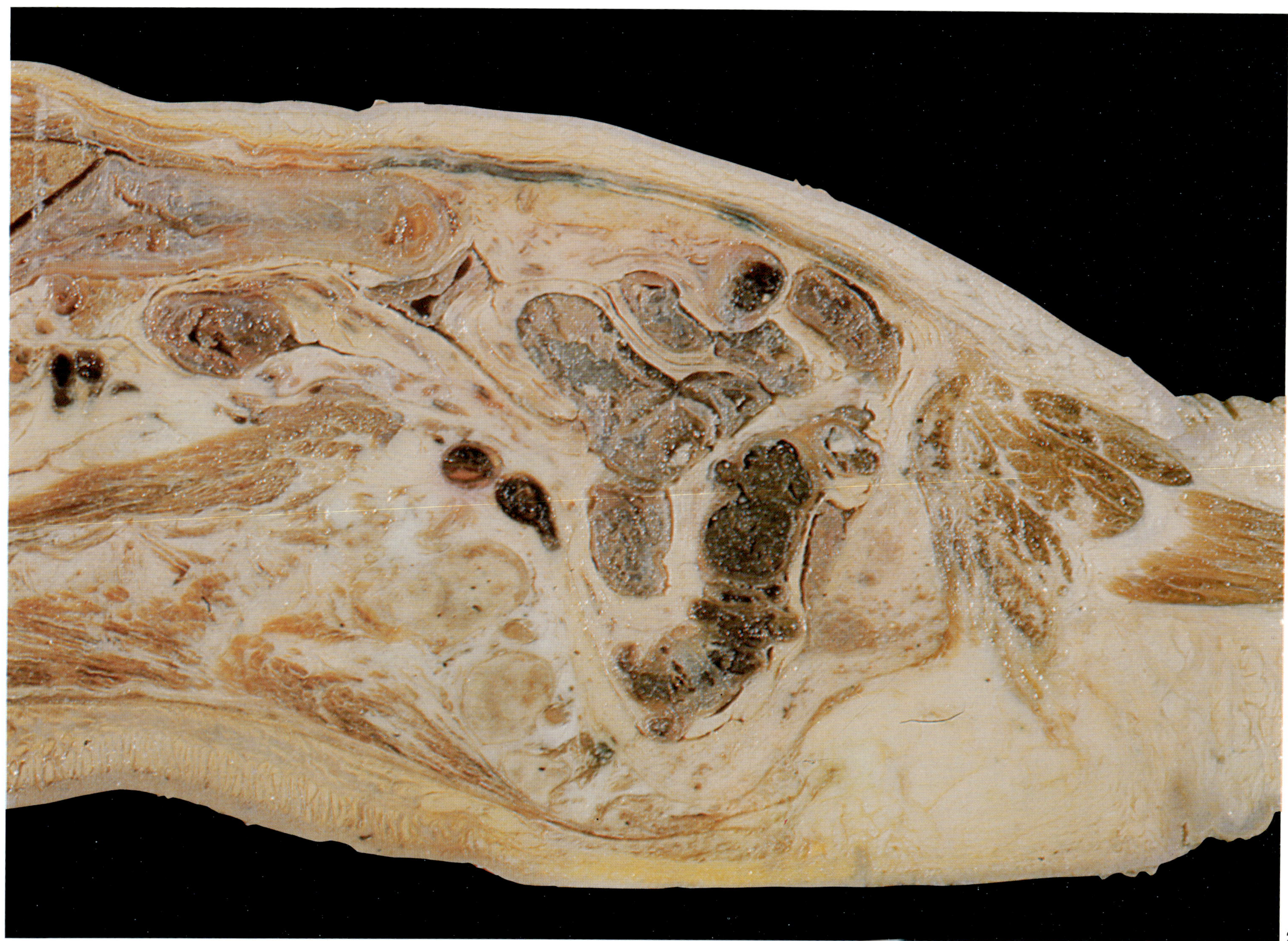

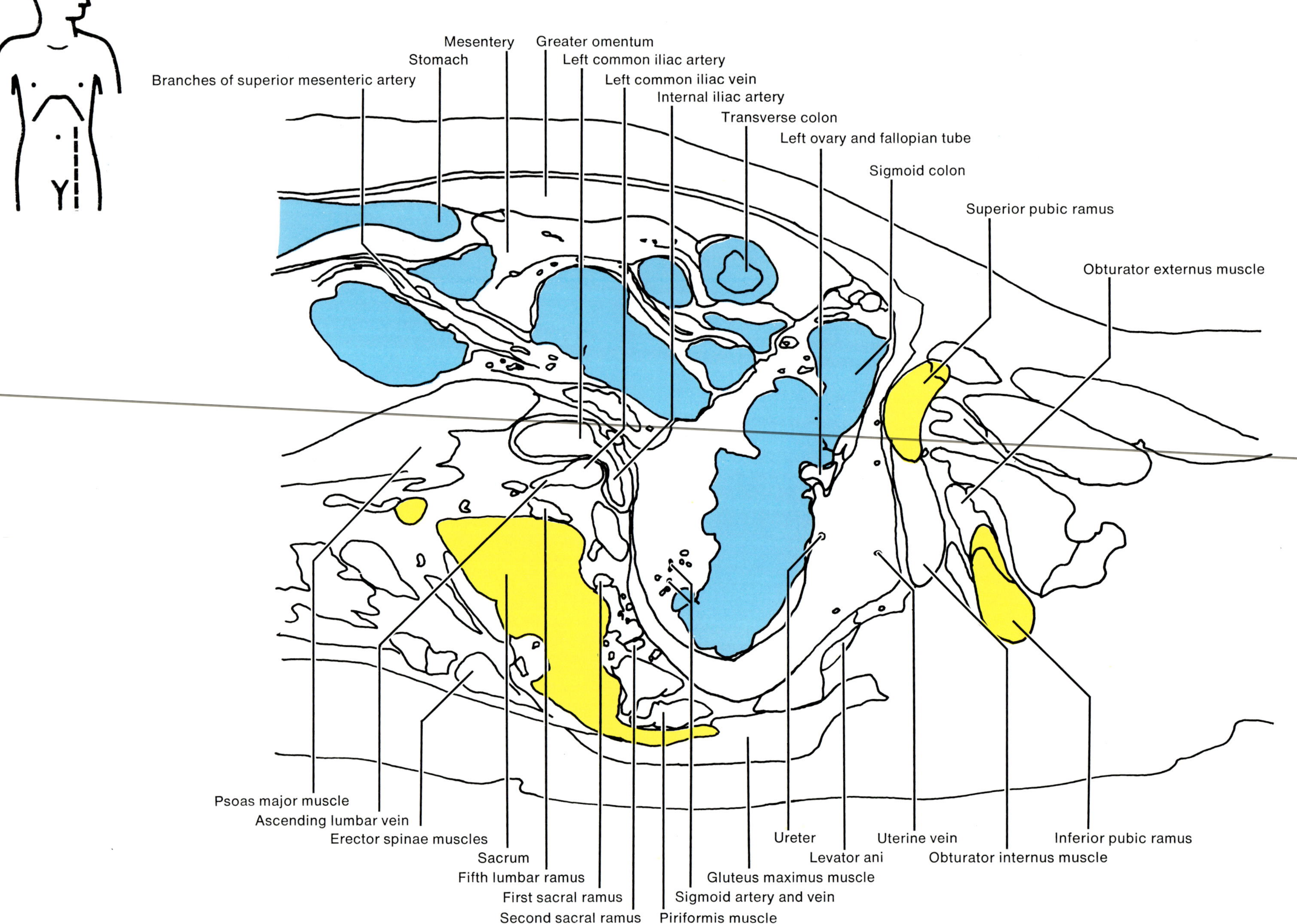
Mesentery
Stomach
Greater omentum
Branches of superior mesenteric artery
Left common iliac artery
Left common iliac vein
Internal iliac artery
Transverse colon
Left ovary and fallopian tube
Sigmoid colon
Superior pubic ramus
Obturator externus muscle
Psoas major muscle
Ascending lumbar vein
Erector spinae muscles
Sacrum
Fifth lumbar ramus
First sacral ramus
Second sacral ramus
Piriformis muscle
Sigmoid artery and vein
Gluteus maximus muscle
Ureter
Levator ani
Uterine vein
Obturator internus muscle
Inferior pubic ramus

PARASAGITTAL **Pelvis—female**

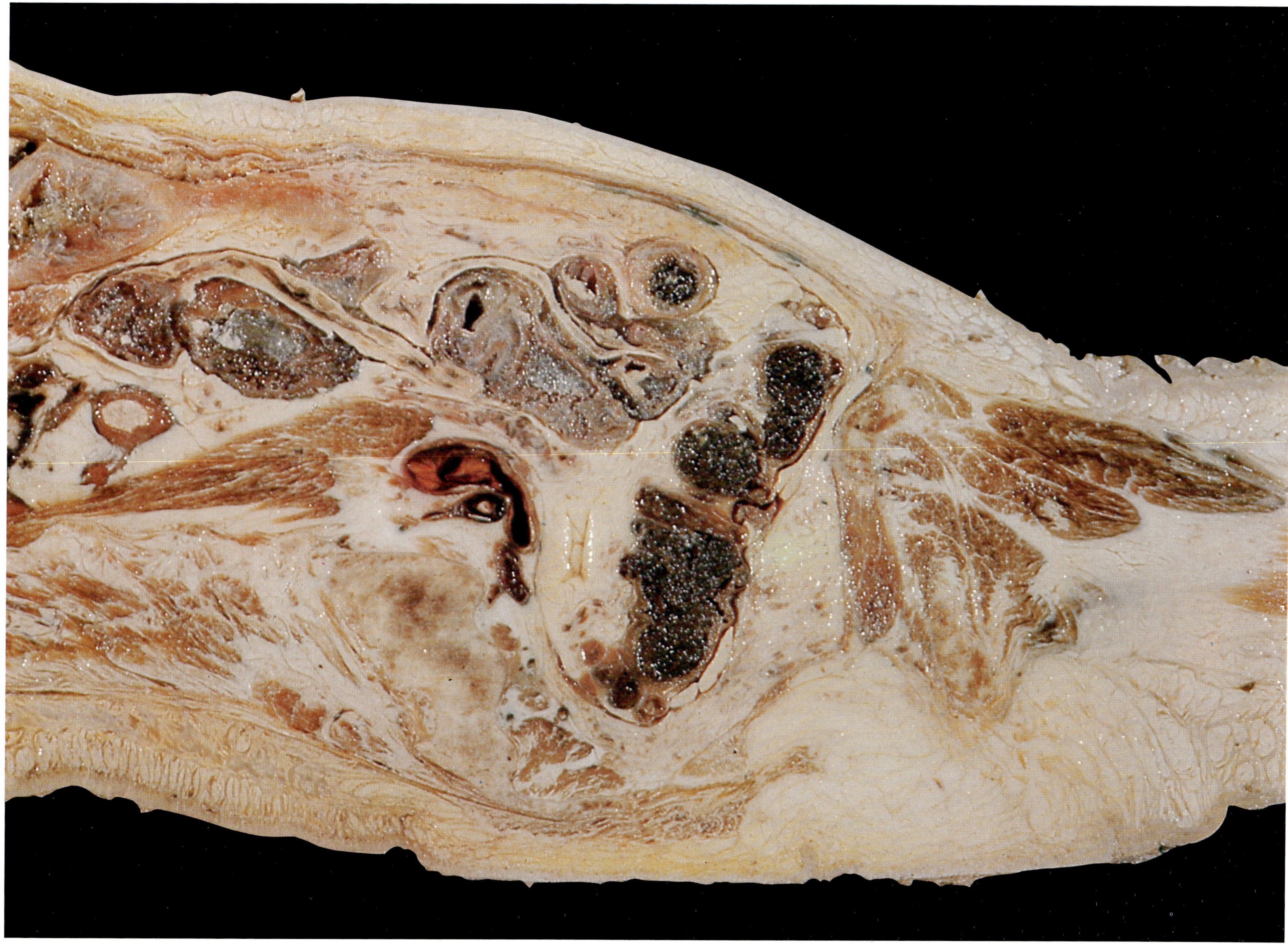

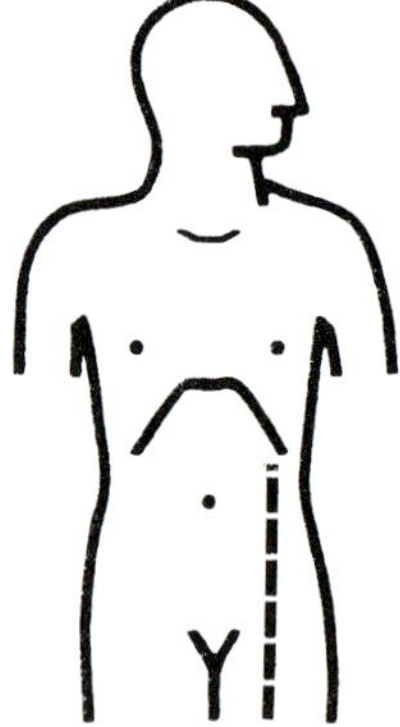

Left kidney
Transverse colon
Small bowel
Psoas major muscle
External iliac artery
Sacral plexus
Sigmoid colon
External iliac vein
Obturator externus muscle
Profunda femoris artery
Fat
Ilium
Interosseous sacroiliac ligament
Sacrum
Sacroiliac joint
Superior gluteal artery and vein
Sacral plexus
Branches of inferior gluteal artery and vein
Piriformis muscle
Gluteus maximus muscle
Inferior gluteal artery and vein
Internal pudendal vein
Ligament of head of femur
Obturator internus muscle
Ischium

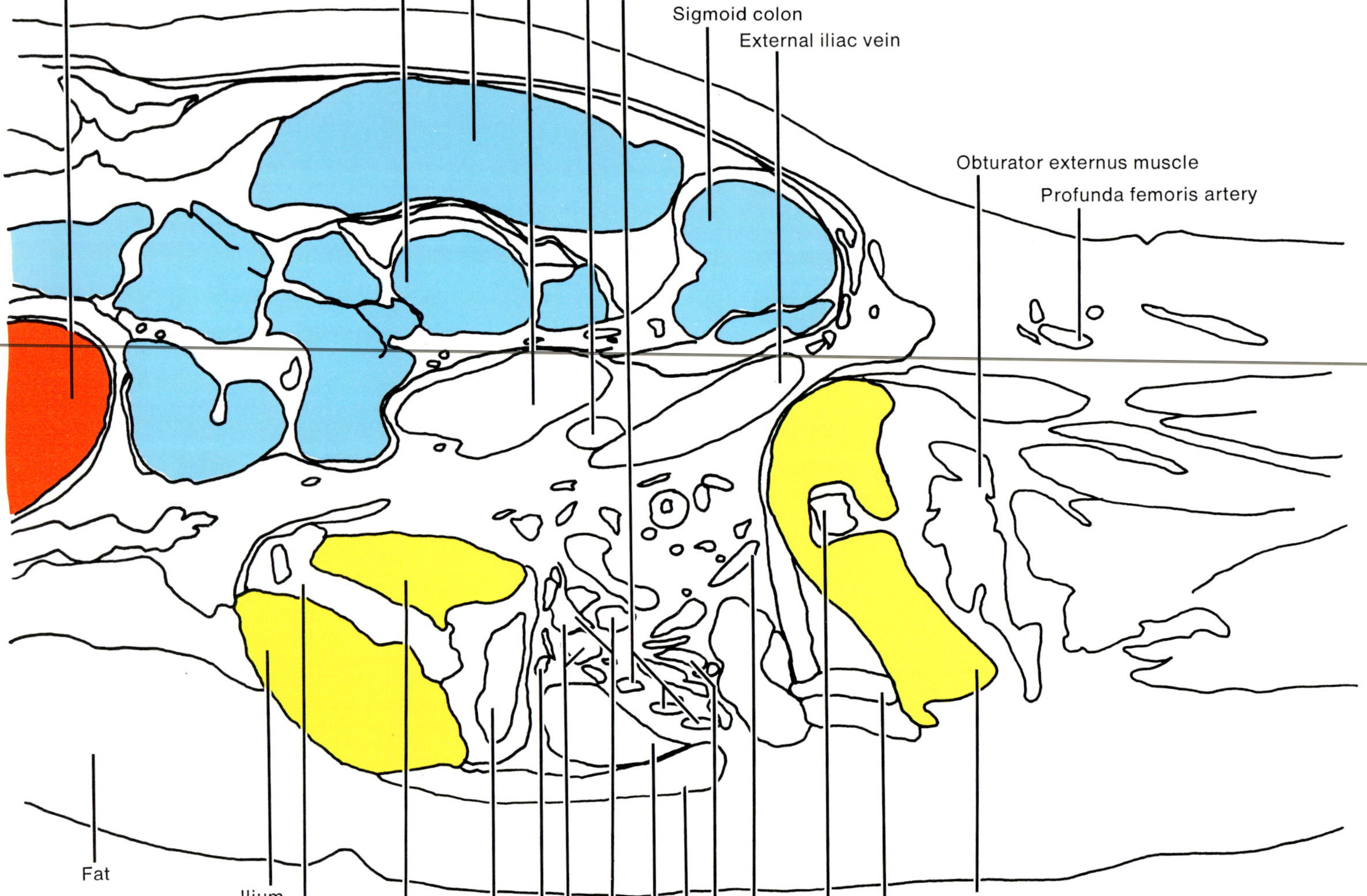

PARASAGITTAL **Pelvis—female**

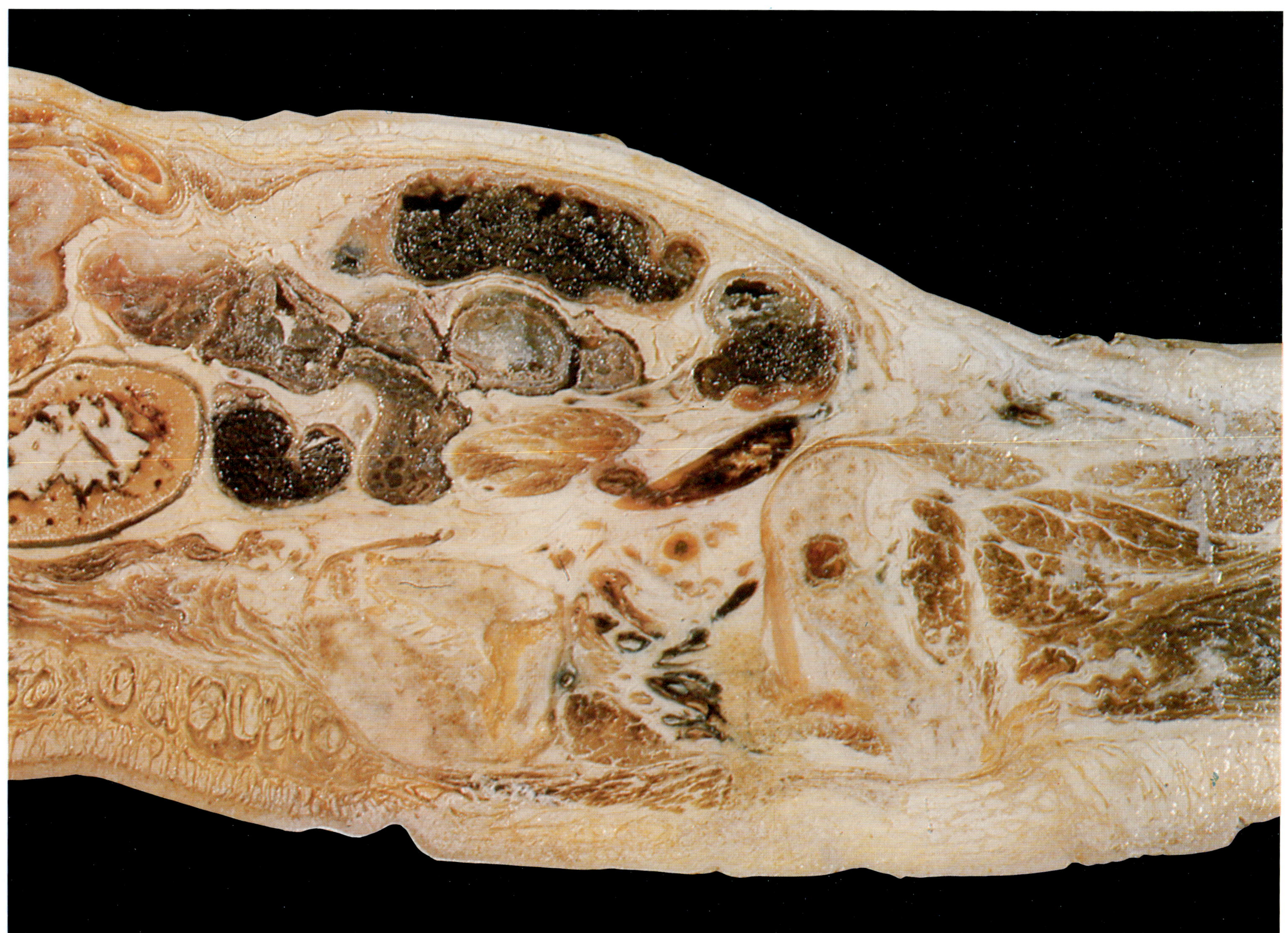

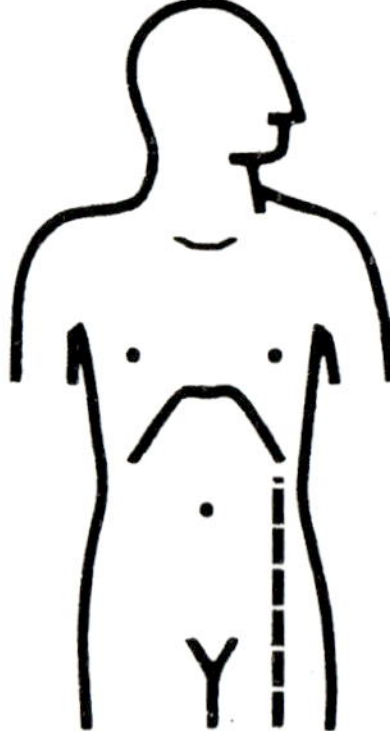

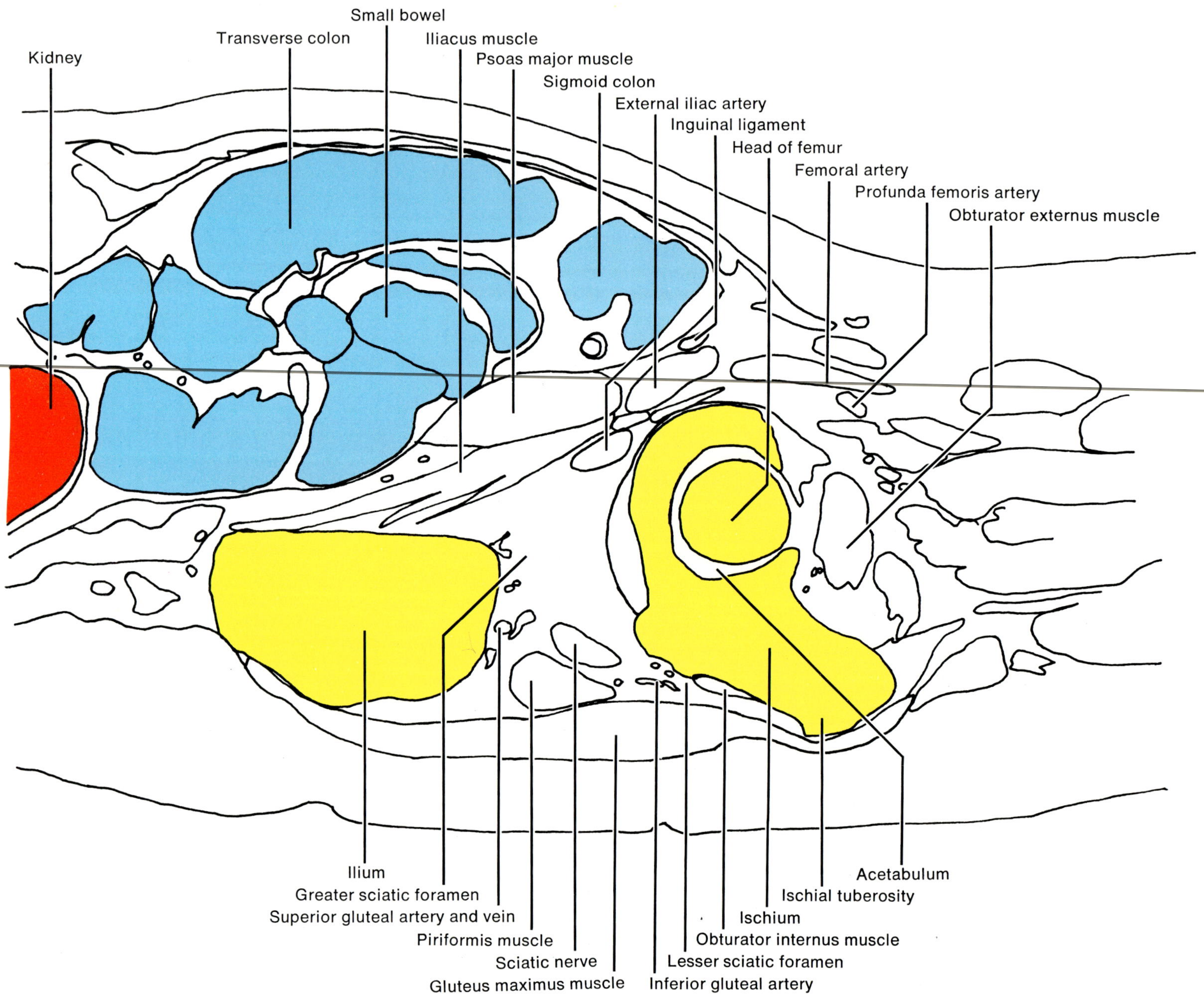

Kidney
Transverse colon
Small bowel
Iliacus muscle
Psoas major muscle
Sigmoid colon
External iliac artery
Inguinal ligament
Head of femur
Femoral artery
Profunda femoris artery
Obturator externus muscle
Ilium
Greater sciatic foramen
Superior gluteal artery and vein
Piriformis muscle
Sciatic nerve
Gluteus maximus muscle
Acetabulum
Ischial tuberosity
Ischium
Obturator internus muscle
Lesser sciatic foramen
Inferior gluteal artery

PARASAGITTAL **Pelvis—female**

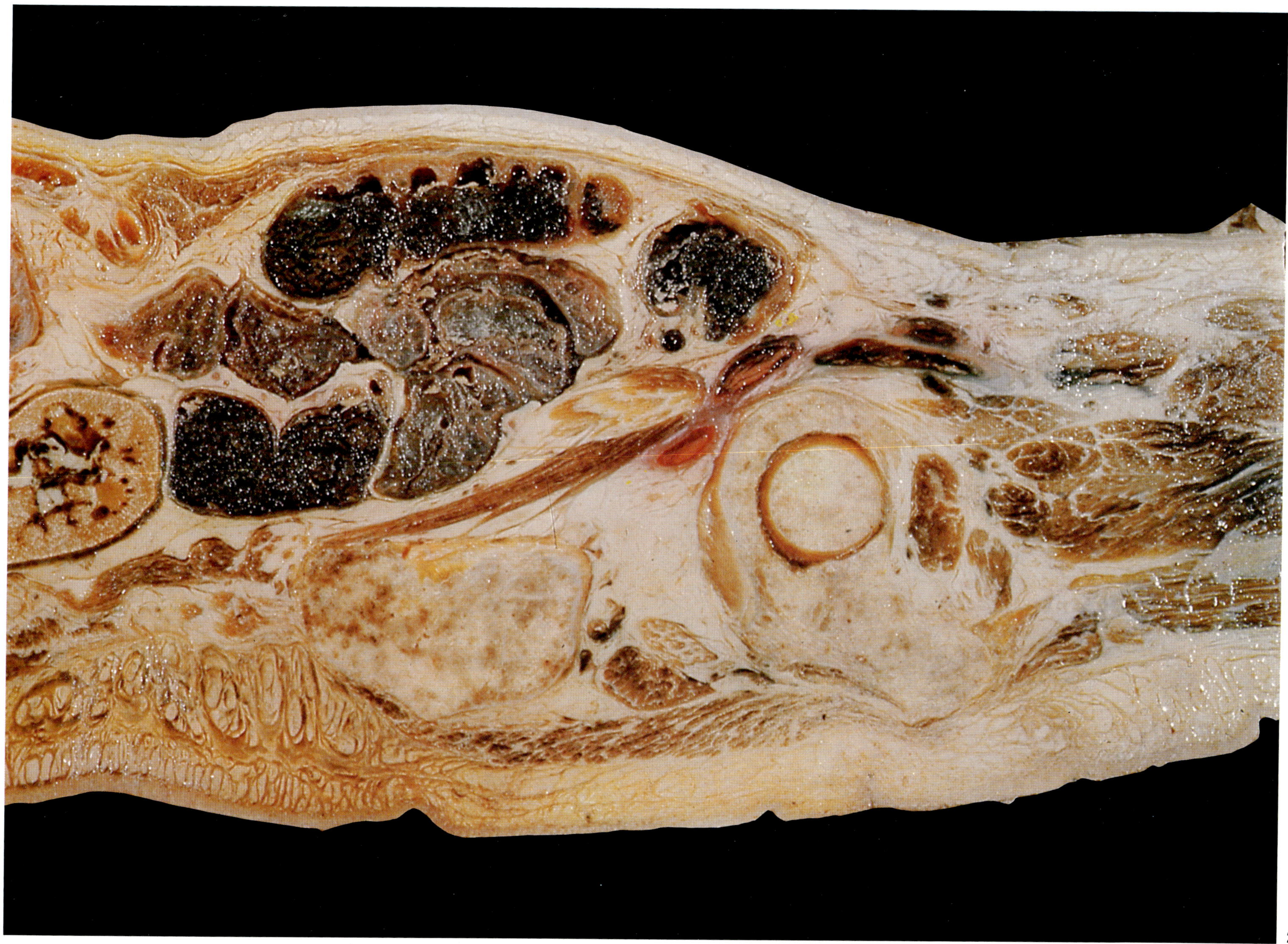

Abdominal aortic aneurysm

PLATES 120-121

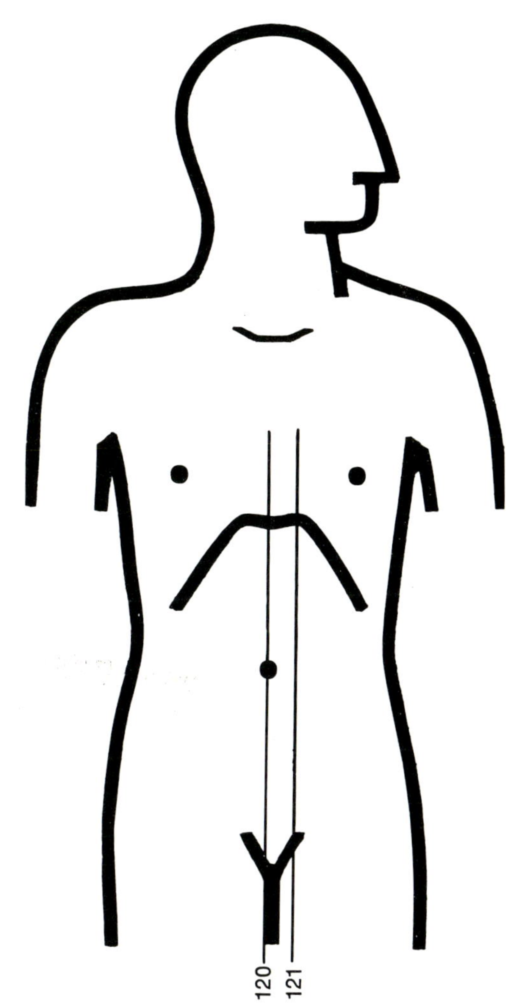

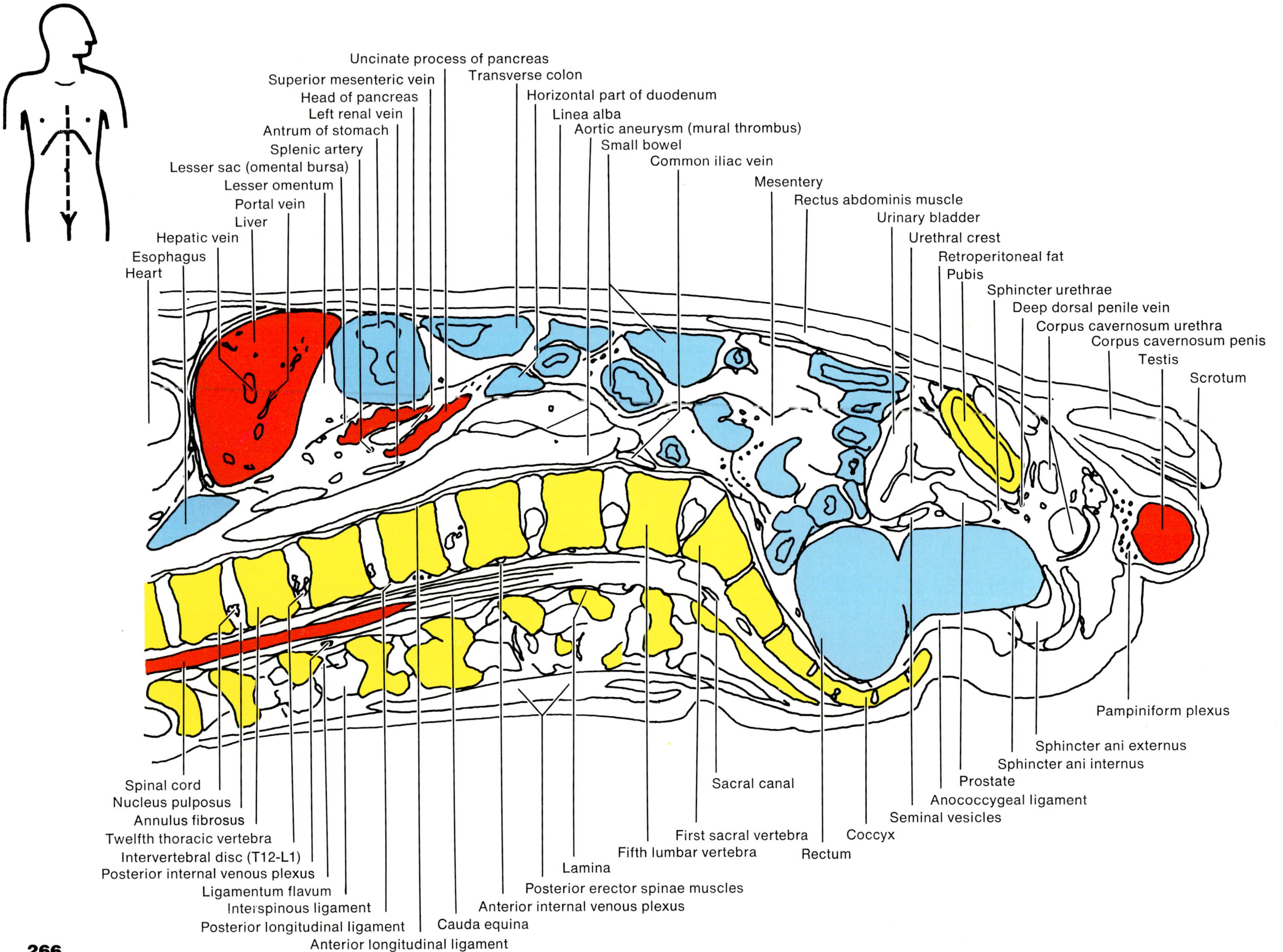

Uncinate process of pancreas
Superior mesenteric vein
Head of pancreas
Left renal vein
Antrum of stomach
Splenic artery
Lesser sac (omental bursa)
Lesser omentum
Portal vein
Liver
Hepatic vein
Esophagus
Heart
Transverse colon
Horizontal part of duodenum
Linea alba
Aortic aneurysm (mural thrombus)
Small bowel
Common iliac vein
Mesentery
Rectus abdominis muscle
Urinary bladder
Urethral crest
Retroperitoneal fat
Pubis
Sphincter urethrae
Deep dorsal penile vein
Corpus cavernosum urethra
Corpus cavernosum penis
Testis
Scrotum
Pampiniform plexus
Sphincter ani externus
Sphincter ani internus
Prostate
Anococcygeal ligament
Seminal vesicles
Coccyx
Rectum
First sacral vertebra
Fifth lumbar vertebra
Sacral canal
Lamina
Posterior erector spinae muscles
Anterior internal venous plexus
Cauda equina
Anterior longitudinal ligament
Posterior longitudinal ligament
Interspinous ligament
Ligamentum flavum
Posterior internal venous plexus
Intervertebral disc (T12-L1)
Twelfth thoracic vertebra
Annulus fibrosus
Nucleus pulposus
Spinal cord

PARASAGITTAL **Abdominal aortic aneurysm**

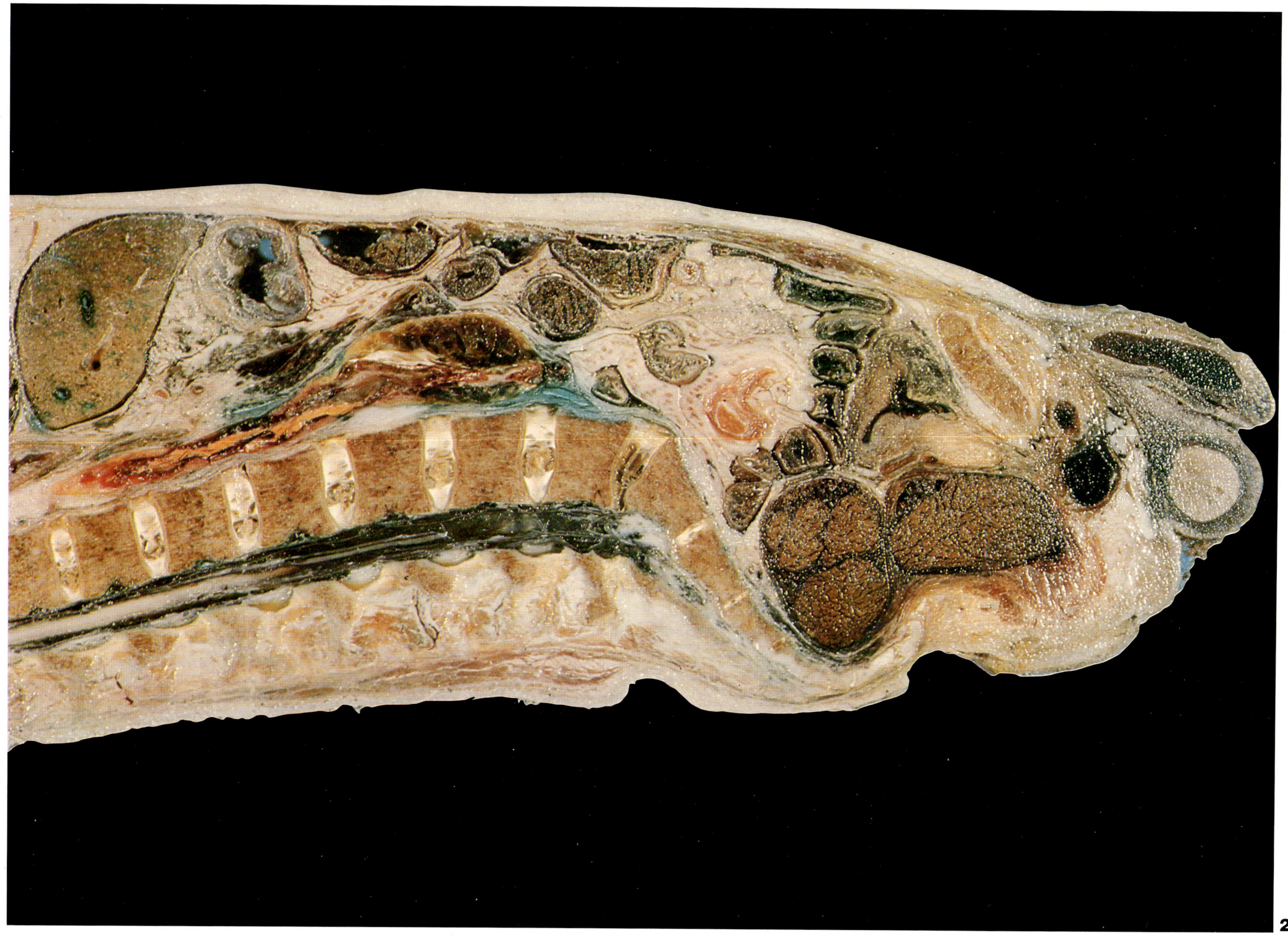

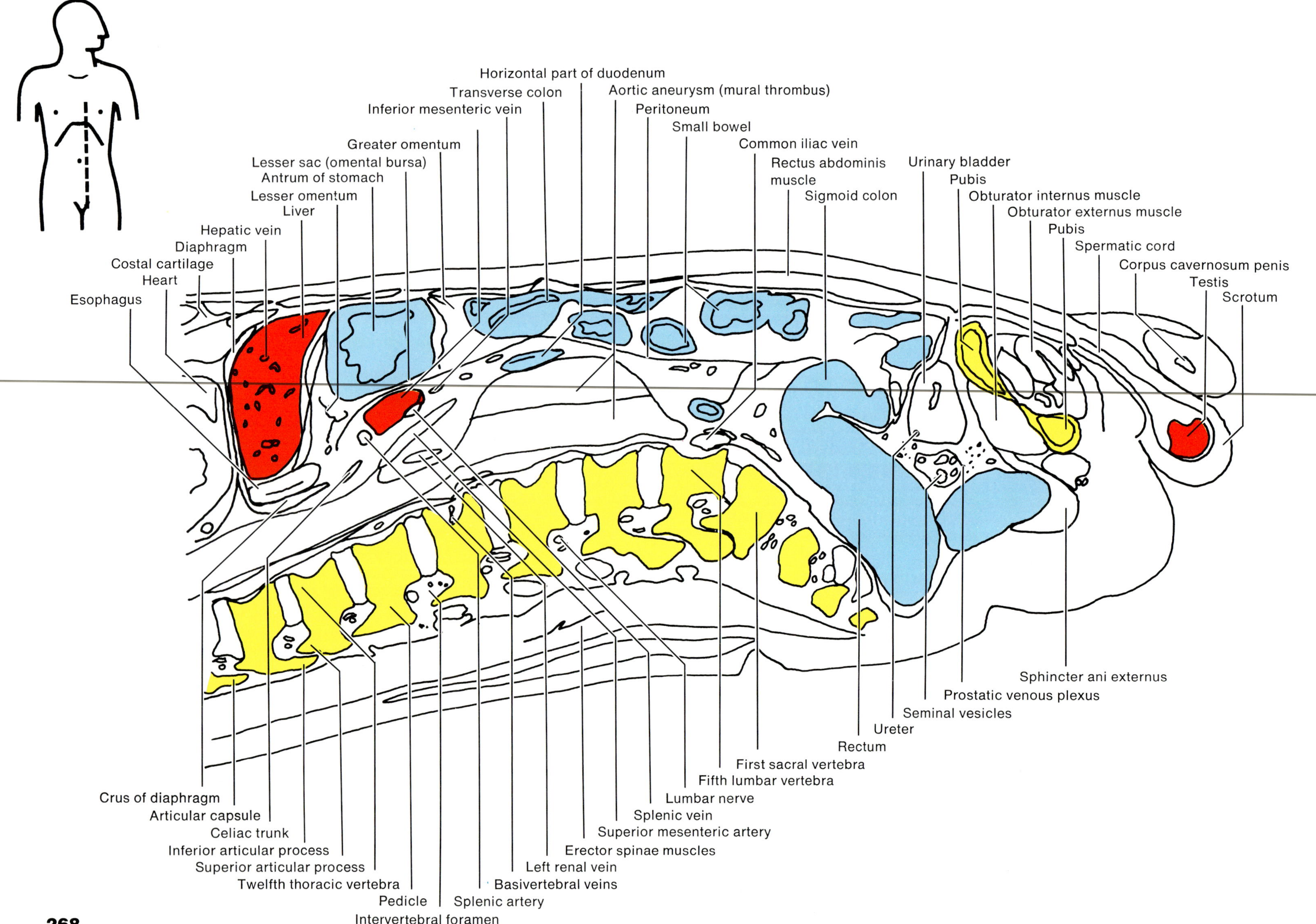

Horizontal part of duodenum
Transverse colon
Inferior mesenteric vein
Aortic aneurysm (mural thrombus)
Peritoneum
Small bowel
Greater omentum
Common iliac vein
Lesser sac (omental bursa)
Rectus abdominis muscle
Urinary bladder
Antrum of stomach
Pubis
Lesser omentum
Sigmoid colon
Obturator internus muscle
Liver
Obturator externus muscle
Hepatic vein
Pubis
Diaphragm
Spermatic cord
Costal cartilage
Corpus cavernosum penis
Heart
Testis
Esophagus
Scrotum
Sphincter ani externus
Prostatic venous plexus
Seminal vesicles
Ureter
Rectum
First sacral vertebra
Fifth lumbar vertebra
Lumbar nerve
Splenic vein
Superior mesenteric artery
Erector spinae muscles
Left renal vein
Basivertebral veins
Splenic artery
Pedicle
Intervertebral foramen
Twelfth thoracic vertebra
Superior articular process
Inferior articular process
Celiac trunk
Articular capsule
Crus of diaphragm

PARASAGITTAL **Abdominal aortic aneurysm**

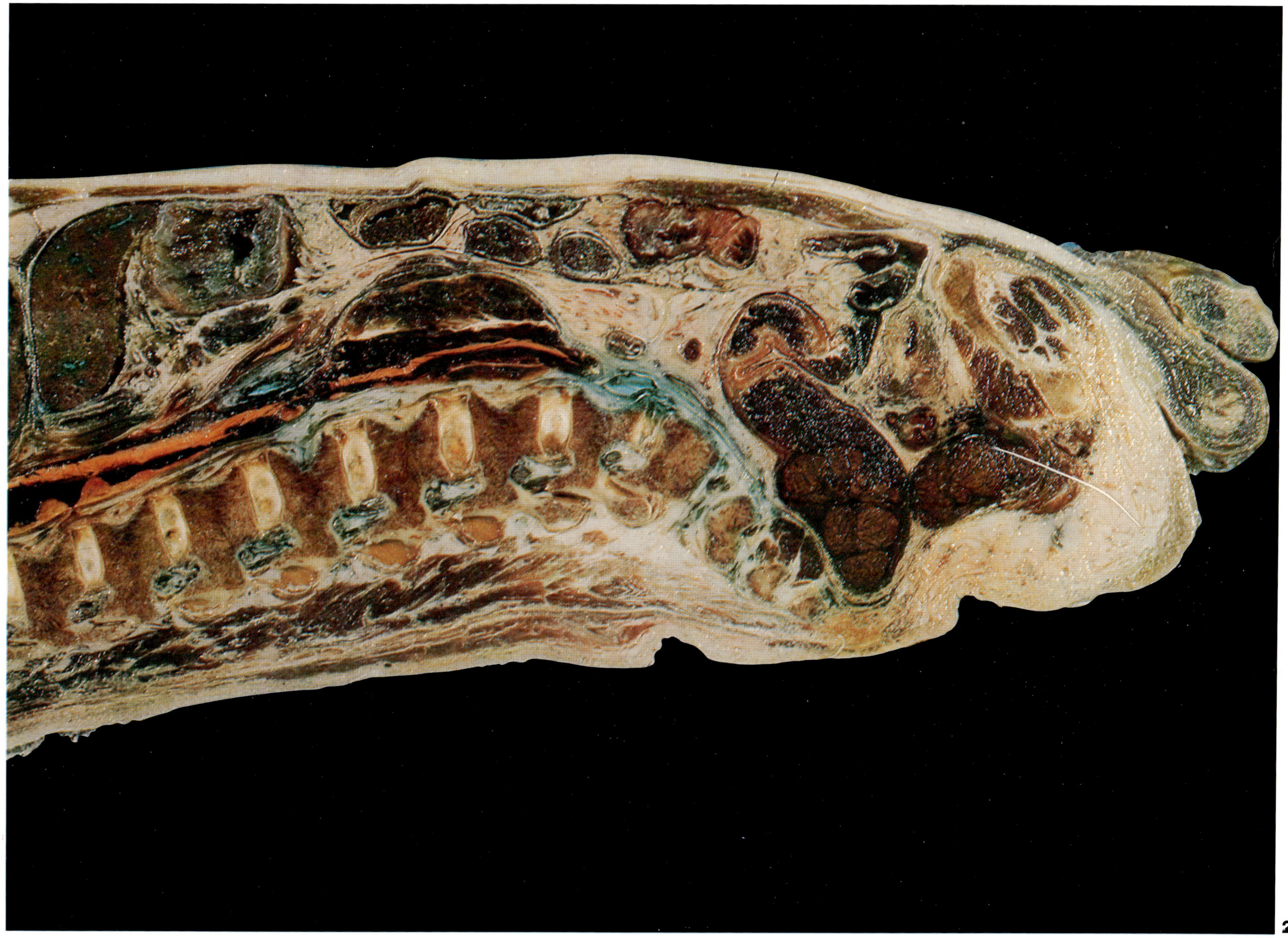

PART THREE

Coronal sections

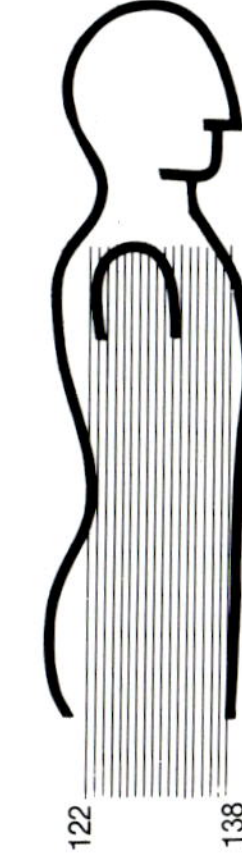

**Chest,
abdomen,
and pelvis**
PLATES 122-138

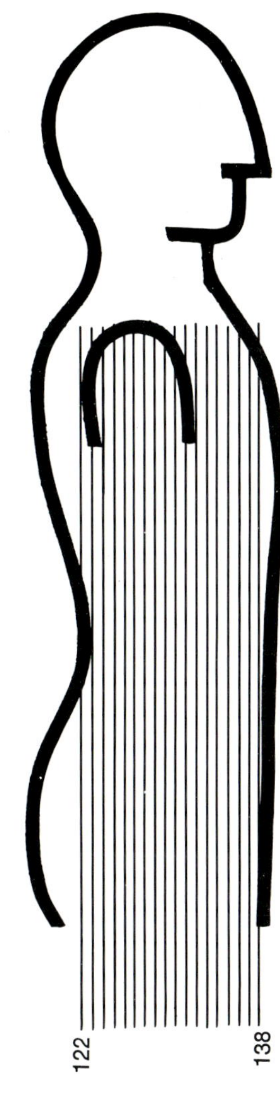

122
138

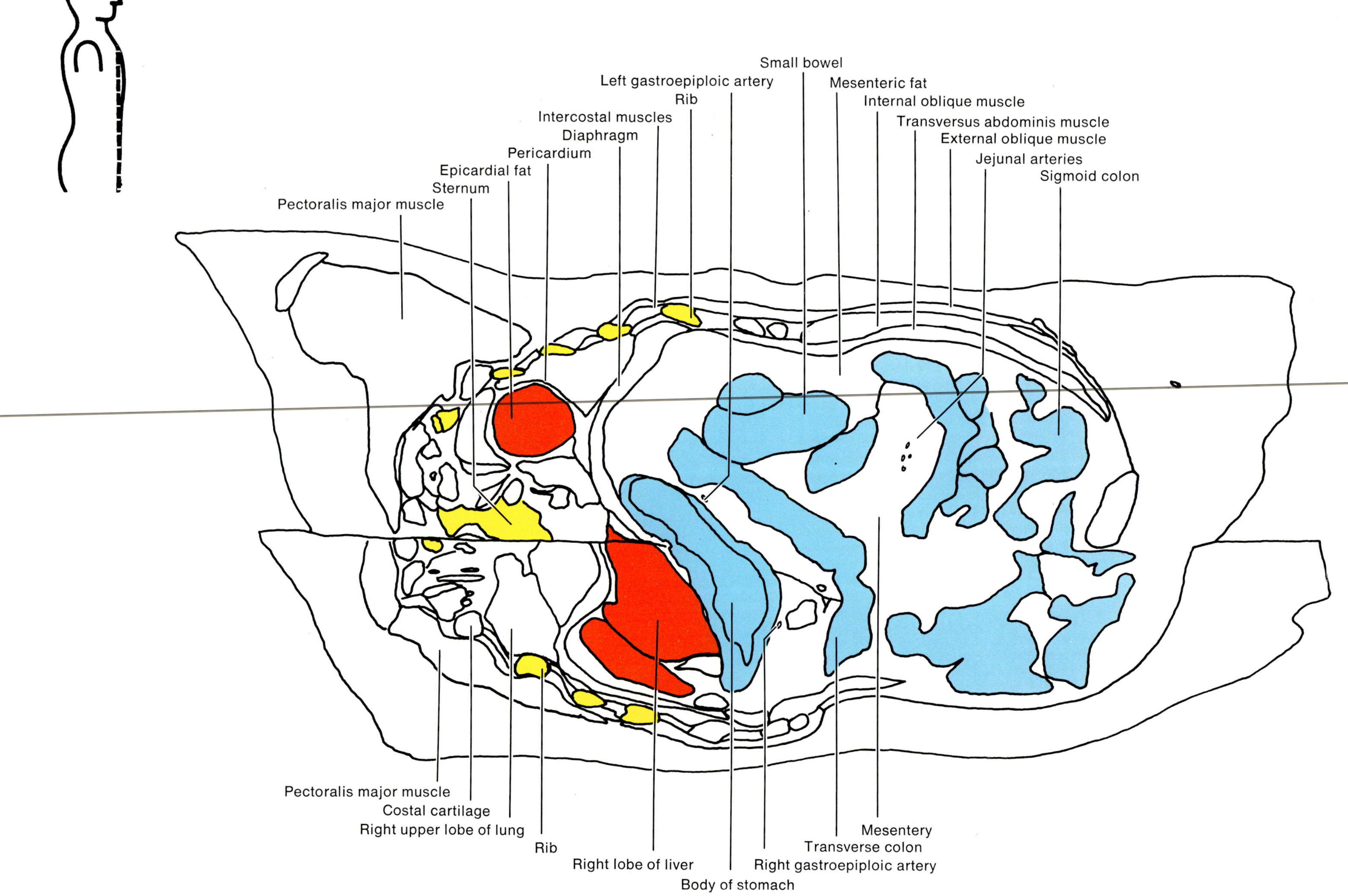

Small bowel
Left gastroepiploic artery
Mesenteric fat
Rib
Internal oblique muscle
Intercostal muscles
Transversus abdominis muscle
Diaphragm
External oblique muscle
Pericardium
Jejunal arteries
Epicardial fat
Sigmoid colon
Sternum
Pectoralis major muscle
Pectoralis major muscle
Costal cartilage
Mesentery
Right upper lobe of lung
Transverse colon
Rib
Right gastroepiploic artery
Right lobe of liver
Body of stomach

CORONAL **Chest, abdomen, and pelvis**

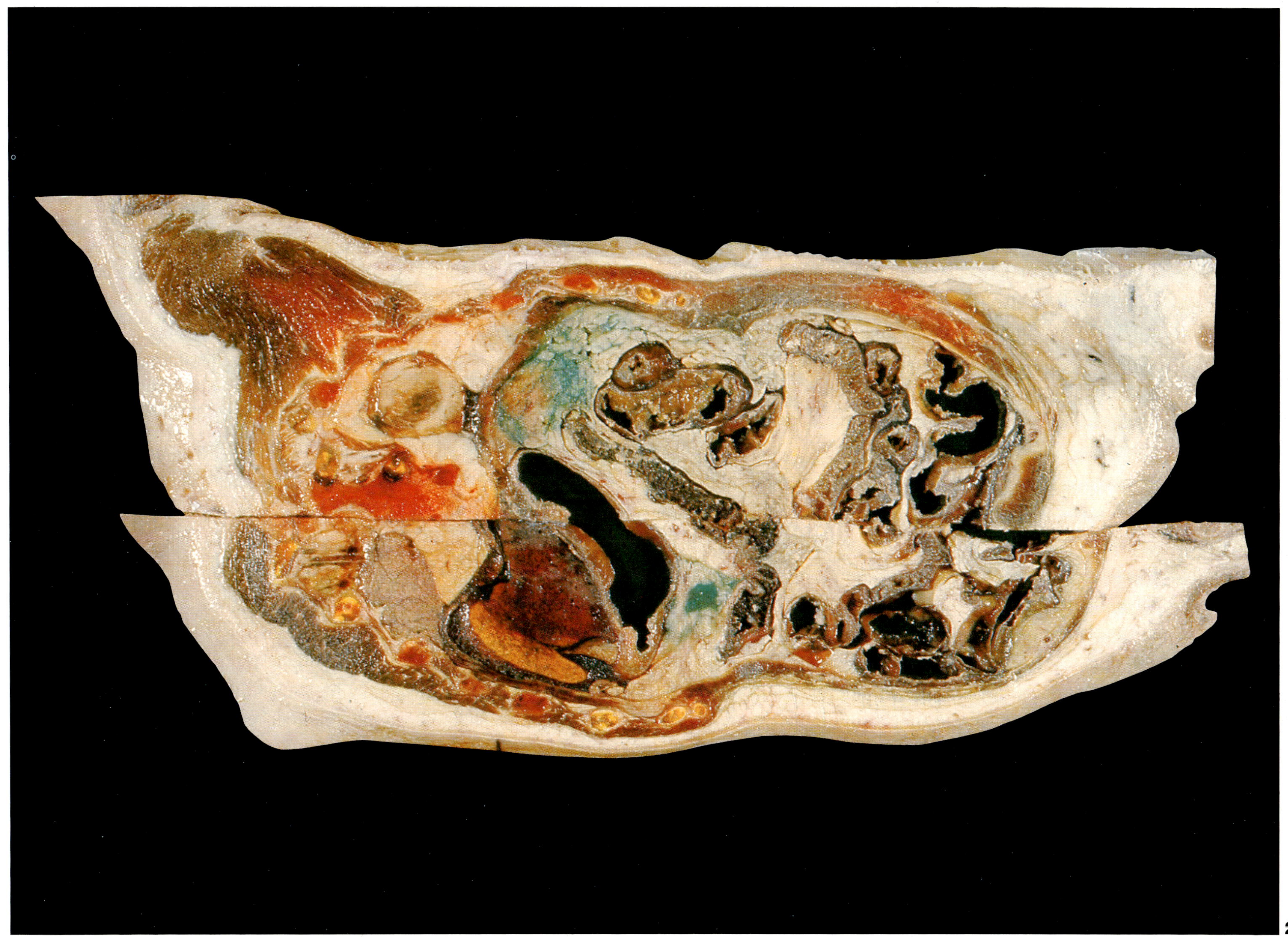

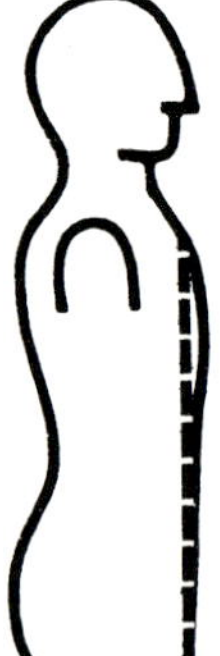

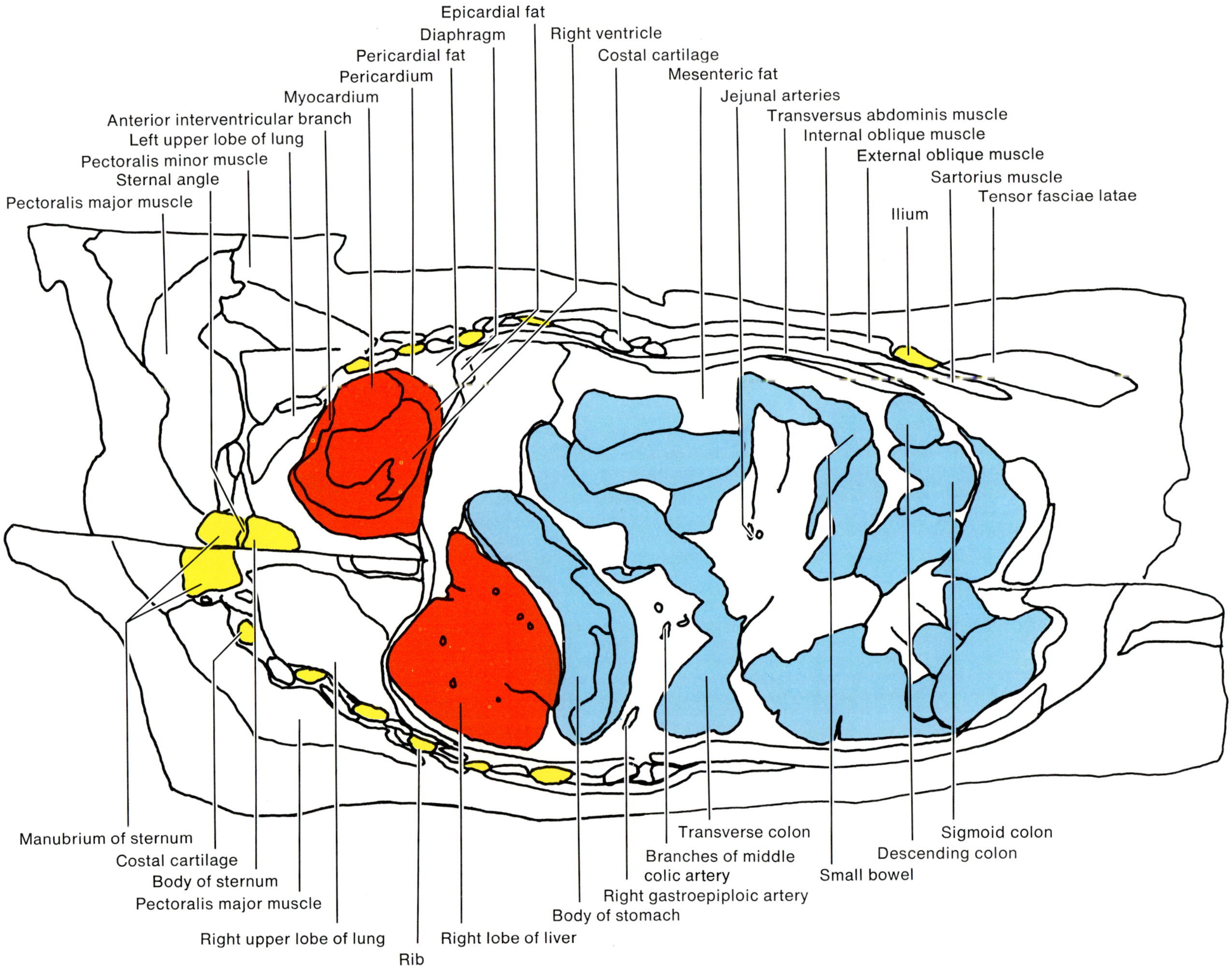

Epicardial fat
Diaphragm
Right ventricle
Pericardial fat
Costal cartilage
Pericardium
Mesenteric fat
Myocardium
Jejunal arteries
Anterior interventricular branch
Transversus abdominis muscle
Left upper lobe of lung
Internal oblique muscle
Pectoralis minor muscle
External oblique muscle
Sternal angle
Sartorius muscle
Tensor fasciae latae
Pectoralis major muscle
Ilium
Manubrium of sternum
Transverse colon
Sigmoid colon
Costal cartilage
Branches of middle
colic artery
Descending colon
Body of sternum
Small bowel
Pectoralis major muscle
Right gastroepiploic artery
Right upper lobe of lung
Body of stomach
Right lobe of liver
Rib

CORONAL **Chest, abdomen, and pelvis**

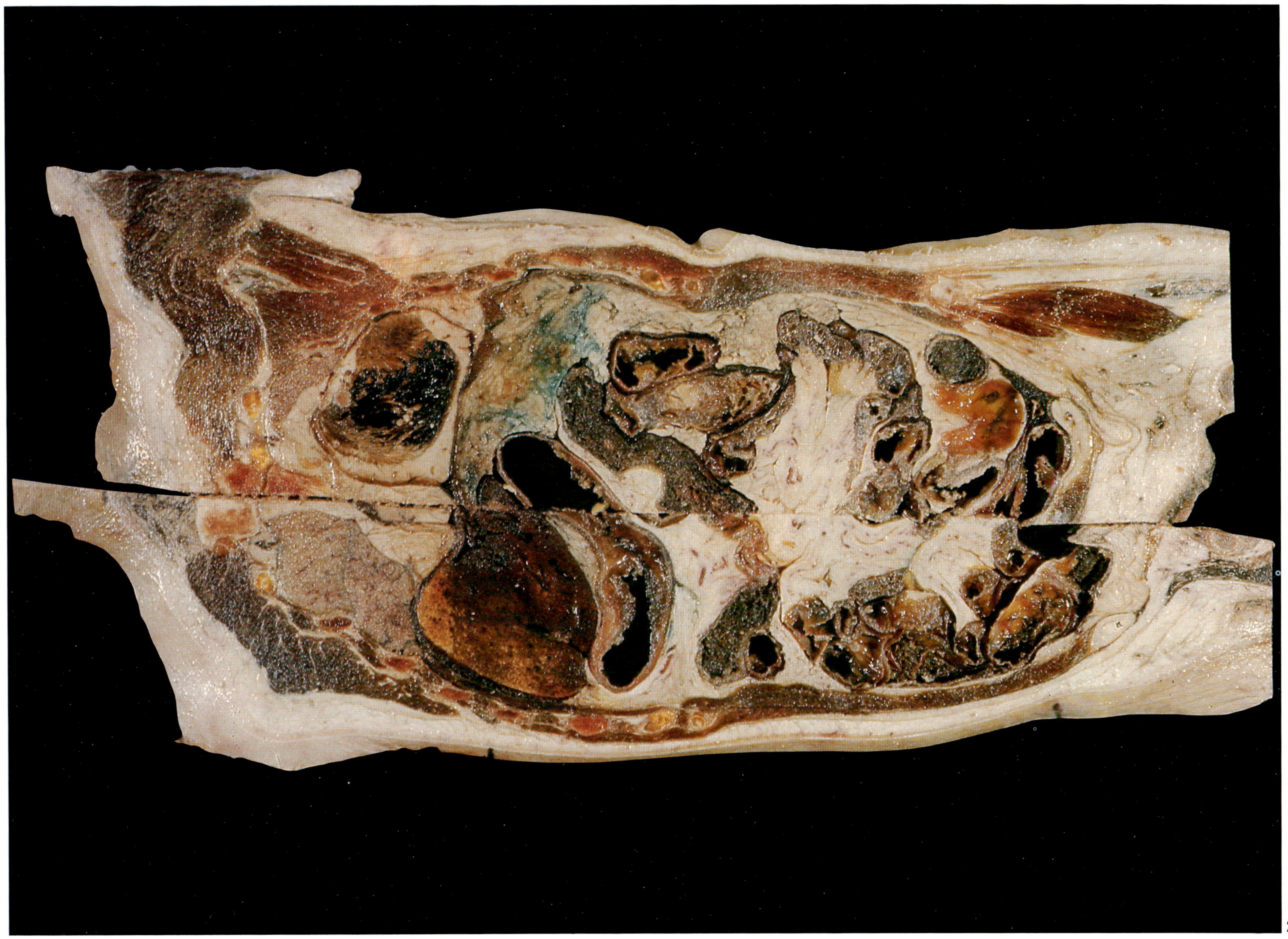

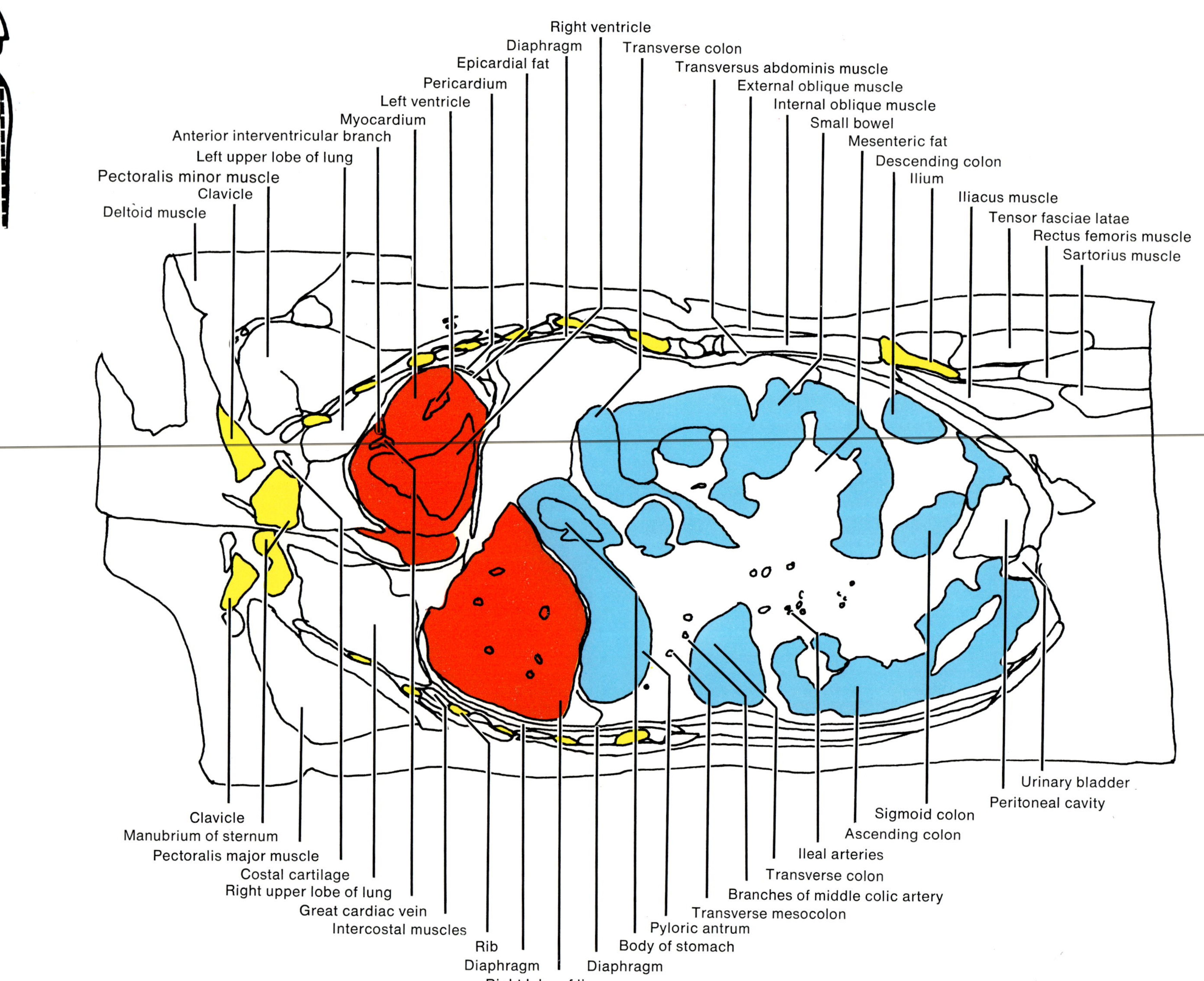

Right ventricle
Diaphragm
Epicardial fat
Pericardium
Left ventricle
Myocardium
Anterior interventricular branch
Left upper lobe of lung
Pectoralis minor muscle
Clavicle
Deltoid muscle
Transverse colon
Transversus abdominis muscle
External oblique muscle
Internal oblique muscle
Small bowel
Mesenteric fat
Descending colon
Ilium
Iliacus muscle
Tensor fasciae latae
Rectus femoris muscle
Sartorius muscle
Clavicle
Manubrium of sternum
Pectoralis major muscle
Costal cartilage
Right upper lobe of lung
Great cardiac vein
Intercostal muscles
Rib
Diaphragm
Right lobe of liver
Diaphragm
Body of stomach
Pyloric antrum
Transverse mesocolon
Transverse colon
Branches of middle colic artery
Ileal arteries
Ascending colon
Sigmoid colon
Urinary bladder
Peritoneal cavity

CORONAL **Chest, abdomen, and pelvis**

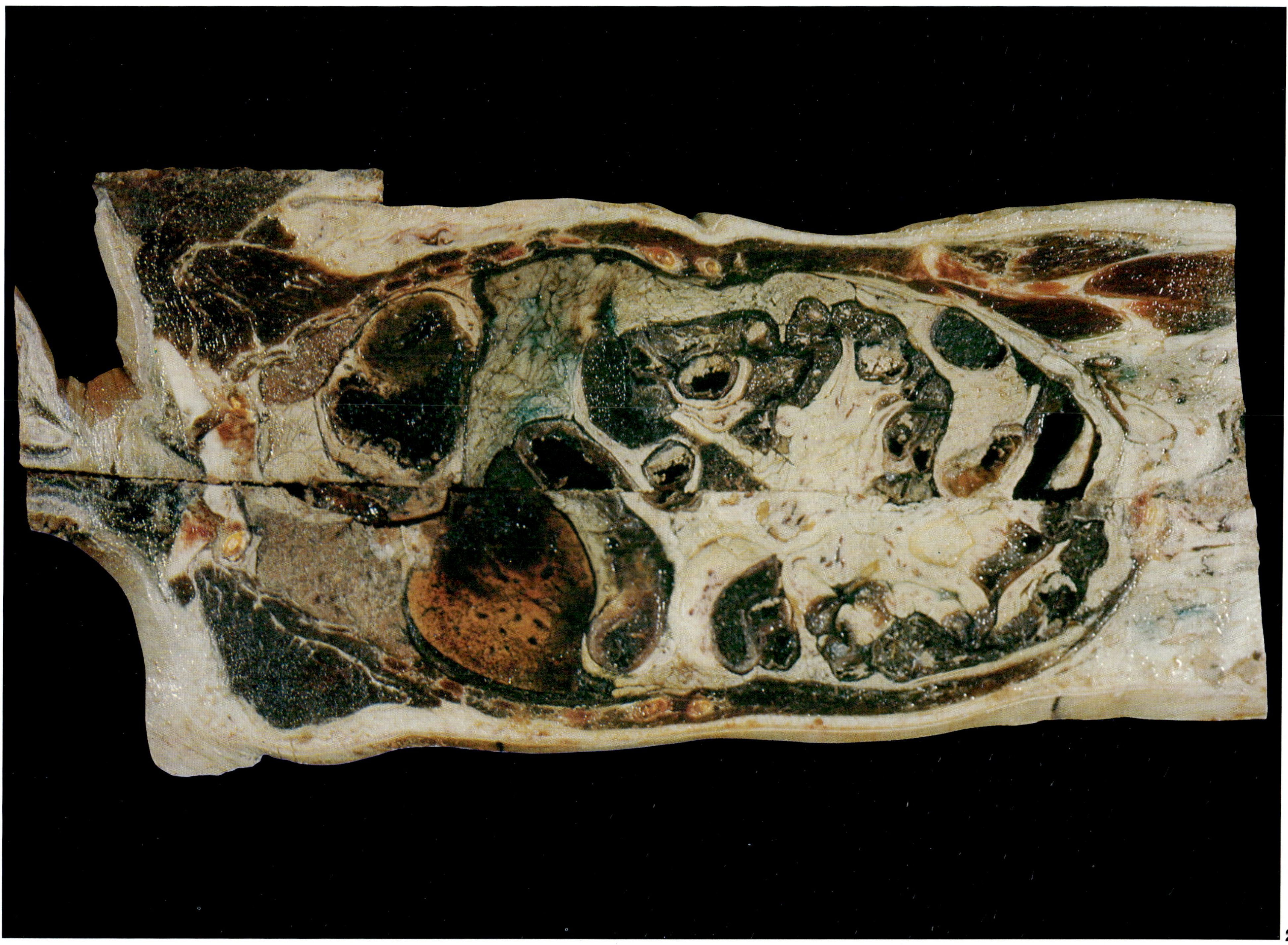

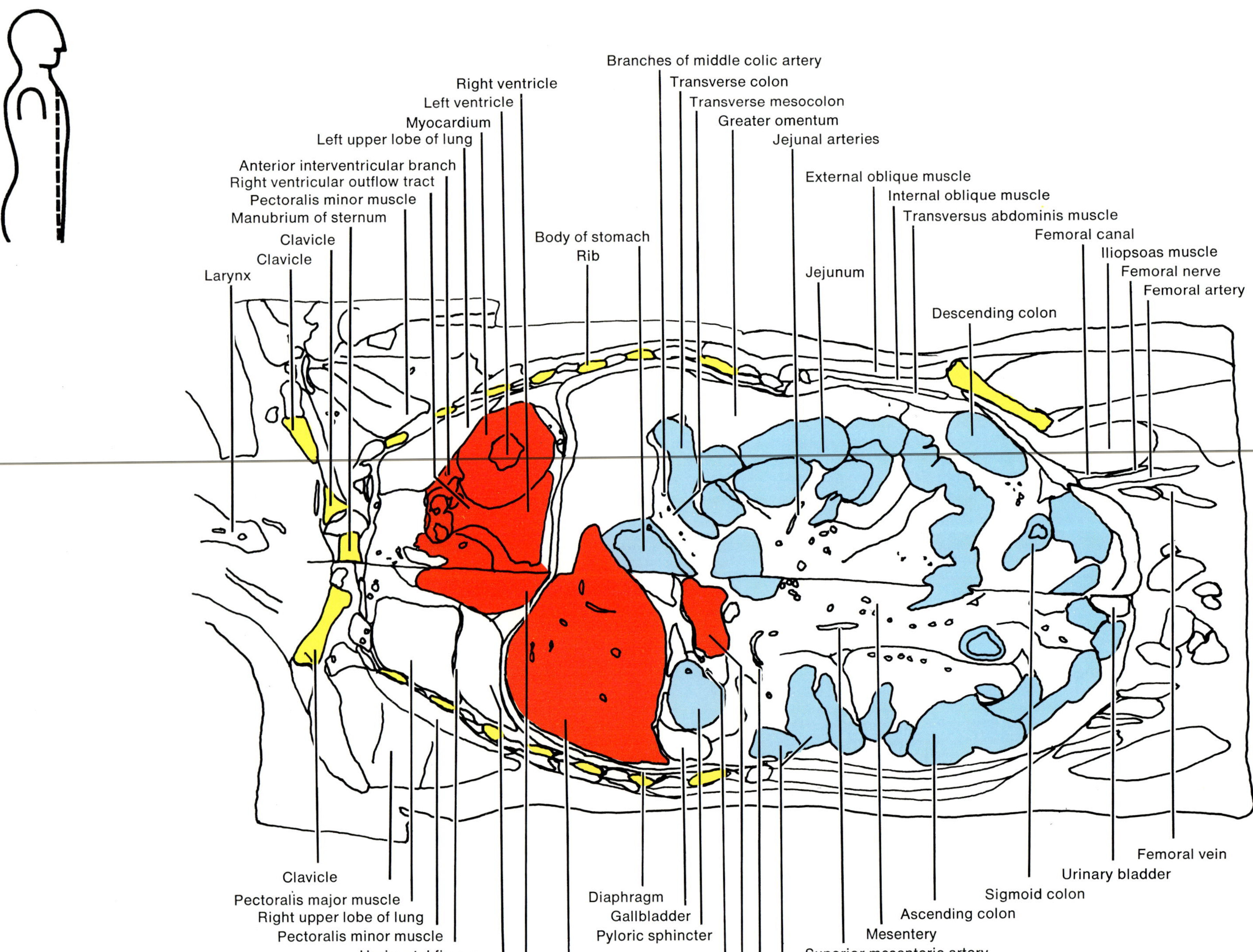

Larynx
Clavicle
Clavicle
Manubrium of sternum
Pectoralis minor muscle
Right ventricular outflow tract
Anterior interventricular branch
Left upper lobe of lung
Myocardium
Left ventricle
Right ventricle
Body of stomach
Rib
Branches of middle colic artery
Transverse colon
Transverse mesocolon
Greater omentum
Jejunal arteries
External oblique muscle
Internal oblique muscle
Transversus abdominis muscle
Femoral canal
Iliopsoas muscle
Femoral nerve
Femoral artery
Jejunum
Descending colon
Clavicle
Pectoralis major muscle
Right upper lobe of lung
Pectoralis minor muscle
Horizontal fissure
Right middle lobe of lung
Right atrium
Right lobe of liver
Diaphragm
Gallbladder
Pyloric sphincter
Right gastroepiploic artery
Head of pancreas
Middle colic artery
Transverse colon
Superior mesenteric artery
Mesentery
Ascending colon
Sigmoid colon
Urinary bladder
Femoral vein

CORONAL **Chest, abdomen, and pelvis**

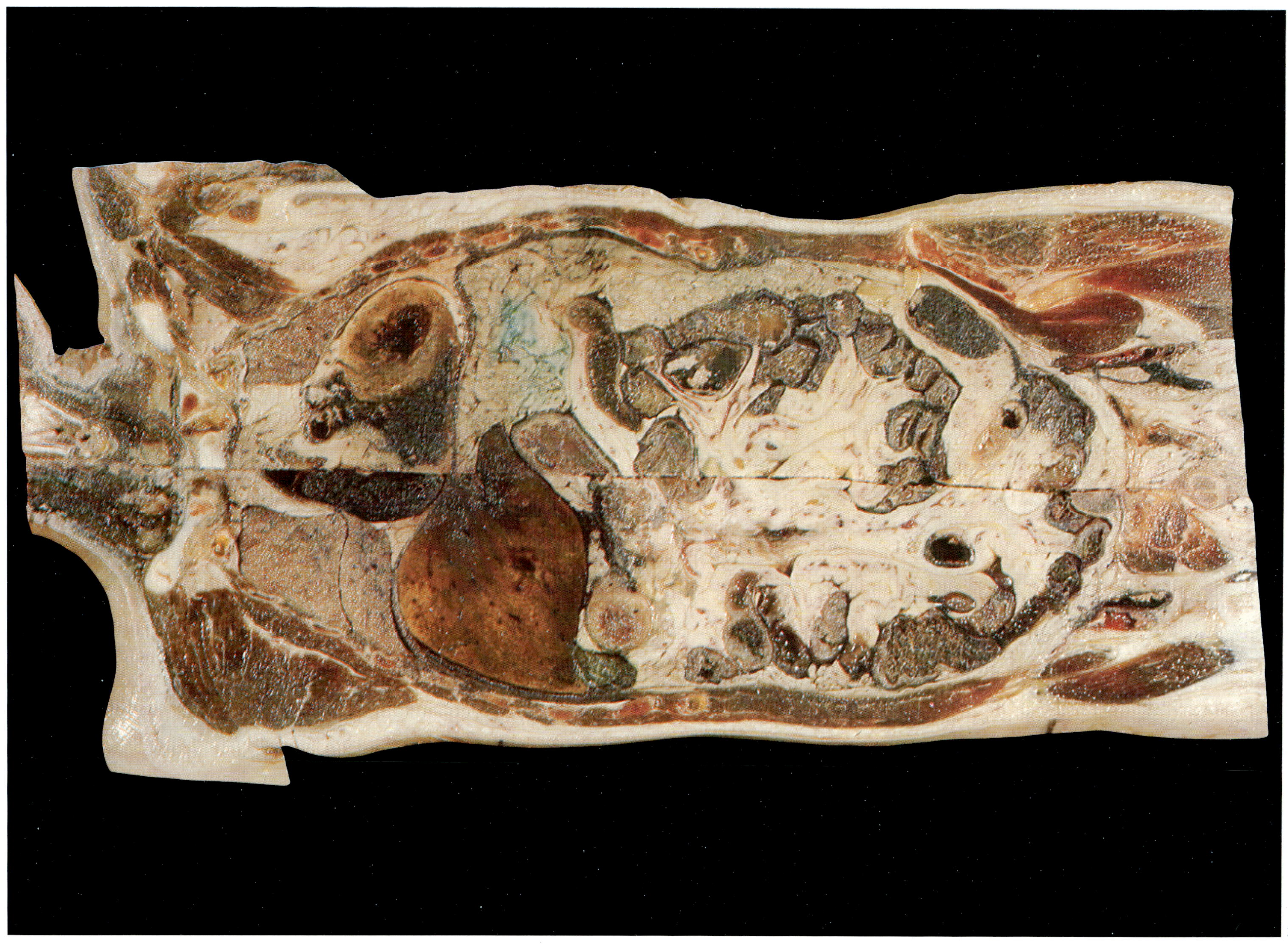

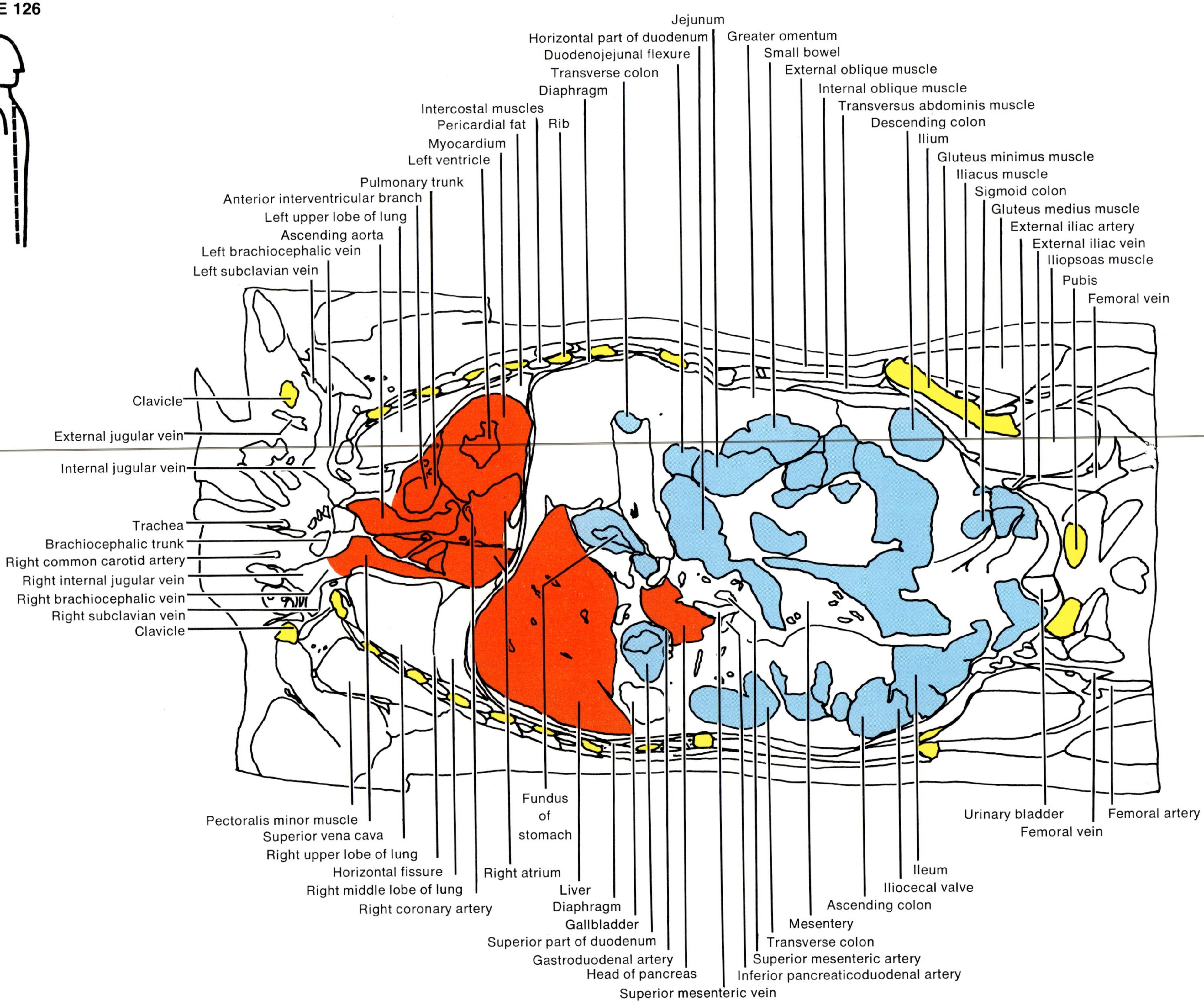

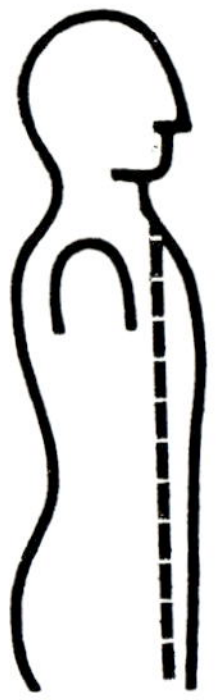

Jejunum
Horizontal part of duodenum
Greater omentum
Duodenojejunal flexure
Small bowel
Transverse colon
External oblique muscle
Diaphragm
Internal oblique muscle
Intercostal muscles
Transversus abdominis muscle
Pericardial fat
Rib
Descending colon
Myocardium
Ilium
Left ventricle
Gluteus minimus muscle
Pulmonary trunk
Iliacus muscle
Anterior interventricular branch
Sigmoid colon
Left upper lobe of lung
Gluteus medius muscle
Ascending aorta
External iliac artery
Left brachiocephalic vein
External iliac vein
Left subclavian vein
Iliopsoas muscle
Pubis
Femoral vein
Clavicle
External jugular vein
Internal jugular vein
Trachea
Brachiocephalic trunk
Right common carotid artery
Right internal jugular vein
Right brachiocephalic vein
Right subclavian vein
Clavicle
Pectoralis minor muscle
Superior vena cava
Right upper lobe of lung
Horizontal fissure
Right middle lobe of lung
Right coronary artery
Fundus
of
stomach
Right atrium
Liver
Diaphragm
Gallbladder
Superior part of duodenum
Gastroduodenal artery
Head of pancreas
Superior mesenteric vein
Superior mesenteric artery
Inferior pancreaticoduodenal artery
Mesentery
Transverse colon
Ascending colon
Iliocecal valve
Ileum
Urinary bladder
Femoral artery
Femoral vein

CORONAL **Chest, abdomen, and pelvis**

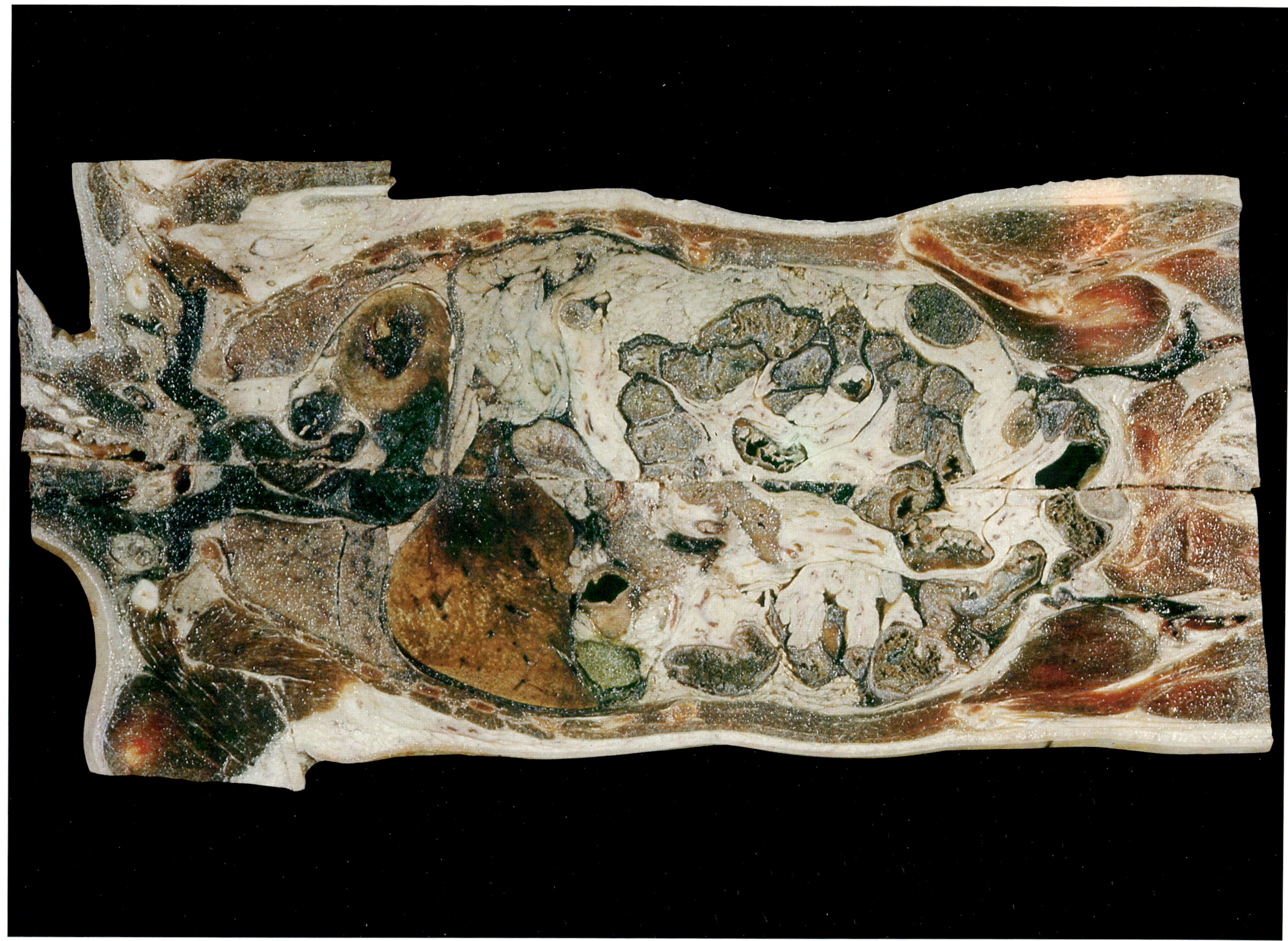

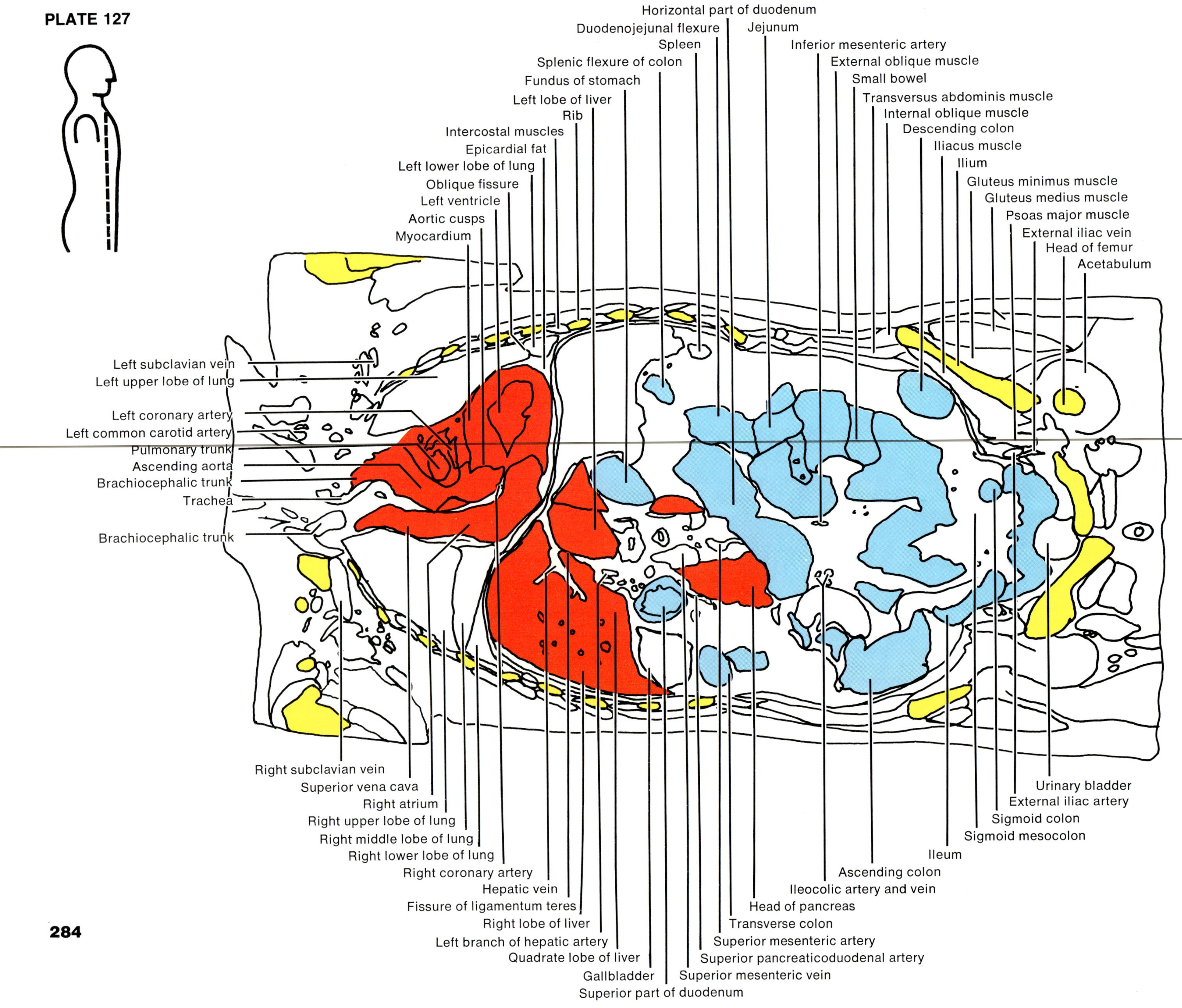
Horizontal part of duodenum
Duodenojejunal flexure
Jejunum
Spleen
Inferior mesenteric artery
Splenic flexure of colon
External oblique muscle
Fundus of stomach
Small bowel
Left lobe of liver
Transversus abdominis muscle
Rib
Internal oblique muscle
Intercostal muscles
Descending colon
Epicardial fat
Iliacus muscle
Left lower lobe of lung
Ilium
Oblique fissure
Gluteus minimus muscle
Left ventricle
Gluteus medius muscle
Aortic cusps
Psoas major muscle
Myocardium
External iliac vein
Head of femur
Acetabulum
Left subclavian vein
Left upper lobe of lung
Left coronary artery
Left common carotid artery
Pulmonary trunk
Ascending aorta
Brachiocephalic trunk
Trachea
Brachiocephalic trunk
Right subclavian vein
Superior vena cava
Right atrium
Right upper lobe of lung
Right middle lobe of lung
Right lower lobe of lung
Right coronary artery
Hepatic vein
Fissure of ligamentum teres
Right lobe of liver
Left branch of hepatic artery
Quadrate lobe of liver
Gallbladder
Superior part of duodenum
Head of pancreas
Transverse colon
Superior mesenteric artery
Superior pancreaticoduodenal artery
Superior mesenteric vein
Ileocolic artery and vein
Ascending colon
Ileum
Urinary bladder
External iliac artery
Sigmoid colon
Sigmoid mesocolon

CORONAL **Chest, abdomen, and pelvis**

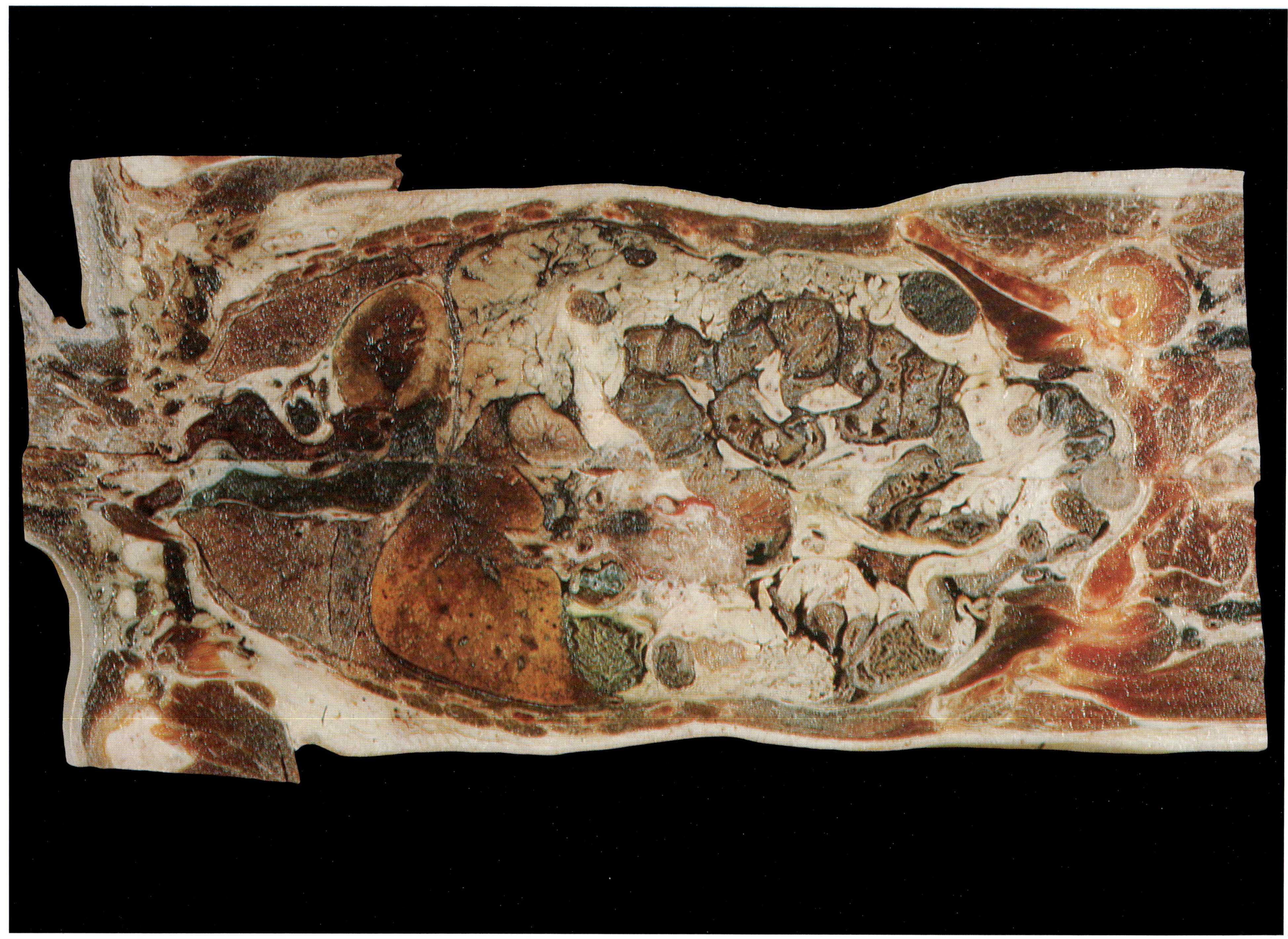

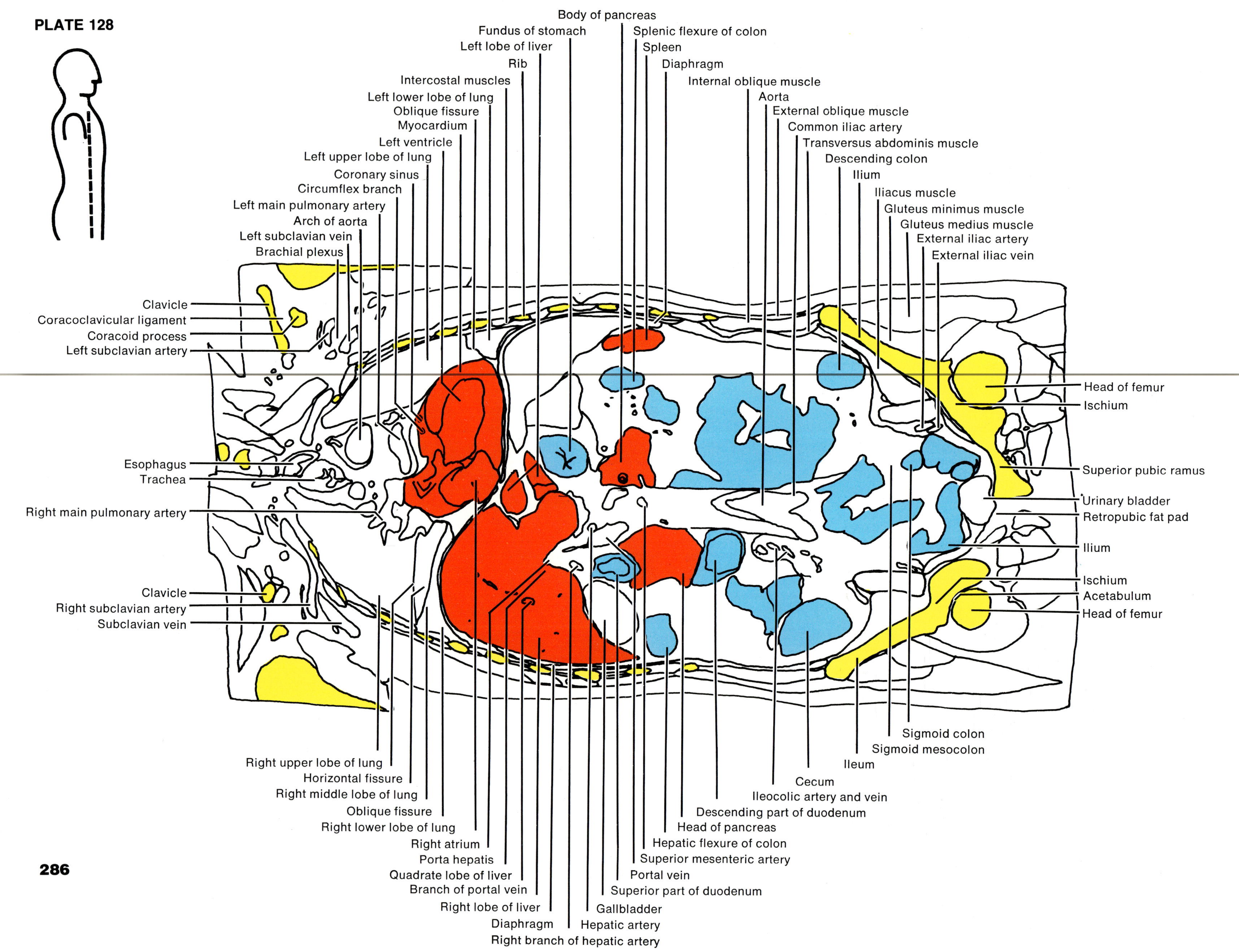
Body of pancreas
Fundus of stomach
Splenic flexure of colon
Left lobe of liver
Spleen
Rib
Diaphragm
Intercostal muscles
Internal oblique muscle
Left lower lobe of lung
Aorta
Oblique fissure
External oblique muscle
Myocardium
Common iliac artery
Left ventricle
Transversus abdominis muscle
Left upper lobe of lung
Descending colon
Coronary sinus
Ilium
Circumflex branch
Iliacus muscle
Left main pulmonary artery
Gluteus minimus muscle
Arch of aorta
Gluteus medius muscle
Left subclavian vein
External iliac artery
Brachial plexus
External iliac vein
Clavicle
Coracoclavicular ligament
Coracoid process
Left subclavian artery
Head of femur
Ischium
Esophagus
Trachea
Superior pubic ramus
Right main pulmonary artery
Urinary bladder
Retropubic fat pad
Ilium
Clavicle
Right subclavian artery
Subclavian vein
Ischium
Acetabulum
Head of femur
Sigmoid colon
Sigmoid mesocolon
Ileum
Right upper lobe of lung
Horizontal fissure
Right middle lobe of lung
Cecum
Oblique fissure
Ileocolic artery and vein
Right lower lobe of lung
Descending part of duodenum
Right atrium
Head of pancreas
Porta hepatis
Hepatic flexure of colon
Quadrate lobe of liver
Superior mesenteric artery
Branch of portal vein
Portal vein
Right lobe of liver
Superior part of duodenum
Diaphragm
Gallbladder
Right branch of hepatic artery
Hepatic artery

CORONAL **Chest, abdomen, and pelvis**

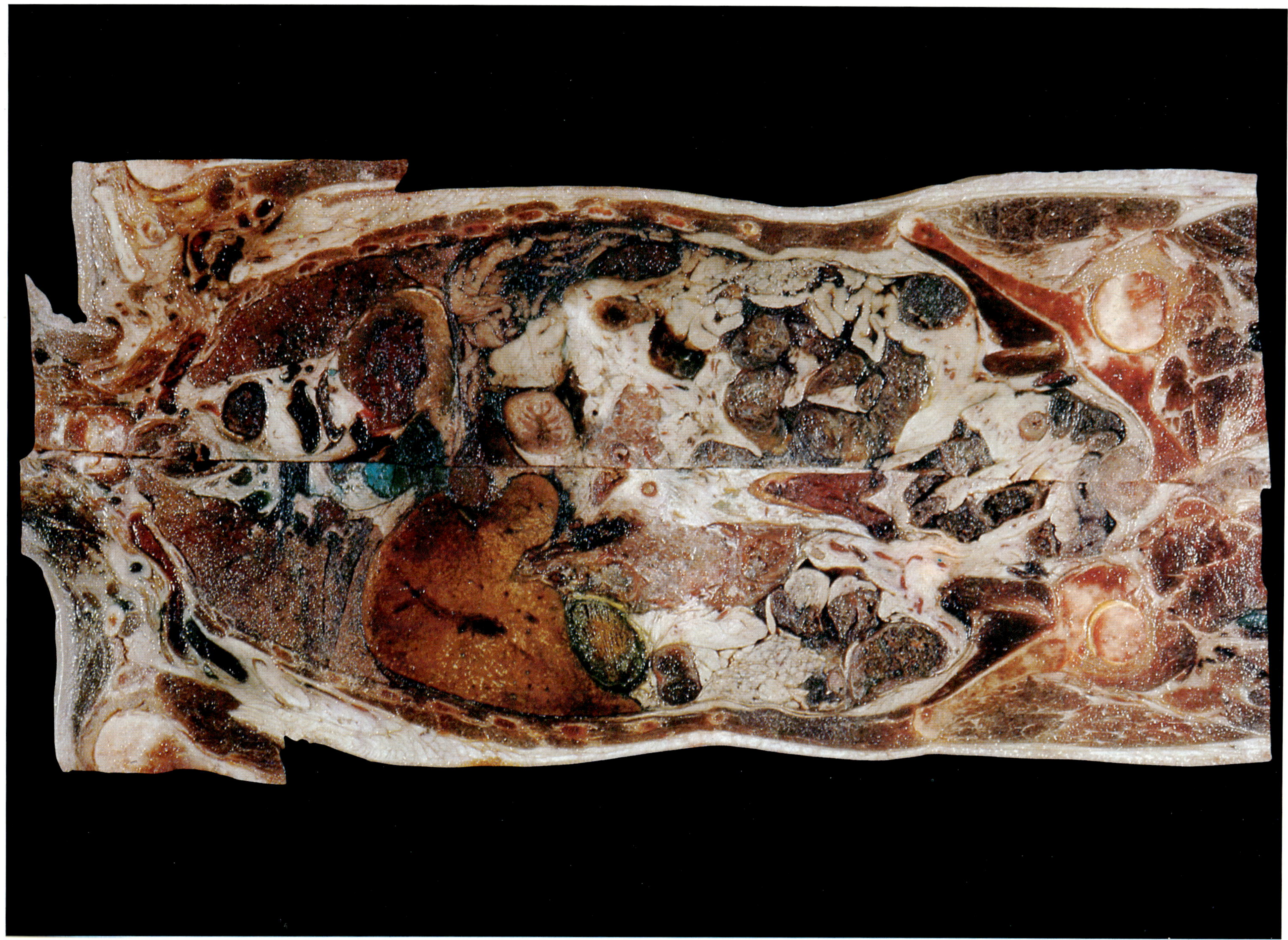

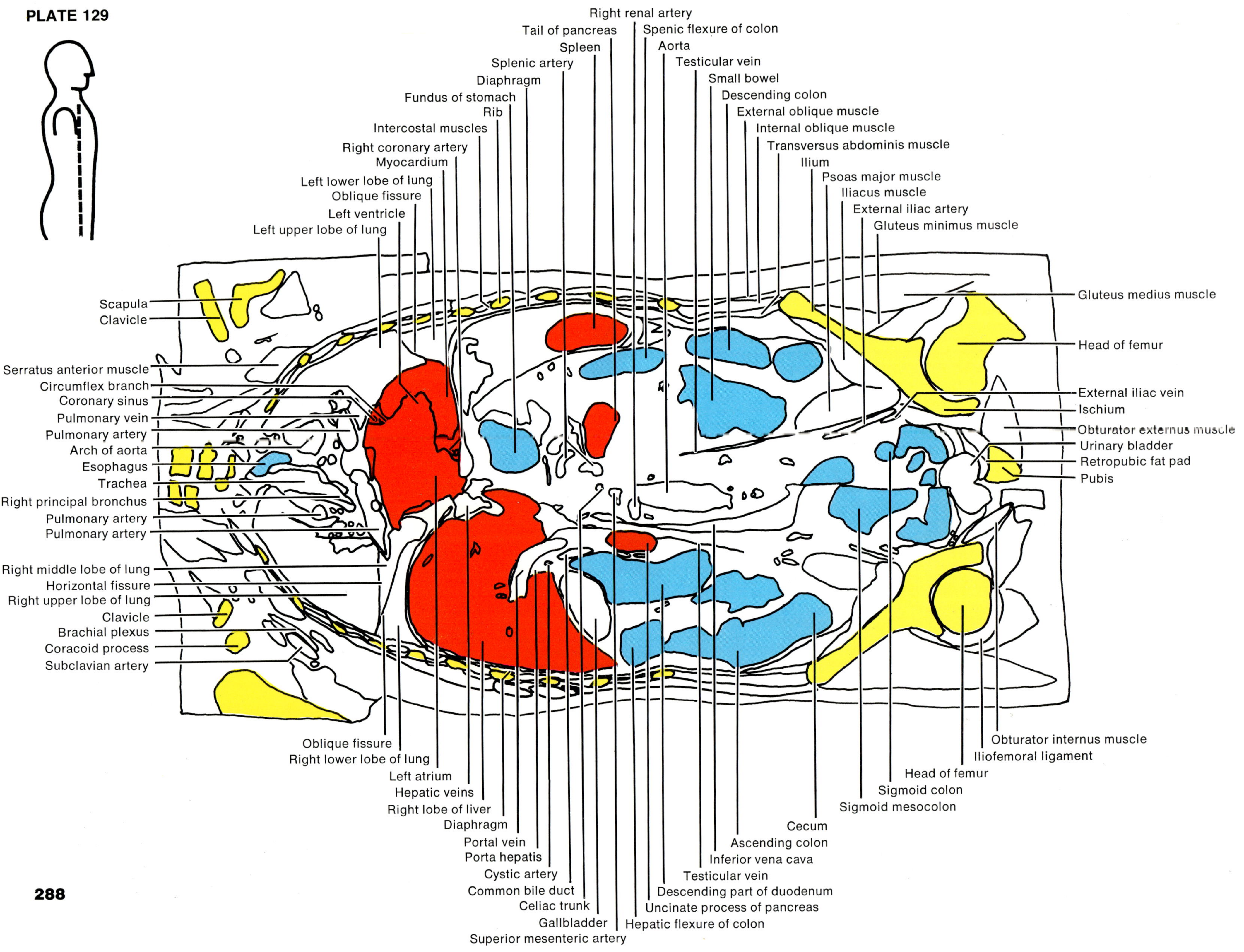
Right renal artery
Tail of pancreas
Spenic flexure of colon
Spleen
Aorta
Splenic artery
Testicular vein
Diaphragm
Small bowel
Fundus of stomach
Descending colon
Rib
External oblique muscle
Intercostal muscles
Internal oblique muscle
Right coronary artery
Transversus abdominis muscle
Myocardium
Ilium
Left lower lobe of lung
Psoas major muscle
Oblique fissure
Iliacus muscle
Left ventricle
External iliac artery
Left upper lobe of lung
Gluteus minimus muscle
Scapula
Gluteus medius muscle
Clavicle
Serratus anterior muscle
Head of femur
Circumflex branch
Coronary sinus
External iliac vein
Pulmonary vein
Ischium
Pulmonary artery
Obturator externus muscle
Arch of aorta
Urinary bladder
Esophagus
Retropubic fat pad
Trachea
Pubis
Right principal bronchus
Pulmonary artery
Pulmonary artery
Right middle lobe of lung
Horizontal fissure
Right upper lobe of lung
Clavicle
Brachial plexus
Coracoid process
Subclavian artery
Obturator internus muscle
Oblique fissure
Iliofemoral ligament
Right lower lobe of lung
Head of femur
Left atrium
Sigmoid colon
Hepatic veins
Sigmoid mesocolon
Right lobe of liver
Diaphragm
Portal vein
Cecum
Porta hepatis
Ascending colon
Cystic artery
Inferior vena cava
Common bile duct
Testicular vein
Celiac trunk
Descending part of duodenum
Gallbladder
Uncinate process of pancreas
Superior mesenteric artery
Hepatic flexure of colon

CORONAL **Chest, abdomen, and pelvis**

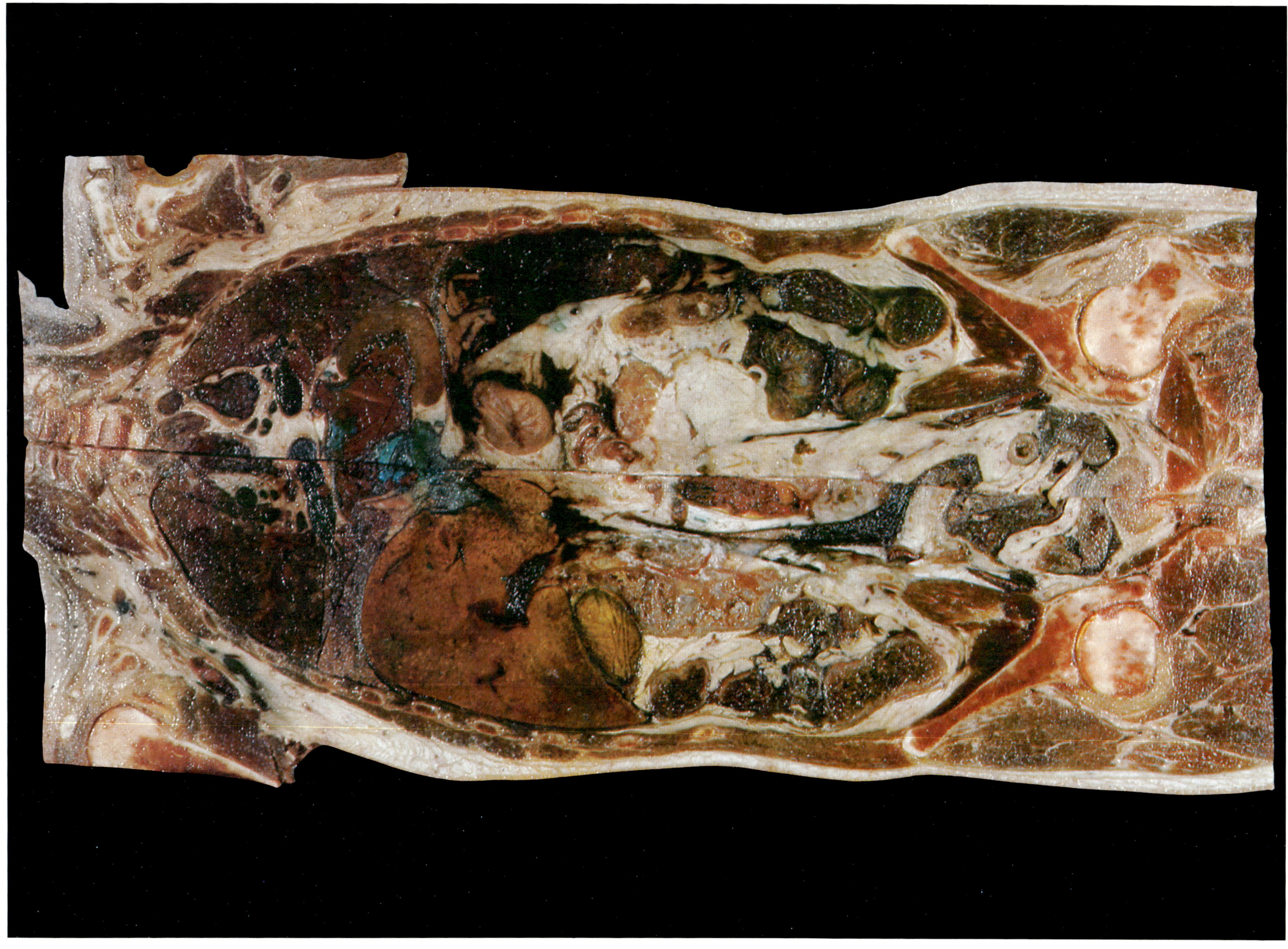

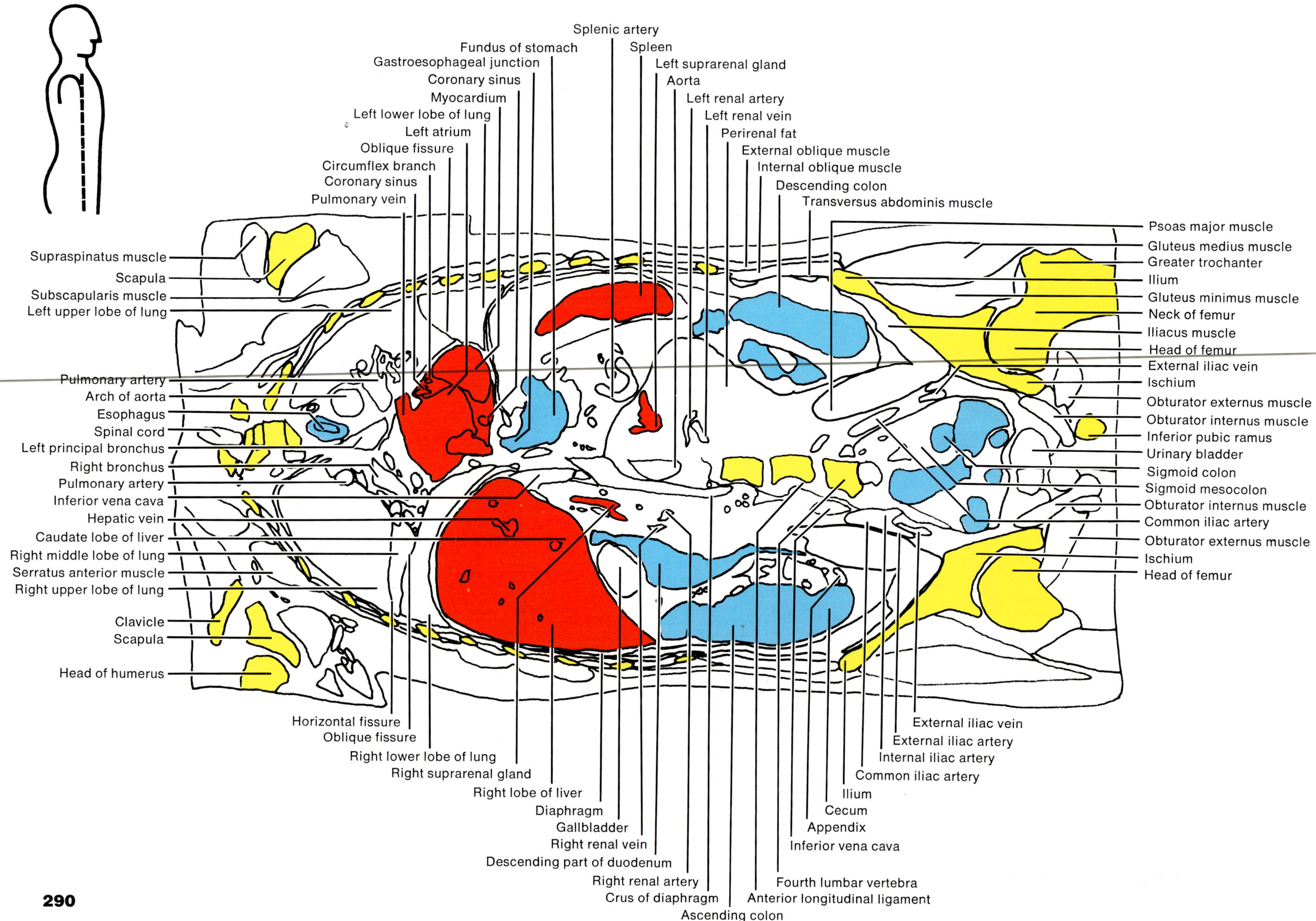
Splenic artery
Fundus of stomach
Gastroesophageal junction
Coronary sinus
Myocardium
Left lower lobe of lung
Left atrium
Oblique fissure
Circumflex branch
Coronary sinus
Pulmonary vein
Spleen
Left suprarenal gland
Aorta
Left renal artery
Left renal vein
Perirenal fat
External oblique muscle
Internal oblique muscle
Descending colon
Transversus abdominis muscle
Supraspinatus muscle
Scapula
Subscapularis muscle
Left upper lobe of lung
Psoas major muscle
Gluteus medius muscle
Greater trochanter
Ilium
Gluteus minimus muscle
Neck of femur
Iliacus muscle
Head of femur
External iliac vein
Ischium
Pulmonary artery
Arch of aorta
Esophagus
Spinal cord
Left principal bronchus
Right bronchus
Pulmonary artery
Inferior vena cava
Hepatic vein
Caudate lobe of liver
Right middle lobe of lung
Serratus anterior muscle
Right upper lobe of lung
Obturator externus muscle
Obturator internus muscle
Inferior pubic ramus
Urinary bladder
Sigmoid colon
Sigmoid mesocolon
Obturator internus muscle
Common iliac artery
Obturator externus muscle
Ischium
Head of femur
Clavicle
Scapula
Head of humerus
Horizontal fissure
Oblique fissure
Right lower lobe of lung
Right suprarenal gland
Right lobe of liver
Diaphragm
Gallbladder
Right renal vein
Descending part of duodenum
Right renal artery
Crus of diaphragm
Ascending colon
External iliac vein
External iliac artery
Internal iliac artery
Common iliac artery
Ilium
Cecum
Appendix
Inferior vena cava
Fourth lumbar vertebra
Anterior longitudinal ligament

CORONAL **Chest, abdomen, and pelvis**

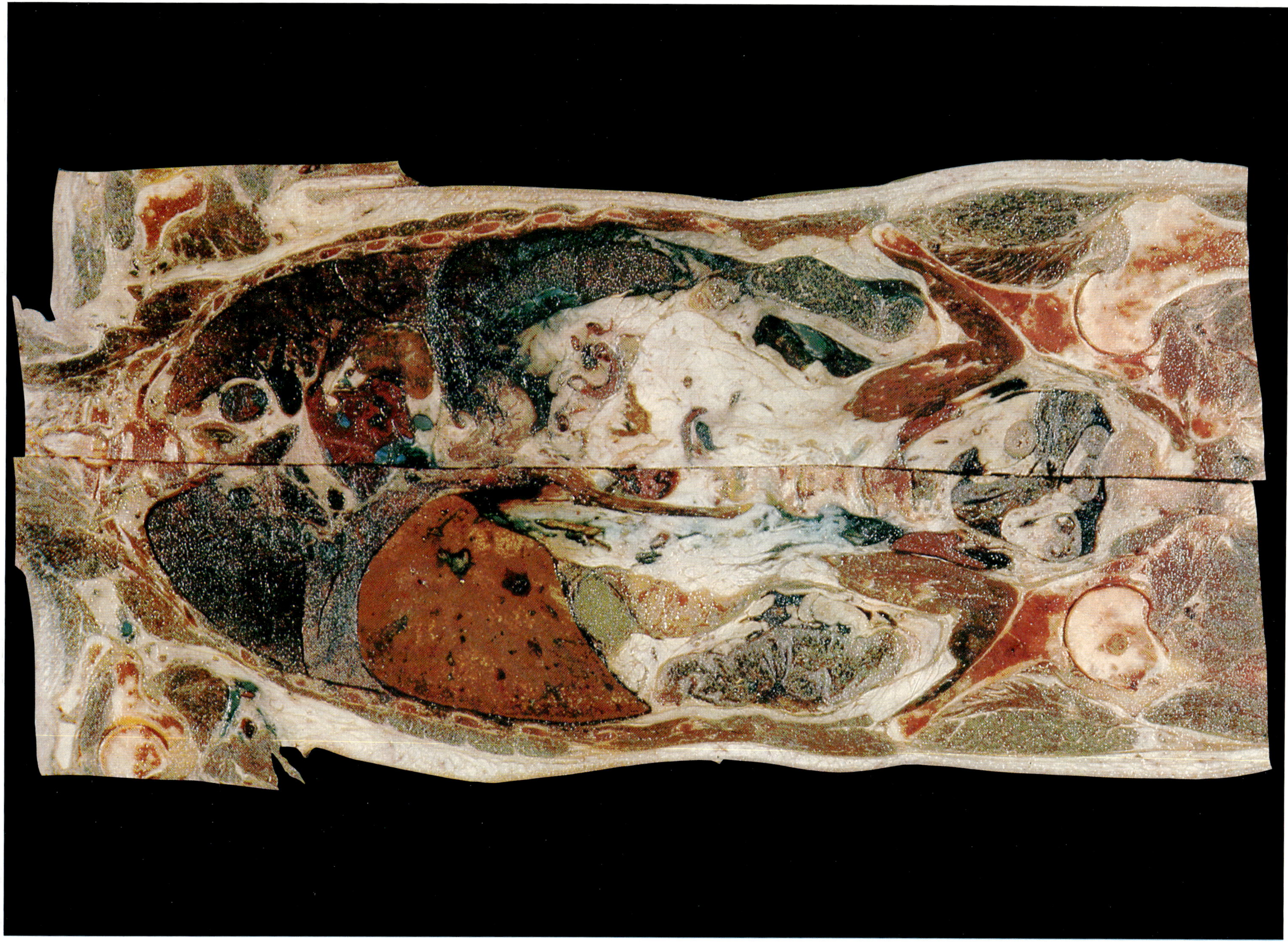

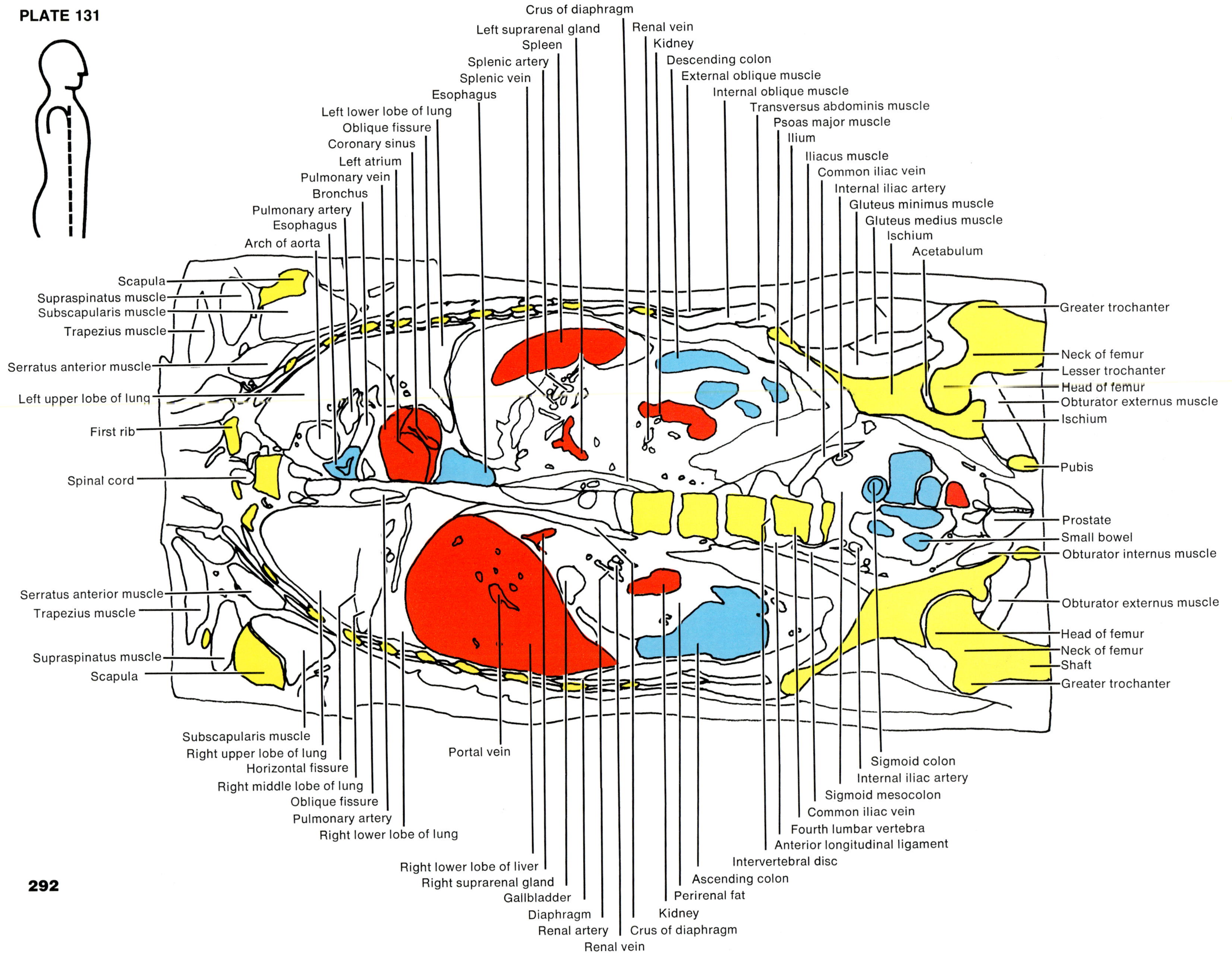

Crus of diaphragm
Left suprarenal gland
Spleen
Splenic artery
Splenic vein
Esophagus
Left lower lobe of lung
Oblique fissure
Coronary sinus
Left atrium
Pulmonary vein
Bronchus
Pulmonary artery
Esophagus
Arch of aorta
Renal vein
Kidney
Descending colon
External oblique muscle
Internal oblique muscle
Transversus abdominis muscle
Psoas major muscle
Ilium
Iliacus muscle
Common iliac vein
Internal iliac artery
Gluteus minimus muscle
Gluteus medius muscle
Ischium
Acetabulum
Scapula
Supraspinatus muscle
Subscapularis muscle
Trapezius muscle
Serratus anterior muscle
Left upper lobe of lung
First rib
Spinal cord
Serratus anterior muscle
Trapezius muscle
Supraspinatus muscle
Scapula
Greater trochanter
Neck of femur
Lesser trochanter
Head of femur
Obturator externus muscle
Ischium
Pubis
Prostate
Small bowel
Obturator internus muscle
Obturator externus muscle
Head of femur
Neck of femur
Shaft
Greater trochanter
Subscapularis muscle
Right upper lobe of lung
Horizontal fissure
Right middle lobe of lung
Oblique fissure
Pulmonary artery
Right lower lobe of lung
Portal vein
Right lower lobe of liver
Right suprarenal gland
Gallbladder
Diaphragm
Renal artery
Renal vein
Crus of diaphragm
Kidney
Perirenal fat
Ascending colon
Intervertebral disc
Anterior longitudinal ligament
Fourth lumbar vertebra
Common iliac vein
Sigmoid mesocolon
Internal iliac artery
Sigmoid colon

CORONAL **Chest, abdomen, and pelvis**

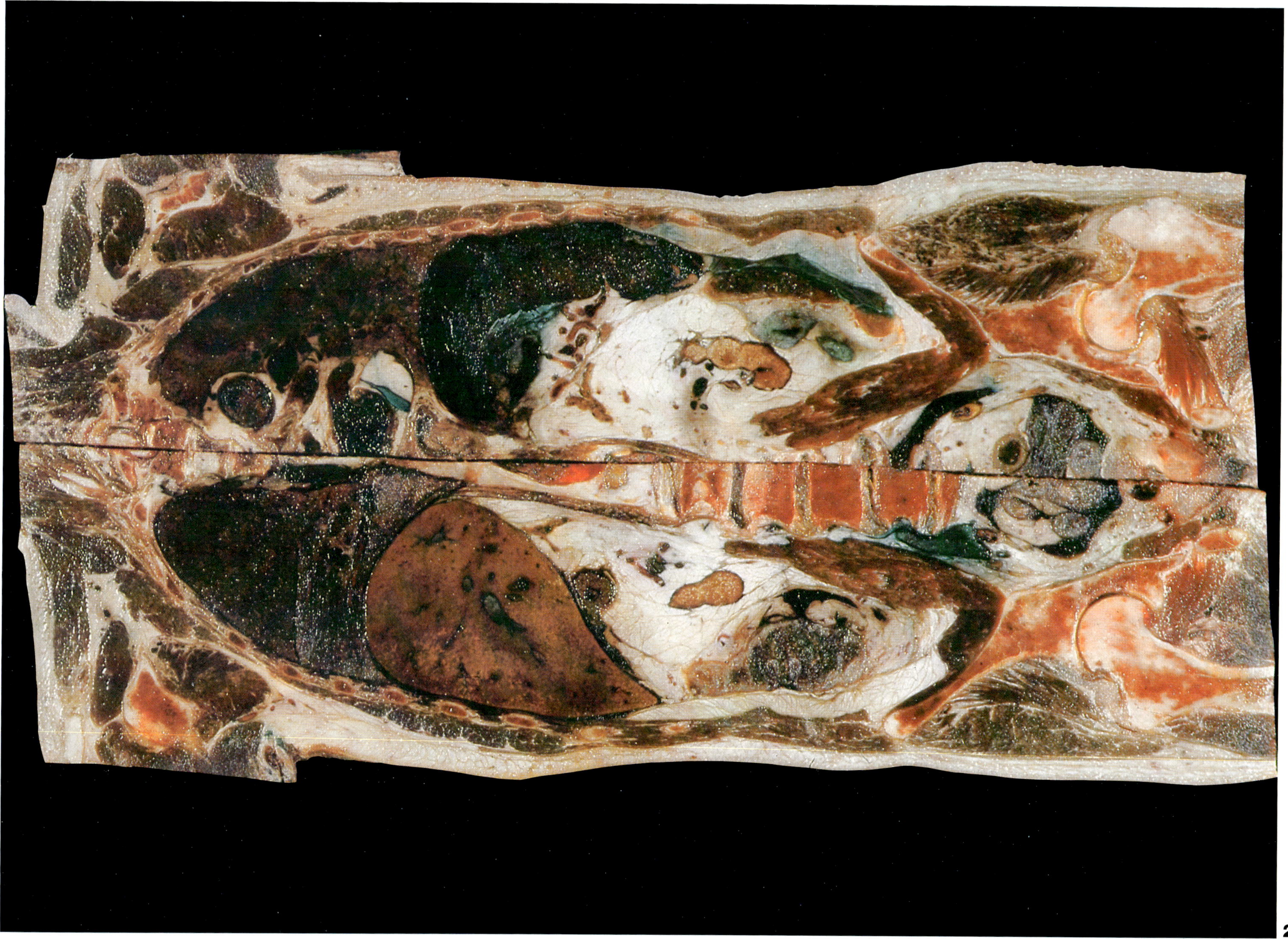

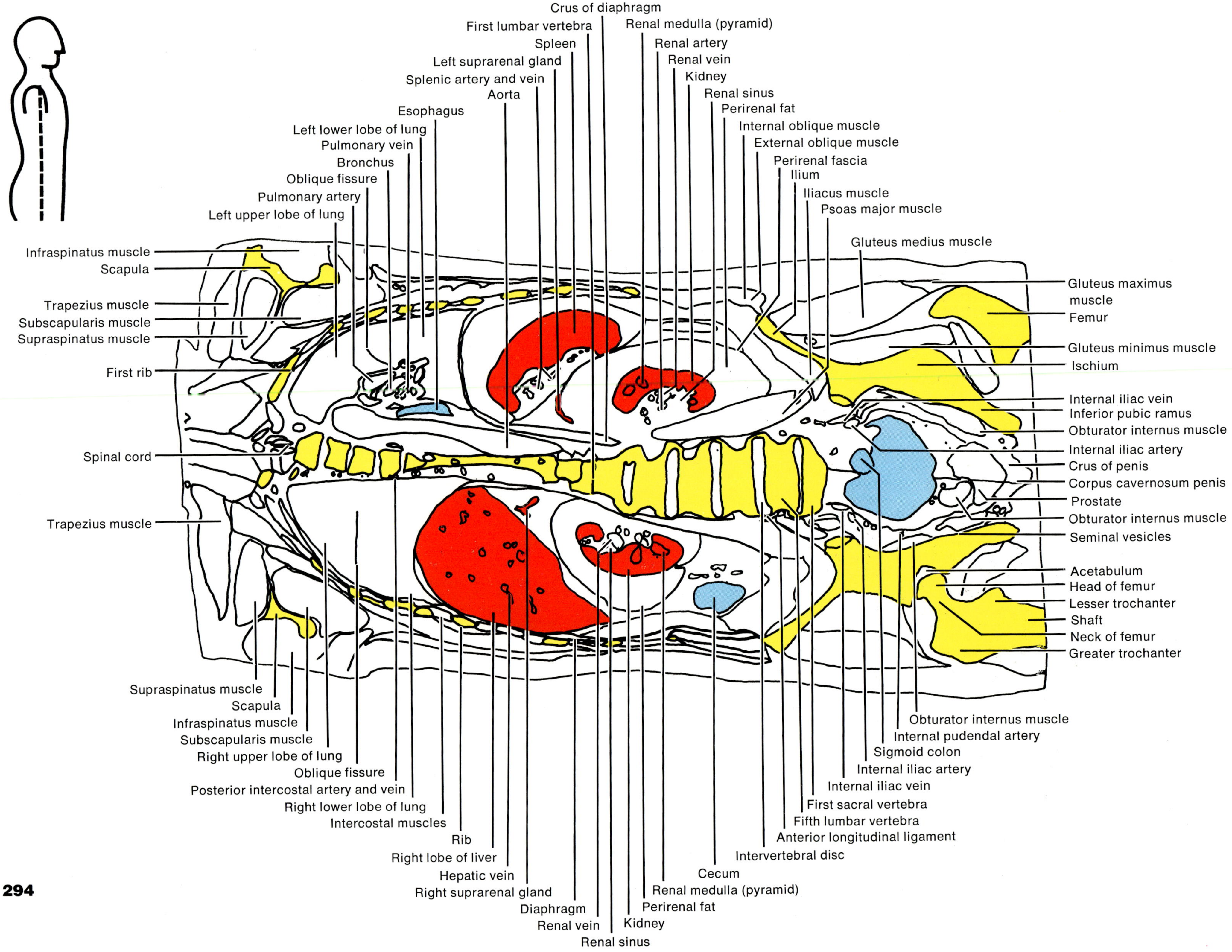

Crus of diaphragm
First lumbar vertebra
Renal medulla (pyramid)
Spleen
Renal artery
Left suprarenal gland
Renal vein
Splenic artery and vein
Kidney
Aorta
Renal sinus
Esophagus
Perirenal fat
Left lower lobe of lung
Internal oblique muscle
Pulmonary vein
External oblique muscle
Bronchus
Perirenal fascia
Oblique fissure
Ilium
Pulmonary artery
Iliacus muscle
Left upper lobe of lung
Psoas major muscle
Gluteus medius muscle
Infraspinatus muscle
Scapula
Gluteus maximus
muscle
Trapezius muscle
Femur
Subscapularis muscle
Supraspinatus muscle
Gluteus minimus muscle
Ischium
First rib
Internal iliac vein
Inferior pubic ramus
Obturator internus muscle
Spinal cord
Internal iliac artery
Crus of penis
Corpus cavernosum penis
Prostate
Trapezius muscle
Obturator internus muscle
Seminal vesicles
Acetabulum
Head of femur
Lesser trochanter
Shaft
Neck of femur
Greater trochanter
Supraspinatus muscle
Scapula
Infraspinatus muscle
Subscapularis muscle
Obturator internus muscle
Right upper lobe of lung
Internal pudendal artery
Oblique fissure
Sigmoid colon
Posterior intercostal artery and vein
Internal iliac artery
Right lower lobe of lung
Internal iliac vein
Intercostal muscles
First sacral vertebra
Rib
Fifth lumbar vertebra
Right lobe of liver
Anterior longitudinal ligament
Hepatic vein
Intervertebral disc
Right suprarenal gland
Cecum
Diaphragm
Renal medulla (pyramid)
Renal vein
Perirenal fat
Kidney
Renal sinus

CORONAL **Chest, abdomen, and pelvis**

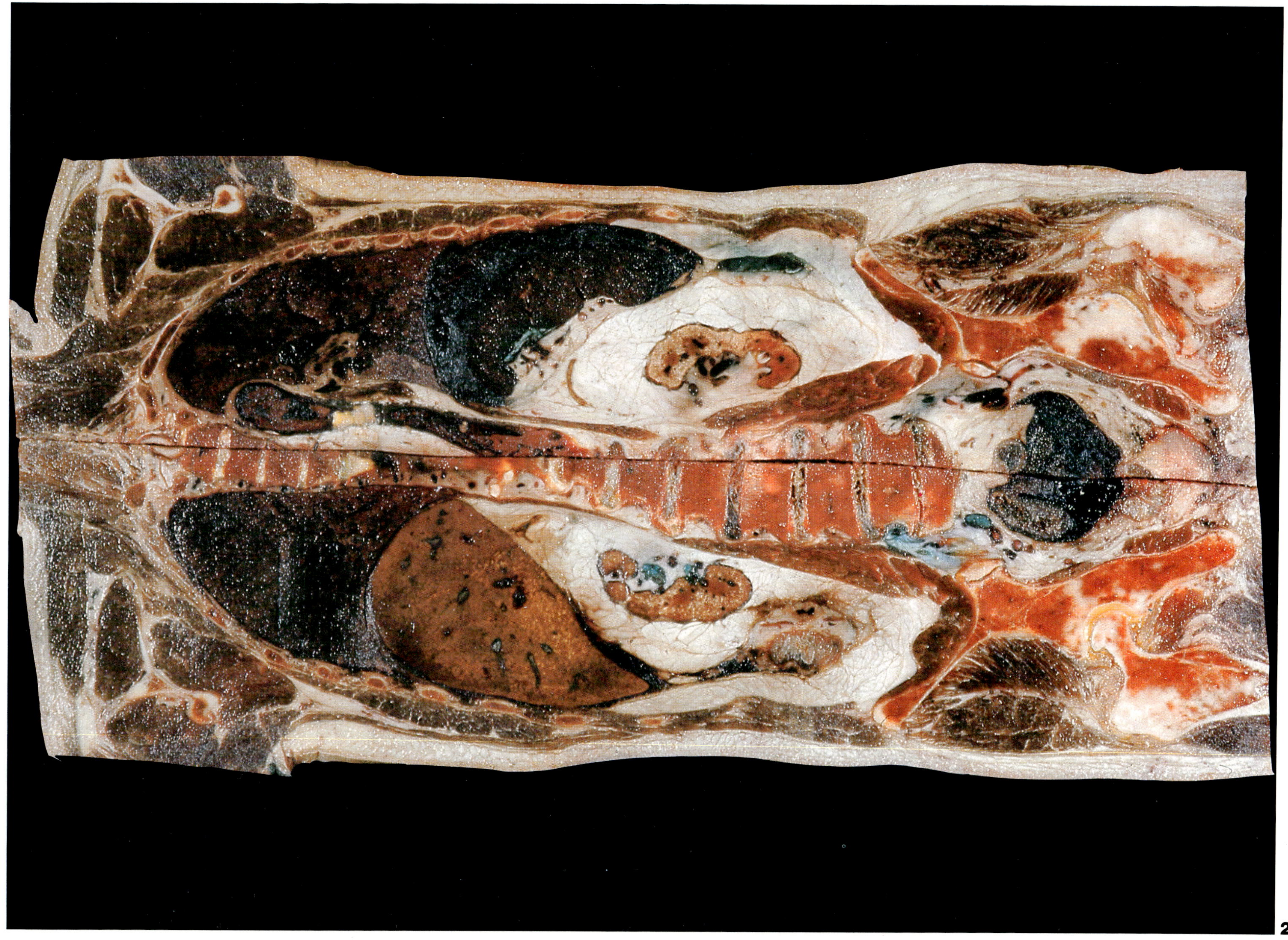

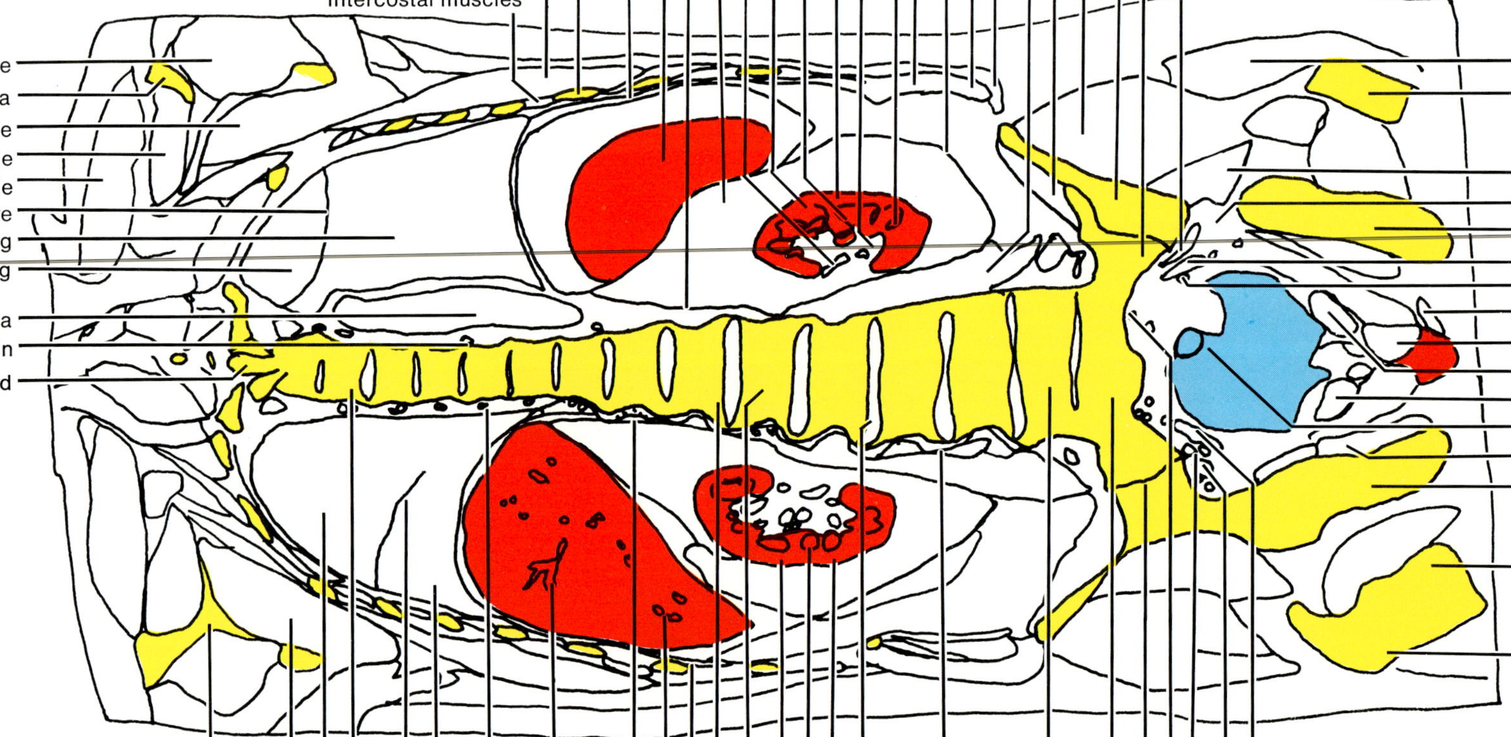

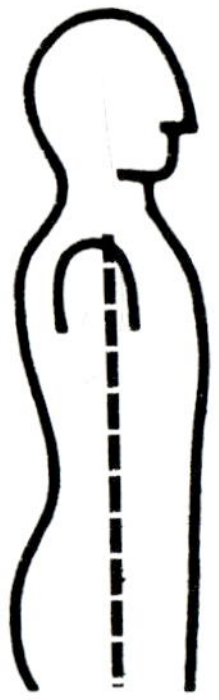

Interlobar vessels
Renal sinus
Renal cortex
Renal medulla
Kidney
Renal artery
Perirenal fat
Crus of diaphragm
Spleen
Diaphragm
Rib
Serratus anterior muscle
Intercostal muscles
Transversus abdominis muscle
Perirenal fascia
Internal oblique muscle
External oblique muscle
Psoas major muscle
Iliacus muscle
Gluteus medius muscle
Ilium
Lateral part of sacrum
Sciatic nerve
Infraspinatus muscle
Scapula
Subscapularis muscle
Supraspinatus muscle
Trapezius muscle
Oblique fissure
Left lower lobe of lung
Left upper lobe of lung
Aorta
Hemiazygos vein
Spinal cord
Gluteus maximus muscle
Greater trochanter
Gluteus minimus muscle
Greater sciatic foramen
Ischium
Internal iliac vein
Internal iliac artery
Crus of penis
Prostate
Seminal vesicles
Seminal vesicles
Sigmoid colon
Obturator internus muscle
Ischium
Lesser trochanter
Femur
Scapula
Subscapularis muscle
Right upper lobe of lung
Fifth thoracic vertebra
Oblique fissure
Right lower lobe of lung
Posterior intercostal artery and vein
Portal vein
Lumbar artery and vein
Right lobe of liver
Diaphragm
Twelfth thoracic vertebra
First lumbar vertebra
Renal cortex
Renal medulla
Kidney
Intervertebral disc
Anterior longitudinal ligament
Fifth lumbar vertebra
First sacral vertebra
Sacroiliac joint
Lateral sacral artery
Superior gluteal artery
Sciatic nerve
Internal iliac vein

CORONAL **Chest, abdomen, and pelvis**

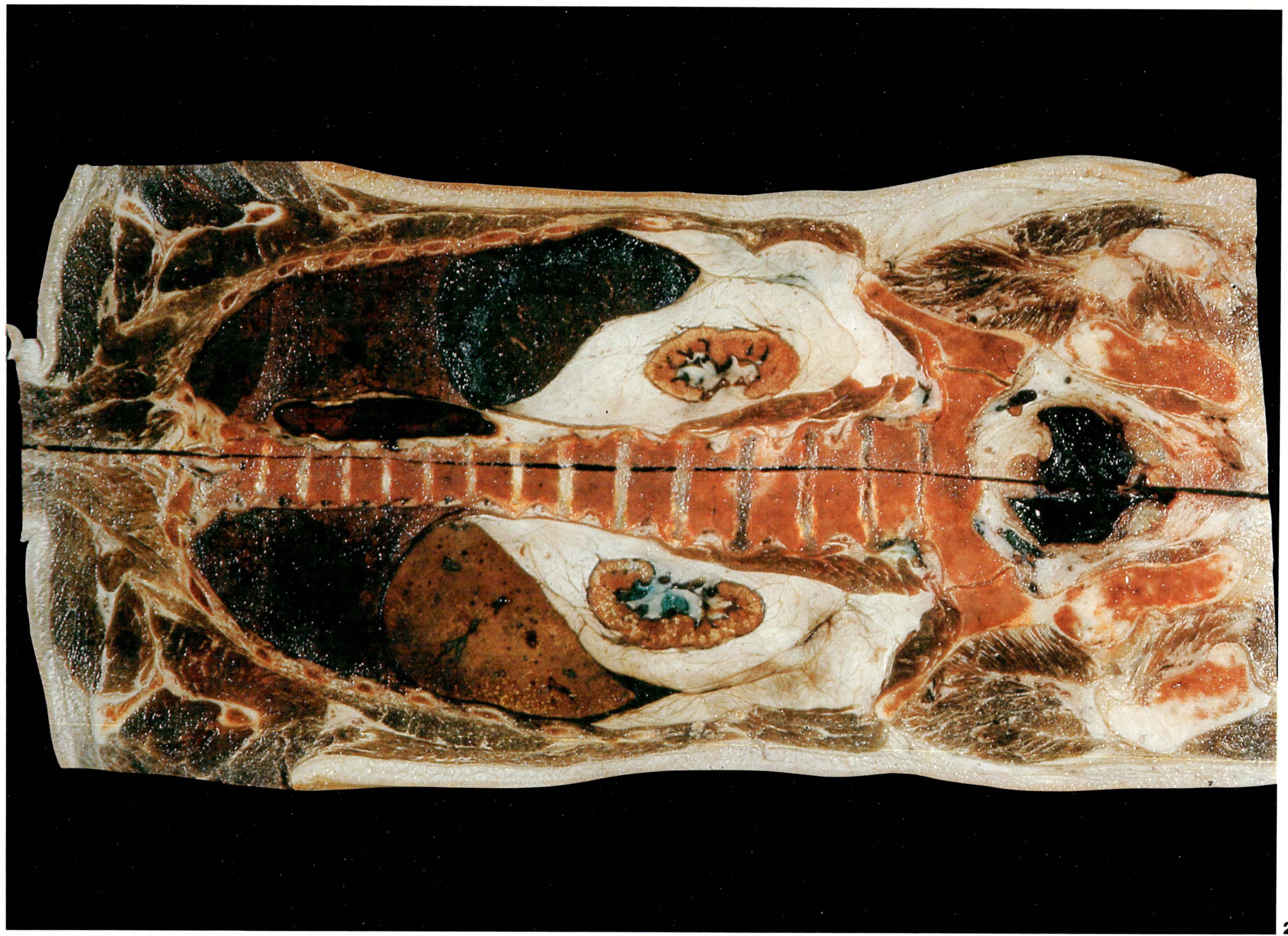

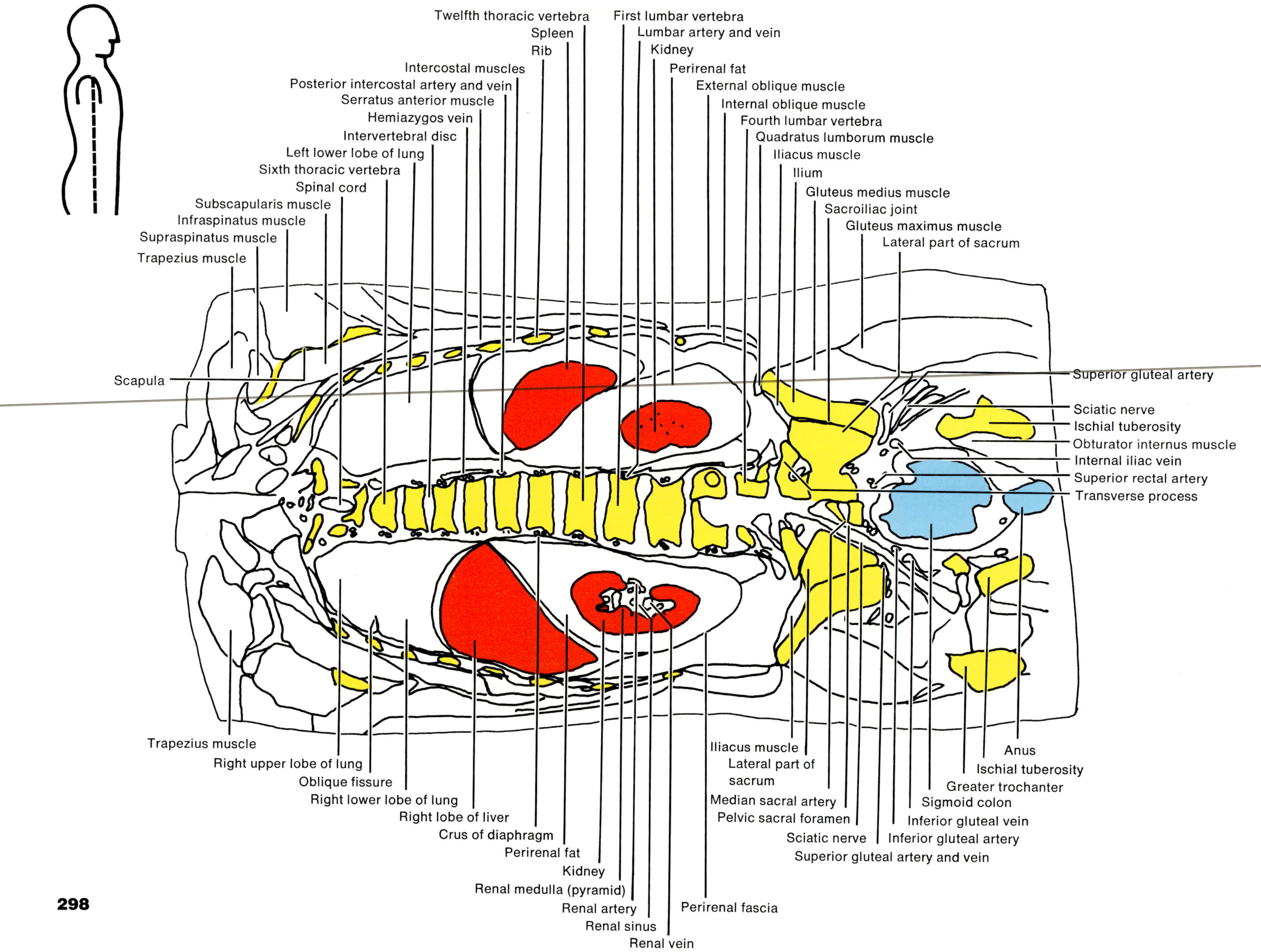

Twelfth thoracic vertebra
First lumbar vertebra
Spleen
Lumbar artery and vein
Rib
Kidney
Perirenal fat
Intercostal muscles
External oblique muscle
Posterior intercostal artery and vein
Internal oblique muscle
Serratus anterior muscle
Fourth lumbar vertebra
Hemiazygos vein
Quadratus lumborum muscle
Intervertebral disc
Iliacus muscle
Left lower lobe of lung
Ilium
Sixth thoracic vertebra
Gluteus medius muscle
Spinal cord
Sacroiliac joint
Subscapularis muscle
Gluteus maximus muscle
Infraspinatus muscle
Lateral part of sacrum
Supraspinatus muscle
Trapezius muscle
Scapula
Superior gluteal artery
Sciatic nerve
Ischial tuberosity
Obturator internus muscle
Internal iliac vein
Superior rectal artery
Transverse process
Trapezius muscle
Right upper lobe of lung
Anus
Oblique fissure
Ischial tuberosity
Right lower lobe of lung
Greater trochanter
Right lobe of liver
Iliacus muscle
Crus of diaphragm
Lateral part of sacrum
Sigmoid colon
Perirenal fat
Median sacral artery
Inferior gluteal vein
Kidney
Pelvic sacral foramen
Inferior gluteal artery
Renal medulla (pyramid)
Sciatic nerve
Superior gluteal artery and vein
Renal artery
Perirenal fascia
Renal sinus
Renal vein

CORONAL **Chest, abdomen, and pelvis**

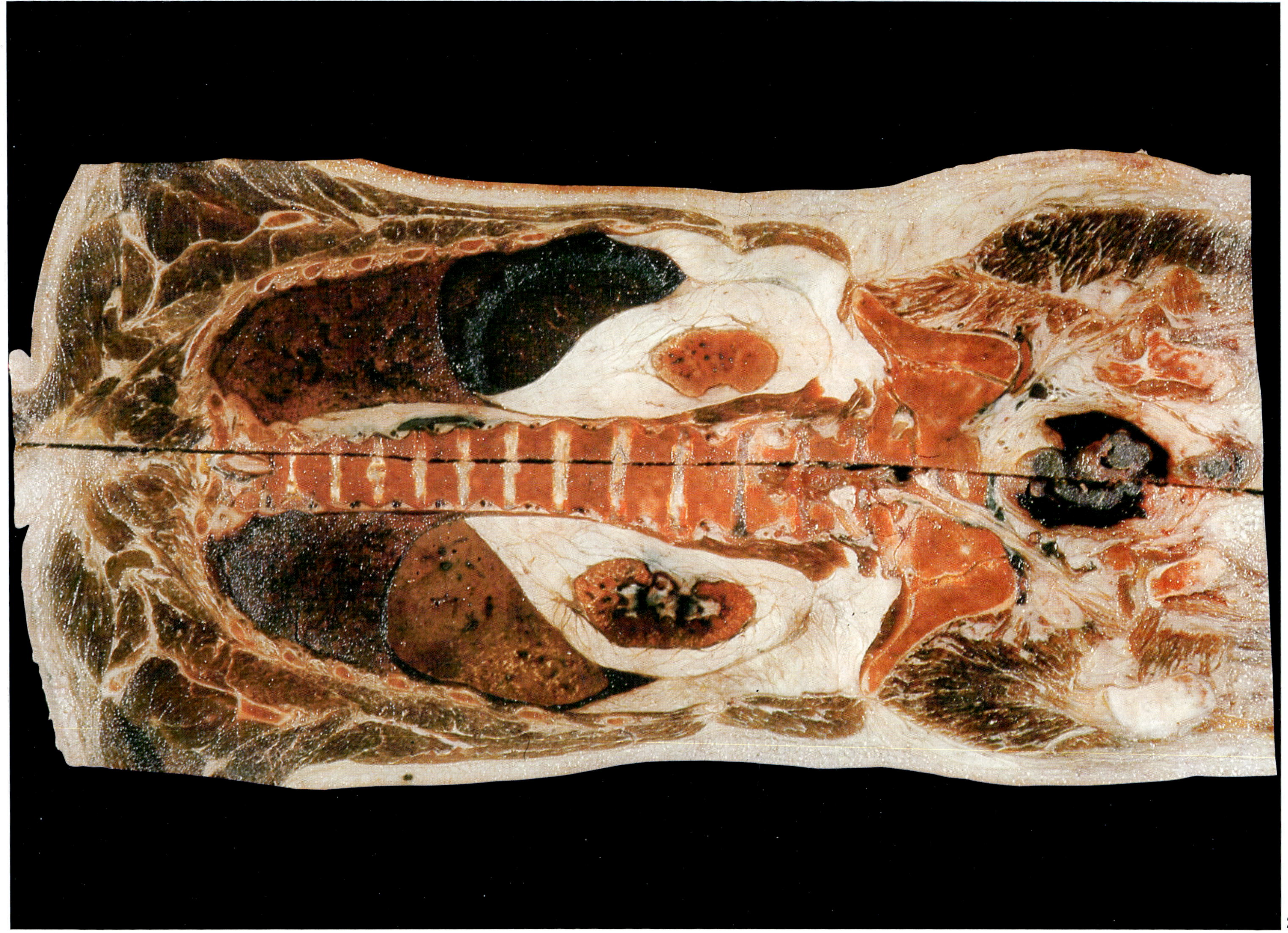

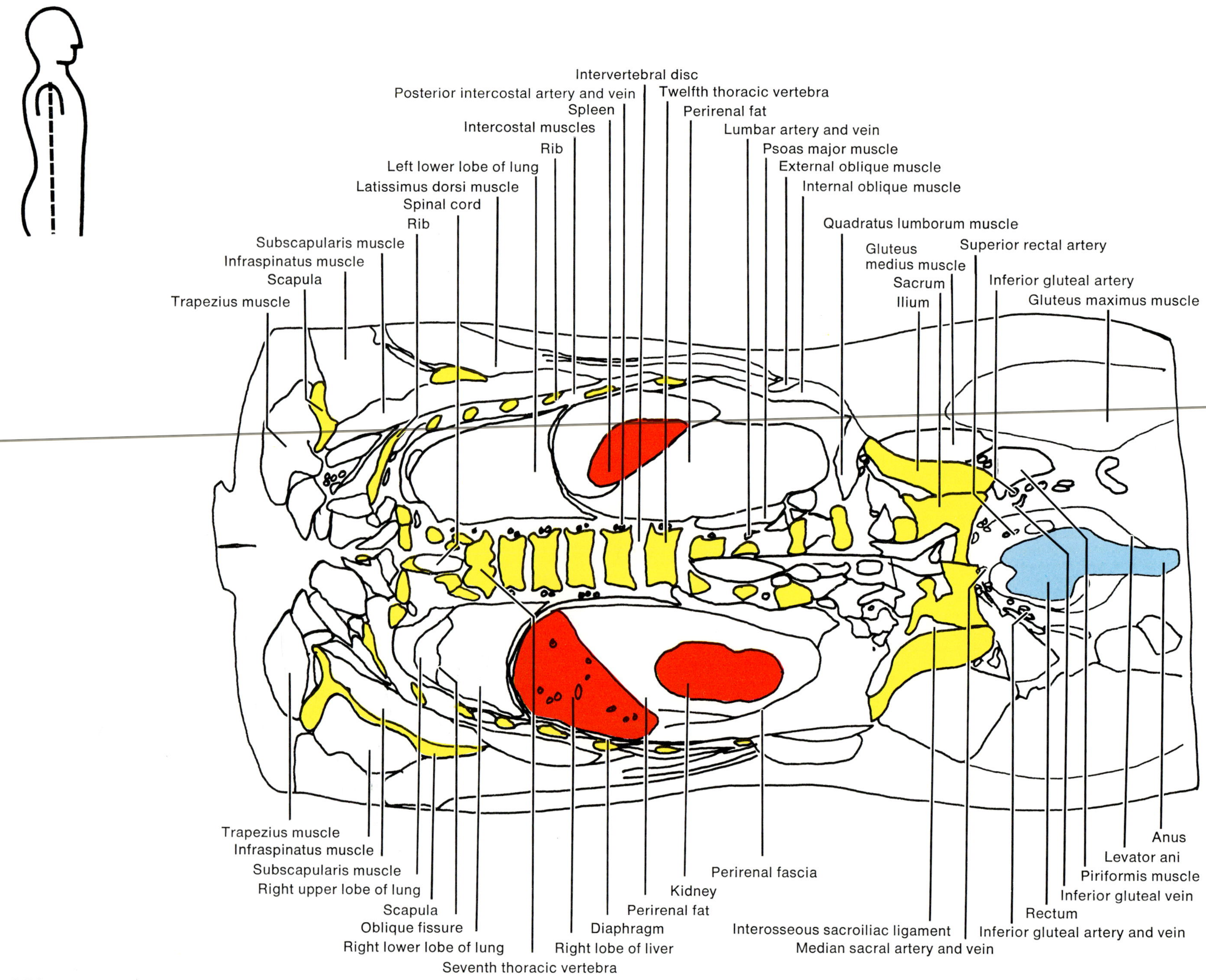

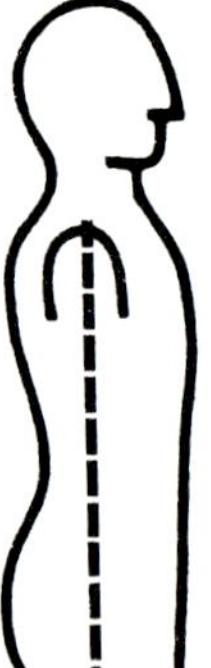

Intervertebral disc
Posterior intercostal artery and vein
Twelfth thoracic vertebra
Spleen
Perirenal fat
Intercostal muscles
Lumbar artery and vein
Rib
Psoas major muscle
Left lower lobe of lung
External oblique muscle
Latissimus dorsi muscle
Internal oblique muscle
Spinal cord
Rib
Quadratus lumborum muscle
Subscapularis muscle
Gluteus
Infraspinatus muscle
medius muscle
Superior rectal artery
Scapula
Sacrum
Inferior gluteal artery
Trapezius muscle
Ilium
Gluteus maximus muscle

Trapezius muscle
Infraspinatus muscle
Anus
Subscapularis muscle
Levator ani
Right upper lobe of lung
Piriformis muscle
Scapula
Perirenal fascia
Inferior gluteal vein
Oblique fissure
Kidney
Rectum
Right lower lobe of lung
Perirenal fat
Inferior gluteal artery and vein
Right lobe of liver
Interosseous sacroiliac ligament
Seventh thoracic vertebra
Diaphragm
Median sacral artery and vein

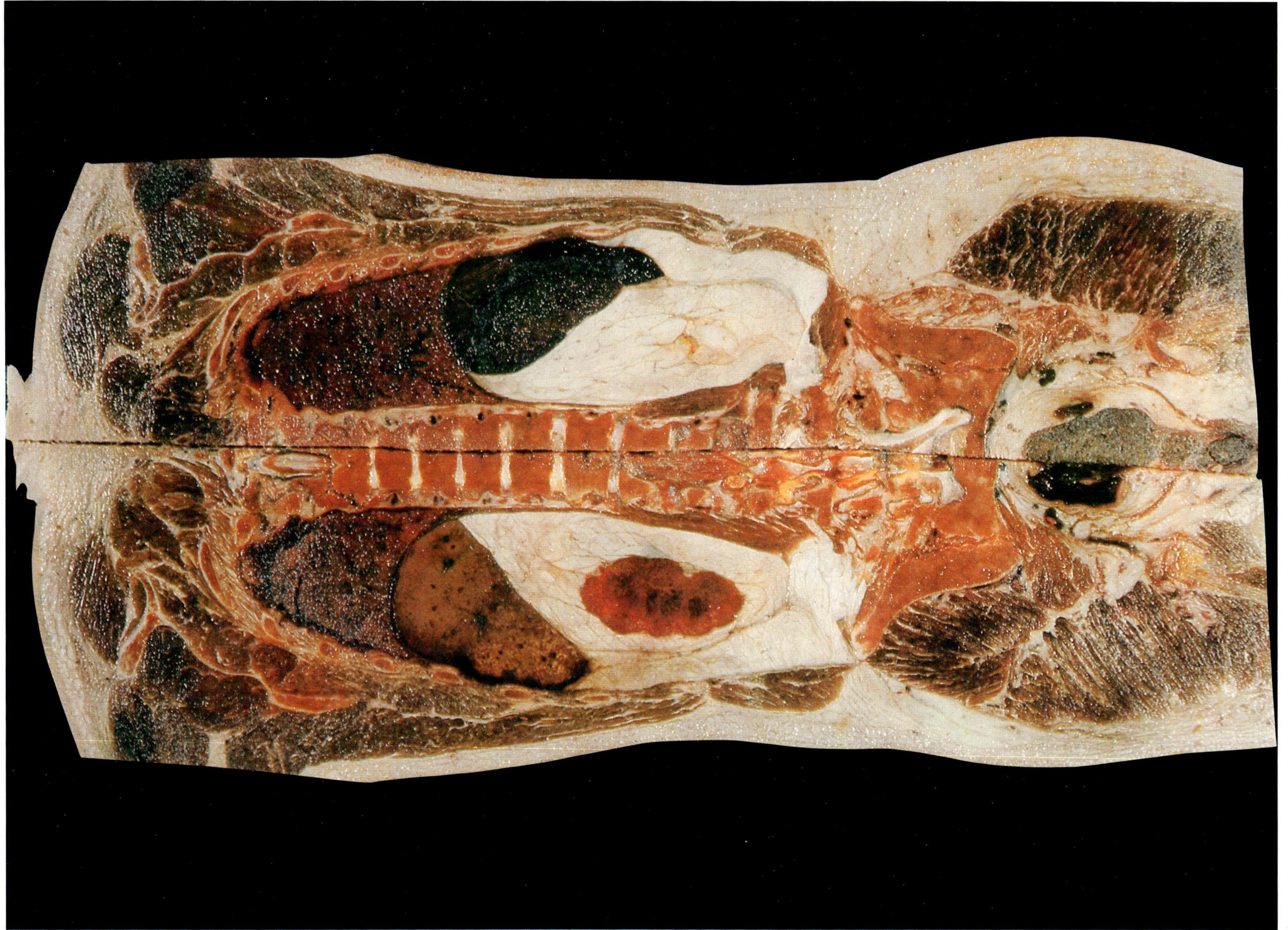

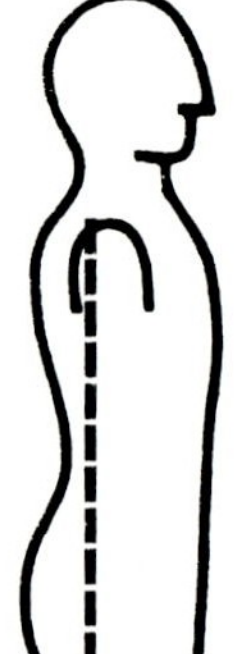

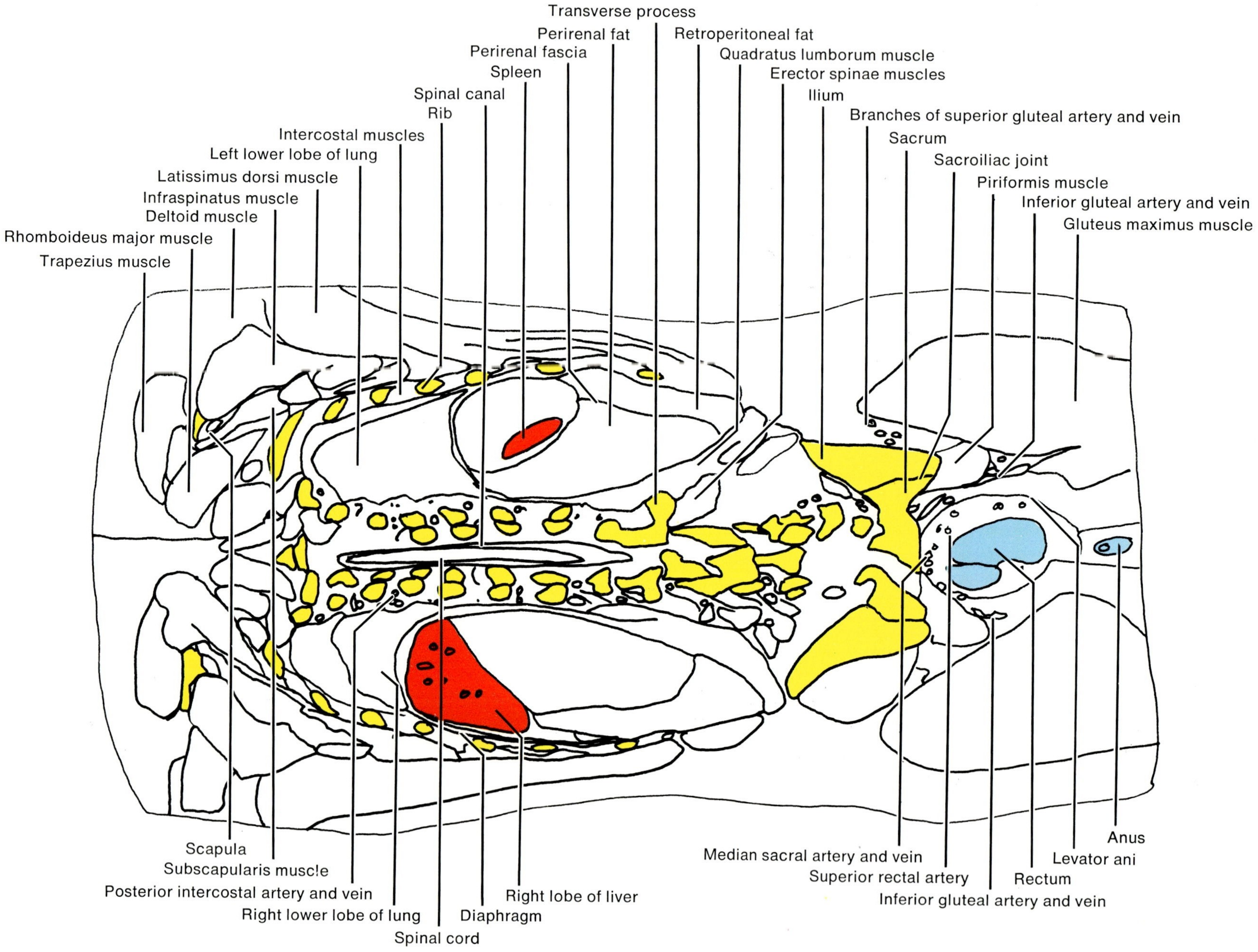

Transverse process
Perirenal fat
Retroperitoneal fat
Perirenal fascia
Quadratus lumborum muscle
Spleen
Erector spinae muscles
Spinal canal
Ilium
Rib
Branches of superior gluteal artery and vein
Intercostal muscles
Sacrum
Left lower lobe of lung
Sacroiliac joint
Latissimus dorsi muscle
Piriformis muscle
Infraspinatus muscle
Inferior gluteal artery and vein
Deltoid muscle
Gluteus maximus muscle
Rhomboideus major muscle
Trapezius muscle
Scapula
Anus
Subscapularis muscle
Levator ani
Median sacral artery and vein
Posterior intercostal artery and vein
Superior rectal artery
Rectum
Right lobe of liver
Right lower lobe of lung
Diaphragm
Inferior gluteal artery and vein
Spinal cord

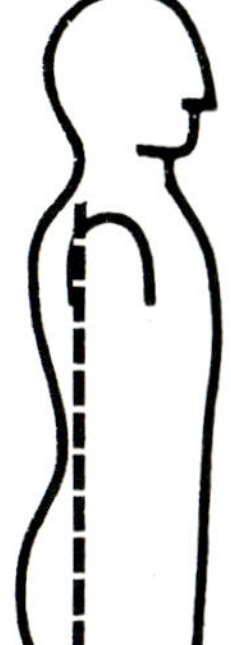

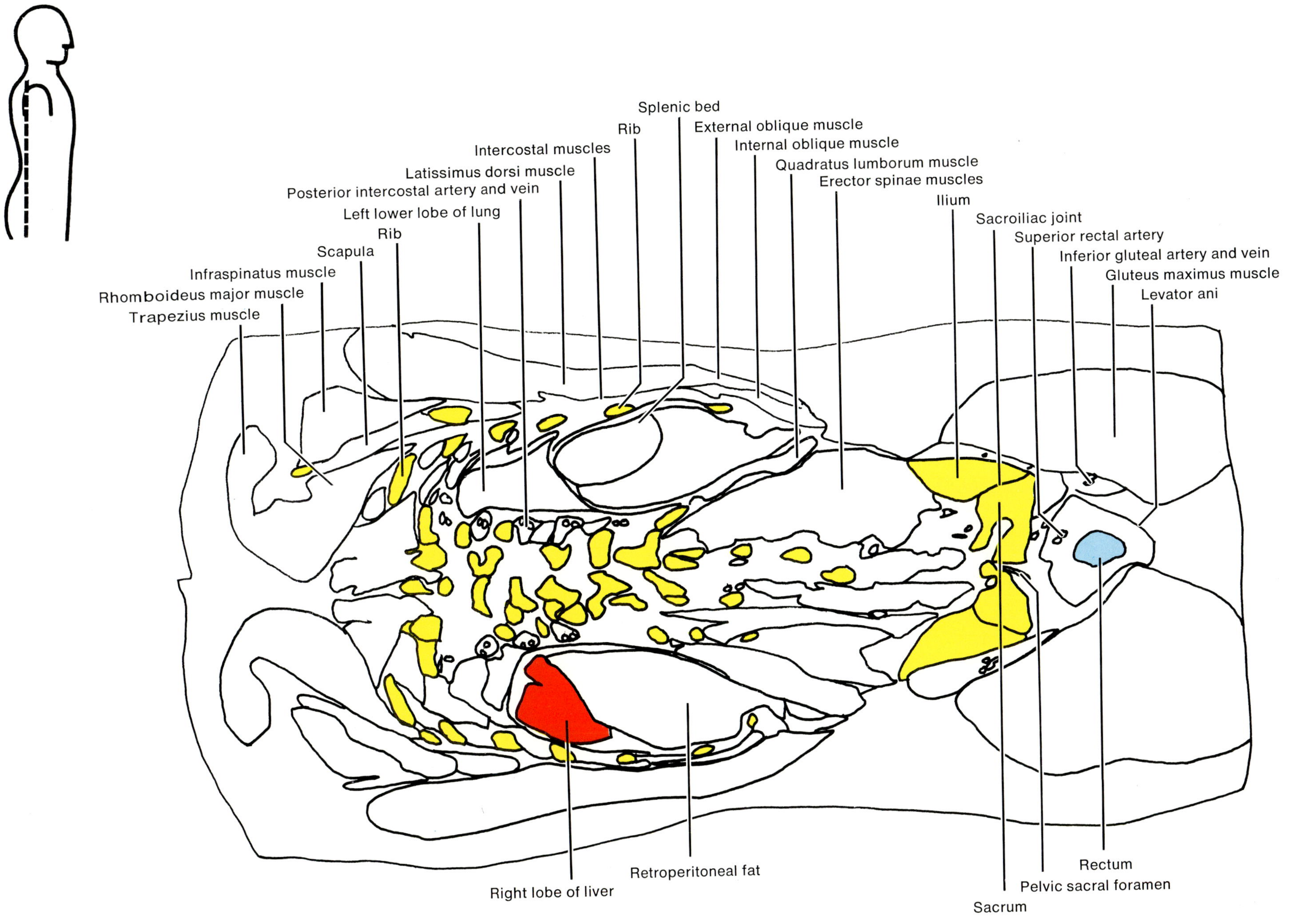

Splenic bed
Rib
External oblique muscle
Internal oblique muscle
Intercostal muscles
Quadratus lumborum muscle
Latissimus dorsi muscle
Erector spinae muscles
Posterior intercostal artery and vein
Ilium
Left lower lobe of lung
Sacroiliac joint
Rib
Superior rectal artery
Scapula
Inferior gluteal artery and vein
Infraspinatus muscle
Gluteus maximus muscle
Rhomboideus major muscle
Levator ani
Trapezius muscle
Retroperitoneal fat
Rectum
Right lobe of liver
Pelvic sacral foramen
Sacrum

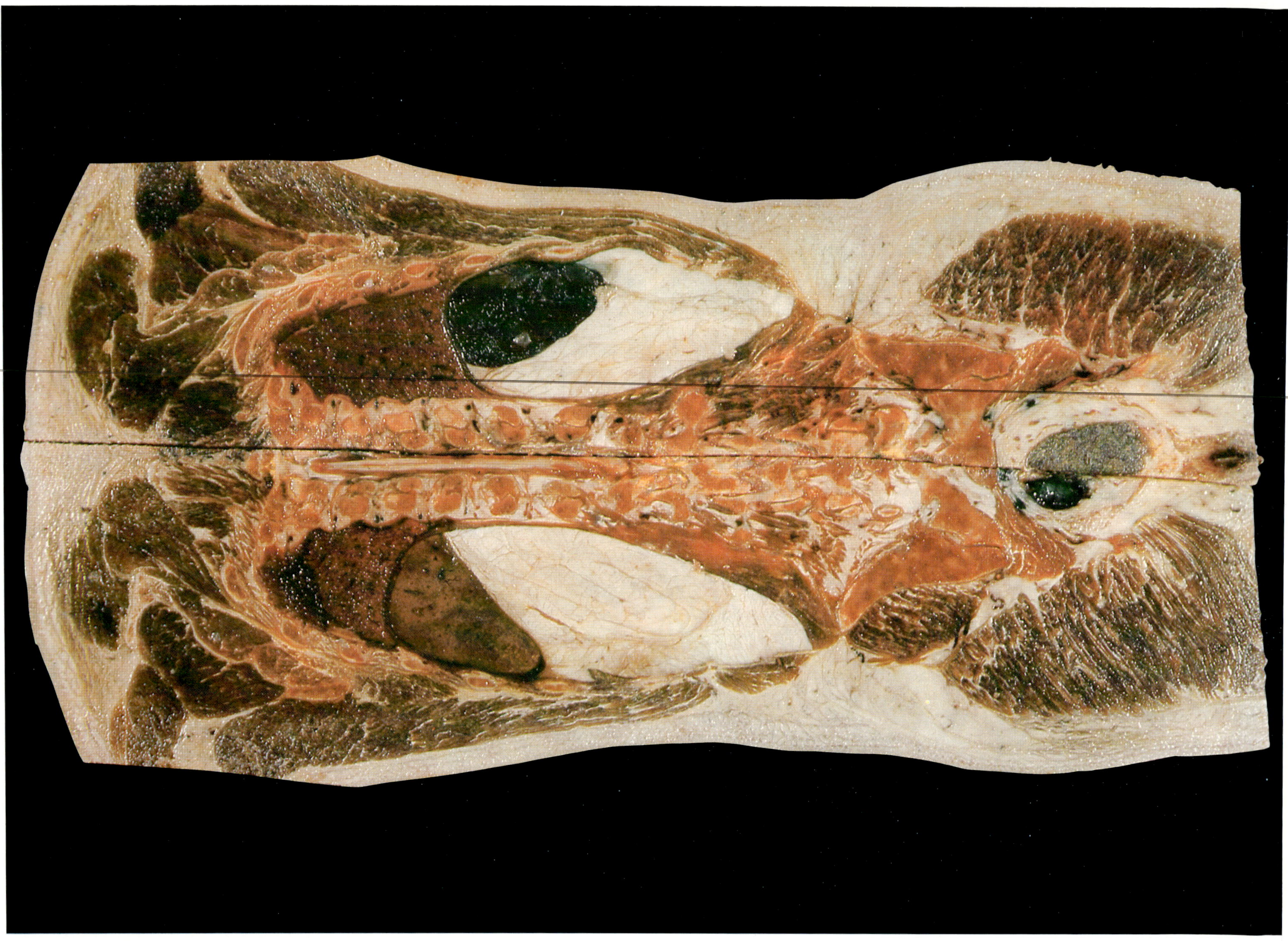

CORONAL **Chest, abdomen, and pelvis**

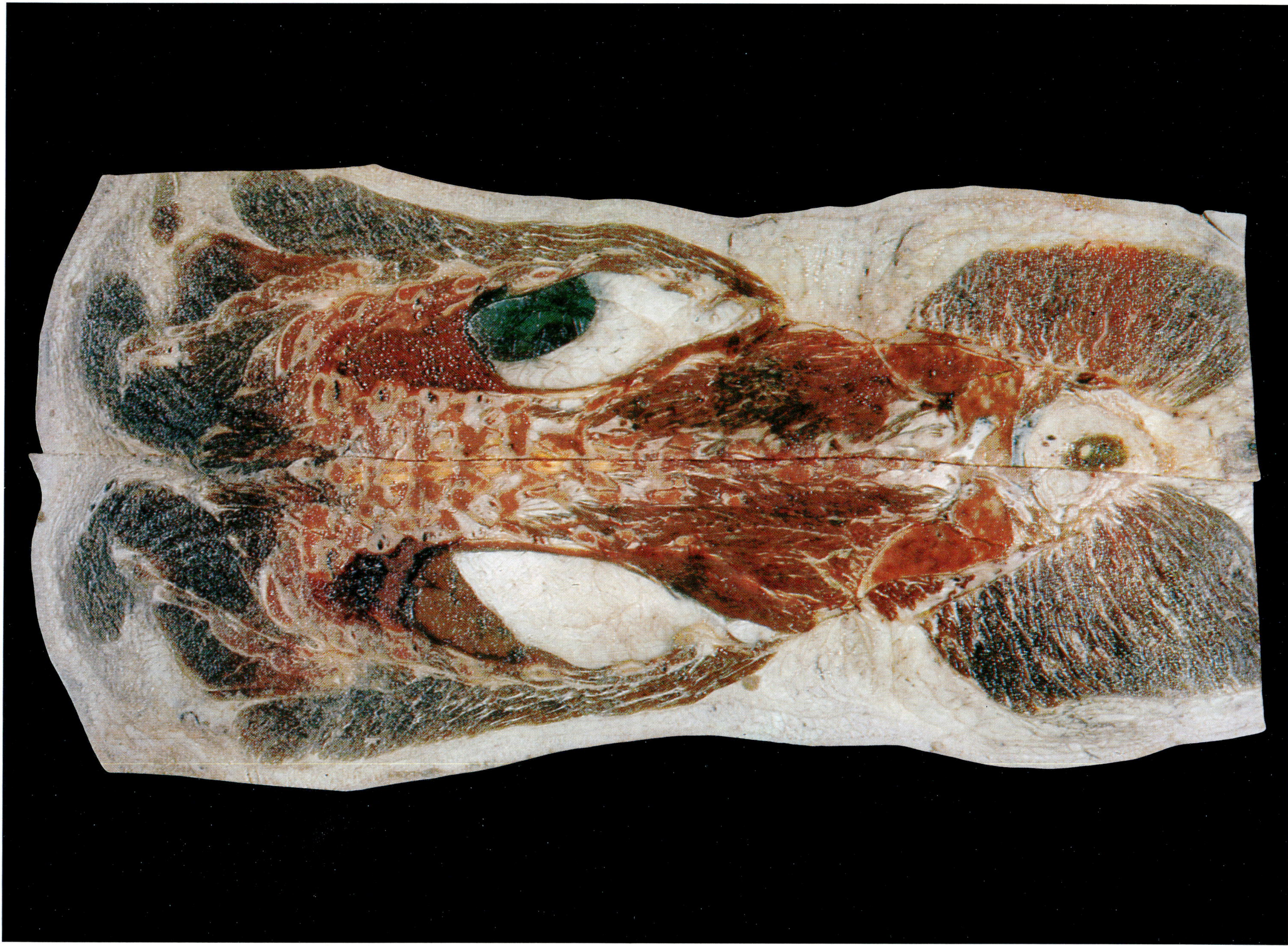

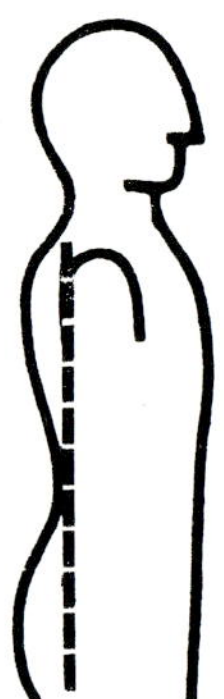

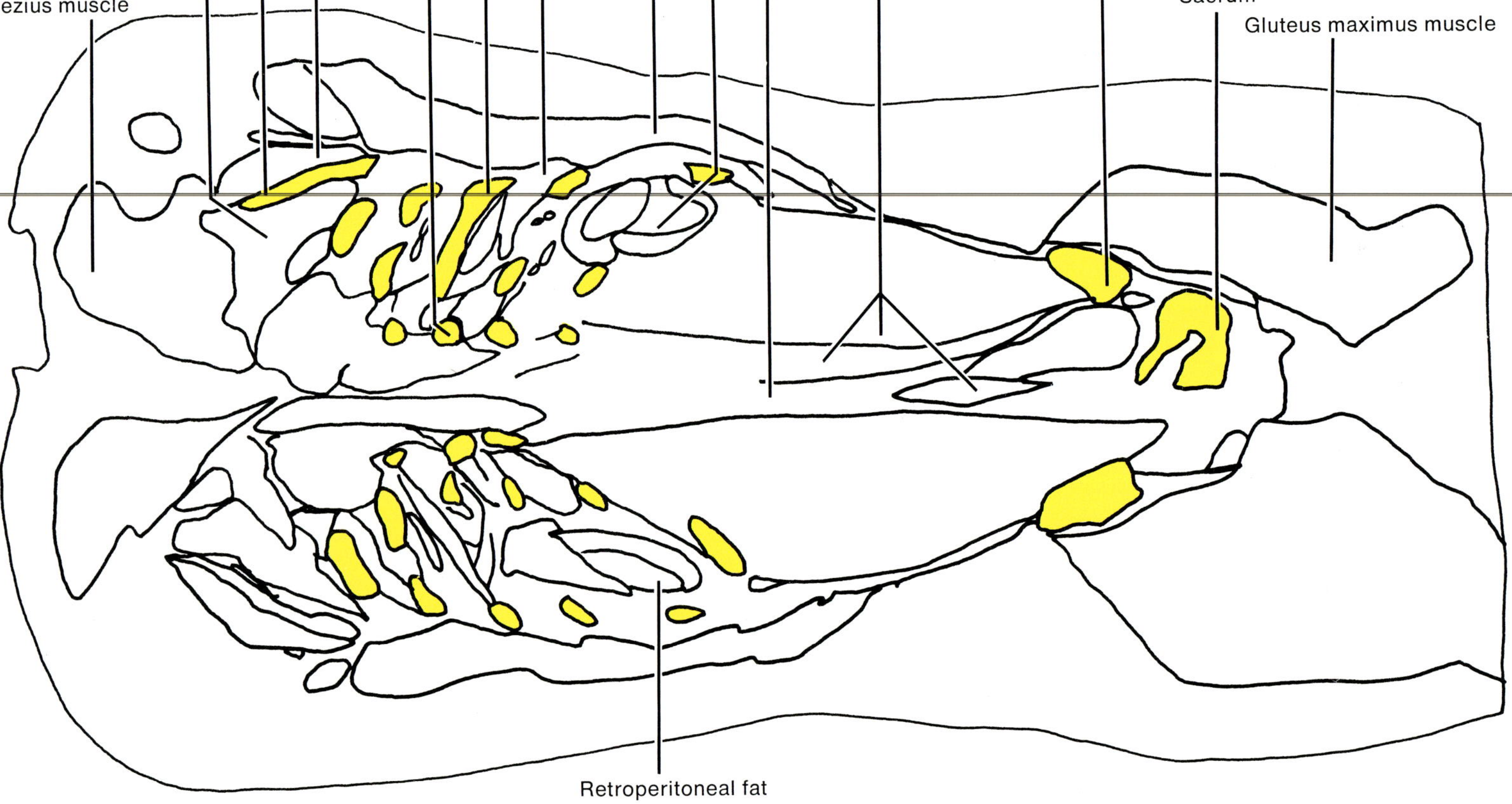

Intercostal muscles
Rib
Latissimus dorsi muscle
Transverse process
Retroperitoneal fat
Infraspinatus muscle
Spinous process
Scapula
Erector spinae muscles
Ilium
Subscapularis muscle
Sacrum
Trapezius muscle
Gluteus maximus muscle
Retroperitoneal fat

CORONAL **Chest, abdomen, and pelvis**

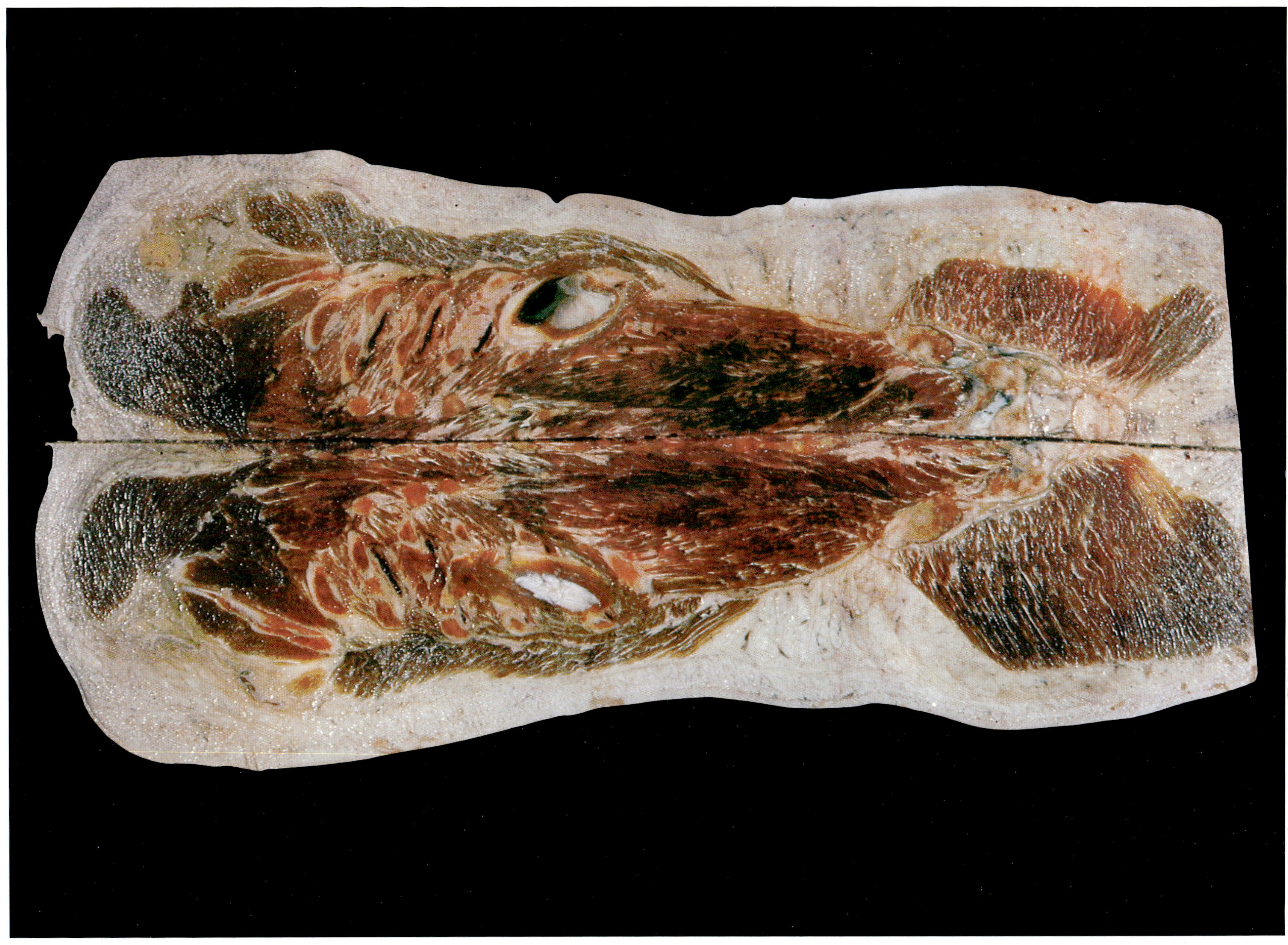

Index

The envelope attached to the inside back cover contains 60 unmounted transparencies in
10 strips of 6 transparencies each. The strips are designed to be cut apart and mounted for use in
a 35-mm slide projector. The transparencies are numbered consecutively
and correspond to the plates in the book as follows:

SLIDE	PLATE			SLIDE	PLATE		
1	2	TRANSVERSE	**Chest**	30	78	PARASAGITTAL	**Abdomen and pelvis—male**
2	3	TRANSVERSE	**Chest**	31	80	PARASAGITTAL	**Abdomen and pelvis—male**
3	4	TRANSVERSE	**Chest**	32	81	PARASAGITTAL	**Abdomen and pelvis—male**
4	5	TRANSVERSE	**Chest**	33	82	PARASAGITTAL	**Abdomen and pelvis—male**
5	6	TRANSVERSE	**Chest**	34	83	PARASAGITTAL	**Abdomen and pelvis—male**
6	7	TRANSVERSE	**Chest**	35	84	PARASAGITTAL	**Abdomen and pelvis—male**
7	9	TRANSVERSE	**Abdomen**	36	85	PARASAGITTAL	**Abdomen and pelvis—male**
8	10	TRANSVERSE	**Abdomen**	37	86	PARASAGITTAL	**Abdomen and pelvis—male**
9	11	TRANSVERSE	**Abdomen**	38	87	PARASAGITTAL	**Abdomen and pelvis—male**
10	12	TRANSVERSE	**Abdomen**	39	88	PARASAGITTAL	**Abdomen and pelvis—male**
11	13	TRANSVERSE	**Abdomen**	40	89	PARASAGITTAL	**Abdomen and pelvis—male**
12	14	TRANSVERSE	**Abdomen**	41	90	PARASAGITTAL	**Abdomen and pelvis—male**
13	15	TRANSVERSE	**Abdomen**	42	91	PARASAGITTAL	**Abdomen and pelvis—male**
14	16	TRANSVERSE	**Abdomen**	43	92	PARASAGITTAL	**Abdomen and pelvis—male**
15	17	TRANSVERSE	**Abdomen**	44	94	PARASAGITTAL	**Abdomen and pelvis—male**
16	18	TRANSVERSE	**Abdomen**	45	96	PARASAGITTAL	**Abdomen and pelvis—male**
17	19	TRANSVERSE	**Abdomen**	46	97	PARASAGITTAL	**Abdomen and pelvis—male**
18	21	TRANSVERSE	**Abdomen**	47	99	PARASAGITTAL	**Abdomen and pelvis—male**
19	26	TRANSVERSE	**Abdomen**	48	102	PARASAGITTAL	**Abdomen and pelvis—male**
20	38	TRANSVERSE	**Pelvis—female**	49	113	PARASAGITTAL	**Pelvis—female**
21	39	TRANSVERSE	**Pelvis—female**	50	114	PARASAGITTAL	**Pelvis—female**
22	40	TRANSVERSE	**Pelvis—female**				
23	41	TRANSVERSE	**Pelvis—female**	51	124	CORONAL	**Chest, abdomen, and pelvis**
24	43	TRANSVERSE	**Pelvis—female**	52	125	CORONAL	**Chest, abdomen, and pelvis**
25	44	TRANSVERSE	**Pelvis—female**	53	126	CORONAL	**Chest, abdomen, and pelvis**
26	46	TRANSVERSE	**Pelvis—female**	54	127	CORONAL	**Chest, abdomen, and pelvis**
27	56	TRANSVERSE	**Pelvis—male**	55	128	CORONAL	**Chest, abdomen, and pelvis**
28	57	TRANSVERSE	**Pelvis—male**	56	129	CORONAL	**Chest, abdomen, and pelvis**
29	58	TRANSVERSE	**Pelvis—male**	57	130	CORONAL	**Chest, abdomen, and pelvis**
				58	131	CORONAL	**Chest, abdomen, and pelvis**
				59	132	CORONAL	**Chest, abdomen, and pelvis**
				60	133	CORONAL	**Chest, abdomen, and pelvis**